A
CHRONOLOGY
OF
NUCLEAR MEDICINE

A CHRONOLOGY OF NUCLEAR MEDICINE

1600 – 1989

A summary of who gave us the ideas for
doing what we do in Nuclear Medicine,
and who gave them their ideas, and
vignettes on why they did it.

Marshall Brucer, M.D.

Edited by Robert R. Buntaine

Certain illustrations, graphs and figures previously
appeared in material published by Mallinckrodt, Inc.
Used here by permission.

Library of Congress
Catalog Card Number 89-82651

ISBN 0-9625674-0-X

Published by Heritage Publications, Inc.
St. Louis, Missouri

Printed in the United States of America

Introduction to
A CHRONOLOGY OF NUCLEAR MEDICINE
1600 – 1989

Ninety percent of what I was taught in medical school 49 years ago is now considered obsolete or false. 90% of what my teachers had been taught was revised before it got to me. I have no reason to believe that what I taught students, or what they are now teaching, is any better. Science is a transient dogma; most of it evaporates within a lifetime. But a durable remnant forms a chronology of concepts explaining some causes of some effects. Predicting measured effects from alleged causes is the red meat of science. On its medical branch a small twig of chronology is called Nuclear Medicine.

Nuclear Medicine is, by definition, the use of radionuclides to diagnose or treat disease. To accomplish this use, some physiological research might precede the diagnosis and therapy. In spite of what academics teach, therapy often precedes diagnosis; research most often is done to explain, not to discover, a therapy. A chronology will help explain why we do what we do.

To compile all the important events that led to Nuclear Medicine would require a history of all science and a lot of gossip. I have limited myself to a double page spread to describe what happened each year. The essential groundwork that preceded the discovery of radioactivity is condensed to a few pages. I have divided the ideas, articles, and events into 30 categories as shown on page vi. This format allows about 100 short sentences plus a coded reference to its origin. A key to the reference code is in the appendix. Full literature references would double the size of the book; I list only first author, journal, in a year. Any librarian can find such a reference. Usually a date in brackets [year] refers to a relevant article in an earlier year so that pathways of ideas can be traced back in time.

Such a condensation of the ideas of 12 generations of scientists requires almost telegraphic writing. For example, the definition of Nuclear Medicine in the style of this chronology is:

<u>Nuc Med = Dx & Rx with °nuclides.</u>

An "°" before a symbol means the radioactive form; hence, °nuclide is read "radionuclide." Slang, jargon, and abbreviations are used, but a glossary is appended. Interspersed between the pages of chronology are vignettes giving some of the gossip on why some things happened.

My selection of items to be included was based largely upon the introduction of ideas that either supported or suppressed Nuclear Medicine — but does not attempt to establish priority. After the 1940s many articles had to be cut out to save space. If any one is hurt by omission of his work, think how I hurt when I cut out most of my own articles to include others obviously more important.

— *MB*

FOREWORD

In each era of Medicine, there are disciplines that stand out above the others, and there are protagonists in these areas — those special people who lead the pack in the development of a specialty. They make, remember, and record the history.

Marshall Brucer, M.D., is our protagonist of Nuclear Medicine. This project, *A Chronology of Nuclear Medicine 1600–1989,* is the culmination of a twenty-year effort by this dedicated and revered scientist. As the unofficial lifetime historian of Nuclear Medicine, Marshall Brucer records the events and applies a unique analytical and personal interpretation. His mixture of science and wit has endeared him to our peers in this relatively young branch of medicine for over three decades.

Marshall's relationship to Jeff Holter and the other founding members of the Society of Nuclear Medicine in the early fifties, and his ascension to the Presidency of the Society in 1957, firmly established a brilliant scientist as our leader and role-model. His appointment as Chairman of the Medical Division of the Oak Ridge Institute for Nuclear Studies (ORINS) from 1948 to 1962 (until his disability retirement) placed him in a position to monitor, support, and guide the tumultuous events that resulted in the unprecedented growth of this new discipline of Nuclear Medicine.

Marshall is blessed with the uncanny ability to take scientific information, perceptions, and plain laboratory gossip and extract the core of truth; to expunge the inevitable accumulation of scientific perceptions and speculations that complicate, retard, and confuse the growth of any scientific endeavour. He would dispatch without mercy, and often with tongue-in-cheek, the pseudoscientific proclamations that circulated the halls of academia, the news rooms of the media, and the government agencies. For this we, his peers, thank him.

This book, as a definitive chronology of Nuclear Medicine, is also a record of the Society of Nuclear Medicine. So many of the names in this chronology are known to our younger colleagues only as names in history, but to many of us they were and are our peers — they are living legends.

To those of us who were privileged to be a part of the meteoric growth of the speciality, this compendium represents a legacy for our peers who will carry the standards of Nuclear Medicine into the next century . . .

Millard N. Croll, M.D.
Historian
Society of Nuclear Medicine

Format for the Chronology Pages

Scientific and Technical Background			Ref.
1. Basic	—	Physical, chemical, biological, and other science theory.	XXX*
2. Obser	—	Some crucial observations that influenced scientists. [year]	**
3. # Nuc	—	How many elements, isotopes, or nuclides?	
4. # Med	—	How many users, medics, licenses, and shipments of °nuclides?	***
Organizations and Internal Politics			
5. Pols	—	Political organizations before 1943 or after 1975.	
or 5. AEC	—	from 1943–75 = MED, AEC, FDA, ICRP, NRC, or other regulatory bodies.	
6. Socs	—	Scientific societies and publications.	
7. Event	—	Some crucial events that made changes occur.	
Instruments, Units of Measurement, and Drugs			
8. Instr	—	Detection, measuring, and recording instruments.	
9. Units	—	Units of measurement, and measures of dose.	
10. Concp	—	Concepts that influenced mensuration.	
11. Drugs	—	Radiochemicals and agents used in Nuclear Medicine.	
Radioiodine, P-32, and Radioactive Therapy			
12. I-Res	—	Physiology and biochemistry in radioiodine research.	
13. I-Dx	—	Diagnostic uses of °I in thyroid disease.	
14. I-Rx	—	Therapeutic uses of °I in thyroid disease.	
15. P-Rx	—	Therapeutic uses of P-32.	
16. Tele	—	Co-60 and other teletherapy and brachytherapy sources.	
17. Other	—	All other radioactive therapy modalities.	
Scans and Other Tests of Function in Various Organs			
18. Brain	—	Tests directed at the central & peripheral nervous system.	
19. Heart	—	Tests directed at the heart and its vascular system.	
20. Liver	—	Tests directed toward hepatic, biliary, and splenic systems.	
21. Lung	—	Tests directed at pulmonary physiology and pathology.	
22. Bone	—	Tests directed at skeletal anatomy and physiology.	
23. Kidney	—	Tests directed to both urine and renal blood flow.	
24. Gut	—	Tests directed at the whole or any part of the gut.	
25. Blood	—	Tests directed at plasma or cells, including water balance.	
26. Other	—	Tests involving other organs or the whole body.	
Radiation Hysteria and Health Physics		* Obituaries*	
27. Hyst	—	Articles that went into the buildup of radiophobia.	
28. React	—	The establishment's reaction to the hysteria.	
29. Respo	—	Articles that tried to correct the hysteria.	
* * *			
30. Obits	—	Obituaries of some who had great influence in Nuclear Medicine.	

*A code of letters gives reference to the statement's origin. [see Key]
**The [year] in brackets is a guide to similar ideas from other years.
***"°" is always read "radio" or "radioactive." (°I reads radioiodine.)
— Jargon & abbreviations are used frequently. A glossary is appended.

Table of Contents

"A Chronology of Nuclear Medicine" tells the complete history in two ways. First, the tabular Chronology pages tell what happened each year. Then the Vignettes, or anecdotal narratives, tell how and why many of these things happened. This sequence is repeated for each period of time. The outline of history is in the Chronology, but it comes to life in the Vignettes.

List of Illustrations

Hand drawn illustrations were originally drawn by Marshall Brucer, M.D.

Necessary alterations for publication were made by C. Merkel, graphic artist.

Photographs were provided from historical records or by the credit shown below the photograph.

Photographs in the Text

Honor Portraits

Margin Index

The Margin Index has been included to make it easier to locate the Chronology pages, which occur at random locations in the text (pages 1–428).

1. To use, place the four fingers of your right hand (palm up) between the back page and the back cover.
2. Place your right thumb near the middle of the edge of a right-hand page.
3. Holding the pages in your right hand, lift your right hand about three inches and move it to the left, bending the book pages almost double.
4. A black bar will show on the edges of the Chronology pages, about an inch from the top. The pages without this marking are the Vignette pages.

PREFACE

WHY
A CHRONOLOGY OF NUCLEAR MEDICINE?
1600 – 1989

(Many subheads have interesting stories. I refer to them by [See Vig1999 .Xx])

Why should anyone try to trace a chronology of Nuclear Medicine back to the beginning of science? Because not a single *new* idea has ever occurred in Nuclear Medicine — or in any other science. Only in religion is there revelation, but even the prophets admitted that some god had the idea first. However, in science, sometimes a slight modification of an older idea appears new. More often, a twist on a combination of older ideas begins a new tack in the direction of a new science.

A good example of a new direction is Blumgart's measurement of circulation time. By reading history backwards, Blumgart's "new" idea can be traced back to Boyle. Of course Boyle's ideas can be traced much further back, but I choose to stay within the field of science.

From Blumgart (1927) to Boyle (1661)

Hermann Blumgart's measurement of the speed of blood flow in 1927 was a combination of unrelated ideas. Blumgart knew that blood flow measurements obstructed blood vessels and hence changed the speed of flow. Heisenberg's 1928 "uncertainty principle" generalized the concept that a measurement can change the thing measured. But Blumgart knew it from an old physiological canon: in the perfect physiological measurement you don't touch the subject. Blumgart could approach this ideal through a new radiation technique. [See Vig1927 .Blu]

Duane Cuts the Cost of Radium Therapy

Radium was important in cancer therapy in 1915 Boston — but very expensive. William Duane had learned that radium was not a therapeutic agent; therapy was done with radium daughters. Why not, Duane said, milk the first daughter, radon, from the radium and use this inexpensive byproduct? He set up a radon extraction plant, the first radium–radon cow, and made radon seeds. After a few days' decay the seeds were too weak for therapy but still contained considerable radon.

Blumgart noticed that Duane detected seeds implanted in a patient without touching the body. Why not inject a bolus of radon into a peripheral vein and measure, from outside the body, the time it takes the bolus to get to the heart? The incredibly small amount of chemical radon would be negligible biochemically and the radiation would be in a harmless background range. He tried it and the procedure worked. We still measure circulation times by a modified Blumgart technique. [See Vig1915 .Cow]

From Rutherford Back to J.J. to Crookes

But was Duane's idea new? He had learned radon separations while working as Marie Curies' lab assistant in 1908. The idea came directly from Rutherford's studies of radium decay in 1899. And how did Rutherford get to the discovery of decay? J.J. Thomson had shoved the interesting 1896 Becquerel phenomenon onto Ernest Rutherford, his graduate student, because he was too busy discovering the 1896 charge unit (now called "electron").
[See Vig1896 .Bq & Vig1898 .ER1]

Crookes Changes Physics With a Toy

Thomson was searching for a unit of charge because Crookes in 1875 had demonstrated a toy called the "radiometer," with vanes that rotated contrary to physical law [See Vig1875 .WC2]. Crookes had stumbled onto the radiometer while building an ultraprecise weighing balance to measure the exact atomic weight of thallium [See Vig1872 .WC1]. He had discovered thallium in 1861, but it couldn't be an official element until its atomic weight was determined. Berzelius had made the atomic (then called "equivalent") weights a part of the definition of a chemical element around 1828 because John Dalton had given atoms a definite quantitative relationship in compounds. [See Vig1815 .WP & Vig1803 .Dal]

In 1803 Dalton made the first weighings of substances Lavoisier had called the 33 "elements" back in 1789. Lavoisier took his definition (any substance that couldn't be further broken down) directly from Robert Boyle's 1661 statement. Before Boyle, chemistry was magic, secret, and Aristotelian nonsense.

[See Vig1794 .Lav]

That's Not the Only Pathway

I could have traced Blumgart's use of batteries back through Faraday to Volta and eventually to Von Guericke, or followed a physiological pathway through Starling back to Magendie. The end point is always around 1600. If, instead, I say that Nuclear Medicine started in 1936 with Robley Evans telling J. Means he could make radioactive iodine [See Vig1936 .°I], the path then stretches back through E. Fermi's 1934 neutron sources to Chadwick's 1932 neutron [See Vig1932 .ER7]. Chadwick was looking for neutrons because his boss, Rutherford, had predicted them in 1919 [See Vig1919 .ER6]. "Neutrons" stemmed from Geiger's protons penetrating gases in 1908, seen with Crookes' 1903 Spinthariscope [See Vig1903 .WC] to see the process of Rutherford's 1899 decay [See Vig1898 .ER1]. Ultimately all paths lead back to a medical student, Galileo, timing the swings of a cathedral chandelier in 1581 Pisa.

Or, you can say that John Lawrence began Nuclear Medicine by treating an adult leukemia patient in 1937 with P-32 [See Vig1937 .JL]. This pathway can be traced through the high energy particle accelerators [See Vig1930 .EL1] and a long history of electricity. It starts with a Chinese sage spinning a piece of lodestone on a flat rock long before recorded history.

Or maybe P-32 should be traced back through Hevesy trying to separate isotopes before their discovery in 1913 [See Vig1911 .GH1]. How can an unknown something be conceptually identified? How can you measure without a standard? — without a unit? Units and standards trace back to Christian Huygens in 1660, when he swung a 1 meter pendulum to beat at 1 second intervals [See Vig1657 .mks]. One standard for two units? Time and space, Huygens implied, are only aspects of a single measurable domain. But the **Conférence Générales des Poids et Mesures** in 1889 required a natural standard for each unit [See Vig1889 .CGP]. My generation's units (1940–1970) were an incoherent mess. We adopted the first coherent system in 1961. [See Vig1977 .SI]

Which Pathway is Most Important?

"Importance" depends upon current fads in scientific discourse. We have just finished suffering through a period of self-mutilating radiation phobia [See Vig1985 .Rum]. Its development can be traced to a group of Health Physicists feathering their nest by exploiting the atom bomb fallout hysteria [See Vig1958 .CC]. Or should it be traced back to Rolf Sievert's first whole body counter (1948) to measure the body burden of radium [See Vig1948 .Bkg] which grew out of A. Krebs' 1940 measurement of radium in crematorium ashes, which followed Robley Evans' 1939 estimate from radon breath analysis of the 1925 radium dial painters? [See Vig1924 .°K & Vig1978 .Bkg]

Gossip May be Just as Important

Was the hysteria started by an outraged professor of biology who was refused a research grant by the AEC — and became a "concerned scientist"? Maybe the phobia can best be traced back to John Lawrence thinking he killed a mouse with a beam of neutrons in a 1935 cyclotron. (The mouse actually was asphyxiated because Paul Aebersold forgot to supply it with air.) [See Vig1935 .NBM]

Was it important to Nuclear Medicine that Robert Stone cured E. Lawrence's mother of a "terminal" pelvic cancer in 1937? He used the new Sloan 2MeV X-ray tube made in Lawrence's lab. The successful therapy flavored cyclotron use for many years [See Vig1930 .EL1]. Was it important that Henry Jaffe cured Glenn Seaborg's mother of thyrotoxic cardiac disease with I-131? (Seaborg discovered I-131.) That cure was as important to Nuclear Medicine as a hundred scientific papers when Seaborg became chairman of AEC [See Vig1938 .Sea]. Joule's honeymoon visit to a waterfall in Scotland is the beginning of the mechanical equivalent of heat [See Vig1847 .Jou]. Prout seeing a snake defecate at a London animal exhibit was the beginning of the Periodic Table [See Vig 1815 .WP]. Crookes' conversion to spiritualism is the beginning of the Atomic Age. [See Vig1872 .WC1]

To compile all the important events that led to Nuclear Medicine would require a history of all sciences and a metric ton of gossip. *— MB*

TRUE HISTORY OF NUCLEAR MEDICINE

The true history of any scientific discipline will show a hundred starts and stops. Most of the brilliant, even Nobel Prize winning, ideas of yesterday never went anywhere. Remember the 1925 prize for the cure of cancer? (You won't find it listed in the Almanac.) Remember the 1928 Kellogg-Briand peace pact that gave Japan three battleships for world war II? History doesn't run in straight lines. A historian must use a little creative selectivity to see relationships and developments. Anybody can imagine a direct line between that Chinese sage who spun a piece of lodestone on a flat rock, and Christopher Columbus. But some things are obvious only when you wear tinted glasses.

I wear tinted glasses that show a direct line between Hevesy's radioactive lead in 1913 and Blumgart's first nuclear medicine procedure in 1927. But Blumgart told me he didn't hear about Hevesy's work until long after his radon studies were completed. William Duane, however, was a connecting link. After Pierre Curie died in 1906, Duane became the technical expert in Marie's laboratory. He invented the radium-radon cow to protect Marie's original radium. Hevesy visited Marie's lab every time he passed through Paris and admired Duane's techniques. In 1926 Duane helped Blumgart salvage radon to use in a Hevesy-type tracer experiment. Blumgart didn't know Hevesy, but Duane is the historical link between them. I will describe, in this book, similar "clear lines" of development between Galileo and last month's journals of nuclear medicine.

— *MB*

Thank You

We acknowledge with deep appreciation the following individuals and organizations who provided funds to help make possible the publication of this book.

Irving M. Ariel, M.D., F.A.C.S., F.A.C.N.M.
The Foundation of Clinical Research

The Houston Institute for Cancer Research, Detection and Treatment

W. R. Konneker, Ph.D.

Mallinckrodt, Inc.

Squibb Diagnostics

* * *

Many other individuals and groups have given encouragement and goodwill, including Chapters and officers of the Society of Nuclear Medicine and affiliates, as well as others who have known or worked with Dr. Brucer.

We are thankful to all.

Section 1

THE BACKGROUND OF NUCLEAR MEDICINE
1600 through 1925

Around 1650 Robert Boyle defined a new intellectual discipline that would eventually be called "Science." Others had similar ideas: Gilbert in England, von Guericke in Germany, Galileo in Italy, Huygens in Belgium, Pascal in France. But Boyle, a compulsive writer, was first to define the field.

The intellectual millieu of the time had three imbedded characteristics: alchemy, secrecy, and mumbo-jumbo religion.

1. Boyle held onto alchemy, but he broke the dogma by defining an "element" in experimental terms: any substance that couldn't be broken down was elementary. He knew of 4 or 5 such substances.
2. Secrecy was a way of life — witness Newton's secret fluxions that had to be reinvented by Leibniz to become the calculus.
3. Boyle was deeply religious, but not in the laboratory; here he was a born-again skeptic. Freedom of science from religious dogma would not occur until the Scopes Monkey Trial in 1925.

Boyle required an experiment (or a carefully controlled observation) in his "Science." The experiment must be reported clearly, completely, and quickly, so that others could repeat and confirm or deny it. The essence of Boyle's new way of thinking was that in "Science" every statement is falsifiable!

After 100 years Lavoisier took Boyle's elements seriously and listed 33 of them. Then Dalton added an essential improvement. He weighed the elements and arrived at an atomic theory of matter. In another 100 years Science had achieved a simplistic "cause & effect" dogma that wasn't broken until, also in 1925, Max Born released science from commutative algebra.

This background to the Chronology of Nuclear Medicine lists the major events in a new emerging dogma called Science:

CNM1600-99 Chemical element defined.
CNM1700-49 Scale required for measures.
CNM1750-99 "Air" is really "airs."
CNM1800-24 There is "order" in elements.
CNM1825-49 Electrolysis defined.
CNM1850-74 Periodic Table of elements.
CNM1875-89 We agree on a meter & kg.
CNM1890-94 Radiometer upsets the atom.
CNM1895 Ionizing radiation discovered.
CNM1896 Radioactivity is discovered.
CNM1897 The electron is discovered.
CNM1898 Radiation hazard is discovered.
CNM1899 "Half-life" is discovered.
CNM1900 Gamma radiation is discovered.
CNM1901 Background radiation is discovered.
CNM1902 "Transmutation" announced.
CNM1903 "Chains" of decay must occur.
CNM1904 Ra cures exophthalmic goiter.
CNM1905 Radiothorium is thorium.
CNM1906 Lo dose radiation stimulates.
CNM1907 Radiation units unsatisfactory.
CNM1908 First "Roentgen" unit cast aside.
CNM1909 Radiation units proliferate.
CNM1910 Brussels conf on rad units.
CNM1911 The nuclear atom announced.
CNM1912 Wilson sees radiation tracks.
CNM1913 Annus Mirabilis in physics.
CNM1914 "Curie" unit accepted.
CNM1915 Radium cow is designed.
CNM1916 Blood cleared of I by thyroid.
CNM1917 Isobars as well as isotopes.
CNM1918 "Threshold erythema dose."
CNM1919 First artificial transmutation.
CNM1920 The Mass Spectrometer.
CNM1921 Protection requires shielding.
CNM1922 Target theory for bioeffect.
CNM1923 Compton scattering proposed.
CNM1924 °Isotope used in animals.
CNM1925 Scopes trial and Max Born free science from religion and mathematics.

CHRONOLOGY OF NUCLEAR MEDICINE — 1600–1699

Scientific and Technical Background

	Year	Event		Ref.
1. Basic	1600	W. Gilbert studies and names magnetic forces "electric."		DSB
	1611	Sartorius first study of metabolism; takes oral body temp.		DSB
	1624	H. Briggs invents method for long division; and changes Napier's Natural logarithms to base 10.	[1614]	DSB
	1629	D. Fermat uses algebra in geometry (analytic geo).	[1637]	DSM
	1636	D. Sennert first defines the modern idea of "Atom."	[1906]	DSB
	1637	R. Descartes introduces analytic geometry.	[1831]	DSM
	1643	E. Torrecelli creates a vacuum; Church says NO, shut up!		DSB
	c1650	R. Boyle defines the field of science.	[1840]	DSB
		THIS MARKS THE BEGINNING OF EXPERIMENTAL SCIENCE		
	1665	I. Newton discovers gravity and laws of motion.	[1906]	Bio
	1671	G. Leibnitz describes "aether" to explain physics.	[1887]	DSB
	1675	G. Leibnitz invents a diff & integral calculus.	[1684]	Bio
	1676	O. Roemer proves that light has a finite velocity.	[1881]	DSB
	1690	C. Huygens postulates a wave theory of light.	[1924]	Bio
2. Obser	1631	W. Oughtred proposes "x" for multiplication.	[1612]	DSB
	1639	N. Cabaeus observes repulsion of "electrons."	[1600]	DSB
	1644	J. Van Helmont coins word "gas" from "chaos" of "airs."		HRC
	1675	Royal Greenwich Observatory set up outside London.	[1986]	EB
3. # Nuc	1661	Boyle element: any substance that cannot be broken down.		DSB
	1670	Newton atom: smallest, hardest, unsplittable, eternal mass.		DSB
	1670	Leibnitz atom: vague, massless, energy center, the monad.		DSB
	1670	H. Brand discovers P in urine; first non-ancient element.		DSB

Organizations and Internal Politics

	Year	Event		Ref.
6. Soc's	1610	J. Beguin writes first chem textbk, "Tyrocinium Chymicum."		DSB
	1614	J. Napier: "Mirifiologariithmorum Canonis Descriptio."		DSB
	1620	F. Bacon writes "Novum Organum," on experimental method.		DSB
	1637	R. Descartes writes "Discourse on Method," "Geometrie."		Bio
	1645	R. Boyle and friends start a scientific society.	[1954]	Bio
	1663	The Royal Society get its first charter (thru Boyle).		DSB
	1661	R. Boyle writes "The Skeptical Chymist."	[1789]	DSB
	1684	G. Leibniz invents & publishes "Calculus" (with symbols).		DSM
	1687	I. Newton writes "Principia."	[1910]	Bio
7. Event	1626	F. Bacon dies, but R. Boyle is born.		Bio
	1642	G. Galileo dies, but I. Newton is born.		DSB
		THIS MARKS THE BEGINNING OF THEORETICAL SCIENCE		
	1654	O. von Guericke demonstrates the Magdeburg hemispheres.		DSB
	1654	Fermat & Pascal introduce probability theory.	[1846]	DSM
	1657	R. Hooke becomes Boyle's scientific assistant.	[1813]	Bio
	1666	I. Newton sees the spectrum of white light.	[1860]	Bio
	1672	O. von Guericke rubs sulfur ball to make electric sparks.		DSB
	1673	A. Leewenhoek describes hundreds of "little animacules."		Bio

Instruments, Units of Measurement, and Drugs

	Year	Event		Ref.
8. Instr	1600	J. Lipdershey invents the telescope.	[1673]	DSB
	1600	G. Galileo makes an astronomical telescope.	[1658]	DSB
	1613	G. Galileo uses a water filled U tube to measure temp.	[1828]	Bio
	1612	A. Neri publishes manual "L'Arte Vetraria." (Glassmaking).		DSB
	1643	E. Torricelli fills Galileo's U tube with mercury.	[1847]	DSB
	1658	A. Kircher is first to use microscope in disease. (Plague).		CDD
	1658	R. Hooke invents balance spring for watches.	[1985]	DSB
	1672	O. von Guericke invents a vacuum pump, first vacuum control.		DSB
	1673	A. Leewenhoek introduces the microscope to science.	[1658]	Bio

9. Units	— 1612	B. Pitislus first to use decimal point (Trig Tables).	[1862]	DSB
	— 1581	Galileo discovers pendulum principle, but doesn't think of it as a time marking device until about 1630.		DSB
	— 1614	J. Napier introduces logarithms.	[1955]	DSM
	— 1630	R. Delamain introduces a log circular slide rule.	[1614]	DSM
	— 1634	S. Stevin introduces decimal fractions.	[1612]	DSM
	— 1642	B. Pascal invents a "metric" calculating machine.	[1855]	DSM
	— 1660	C. Huygens finds 1 meter pendulum beats 1 second.	[1581]	Bio
	— 1661	C. Huygens invents manometer for elastic force of gas.	[1613]	Bio
	— 1673	J. Wallis introduces imaginary numbers.	[1675]	DSM
10. Concp	— 1605	G. Bauhin begins modern Anatomy.	[1964]	CDD
	— 1610	Galileo finds it necessary; test ALL assumptions. (1985 Sc)		
	—c1625	R. Descartes adopts a mechanistic biology.	[1896]	DSB
11. Drugs	— 1625	J. Glauber discovers a cathartic sodium sulfate salt.		CDD

Radioiodine, P-32, and Radioactive Therapy

12. I-Res	— 1602	Paracelsus describes cretinism & endemic goiter.	[1983]	CDD
	— 1657	W. Hoefer relates strumae to Alpine drinking water.	[1907]	CDD
14. I-Rx	— 1623	Augustana Pharmacopoeia Rx for goiter is burnt sea sponge.		V91

Scans and Other Tests of Function in Various Organs

18. Brain	— 1662	R. Descartes deduces reciprocal enervation of eye muscle.		CDD
19. Heart	— 1628	W. Harvey pubs "Exercitation de Moto Cordis et Sanguinas."		Bio
	— 1646	R. Wiseman describes aneurisms of large vessels.	[1958]	CDD
	— 1658	J. Wepfer says apoplexy cause is cereb hemorrhage.	[1963]	CBB
	— 1661	M. Malpigi describes capillaries and circulation.	[1894]	DSB
	— 1661	Earl Clarendon's death described as Angina Pect.	[1916]	CDD
	— 1663	N. Steno teaches the heart is a muscle.	[1625]	DSB
20. Liver	— 1650	D. Sennert describes gall-bladder stones, says they were found on first recorded autopsy in 1341.	[1980]	CDD
	— 1654	F. Glisson describes "swelling" (stones) bile duct.	[1650]	CDD
	— 1685	J. Brown describes a "scirrhus" liver.	[1968]	PTRS
21. Lung	— 1669	R. Lower proves lungs make bright red blood.	[1960]	CDD
24. Gut	— 1554	J. Fernes is first to describe "appendicitis."	[1886]	CDD
	— 1679	T. Willis notes sweet taste of diabetic urine.	[1925]	CDD
25. Blood	— 1658	J. Swammerdam first describes Red Blood Cells.	[1926]	CDD
26. Other	— 1642	J. Bontius describes Beri-Beri (Vit B deficiency).	[1950]	CDD
	— 1645	D. Whistler describes Rickets (Vit D deficiency).	[1938]	CDD
	— 1650	F. Glisson gives classical description of Rickets.	[1645]	CDD
	— 1672	V. Ketelar describes Sprue (non-trop) (Vit B def).	[1650]	CDD

Radiation Hysteria and Health Physics * Obituaries *

27. Hyst	— 1616	Cath church prohibits Galileo from any scientific work.		Bio
	— 1621	Catholic church bans Kepler's "Epitome."		DSB
29. React	— 1646	A. Kircher invents the "Magic Lantern."	[1879]	DSB

* * *

30. Obits	— W. Gilbert (1544–1603) Eng physics, physiol; magnetism.	DSB
	— F. Bacon (1561–1626) Eng philos; experiment "scientific" method.	DSB
	— Sartorius (1561–1636) It physician; body metabolism.	DSB
	— G. Galileo (1564–1642) It physics; math in "scientific" method.	DSB
	— J. Helmont (1577–1644) Belg chem; "gas."	DSB
	— E. Torricelli (1608–1647) It physics; atmospheric pressure.	DSB
	— R. Descartes (1596–1650) Fr math, physics; philos of science.	Bio
	— W. Harvey (1578–1657) Eng physician; circulation of blood	Bio
	— R. Boyle (1627–1691) Eng physics, chem; first exper "scientist."	Bio
	— C. Huygens (1629–1695) Dutch physics; wave theory of light.	DSB
	— H. Brand (1630–16??) Ger chem; first new element.	DSB

CHRONOLOGY OF NUCLEAR MEDICINE — 1700–1749

				Ref.
Scientific and Technical Background				
1. Basic —	1729	S. Gray transmits electricity over metal wires.	[1600]	DSB
—	1745	E. von Kleist invents the Leyden Jar.	[1672]	DSB
—	1747	B. Franklin names electric fluids positive and negative.		DSB
—	1748	Abbe Nollet makes an "electric egg."	[1671]	DSB
2. Obser —				
3. # Nuc —	1718	E. Geoffroy publishes table of chem affinities.	[1661]	DSB
4. # Med —				
Organizations and Internal Politics				
5. Pols —	1700	G. Leibnitz is first pres of new Berlin Acad Science.	[1663]	Bio
—	1703	I. Newton elected pres of Royal Society.	[1663]	Bio
—	1725	St. Petersburg academy of science founded.	[1663]	EB
6. Socs —	1738	D. Bernoulli publishes "Hydrodynamics."	[1643]	DSB
—	1704	I. Newton publishes secret fluxions (calculus).	[1684]	Bio
—	1724	H. Boerhaave pubs clinical "Elemente Chemicae."	[1661]	DSB
7. Event —	1705	E. Halley predicts correct return of comet in 1778.	[1682]	DSB
Instruments, Units of Measurement, and Drugs				
8. Instr —	1707	G. Fahrenheit uses Hg for his thermometer fluid.	[1613]	DSB
—	1707	J. Floyer invents watch second hand (pulse count).	[1658]	CDD
—	1714	D. Anel invents fine-pointed syringe for surgeons.	[1960]	EB
—	1727	J. Schultze mixes AgCl in chalk paste, it darkens in sun.		EB
—	1730	R. Reaumur makes alcohol thermometer, with scale.	[1707]	DSB
—	1733	C. Dufay uses pith balls to tell vitreous from resinous electricity.		DSB
—	1746	J. Canton suspends 2 pith balls for first electrometer.		DSB
9. Units —	1701	I. Newton sets temp scale: 0 = ice water, 12 = body temp. ESTABLISHES PRINCIPLE: MEASURING DEVICES MUST HAVE A SCALE		Bio
—	1708	G. Fahrenheit sets temp scale: 0 = salt water ice.	[1613]	DSB
—	1742	A. Celsius sets temp scale: 0 = boiling water, 100 = fresh ice.		DSB
—	1748	C. Linnaeus reverses Celsius' scale to 0 = Fresh water ice.		Bio
10. Concp —	1706	W. Jones first uses symbol "π" (a circle ratio).	[1612]	DSM
—	1733	A. DeMoivre devises first formula for "normal curve."	[1654]	DSM
11. Drugs —	1724	J. Lowitz prepares first ethyl alcohol.	[1947]	DSB
—	1700	J. Tournefort discovers ammonium chloride.	[1625]	DoE

Radioiodine, P-32, and Radioactive Therapy

12. I-Res —				
13. I-Dx —				
14. I-Rx —				
15. P-Rx —				
16. Tele —				
17. Other —				

Scans and Other Tests of Function in Various Organs

18. Brain —				
19. Heart —	1705	W. Cowper describes ossification of aortic valves.	[1663]	CDD
—	1707	J. Floyer introduces counting of pulse.	[1628]	EB
—	1708	A. van Leeuwenhoek says there is palpable "pulse."	[1628]	DSB
—	1715	R. Vieussens describes mitral stenosis & aortic insuff.		CDD
—	1725	S. Hales measures the blood pressure of a horse.	[1663]	DSB
—	1749	J. de Sénac treats palpitation with quinine, writes text.		Bk
20. Liver —				
21. Lung —				
22. Bone —	1740	J. Freke describes first pt with myositis ossificans.	[1974]	CDD
—	1745	T. Cadwalader describes osteomalacia.	[1963]	CDD
23. Kidney —				
24. Gut —	1711	L. Heister gives classic descript of appendicitis.	[1554]	CDD
—	1736	C. Aymand performs first success appendectomy.	[1711]	CDD
25. Blood —				
26. Other —	1717	M. Montague introduces inoculation against smallpox.		CDD
—	1737	J. Hunter inoculates his penis to prove syphilis contag.		CDD
—	1740	J. Freke advises remove large lymph nodes in breast ca.		CDD
—	1748	J. Fothergill describes diphtheria in England.	[1876]	CDD

Radiation Hysteria and Health Physics * Obituaries *

27. Hyst —	1700	F. Platter sees enlarged thymus, stridor & death.	[1913]	CDD
—	1700	Joachimsthal mined for silver from 1516 to 1700.	[1932]	AJC
28. React —	1729	Emperor Yung Cheng prohibits opium smoking.	[1986]	EB
—	1740	Frederick: freedom of press & worship in Prussia.	[1650]	EB
29. Respo —	1714	Witch trials abolished in England, Prussia.	[1621]	EB
—	1717	School attendance made compulsory in Prussia.	[1650]	EB

* * *

30. Obits —	G. Leibnitz (1646–1719) Ger math phil; philosophy of science.	DSB
—	A. Leewenhoek (1632–1723) Dutch biol; introduced microscopy.	Bio
—	I. Newton (1642–1727) Eng math physics; gravity, laws of motion.	Bio
—	G. Fahrenheit (1686–1736) Dutch inst maker; thermometry.	Bio

CHRONOLOGY OF NUCLEAR MEDICINE — 1750–1799

Scientific and Technical Background

1. Basic	— 1761	G. Morgagni publishes results of 640 autopsies.	[1661]	DSB
	— 1783	A. Lavoisier doubts the phlogiston theory.	[1610]	Bio
	— 1789	A. Lavoisier ANNOUNCES CONSERVATION OF MASS LAW.	[1847]	DSB
	— 1785	L. Galvani's bimetal contact twitches frog muscle.	[1843]	DSB
	— 1793	J. Richte announces principles of stoichiometry.	[1661]	DSB
	— 1794	E. Darwin states: sex selection guides evolution.	[1859]	Bk
2. Obser	— 1750	J. Black distinguishes fixed (CO_2) from normal air.	[1644]	DSB
	— 1766	H. Cavendish weighs fixed air at 1.47 normal air.	[1940]	DSB
	— 1766	H Cavendish inflammable air (H) 11 × lighter than air.	[1886]	DSB
	— 1772	J. Priestly adds 8 more different kinds of air.	[1650]	DSB
	— 1779	T. Bergman knows composition of 8 different gases.	[1750]	DSB
3. # Nuc	— 1758	Boscovich atom: point size mass, ringed by force.	[1670]	WoA
	— 1766	H. Cavendish discovers H, is first to make H_2O.	[1951]	DSB
	— 1772	J. Priestly discovers an "air" later called N.	[1644]	Bio
	— 1774	J. Priestly discovers fixed air (CO_2), then O.	[1929]	Bio
	— 1774	A. Lavoisier coins names for H and O.	[1789]	Bio
	— 1774	J. Gahn isolates manganese.	[1718]	DSB
	— 1778	L. Vauguelin discovers chromium.	[1954]	DOE
	— 1789	A. Lavoisier element: substance cannot be degraded.	[1661]	DSB
	— 1789	M. Klaproth discovers uranium (really an oxide).	[1985]	DOE
	— 1789	A. Lavoisier says: 33 "elements" (11 are oxides).	[1661]	HRC
	— 1794	J. Gadolin discovers first rare earth, Yttria (Y).	[1942]	DSB

Organizations and Internal Politics

5. Pols	— 1751	Ecole Supérieure founded in Paris.	[1661]	EB
	— 1759	Bavarian Academy of Science founded.	[1898]	DSB
6. Soc's	— 1761	G. Morgagni publishes "Seats and Causes of Disease."	[1650]	CDD
	— 1789	A. Lavoisier writes a "Treatise of Chemistry."	[1610]	Bio
	— 1792	First Chemical Society founded in Philadelphia.	[1663]	DSB
	— 1768	First of weekly issues of Encyclo Britannica pub.	[1621]	EB
7. Event	— 1751	Jan 1 established as New Year's day by Brit Parl.	[1687]	EB
	— 1752	B. Franklin charges a Leyden jar with lightning.	[1745]	Bio
	— 1754	First female gets MD from U of Halle (Ger).	[1905]	EB
	— 1762	Carron Ironworks casts first malleable cast iron.	[1953]	EB
	— 1766	J. Priestly discovers carbon conducts electricity.	[1729]	DSB
	— 1783	P. de Rozier makes first free balloon flight.	[1913]	EB
	— 1783	Montgolfier brothers ascend in first free balloon.	[1911]	DSB
	— 1783	Pres Roy Soc: balloon flights have no scientific value.		SA
	— 1783	J. Watt improves steam engine, starts indust revolution.		DSB
	— 1786	J. Jeffries, first to study bio effects in balloon.	[1918]	Bk

Instruments, Units of Measurement, and Drugs

8. Instr	— 1752	B. Franklin invents the lightning conductor.	[1745]	Bio
	—c1753	J. LeRoi invents the electrometer.	[1746]	DSB
	— 1777	C. Coulomb invents torsion balance.	[1889]	DSB
	— 1783	J. Watt measures a horse's power at 550 ft lbs.	[1764]	Bio
9. Units		WEIGHTS AND MEASURES BECOME A PROPER FUNCTION OF GOVERNMENTS.		
	— 1761	J. Süssmilch initiates study of statistics.	[1624]	DSB
	— 1781	Continental Congress considers problem of weights.	[1875]	V101
	—c1786	T. Jefferson recommends metric system coins & wts.	[1795]	Bio
	— 1789	U.S. Constitution Art. 1: Congress will set measures.	[1901]	V101
	— 1790	J. Watt suggests std volume to Tallyrand (liter).	[1901]	Bio
	— 1795	J. Lagrange's comm recommends the metric system.	[1875]	DSB
	— 1795	French Acad Science establishes universal metre.	[1889]	V101

10. Concp — 1768 L. Spallanzani starts argument on spontaneous generation. DSB
— 1798 C. Wessel uses a "direction vector" with complex numbers. DSM
11. Drugs — 1767 O.Bergmann examines the "chemical affinities". [1789] DSB
— 1775 J. Priestly discovers HCl and H_2SO_4. [1824] DSB
— 1775 W. Withering uses digitalis as diuretic in dropsy. [1960] CDD
— 1785 W. Withering: digitalis for Rx of congest failure. [1960] CDD

Radioiodine, P-32, and Radioactive Therapy

12. I-Res — 1786 C. Perry sees goiters with cardiac hyperactivity. [1602] CDD
17. Other — 1774 P. Favre treats ulcers with sunlight. [1896] GSR
— 1776 A. LeCompte treats wounds and inflammation with sunlight. GSB

Scans and other tests of function in various organs

18. Brain — 1761 G. Morgagni shows R-lesion yields L-side effect. [1662] DSB
— 1766 A. Waller says nerves are not hollow, all lead to brain. DSB
19. Heart — 1755 A. Haller sees adhesive pericarditis & hard valves. [1705] CDD
— 1761 L. Auenbrugger describes fluid in the pericardium. [1964] CDD
— 1761 L. Auenbrugger reports on percussion of heart. [1905] Bk
— 1761 G. Morgagni describes coronary calcification. [1661] DSB
— 1768 W. Heberden describes angina pectoris as a disease. [1661] DD
21. Lung — 1777 A. Lavoisier says O_2 is a respiratory gas. [1644] CDD
22. Bone — 1776 H. Thomas describes a patient with soft bones. [1745] CDD
—c1791 S. Soemmerring describes achondroplasia. [1961] CDD
(He also invents an electric telegraph.) [1745] CDD
24. Gut — 1750 G. Cassal describes pellagra. [1755] CDD
— 1753 J. Lind recommends lemon juice to prevent scurvy. [1642] CDD
— 1755 F. Thiery describes pellagra. [1750] CDD
— 1759 W. Hillary gives first known description of sprue. [1965] CDD
— 1776 M. Dobson demonstrates sugar in urine of diabetics. [1679] CDD
26. Other — 1785 L. Spallanzani: first artificial insemination (dog). [1658] DSB

Radiation Hysteria and Health Physics * Obituaries *

27. Hyst — 1770 H. Scheffer sees lung dis in Joachimsthal miners. [1700] AJC
— 1774 A. Mesmer uses first hypnosis for medical purpose. [1895] EB
— 1784 J. Haygarth suggests isolation stops spread of infection. CDD
— 1794 A. Lavoisier's head chopped off by science rival. [1789] Bio
— 1796 Population of China estimated at 275 million. [1960] EB
29. Rep — 1771 S. Bard states laws of medical innovation:
a. New names are ALWAYS deceiving.
b. New theories are usually false or useless.
c. New remedies may be dangerous. CDD

* * *

30. Obits — G. Morgagni (1682–1771) It pathol; anatomic pathology. DSB
— C. Linnaeus (1707–1778) Swe botany; reverses Celsius' scale. Bio
— B. Franklin (1706–1790) Am physics; electricity, politics. DSB
— A. Lavoisier (1743–1794) Fr chem; 33 chemical elements exist. DSB
— L. Spallanzani (1729–1799) It biology; no spontan generation. DSB

GASPARO BERTI DISCOVERS A VACUUM

Galileo did not believe, in 1642, that air was under pressure, but he wavered on the idea. A group of physicists in Rome devised an experiment to convince him. The subject concerned suction pumps and getting water to the second floor — very practical in multi-storied Italian cities.

Gasparo Berti attached a lead pipe to the side of his house in Rome. At the top, next to the tower window, he hermetically sealed a large glass bottle with a screw cap on top. The bottom of the pipe was closed with a stopcock under water in a half filled rain barrel. Berti filled the bottle and pipe with water and sealed the screw cap.

In the presence of physicist friends and a few Jesuits (the church trusted none of Galileo's witchcraft) Berti opened the stopcock. The water disappeared from the bottle on top of the pipe with a plop, but the rain barrel below did not overflow. How much water was standing in the pipe? Berti closed the stopcock to prevent further water drainage, then rushed up to the tower to lower a sound into the pipe to measure the water level. As he unscrewed the cap even the Jesuits below heard the air rush in with a hiss. The water level stood at 18 *braccia* (about 33 ft), exactly where Galileo had predicted it would stand. Ergo, said Berti, a vacuum in the bottle holds up 18 *braccia* of water.

No! thundered the Jesuits. Aristotle said, *"Nature abhors a vacuum."* He didn't do silly experiments but proved truth with impeccable logic. Light shines through things. No light comes through nothing; hence, a vacuum, being nothing, must be opaque. We could see through the bottle, hence there was no vacuum. Amen.

"But we all heard the hiss of air ..." began Berti, but friends restrained him. The church owned all the matches in Rome and had the nasty habit of lighting them under people who won arguments. And so the results of the experiment were never published. But Torrecelli heard of it by word of mouth.

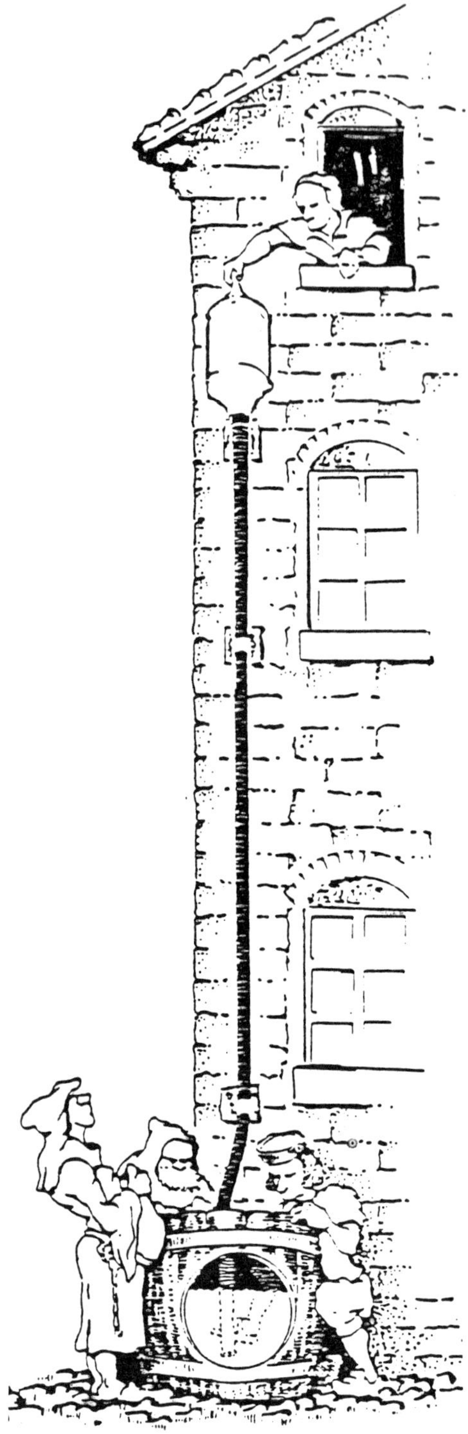

Gasparo Berti produces the first experimental vacuum (c1640) to convince Galileo. "No!" thundered the church, "it is written that Nature abhors a vacuum." Berti did not publish.

[See Vig1644 .Tor]

TORRECELLI EXPLAINS AIR PRESSURE

Three months before he died in 1642 Galileo asked Evangelista Torrecelli to move to Florence as his associate. He had heard of the experiment Berti had conducted in Rome and would allow Torrecelli to repeat and improve many of the technical details. Torrecelli made some glass bottles with necks about 2 ells long (about 1 meter) and filled them with quicksilver.

Stoppering their mouths with his thumb Torrecelli inverted the bottles in a vase half filled with mercury. In every case, no matter what size bottle or neck, the result was the same. Each bottle emptied upon inversion but quicksilver remained in the bottle neck at the same height above the mercury level in the vase.

The bottles, he said, now contained nothing; hence, a vacuum. To demonstrate this further he added a layer of water over the mercury in the vase. When he raised the mouth of a bottle into the water layer, *"the quicksilver in the neck came down and the water rushed in with horrible violence and filled the vessel completely."*

The weight of fifty miles of air above us presses down on the mercury in the vase, explained Torrecelli; it pushes its weight of mercury up into the neck. There is no opposing weight in the vacuum. *"We live submerged at the bottom of an ocean of air."*

There is NO vacuum, thundered the Church. Torrecelli was looking at what the Church did to Galileo. The experiment was never published.

The quotations above are from letters Torrecelli wrote to friends in Rome. These friends wrote to friends in Paris who wrote to friends in Stockholm who wrote to friends in England who wrote to friends in Poland. Finally, 4 years later, a letter was delivered in Rouen to a friend of Blaise Pascal. The famous French mathematician delighted in disproving anything Aristotle had written, and was not, at the time, influenced by Church doctrine.

PASCAL DISCOVERS HOW TO CLIMB A MOUNTAIN

When told the story of Torrecelli's novel experiment Blaise Pascal was delighted. He had long believed that a vacuum, if such a thing existed, must be the physical equivalent of "zero" in mathematics. He repeated the experiment on a grand scale with wide and thin bottle necks and with water, wine, and with 40–60 lbs of mercury. He often demonstrated in public, and demolished Aristotle's concept of the vacuum with glee.

Was Torrecelli correct that 50 miles of air pressed down on us and pushed the mercury column up? There was one decisive test: take a Torrecellian tube to the top of a mountain where there was a mile less air. He wrote to his brother-in-law in Cleremont, at the foot of Puy-de-Dome (a 4080 ft mountain).

After some persuasion, on 19 Sep, 1648, his brother-in-law and four friends (Blaise was not in the party) backpacked two fifty pound mercury barometers to a monastery in the foothills. After teaching a monk how to record the barometer readings hourly, they climbed the mountain. At the summit, throughout the day their mercury column stood at 23 inches 2 lines (12 lines/inch then). Returning to the monastery they read 26 inches 3+ lines which checked with the monk's reading on his instrument. Torrecelli's explanation was confirmed. Pascal published his results without asking the Church's approval.

For centuries barometric (from Greek *baros* for weight) or air pressure was measured in inches of water or mmHg. In 1971 the CGPM (Conf Genrale des Poids et Mesures) substituted a coherent unit. A newton of 1 kg acting on 1 cm^2 of surface area became the derived unit of pressure. They named the unit a pascal (Pa), not because Pascal discovered "pressure," but because any man who can talk his brother-in-law into packing 50 lbs up a mountain deserves accolade. In Science it is not good enough to be merely correct; you must also convince others that you are correct.

THE FIRST HINT OF A METRIC SYSTEM
(Huygens & Mouton Invent a Metric System)

Gabriel Mouton (1618–1694), Vicar of St Paul's at Lyons, France, had a special interest in establishing Lyons' precise geometrical position on earth: the sometimes bloody disagreements on how far Lyons was from Paris. Every province in France had its own unit of distance and was wedded to its logic, antiquity and irreplacability. As a part time mathematician and astronomer, he knew that any unit of length could be used so long as we all agreed upon the unit.

Mouton tried to find a universally acceptable unit for the measurement of distance or length. To the North, at about the same time, a Dutchman was trying to find a unit for the measurement of a second of time. They both soon discovered that they could be satisfied with the same tool: a pendulum.

Huygens and the Meter-Second Pendulum

Around 1657 Mouton heard of Christian Huygens' meter-second pendulum and was impressed. A few years earlier Huygens had discovered that the time period of a pendulum is not totally independent of its amplitude as Galileo had said. (Galileo had missed the pendulum-clock connection.) But the error was small at small amplitudes. Huygens found a way to correct the error. The pendulum bob was slightly distorted to swing a cycloidal pathway. Amplitude independence was restored and a tautochronus beating pendulum achieved. Huygens added falling weights to his grandfather clocks to transfer just enough energy to keep the pendulum beating.

From ancient times the heart beat has been the unit of time. It is so highly variable that some natural oscillator had to be used to mark a standard heart beat duration. The Babylonian double-12 hours/60 minutes/60 second convention persisted. (Nobody knows why.) Huygens found the length of pendulum required to beat at one second intervals was a "meter," the Greek noun for "measure." It was very close to our 1980s "meter," which was not defined for another 140 years — 1795.

[See Vig1810 .1SI]

Mouton Invents the Metric System.

Even Frenchmen tended to agree upon the length of the day and a "second." (Modern "time" uncertainties did not exist then.) With a known "second" everybody could now make his own "metre," and all "metres" would be the same. Gabriel Mouton, as a pioneer metrologist, read with growing interest reports on the variations in length of Huygens' pendulum with latitude. He calculated what the length would be at the equator. From this position the length of a meridian, pole to equator, could be calculated. Some fraction of this was the obvious natural fundamental unit of length.

Mouton selected, but as an example only, 1/600,000 of his calculated meridian as a "geometric foot." He constructed a pendulum a geometric foot long and counted 3659.2 oscillations in 30 minutes. only 1% off of a true 3600. Multiples and submultiples of this unit written in a decimal notation would give large and small sub units of convenient size. All numbers could be written around a decimal point that indicated zero place in magnitude. He called a degree of arc *"mille."* Multiples or fractions were *mille* or *millesima, centuria* or *centesima, decuria* or *decima.*

Thus Gabriel Mouton, Vicar of St. Paul's in Lyons, invented the decimal or metric notation. "Metric" was from Greek for a "measure" and was not our "meter of length." He published his only book, *Observationes Diametrorum,* in 1670. His universal standard of length was based on the pendulum. But his meridian suggestion would not bear fruit for 120 years. In 1794 the French Academy discarded the pendulum for triangulation of a large segment of Mouton's meridian.

The metric idea is so simple that Christian Huygens immediately adopted it in his formal paper on the isochronous pendulum in 1673. The system of notation became popular in tables of logarithms and trigonometric functions. Such tables were the daily bread of astronomers, navigators, surveyors, artillerists. Within a generation the metric or decimal system had become, not the exclusive, but the easiest accepted way of writing large and small numbers.

[See Vig1790 .Wat; Watt's volume]

THESE MEN MADE NUCLEAR SCIENCE A POSSIBILITY

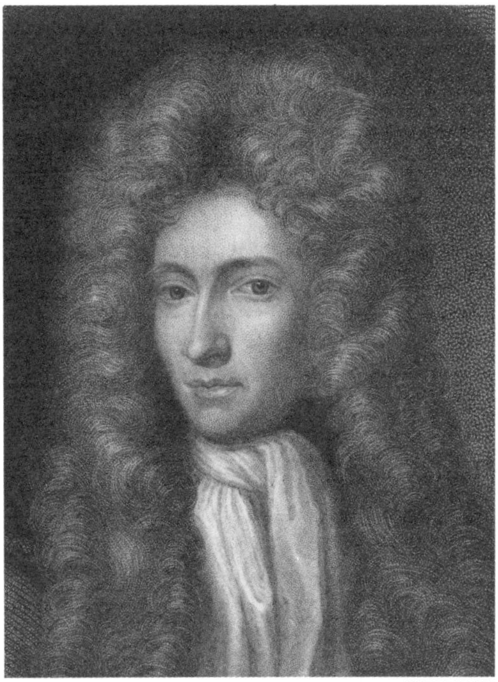

BETTMAN ARCHIVE

Robert Boyle, 1627–1691

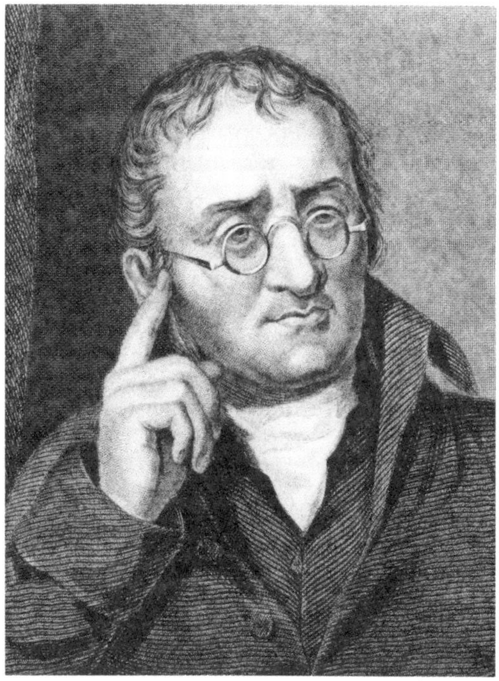

BETTMAN ARCHIVE

John Dalton, 1766–1844

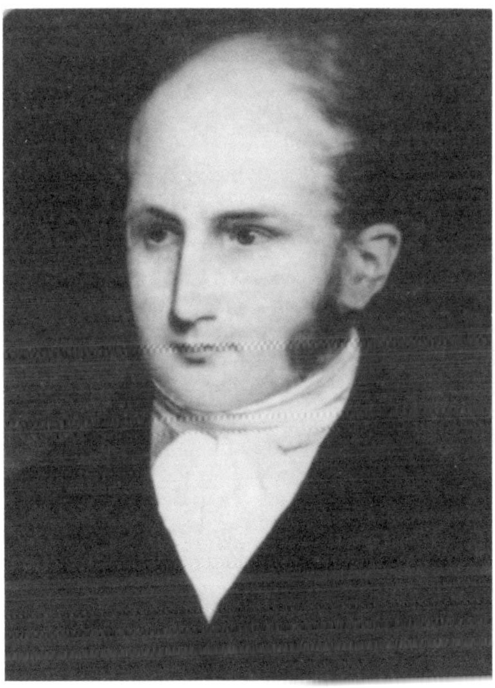

William Prout, M.D., 1785–1850

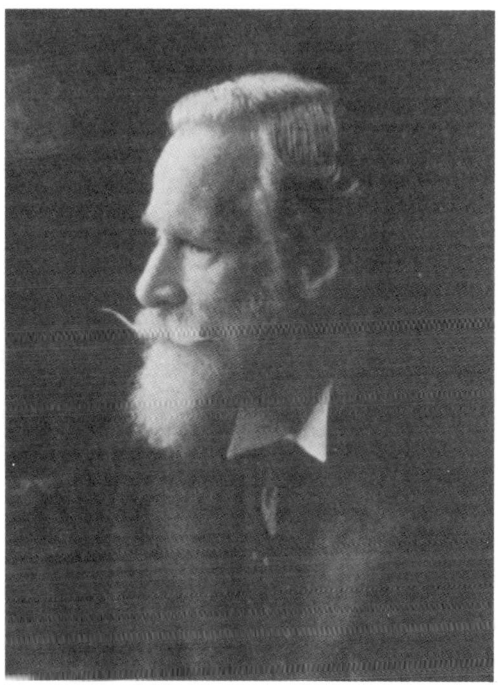

William Crookes, 1832–1919

FAHRENHEIT ESTABLISHES A LOUSY SCALE
(Celsius Corrects it — but Upside Down)

In 1613 Galileo bent a glass tube into a "U" shape, sealed one end and filled it with water. Upon inversion, under water, the length of the air space in the sealed end varied with pressure on the open end. As he used the U tube for measuring water pressure in hydraulic problems for many years he noticed that room air temperature affected his measurements. Also, red wine in the tube — cleaner and more reliable than most water at the time — changed more actively than water.

In 1637, working on hydraulics in pipes, he needed to compare the effect in cold and warm air. He sealed a length of glass tubing at one end, filled it with wine, stoppered the open end with a finger and inverted it into a bottle of wine. The level of wine in the vacuum at the sealed end was low inside his house but climbed rapidly out in the sun.

Galileo didn't believe vacuums could exist — that was Torrecelli's (his assistant) great discovery five years later — but the wine level was so sensitive to perceptible changes in room temperature that the device became an instant popular toy.

Soon Italian glass blowers made many "Galileo tubes," but with a small bulb at the bottom instead of a bottle. They added colored glass beads to mark arbitrary levels of warm and cool. They made long spirals and intricate examples of the glassblower's art, but nobody, not even Torrecelli, thought to add a standardized "cold" signal. These toys were thermo-*scopes,* not *-meters.*

Newton makes a thermo-meter

In 1701 Isaac Newton had a thermoscope blown for his own use. He wanted a practical tool, not fancy art work. Rather than the volatile alcohol he filled his glass tube with a more stable linseed oil. As Master of the Mint, and a confirmed bureaucrat, he also wanted numbers to record.

In order to establish a natural and easily available benchmark for "cold" he packed some fresh snow around the bulb of his thermoscope. Scratching a line on the glass to mark the oil level, he called it "0."

Packing the snow around the tube made his hands cold. He put them in his armpits to get warm, which gave him the idea for a natural and always available benchmark for "warm." He put the bulb of is thermoscope into his armpit to get warm and looked at his clock to see how long it would take. The upper end of the scale on the clock face was 12 and when he scratched the new oil level on the glass tube he marked it "12."

Newton scratched 12 equal divisions between cold and warm. They had nothing to do with "hours" so he called them "degrees" of temperature. Although Galileo gets the credit for the thermoscope, Newton actually invented the thermo*meter.* But it was not a precision instrument.

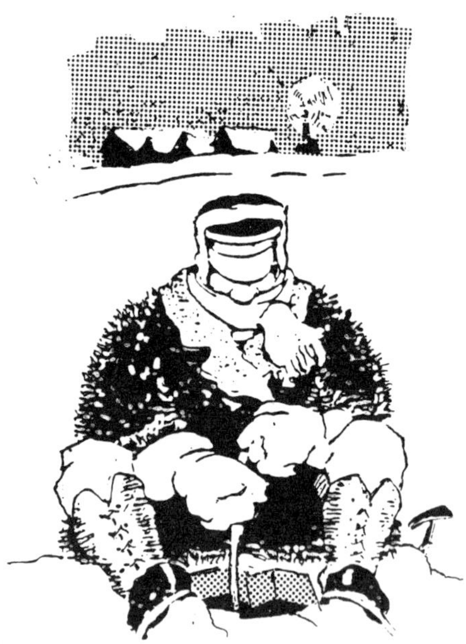

Fahrenheit adds precision

Across the Channel a Dutch instrument maker (a craftsman, not a scientist) named Gabriel Fahrenheit, was delighted with Newton's crude thermometer but thoroughly dissatisfied with its craftsmanship. The tube's bore was not uniform and oil crept up its inside surface to obscure its exact level. He had often seen quicksilver used as a fluid, but it was a dirty material and stained the insides of hand blown glass tubing.

Fahrenheit knew the first principle of precision instrument making: *KEEP IT CLEAN*. He devised a way to clean quicksilver — he filtered it through chamois leather — and to clean-dry narrow glass tubing. Quicksilver froze (−36°F) and boiled (+673°F) beyond the range of his requirements.

In the winter of 1714 Fahrenheit made his first thermoscope and looked around for a way to calibrate it into a thermometer. Copying Newton he found a "coldest thing" outside his door in the frozen canals of Holland: chipped salt water ice. He marked its mercury level as "0." He put the bulb in his armpit and marked the level as Newton's "12."

However, he could read the mercury column much more accurately than Newton could read linseed oil, so he divided Newton's scale of 12 in half, then in half again, and again; hence body temperature became 96°. (Remember this was armpit, not oral temperature.)

A New "Hot" is Required

Newton's "0," fresh water ice, now became 32°F. But, to be consistent with Newton's "coldest" he looked for a "hottest." It had to be easily available and reproducible, but non-destructive to glass. The hottest substance he could find was the steam over a kettle of boiling water. His thermometer read 212° on the modified Newton scale. He wrote up his technique and sent it to the Royal Society in London.

Newton was impressed. As president of the Royal Society (and *Sir* Isaac since 1705) he had Fahrenheit elected to fellowship in 1724 based upon this one scientific (really technical) report. Because of Newton's tremendous reputation, all English speaking countries, until a few years ago, were stuck with the queer 32°–212° scale.

Celsius makes an upside-down correction

A young Swedish astronomer, Anders Celsius, though teaching Newtonian physics, wasn't intimidated by Newton's mathematics. His father and grandfather were both noted mathematicians. When, as professor of astronomy at Uppsala, he was put in charge of their new observatory he rebelled against the necessity for making temperature corrections on a 32°–212° scale. His first measurements of the magnitude of stars by light intensity involved temperature corrections. Why not simplify things with a 100° or centigrade scale? He proposed that the scale read boiling water = 0° and freezing fresh water = 100°.

The Scale is Upside Down

Another thing Celsius had done was to take a financially strapped botany student, Carl Linné, into his home. (Celsius' uncle was professor of botany at Uppsala.) With his name Latinized to "Linnaeus," the student had become the founder of modern Taxonomy, and was a fanatic on the proper and exact use of words. When Linnaeus heard of Celsius' proposed new temperature scale, he screamed in taxonomic pain. *"That's upside down."* Flowers grow from the cold earth up to the hot sun. Cold is 0° and hot is 100°. The inverted centigrade scale was slowly adopted by most scientists and in worldwide commerce (except in the commercially chauvinistic US).

In 1944, after two centuries of centigrade temperatures, the International Commission on Weights and Measures (CGPM) made it official: the temperature interval (not "heat," it is only a scale of temperature *change*) will be 1/100 of the range from freezing fresh water at sea level, 0°C, to boiling fresh water at sea level, 100°C. The °C, they said, stands for degrees celsius.

[See Vig1847 .Jou; Joule]

MORGAGNI'S WARNING ON "CAUSES OF DEATH"

("Cancer," Once a Disease, is now a Journalists' Favorite Buzz Word)

After 1959, radiation hysteria in the U.S.A. climbed a sigmoid growth curve. It climaxed in 1979 at Three Mile Island: a biologically trivial, almost unmeasurable, release of fission °iodine was fanned into a newsmedia frenzy by an irresponsible NRC (Nuc Reg Commis), some crafty politicians, and incredibly incompetent reactor safety personnel.

The Chairman of the Senate Sub-Comm on Nuclear Regulation ordered (against expert advice) evacuation of a large population because "radiation caused leukemia." One percent of humans exposed to over 200 rads will have a delayed leukemic death. But the assumption that leukemia occurs after low level exposure has been proved false repeatedly. This politician, who could not distinguish between no risk and low risk, was, eight years later, dropped from a bid for the presidency of the U.S. because he could not see the risk in pre-election adultery.

The Secretary of HEW ordered (against expert advice) potassium iodide for the entire population because radioiodine causes thyroid cancer. (But no °iodine was detected in anybody's thyroid gland, and °iodine was known to prevent, not to cause, thyroid cancer.) His announcement was followed on one TV news program by a teenager crying, *"I don't want to die."* The histrionics were staged to compensate for the lack of blood & gore at Three Mile Island. [See Vig1979 .TMI]

Koch Proves a "Cause" of Disease

"Cause of death" is the most difficult decision an honest pathologist makes. Contributing causes may abound in postmortem examination of any death, but a single cause, except in obvious traumatic events, is hard to pin down. Robert Koch proved in 1876 that specific bacteria could "cause" a disease. He soon noted that fly-by-night scientists were implicating various bacteria as the cause of every disease. Before the turn of the century he tried to foil a developing bacteriophobia by devising five tests that had to be run before any germ could be implicated as a "Cause-of-a-Disease." The bacteria had to be isolated in pure culture from *every* case of the disease, and injected into another animal to cause the disease. Written as "five postulates," these are a satisfactory proof of "cause." They enforce the scientific requirement that only a 100% association can justify the consideration of cause & effect. Not until after Max Born and Quantum Mechanics in 1925 was a statistical probability acceptable as a "cause." Quantal statistics apply only in the picoworld of atoms.

[See Vig1925 .MB1]

In the macroworld of 1930s science, a strong statistical association, say 60% or 70%, was a reason for further research to look for a cause — and almost was proof of non-"cause." The "few-more-than-expected" associations were treated as scientific trivia until politics took the place of science in the 1959 cranberry crisis. [See Vig1959 .GCC] Establishment scientists then learned that "cause-of-disease," and especially "cause-of-death," was a manipulatable variable. "Death," according to the politically inspired, *"MAY"* be caused by anything you can get into newsprint.

Cause-of-Death of the Month Club

Egg yolks, strong coffee, burnt steak, smoking, any you care to mention, have a weak statistical association with diseases that cause death. They all are associated with human beings who, so far, have also always died. Flip a coin a few times and eventually you will come up with four heads in a row. Learn how to cheat just a little, like not keeping records, and it is surprising how often you can get five heads in a row. "Death" according to the politically inspired, "MAY" be caused by anything.

In 1936 a physician, Aaron Arkin, at Cook County Hospital in Chicago, said that most of his bronchogenic carcinoma patients had smoked cigarettes. By 1956 a few physicians convinced the American Cancer Society that this was a strong association, and funds were granted to search for evidence. They never found any, but something more convincing than science was substituted: a mesmeric constant

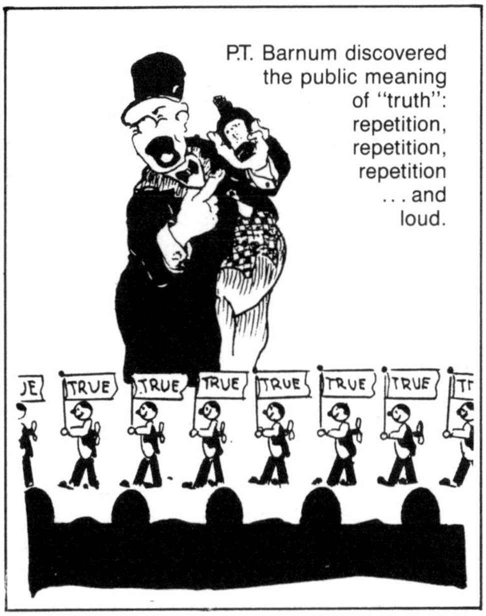

repetition of words. By 1966 cigarette smoking was associated in the newspapers with *"lung cancer"* which became *"deadly lung cancer,"* to *"may cause lung cancer"* and by 1976 *"causes lung cancer."* By 1986 the Surgeon General made it official: *"all* lung cancer is caused by cigarette smoke." But he reckoned without the anti-radon zealots. It is inevitable that in due course, uranium miners who smoke will each have to develop two lung cancers.

Two cancers per person may soon be insufficient in advanced societies. Too much of almost anything, sometimes too little, has become a prime cause of death among newspaper experts. Too much, too little, or improper exercise, or the wrong kind of food, drink, or any chemical, *may* cause disease or death. It is statistically more honest to say *may not* cause anything, but you forfeit your place on the evening TV news.

Risk is assessed by statisticians, politicians, and popular musicians. It is a prediction. Any scientist who makes a prediction that he knows cannot be verified is a liar. Cause-of-death is not a casual prediction, it comes from the *recorded* observations of many similar past events. This, one of the verities of science, has been known since 1771.

Morgagni Seeks a Cause-of-Death

Giovanni Battista Morgagni (1682–1771) was an Italian anatomist at a time when anatomy included much physiology and some clinical medicine. Before appointment as professor at the U of Padua at age 30 (which he held until death at age 90) he had published a book on the anatomy of diseases of the ear that gave him an international reputation. His interest had been, and continued to be, the anatomy of diseased bodies. Meticulous notes on post-mortem dissections made him the father of Pathology.

At age 80, in 1761, he published *"The Seats and Causes of Disease,"* the results of the 640 post-mortems he had performed. After a long career he was trying to explain the disease process, and the already legally important "Cause of Death." If he disregarded the obvious traumatic events, hemorrhages from knife wounds, crushed heads, etc., he was disillusioned by his lack of success. As with modern pathologists, he was appalled by bureaucratic acceptance of simplistic "causes" that had no basis in fact. His summary in 1761 is most applicable to the 1986 U.S. Government publications on "Risk vs Benefit": *". . . is dangerous to your health," ". . . may cause cancer,"* are predictions that cannot be verified.

"Those who have dissected many bodies have at least learned to doubt [the causes of disease]; while others who are ignorant of [pathology] and do not take the trouble to attend to it, are in no doubt at all." (Morgagni, 1761) You do not have to be a pathologist to realize that most causes of death are political, not scientific statements. The next time you hear a TV newsreader say, *"may cause cancer,"* ask yourself, "who makes money on cancer?"

In their *1968 Cancer Facts and Figures,* the American Cancer Society revealed the true cause of lung cancer. From 1950 to 1965, the lung cancer death rate per 100,000 U.S. male population increased in direct proportion to the funds collected in the Annual Cancer Crusade — an almost 100% statistical association. For every additional $500 collected by the Society, another man died of lung cancer.

WATT INVENTS A LITER-KILOGRAM

James Watt (1736–1819), best known because his name is on every light bulb, had nothing to do with electricity; but a lot to do with power. In his day it was common to refer to a man as "strong as a horse." Watt wanted to advertise his steam engines as strong as many horses. He wondered: how strong is a horse? He rented the biggest horse in a livery stable down the road, rigged its harness through a pulley, and lifted a 1500 pound mass 4 feet off the ground. By his calculations the horse had lifted 550 foot pounds in a second. He then declared 550 fp/s a unit of "horse-power." The unit is still in use. (But we use SI units, $kg \cdot m^2/s^3$.) [See Vig1847 .Jou]

Watt Invents Practical Power

How did Watt get into the esoteric (in 1760) power business? He was born in Scotland to a family selling nautical instruments. After apprenticeship Watt became an instrument maker at the University of Glasgow. In 1764 the University held an exhibition of technical marvels. Their working model of a Newcomen steam engine had been returned from London instrument makers as irreparable. They asked Watt to at least put it into displayable condition. Watt not only repaired the model, but had it pumping water for the exhibit.

Watt Re-invents the Steam Engine

Watt was appalled at the inefficiency and waste of heat in a Newcomen engine. He added a cold condenser chamber so that the hot cylinders did not have to be cooled in their power cycle. By 1769 he had built his own steam engine. Its performance was so much faster and power-efficient that he patented the idea, raised money, and went into business by 1774.

Watt added, and patented, many improvements: gear chains to convert pumping to rotary motion, or to power bellows, or crush ore. Centrifugal governors automatically shut off the steam when the pressure exceeded safety levels. Thus Watt invented "automatic feedback controls."

By 1800 over 500 Watt steam engines powered the Industrial Revolution in England. Watt received an honorary doctorate from U of Glasgow and was elected to the Royal Society. 150 years later he received his greatest honor: the SI unit of power was named the watt:

$$1 \text{ horsepower} = 746 \text{ watts.}$$

The Liter Could Be a Unit of Weight

Sought after in Glasgow and London society as a raconteur, Watt came to know Charles de Talleyrand (just appointed to the Ministry of Finance in Paris). Talleyrand complained at a dinner party of the difficulty of taxing many items due the lack of a standard unit of weight. Each village had its own "unit" that got leaner at tax time. An easily standardized "weight" was needed.

After thinking about the subject, Watt wrote a letter to Talleyrand with a simple solution. The French government was about to adopt a standard "metre." Make a container some handy fraction of a meter long, wide and deep. Fill this container with something available to everybody: water, and call its mass the "Unit of weight."

Upon receiving the suggestion, Talleyrand, being a politician, called a committee meeting. They settled on a container 1/10th of a meter long, wide, and deep and called it a "litre." It is such a handy unit of volume that the liter became the first metric unit to be accepted by the public.

Before a liter of water could be Watt's weight unit, many details: temperature, pressure, purity, had to be ironed out. The CGPM accepted the "weight" of a liter of water as the "Kilogram" in 1889, but abrogated this decision in 1903. (It is a unit of "mass," not "weight.") Because of the liter's widespread popularity, they accepted it as a unit of "volume" in 1903. They had to abrogate it again in 1964 (0.001 m^3 is incoherent in SI). It is now accepted as a special unit of volume. [See Vig1821 .kg]

LAVOISIER GETS HIS HEAD CUT OFF

Antoine Laurent Lavoisier (1743–1794) was born of a well-to-do family. His head was cut off 53 years later for a good reason. Titled aristocrats were obnoxious trivia to be swept away. Lavoisier's father had purchased a minor hereditary title — almost required of the wealthy in spendthrift France. But Lavoisier, in contrast to King and attending clowns, was one of the real evils that justified revolution. He was "earning" about 100K francs/year on a tax scheme that made him a perfect target for political murder.

Lavoisier's Work Required a Rich Man

In 1764 Lavoisier published his first important work: a study of the composition of the mineral gypsum. He was already looking for "elements" in the sense that Robert Boyle had defined the term around 1650. He fortified Boyle's idea that an "element" was a substance that always gains and never loses weight upon chemical manipulation. (He gave no credit to Boyle.) He discovered and named oxygen (but gave no credit to J. Priestly who made the real break with phlogiston). He was the first to see air as two separate gases. He discovered and named hydrogen (without giving credit to the Cavendish contribution).

In 1787 Lavoisier published a system of chemical nomenclature in which a compound's name would be a combination of the elements in it: hence sodium-chloride, or hydrogen-oxide (valence couldn't be considered until Dalton began weighing stuff in 16 more years). His nomenclature demanded knowing all of the elements. In 1789 he published his famous *Elementary Treatise on Chemistry* that contained a list of all 33 known "elements" (11 we now know are oxides). This landmark began modern chemistry.

By 1789 Lavoisier was only a part time scientist. He devoted from 6–8 am and 7–10 pm, plus one full day each week, to science. The rest of the day went to scientific and financial politics. As a typical knee-jerk liberal he even joined a revolutionary Society of 1789. Many friends considered him a financial genius who dabbled in chemistry, but his money grew directly out of interest in science.

Taxation is the Best Way to Raise Money

In 1768 Lavoisier needed a "laboratory" — practically unheard of in those days. Only a rich man could afford the high (for its day) technology and what Lavoisier was now adding, high (for its day) precision equipment. He had to build his own laboratory, and with his tastes it cost a lot of money. To pay for it he invested large sums in "Ferme générale." Three years later (1771) he married the daughter of a director of the "Ferme." Both were good investments except for a minor detail to which he paid no attention.

The Ferme générale was a private group of thugs hired by the King to collect taxes. These "tax farmers" could keep every thing collected over the legal rate. Because of a tendency to extract taxes forcibly they made lots of money and quite a few enemies. Although Lavoisier used all of his profits to equip and run a world famous laboratory that was the pride of France, tax-gouging hurt quite a few people. (It is surprising to learn how many people don't care that a diamond when burned in air forms CO_2.)

In 1780, as a member of the French Academy of Science (he had been a member since 1768 at age 23), he blackballed an incompetent who considered his journalism scientific. The journalist was Jean-Paul Murat. It turned out that Murat had a very good memory.

By 1792 radical anti-monarchists were in control of France. After declaring France a republic they beheaded a few royalists, but quickly turned to their real hate, the "tax farmers." At the head of one revolutionary tribunal Jean-Paul Murat was eager to give a fair trial to anybody who was going to the guillotine. Lavoisier was charged with, among other things, watering the People's tobacco, which carried the death penalty. On 8 May 1794 his head was cut off. Two months later the Reign of Terror was overthrown and a new government proclaimed him a great Frenchman, which he was — if you don't look too close.

[See Vig1803 .Dal]

CHRONOLOGY OF NUCLEAR MEDICINE — 1800–1824

Scientific and Technical Background

		Event		Ref.
1. Basic	— 1800	A. Volta invents the battery for galvanic current.	[1785]	DSB
	— 1800	W. Herschel discovers temperature in the IR region.	[1666]	DSB
	— 1801	J. Ritter discovers activity in the UV region.	[1666]	DSB
	— 1803	T. Young introduces wave theory of light.	[1690]	DSB
	— 1804	T. Grotthus law: only absorbed rays produce photo effect.		DSB
	— 1807	J. Proust announces law of definite proportions.	[1793]	DSB
	— 1808	J. Dalton writes law of multiple proportions.	[1767]	DSB
		J. Dalton POSTULATES THE ATOMIC THEORY.		Bio
	— 1808	L. Gay-Lussac writes law on volumes of gases.	[1661]	DSB
	— 1815	W. Prout postulates a primordial "protyle" atom (H).	[1803]	V92
		W. Prout says ALL ATOMIC WEIGHTS ARE WHOLE NUMBERS.	[1922]	V92
	—	(S. Glasstone reviews the Prout Whole-Number controversy.	1947	JCE)
	— 1819	E. Mitscherlich discovers isomorphism.	[1767]	DSB
	— 1820	P. Laplace can predict history of universe IF he knows the position and velocity of any particle.	[1926]	DSB
	— 1821	T. Szebeck misinterprets solidstate thermoelectric.	[1947]	DSB
	— 1821	M. Faraday invents electric generator & transformer.	[1729]	Bio
	— 1821	A. Ampere separates rate-of-current-passage from voltage.		DSB
	— 1823	A. Ampere founds science of electrodynamics.	[1729]	DSB
2. Obser	— 1802	G. Treviranus coins the word "Biology."	[1644]	DSB
	— 1803	J. Dalton weighs some elements (equivalent weights).	[1789]	Bio
	— 1808	H. Davy demonstrates electrochem to Royal Inst.	[1745]	DSB
	— 1809	H. Davy first use of "Radiant matter" requires high speed.		Bio
	— 1813	H. Davy makes his most important discovery: M. Faraday.	[1657]	DSB
	— 1813	J. Berzelius changes chemical notation to H, O, etc.	[1789]	Bio
	— 1816	M. Faraday: "transmutation can now be investigated."	[1919]	Bio
	— 1822	J. Lamarck coins word "vertebrate," uses "biology," but makes a mistake on evolution & is discredited.	[1802]	DSB
3. # Nuc	— 1803	J. Dalton says atoms of same element have equal weight.		Bio
	— 1805	J. Dalton publishes first table of 6 atomic weights.	[1766]	PML
	— 1808	J. Dalton publishes second table of 20 atomic weights.	[1869]	PML
	— 1804	H. Davy adds 10 more elements to Lavoisier's list of 33.		DoE
	— 1807	H. Davy isolates sodium and potassium.	[1789]	DoE
	— 1808	H. Davy isolates Ba, Bo, Ca, Mg, Sr, corrects Lavois oxides.		DoE
	— 1804	W. Wollaston discovers palladium & rhodium.	[1869]	DSB
	— 1814	W. Wollaston writes "Synoptic Table of Equivalents."	[1803]	DPL
	— 1811	A. Avogadro distinguishes atoms from molecules.	[1808]	DSB
	— 1811	B. Courtois discovers iodine.	[1934]	V91
	— 1815	J. Berzelius gives table of 43 At Wts (48 known elements).		DSB
	— 1817	J. Dobereiner groups triads of similar elements.	[1767]	APg

Organizations and Internal Politics

		Event		Ref.
5. Pols	— 1819	W. Wollaston blocks Metric System in UK for Imperial Sys.		DSB
	— 1821	J.Q. Adams (Sec of State) reports on Wts & Measures mess.		FR
	— 1824	J. Berzelius measures At Wt of Cl at 35.4 — Prout wrong.		DSB
6. Socs	— 1800	Royal College of Surgeons founded in London.	[1751]	EB
	— 1808	J. Gay-Lussac writes "The Combination of Gases."	[1644]	DSB
	— 1814	M. Orfila publishes "Toxicologie Generale."	[1761]	DSB
	— 1820	P. Laplace publishes "Celestial Mechanics."	[1927]	DSB
	— 1823	Brit Med J "Lancet" begins publication.	[1880]	La
7. Event	— 1800	M. Bichat introduces the word "tissue" = organized cells.		DSB
	— 1811	N. Appert: food preservation by heat in glass bottles.	(1985	NEJM)
	— 1815	Brit Apothecaries Act forbids "practice w/o a license."		La

Instruments, Units of Measurement, and Drugs

8. Instr	— 1801	R. Fulton makes first submarine "Nautilis."	[1954]	EB
	— 1802	H. Davy introduces the electric arc into chemistry.	[1745]	DSB
	— 1802	H. Davy makes photoprints of leaves by Schutz tech.	[1727]	Bio
	— 1804	H. Davy uses voltaic electricity as a chemical tool.	[1800]	Bio
	— 1821	A. Ampere invents the galvanometer.	[1785]	DSB
	— 1816	R. Laennec invents ascultation with stethoscope.	[1761]	CDD
9. Units	— 1823	M. Faraday finds a temperature below 0°F.	[1708]	Bio
	— 1817	J. Berzelius pubs mol weights of 2000 compounds.	[1808]	DSB
10. Concp	— 1803	T. Young introduces the word "energy."	[1690]	DSB
	— 1805	A. Legendre publishes method of least squares.	[1733]	DSM
	— 1812	J. Fourier theorizes on periodic harmonic functions.		DSB
	— 1805	W. Congreve introduces rockets into British Army.	[1644]	EB
	— 1819	E. Mitscherlich discovers isomorphism.	[1718]	DSB
11. Drugs	— 1805	F. Sarturner isolates morphine.	[1785]	CDD
	— 1810	W. Wollaston finds second amino acid (cystine) in bladder.		

Radioiodine, P-32, and Radioactive Therapy

12. I-Res	— 1811	B. Courtois' iodine from seaweed suggests thyroid.	[1934]	V90
	— 1821	J. Coindet recognizes I-induced hyperthyroidism.	[1637]	V90
14. I-Rx	— 1816	W. Prout starts iodine Rx of goiter at St Thom London.		V90
	— 1820	A. Coindet pubs first paper on iodine Rx of goiter.	[1623]	V90
	— 1824	A. Coindet causes toxic nod goiter with iodine Rx.	[1657]	V90

Scans and Other Tests of Function in Various Organs

18. Brain	— 1810	Gall & Spurzheim pub "Anat et Physiol du Syst Nerveux."		DSB
	— 1811	C. Bell sees function of spinal ant & post roots.	[1766]	CDD
19. Heart	— 1806	J. Corvisart describes stenosis of valves.	[1755]	Bk
	— 1815	J. Hogson pubs textbk on dis of arteries & veins.	[1661]	Bk
	— 1811	W. Wells finds albuminous urine in pts with dropsy.	[1785]	CDD
	— 1816	W. Wells describes complications of rheumat fever.	[1715]	CDD
	— 1815	J. Hodgson note syphilitic aortitis & insufficien.	[1761]	CDD
	— 1818	J. Cheyne describes Cheyne-Stokes respiration.		Bk
23. Kidney	— 1822	R. Bright studies diseases of kidney, esp nephritis.		Bk
24. Gut	— 1824	W. Prout discovers HCl in normal stomach.	[1775]	PTRS
25. Blood	— 1826	J. Combe describes a patient with Anemia.	[1658]	CDD
26. Other	— 1824	J. Prevost proves sperm required for fertilization.	[1785]	DSB

Radiation Hysteria and Health Physics * Obituaries *

27. Hyst	— 1800	J. Spurzheimer becomes pupil of F. Gall in phrenology.		DSB
	— 1802	F. Gall "reads" brain from depressions in skull.	[1931]	DSB
	— 1802	Church orders F. Gall to stop lecturing on phrenology.		DSB
	— 1805	F. Gall's phrenology is rage of Paris.	[1802]	DSB
	— 1810	J. Spurzheim divides brain into 36 phrenological patches.		DSB
	— 1824	55 books published (1803–57) on phrenology "science."		DSB
	— 1814	-. Pansa sees lung disease in Joachimsthal miners.	[1770]	AJC
28. React	— 1810	S. Hannemann founds Homeopathy — a harmless foolishness that stops stupid medical phlebotomy.	[Kaufman 1971]	Bk

* * *

30. Obits	— J. Priestly (1733–1804) Eng chem; electrical chemistry.	DSB
	— H. Cavendish (1731–1810) Eng physics; gas physics.	DSB
	— J. LaGrange (1736–1813) Fr math; first Comm on Poids et Mesures.	DSB
	— M. Klaproth (1743–1817) Ger physics; first analytical chemist.	DSB
	— J. Watt (1736–1819) Scot physics; steam energy, horsepower.	DSB

CHRONOLOGY OF NUCLEAR MEDICINE — 1825–1849

		Scientific and Technical Background		Ref.
1. Basic	— 1832	M. Faraday states the laws of electrolysis.	[1808]	Bio
	— 1829	J. Dobereiner repeats triad similarities.	[1817]	DSB
	— 1830	Prout's reception by his peers reviewed (O. Benfey;	1952	JCE)
	— 1831	J. Henry invents the electric motor.	[1821]	DSB
	— 1835	J. Henry invents the electric relay.	[1821]	DSB
	— 1833	C. Babbage builds steam calculator analytic engine.	[1642]	DSB
	— 1838	M. Faraday repeats Abbe Nollet's "electric egg."	[1748]	Bio
	—c1840	F. Magendie founds sciences of physiol & pharmacol.	[1810]	DSB
	— 1842	J. Mayer announces law of "conservation of energy."	[1784]	DSB
	— 1847	H. Helmholtz announces "conservation of energy" law.	[1842]	Bio
	— 1844	M. Faraday suggests lines-of-force in mag field.	[1733]	Bio
	— 1849	J. Joule announces "mechanical equivalent of heat."	[1803]	DSB
2. Obser	— 1825	T. Drummond invents "lime light": H flame on lime sticks.		HRP
	— 1831	R. Brown recognizes and names the cell nucleus.	[1800]	DSB
	— 1837	R. Brown observes "Brownian" motion in water.	[1905]	DSB
		BROWNIAN MOTION IS FIRST *OBSERVED* EVIDENCE OF ATOMS		
	— 1838	M. Faraday sees "dark space" in low pressure tubes.	[1752]	HRP
	— 1839	J. Perkinje introduces the term "protoplasm."	[1802]	DSB
	— 1849	J. Joule finds loss of energy balanced by heat.	[1803]	DSB
3. # Nuc	— 1829	J. Berzelius discovers thorium (Th #90).	[1789]	DOE
	— 1840	C. Schoenbein discovers and names Ozone.	[1774]	DSB
		Organizations and Internal Politics		
5. Pols	— 1825	Hungarian Academy of Science founded in Budapest.	[1759]	EB
6. Socs	— 1836	A. Gray publishes first "Textbook of Botany."	[1789]	DSB
	— 1847	Am Medical Assoc has first meeting in Philadelphia.	[1792]	JAMA
	— 1847	G. Boole writes first text on symbolic logic.	[1704]	DSB
	— 1850	W. Talbot publishes first book with photographs.	[1831]	DSB
7. Event	— 1825	M. FARADAY INVENTS "ELECTROLYSIS," = + & − IONS.	[1808]	Bio
	— 1840	W. Whewell coins the name "Scientist" (thinking of Faraday).		Bio
	— 1840	W. Whewell first uses "normal" in its scientific sense.	[1733]	OED
	— 1842	C. Long first uses ether anesthesia.	[1805]	CDD
	— 1846	W. Morton introduces ether anesthesia in public.	[1842]	CDD
	— 1846	W. Thomson (Kelvin) calculates earth's age @ 100 My.	[1980]	DSB
		Instruments, Units of Measurement, and Drugs		
8. Instr	— 1829	J. Niepce makes first AgCl photograph.	[1802]	DSB
	— 1830	J. Perkinje is first to use "Microtome" for thin slices.		DSB
	— 1831	Niepce & Daguerre make permanent prints with AgCl.	[1829]	EB
	— 1838	M. Faraday passes current thru low pressure gas.	[1895]	Bio
	— 1840	J. Herschel introduces "hypo" fixing of photos.	[1831]	EB
	— 1841	W. Talbot introduces the photographic negative.	[1829]	EB
	— 1850	W. Talbot deciphers the cuneiform tablets of Nineveh.		DSB
	— 1847	K. Ludwig invents the Kymograph.	[1643]	DSB
9. Units	— 1828	J. Berzelius writes first Table of Atomic Weights.	[1815]	DSB
	— 1829	N. Lobachevsky derives first non-Euclidean geometry.	[1637]	DSB
	— 1831	J. Bolyai derives a similar non-Euclidean geometry.	[1829]	DSB
	— 1832	J. Gauss conceives a coherent system based upon . . . length, mass, time, and combinations.	[1962]	Bio
	— 1841	Grotthuss & Draper Law: "absorbed" energy is dose.	[1804]	PM
	— 1845	T. Andrews discovers the "critical point" in temp.	[1823]	DSB
	— 1845	L. Traub introduces clinical "bedside" thermometry.	[1701]	CDD
	— 1846	W. Weber devises logical electricity units.	[1832]	DSB

10. Concp	— 1835	L. Quetelet: first statistical study of human bodies.	[1654]	DSB
	— 1846	L. Quetelet applies Gaussian "bell curve" in vital stats.	[1733]	Bio
	— 1837	P. Bretonneau sees specificity in infect disease.	[1673]	CDD
	— 1838	T. Schwann tries to disprove "spont generation."	[1768]	DSB
	— 1839	T. Schwann proclaims all living things made of cells.	[1800]	DSB
	— 1840	F. Henle postulates: microorganisms cause disease.	[1897]	DSB
	— 1845	R. Remak names embryo layers ecto, meso, endoderm.	[1800]	DSB
	— 1847	J. Gerlach "labels" a cell's nucleus with carmine.	[1912]	CDD
	— 1849	H. Helmholtz destroys religious concept of "Vital Force."		DSB
11. Drugs	— 1828	F. Woehler makes first organic (urea) from inorganic.	[1810]	DSB
	— 1844	F. Magendie teaches pharmacology to Claude Bernard.	[1761]	DSB

Radioiodine, P-32, and Radioactive Therapy

12. I-Res	— 1825	C. Perry publishes hyperthyroidism description.	[1786]	CDD
13. I-Dx	— 1835	R. Graves describes exophthalmic goiter symptoms.	[1825]	CDD
	— 1840	K. Basedow describes 4 exophthalmic goiter pts.	[1835]	V90
17. Other	— 1840	R. Remak treats nerve disease by "Electrotherapy."	[1776]	DSB

Scans and Other Tests of Function in Various Organs

18. Brain	— 1837	M. Hall proves nerves are either sensory or motor.	[1811]	CDD
	— 1843	E. DuBois-Reymond times nerves, first electrophysiol.	[1766]	DSB
19. Heart	— 1828	J. Poiseuille uses Hg U tube for blood pressure.	[1613]	DSB
	— 1831	J. Hope details minute pulse characteristics.	[1872]	CDD
	— 1832	D. Corrigan describes pulse in aortic regurgitat.	[1806]	Bk
	— 1840	J. Bouillaud pubs textbook on rheumatic fever.	[1816]	Bk
	— 1846	K. Ludwig perfuses the isolated mammalian heart.	[1976]	DSB
20. Liver	— 1826	R. Laennec names "cirrhosis" after color of liver.	[1685]	CDD
21. Lung	— 1839	J. Skoda pubs textbook: auscultation & percussion.	[1761]	Bk
23. Kidney	— 1827	R. Bright describes a chronic nephritis.	[1822]	CDD
	— 1843	C. Ludwig notes glomerular and tubular urine excretion.		DSB
	— 1846	F. Henle describes kidney microanatomy.	[1964]	DSB
	— 1849	T. Addison describes suprarenal capsule disease.	[1867]	CDD
24. Gut	— 1826	W. Beaumont sees motion and digestion in stomach.	[1824]	CDD
24. Gut	— 1834	T. Schwann discovers stomach "pepsin," first enzyme.	[1824]	DSB
25. Blood	— 1832	T. Hodgkin describes spleen and lymph node disease.	[1968]	CDD
	— 1838	G. Valentin measures blood volume by dilution.	[1928]	RAP
	— 1845	R. Virchow is first to describe leukemia.	[1638]	DSB
	— 1845	J. Bennett describes "suppuration of blood" (leukemia).		CDD
26. Other	— 1840	T. Schwann studies and coins name "metabolism."	[1630]	DSB

Radiation Hysteria and Health Physics * Obituaries *

27. Hyst	— 1844	J. Mayer originates myth that all energy comes from sun.		DSB
	— 1832	J. Spurzheim founds Phrenology as science at Yale.	[1802]	BMSJ
	—	Reading "bumps-on-the-head" is the scientific fad 1830–c1885.		EB
	— 1848	Immigrant writes family in Ireland, Boston cat has 6 toes. First mention of polydactyl cats, now 15% in Boston. (NatHist 1986)		

* * *

30. Obits	—	A. Volta (1745–1827) It physics; Voltaic pile (battery).	DSB
	—	W. Wollaston (1766–1828) Eng chem; equivalent numbers.	DSB
	—	T. Young (1773–1829) Eng physics; wave theory of light.	Bio
	—	H. Davy (1778–1829) Eng chem; electrochemistry.	DSB
	—	J. Niepce (1765–1833) Fr inventor, first photography.	DSB
	—	A. Ampere (1775–1836) Fr math physics; electrical currents.	DSB
	—	B. Courtois (1777–1838) Fr indust chem; discovered iodine.	DSB
	—	J. Dalton (1766–1844) Eng chem; the atomic theory.	Bio
	—	J. Berzelius (1779–1848) Swed chem; first Table of Atomic Wts.	DSB
	—	J. Dobereiner (1780–1849) Ger chem; Law of Triads.	DSB

CHRONOLOGY OF NUCLEAR MEDICINE — 1850–1874

		Scientific and Technical Background		Ref.
1. Basic	— 1850	R. Clausius: "Entropy always increases" (closed sys).	[1842]	DSB
	—c1850	R. Virchow introduces microscopy & cells to path.	[1673]	DSB
	— 1860	R. Virchow says, "All cells arise from cells."	[1839]	Bio
	— 1854	G. Riemann introduces non-Euclidean surfaces.	[1831]	DSM
	— 1858	K. Ludwig requires phys/chem evidence in physiol.	[1844]	DSB
	— 1860	Avogadro's law reborn by Cannizzaro at Karlsruhe.	[1811]	WoA
	— 1860	J. Stas says Prout's hypothesis "a pure illusion."	[1818]	BAR
	— 1860	R. Bunsen (& Kirchoff) invents spectroscopy as chem tool.		DSB
	— 1862	L. Euler uses "e" for 2.718 . . . base natural logs.	[1614]	DSM
	— 1862	G. Kirchhoff describes a perfect "Black Body."	[1900]	DSB
	— 1864	W. Crookes changes "equivalent" to "atomic" weights.	[1828]	CN
	— 1864	L. Pasteur disproves spontaneous generation.	[1838]	DSB
	— 1865	L. Pasteur establishes "Germ Theory" of disease.	[1840]	Bio
	— 1873	J. Maxwell converts Faraday's "lines" into math emf.	[1844]	Bio
	— 1873	J. Maxwell postulates light is oscillating charge.	[1803]	Bio
2. Obser	— 1854	P. Berthelot makes organic compound; no vital force.	[1849]	DSB
	— 1861	T. Graham notes & names "colloids" (vs crystaloids).	[1861]	DSB
	— 1865	A. Butlerov sees "chemical structure" of compounds.	[1828]	DSB
	— 1869	J. Hittorf casts a shadow in cathode ray beam.	[1858]	V93
	— 1874	G. Stoney coins word "electron" for electric unit.	[1891]	PM
3. # Nuc	— 1853	J. Gladstone first to arrange elements by At Wt.	[1829]	PM
	— 1857	J. Dumas finds At Wt periodicity, believes Prout.	[1824]	CRS
	— 1861	W. Crookes discovers thallium (Tl #81).	[1975]	Bio
	— 1862	D. Chancourtois shows "telluric screw" periodicity.	[1829]	DSB
	— 1863	W. Crookes finds elements have similar properties.	[1829]	CN
	— 1865	J. Newlands finds a "law of octaves" periodicity.	[1829]	CN
	—	(J. Spronson: did Newlands invent the Periodic Table?	1959	JCE)
	— 1869	D. MENDELEEV BUILDS PERIODIC TABLE OF 64 ELEMENTS.	[1815]	JRC
	— 1869	D. Mendeleev leaves 35 empty spaces, predicts filling.	[1875]	DSB
	— 1870	L. Meyer constructs Periodic Table, no predictions.	[1869]	AC

		Organizations and Internal Politics		
6. Socs	— 1854	G. Boole writes "Investigation of Laws of Thought."	[1831]	DSB
	— 1856	A. Fleck publishes "Medical Physics."	[1843]	DSB
	— 1856	J. Maxwell publishes "On Faraday's Lines of Force."	[1844]	DSB
	— 1859	C. Darwin publishes "The Origin of Species."	[1840]	Bk
		SEPARATION OF SCIENCE FROM RELIGION BECOMES PUBLIC	[1871]	
	— 1859	W. Crookes begins publication of Chemical News (London).		CN
7. Event	— 1871	J. Maxwell is first Cambridge prof of experimental physics.		Bio
	— 1872	J.J. Thomson is 1 of 4 students to take Maxwell lectures.		Bio
	— 1872	E. Hoppe-Seyler starts Biochemistry & first Journal.	[1823]	DSB

		Instruments, Units of Measurement, and Drugs		
8. Instr	— 1851	Collodian photosens glass "wet plates" introduced.	[1831]	EB
	— 1855	R. Bunsen mixes gas with air in new "Bunsen Burner."	[1825]	DSB
	— 1855	H. Geissler first to seal metal wires in glass.	[1838]	HRC
	— 1855	H. Geissler invents the mercury vacuum pump.	[1672]	HRC
	— 1855	H. Geissler makes first cathode ray tube for Plücker.	[1895]	HRC
	— 1857	W. Thompson (Lord Kelvin) devises an electrometer.	[1746]	Bio
	— 1858	J. Plücker discovers fluorescence in wall of tube.	[1838]	HRC
	— 1859	W. Crookes makes first autoradiogram (of U in rock).	[1955]	CN
	— 1866	M. Coulier discovers supersaturated air in clouds	[1896]	DSB
	— 1867	N. de St Victor finds U Nitrate will expose film.	[1859]	CN
	— 1869	J. Hittorf puts shadow shield in a Geissler tube.	[1858]	HRC

9. Units	— 1860	J. Stas adopts Oxygen as standard for At Wt of 16.	[1828]	DSB
	— 1860	G. Mendel notes math basis of hereditary markings.	[1925]	DSB
10. Concp	— 1856	K. Ludwig removes organs, keeps viable by perfusion.	[1846]	DSB
	— 1856	C. Bernard discovers anabolism + catabolism.	[1844]	DSB
	— 1868	J. Lockyer discovers & names Helium (Gr = sun).	[1896]	DSB
	— 1869	F. Galton says many variables fall on bell curve.	[1846]	DSB
	— 1871	J. Maxwell says Heat is not an imponderable fluid.	[1819]	Bio
	— 1871	J. Maxwell says Heat is stat average of molecular motion.	[1849]	Bio
	— 1867	P. Chebyshev publishes a theory of "mean" value.	[1835]	DSM
	— 1867	W. Waldeyer describes genesis and spread of ca.	[1851]	CDD
11. Drugs	— 1857	M. Faraday scales first particles with AuCol color.	[1952]	RSPT

Radioiodine, P-32, and Radioactive Therapy

12. I-Res	— 1850	T. Curling notes "absence" of thyroid in myxedema.	[1840]	CDD
	— 1852	A. Chatin says goiter due to iodine lack in soil.	[1657]	CRS
	— 1866	K. Voit builds human calorimeter for O_2, CO_2 & Heat.	[1871]	DSB
13. I-Dx	— 1873	W. Gull considers thyroid in adult female cretins.	[1850]	V91
14. I-Rx	— 1867	R. Smith: clinical trial of I-127 doses in toxics.	[1824]	BMJ

Scans and Other Tests of Function in Various Organs

18. Brain	— 1861	P. Broca localizes a "speech" area in brain.	[1658]	DSB
19. Heart	— 1854	A. Trousseau discusses pericard fluid and Rx.	[1761]	Bk
	— 1862	M. Raynaud studies vaso-spastic diseases of limbs.	[1815]	Bk
	— 1867	T. Brunton introduces amyl nitrate Rx of angina.	[1761]	Bk
	— 1870	A. Fick devises a cardiac output method.	[1847]	DSB
	— 1872	L. Traub records the pulse with kymograph.	[1831]	CDD
20. Liver	— 1856	C. Bernard discovers glycogen in liver.	[1826]	DSB
25. Blood	— 1850	C. Lehmann drains blood post-execution for blood volume.		LPC
	— 1856	T. Bischoff drains blood post-execution for volume.	[1959]	V44
	— 1854	H. Welcker measures Hb to estimate blood volume.	[1850]	AAF
	— 1855	T. Addison describes Pernicious Anemia in Guy's.	[1826]	V48
	— 1862	C. Bernard explains poison action of CO in blood.	[1774]	DSB
	— 1856	C. Bernard finds CO_2 displaces O_2 in hemoglobin.	[1777]	DSB
	— 1862	E. Hoppe-Seyler prepares crystalline hemoglobin.	[1855]	DSB

Radiation Hysteria and Health Physics * Obituaries *

27. Hyst	— 1851	W. Marsden reports alarming increase in ca mortality; 1839 — 463 ca deaths in London district, 1850 — 889 ca deaths in London district, thus the first ca hospital was built by scaring politicians.		BMJ
	— 1850–1890s	Spiritualism slowly gains "scientific" popularity.		EB
	— 1870	C. Bernard is first target of antivivisectionists.	[1856]	DSB
	— 1860	Bishop Wilberforce: was your grandmother an ape?	[1859]	DSB
28. React	1860	T. Huxley: better an ape than a Bishop who lies.	[1925]	DSB
	— 1860	R. Virchow rejects Pasteur's germ theory.	[1840]	DSB
	— 1869	F. Galton measures efficacy of prayer with statistics.		Bio
29. Respo	— 1865	M. Pettenkoffer swallows cholera culture to disprove Germ Theory and gets away with it.		DSB

* * *

30. Obits	—	W. Prout (1785–1850) Eng physician, chem; whole number rule.	V92
	—	L. Daguerre (1789–1851) Fr inventor; photography.	DSB
	—	G. Ohm (1787–1854) Ger physics; electrical resistance.	DSB
	—	K. Basedow (1799–1854) Ger physician; exophthalmic goiter.	EB
	—	F. Magendie (1783–1855) Fr physiol; first physiol pharmacologist.	DSB
	—	A. Avogadro (1776–1856) It physics; atoms vs molecules.	DSB
	—	N. Lobachevsky (1792–1856) Pol math; non-Euclidean geometry.	DSB
	—	M. Faraday (1791–1867) Eng phys, chem; fields of force.	DSB
	—	L. Quetelet (1796–1874) Belg math; first biological statistics.	DSB

CHRONOLOGY OF NUCLEAR MEDICINE — 1875–1889

				Ref.
		Scientific and Technical Background		
1. Basic	— 1875	W. CROOKES DISPLAYS RADIOMETER TO ROY SOC.	[1855]	Bio
	— 1875	W. Clifford says every atom has electric current.	[1873]	CN
	— 1876	R. Koch discovers anthrax bacillus.	[1865]	CDD
	— 1876	R. Koch is first to use stain to see bacteria.	[1913]	CDD
	— 1883	R. Koch devises inoculation to prevent anthrax.	[1865]	DSB
	— 1879	W. Crookes postulates fourth (radiant) state of matter.	[1809]	CN
	— 1880	P. Curie discovers piezoelectricity.	[1857]	DSB
	— 1881	A. Michelson measures speed of light, 3×10^8 m/s.	[1873]	Bio
	— 1887	A. Michelson says "aether," if any, is unmeasurable.	[1671]	Bio
	— 1881	A. Helmholtz postulates "atoms" of electricity.	[1874]	CN
	— 1881	J.J. Thomson hints cathode rays are "corpuscles."	[1873]	PM
	— 1885	J. Balmer gets empirical formula for H spectrum.	[1860]	DSB
	— 1886	E. Goldstein finds (& names) "+" kanalstrahlen.	[1858]	BB
	— 1886	P. LaPlace derives the "Gaussian" law of errors.	[1846]	DSM
	— 1887	J. Stas repeats, "Prout's law a complete illusion."	[1860]	JCE
	— 1888	H. Hertz builds an oscillating electric circuit; finds electricity travels at speed of light.	[1881]	Bio
2. Obser	— 1876	E. Goldstein finds Hittorf's shadows are not sharp.	[1869]	V93
	— 1877	L. Cailletet: compressed gases cool on expansion.	[1896]	DSB
	— 1877	W. Crookes invents "Crookes Tube," first X-ray device.	[1855]	V93
	— 1879	W. Crookes puts paddle wheel in cathode ray beam.	[1858]	V93
	— 1880	C. Pierce says elec circuits emulate Boolean logic.	[1854]	FV
	— 1881	C. Finlay says mosquitos transmit yellow fever.	[1837]	CDD
	— 1883	A. King lists 19 facts: mosquitos carry malaria.	[1881]	CDD
	— 1884	S. Arrhenius divides electro from non-electrolytes.	[1875]	DSB
	— 1885	H. Marquand designs an electrical logic machine.	[1833]	FV
	— 1889	A. Righi shows hertz same as visible light waves.	[1873]	DSB
	— 1882	J. Strutt (third Rayleigh) checks Prout's hypothesis.	[1815]	DSB
	— 1896	J. Strutt is impressed and leads to inert gas discoveries.		DSB
3. # Nuc	— 1875	L. Boisbaudrau discovers first predicted element, Ga.	[1869]	DSB
	— 1882	F. Clarke recalculates 66 At Wts, says Prout right.	[1860]	SIP
	— 1885	K. Auer gets neo (#60) & praseo (#59) from didynium.	[1898]	DSB
		K. Auer patents "Welsbach" Th + Ce gas mantle. (First RE use.)	[1869]	DSB
	— 1885	W. Crookes' "metaelements" have mean At Wt value.	[1863]	CN
	— 1886	W. Crookes introduces "protyle" (H) in element's genesis.	[1815]	CN
	— 1886	W. Crookes says 70 elements are known, others probable.	[1869]	CN
	— 1886	G. Stokes redefines "element" as specif spect lines.	[1789]	CN
		Organizations and Internal Politics		
5. Pols	— 1875	Diplomatic Conf signs Treaty of Metric Convention.	[1795]	NBS
	— 1883	Bismarck introduces sickness insurance in Germany.	[1761]	EB
6. Socs	— 1884	I. Mechnikov publishes "Theory of Phagocytes."	[1860]	DSB
	— 1887	W. Ostwald, first prof of "physical chemistry," starts "ZPC."		ZPC
	— 1879	"J American Chem Soc" begins publication.	[1859]	JACS
	— 1880	"Science" weekly magazine begins publication.	[1823]	Sc
	— 1883	"JAMA" begins publication.	[1847]	JAMA
	— 1889	G. Peano pubs "A Logical Exposition of Geometry."	[1847]	DSB
7. Event	— 1876	R. Koch proves anthrax caused by specific organism.	[1840]	DSB
	— 1879	T. Edison, J. Swan (Eng) invent electric light bulb.	[1821]	Bio
	— 1881	L. Pasteur immunizes some sheep against anthrax.	[1865]	DSB
	— 1882	R. Koch proves tuberculos caused by specif bacty.	[1876]	Bio
	—c1885	R. Koch BEGINS TO DEVELOP "KOCH'S POSTULATES" ON "CAUSE."		Bio
	— 1888	H. Hertz builds electromagnetic wave oscillator.	[1873]	DSB
	— 1888	W. Roentgen appointed prof physics, U of Würzburg.	[1895]	GSR

Instruments, Units of Measurement, and Drugs

8. Instr	— 1880	J. Aitken: air expansion causes H_2O saturated cloud.	[1866]	DSB
	— 1881	A. Michelson invents the "interferometer."	[1873]	Bio
	— 1881	S. Basch builds an early sphygmomanometer.	[1767]	Bk
	— 1883	K. Auer says Pt mantle on lime light is brilliant.	[1825]	DSB
	— 1885	E. Marey writes textbk on graphic data recording.	[1847]	Bk
	— 1889	G. Eastman invents celluloid-backed photo film.	[1851]	Bio
9. Units	— 1875	Bureau Int des Poids et Mesures (BIPM) founded.	[1795]	V101
	— 1861	First Cong (pre-CGPM) adopts Weber's elec units.	[1846]	NBS
	— 1889	First Conf Gen des Poids et Mes (CGPM) defines meter & kg.		V101
10. Concp	— 1875	TREATY OF THE METER, 17 NATIONS CREATE THE BIPM.	[1795]	EB
	— 1881	S. Langley's .001° bolometer — 1 cal/cm^2 = 1 Langley.	[1748]	DSB
11. Drugs	— 1877	A. Downes: UV rad in sunlight is bactericidal.	[1801]	PRSL
	— 1879	A. Kossel discovers & names nucleic acid.	[1828]	DSB
	— 1884	C. Koller develops cocaine as local anesthetic.	[1809]	DSB
	— 1889	-. Widmark implicates UV in producing erythema.	[1877]	DSB

Radioiodine, P-32, and Radioactive Therapy

12. I-Res	— 1876	K. Voit uses human calorimeter to measure BMR.	[1866]	DSB
	— 1884	M. Rubner uses BMR, shows food energy thermodynamic.	[1876]	DSB
14. I-Rx	— 1889	J. Hutchinson's Rx for Graves Dis is mountain air.	[1867]	As

Scans and Other Tests of Function in Various Organs

18. Brain	— 1882	P. Erlich studies eye's fluid with fluorescein.	[1847]	V10
	— 1886	P. Marie notes acromegaly with pituitary lesion.	[1837]	CDD
19. Heart	— 1875	E. Galvagni studies adhesive pericarditis.	[1854]	Bk
	— 1875	C. Rokitansky writes bk on Path of Heart & Vessels.	[1850]	DSB
	— 1876	J. Cohnheim describes embolism, pulm edema, amyloid.	[1875]	Bk
	— 1878	A. Hammer diagnoses a coronary occlusion.	[1768]	WMW
	— 1883	O. Schmiedeberg does experiments with digitalis.	[1785]	DSB
	— 1888	E. Fallot describes the causes of "blue babies."	[1973]	DSB
21. Lung	— 1888	G. Steel brings up question of pulmonary embolism.	[1969]	CDD
22. Bone	— 1876	J. Paget describes a chronic "Osteitis Deformans."	[1985]	CDD
24. Gut	— 1881	C. Voit's "Science of Nutrition" starts food studies.	[1876]	CDD
	— 1886	R. Fitz names "appendicitis" on review of 157 pts.	[1711]	CDD
	— 1889	O. Monkowieki: no pancreas in dog causes diabetes.	[1776]	CDD
26. Other	— 1884	H. Gram develops iodine stain for some bacteria.	[1847]	DSB

Radiation Hysteria and Health Physics * Obituaries *

27. Hyst	—c1875	Lodge, Crookes, Wallace, many others sold on spiritualism.		Bio
	— 1879	P. Harting: no lung ca in Joachimsthal miners.	[1700]	AJC
	— 1882	J. Cohnheim: no lung ca in Joachimsthal miners.	[1814]	AJC
	— 1884	-. Anzke finds no lung ca in Schneeberg miners.	[1814]	AJC

* * *

30. Obits	— W. Talbot (1800–1877) Eng inventor; photography.	DSB
	— J. Henry (1797–1878) Am physics; electricity, the motor.	DSB
	— C. Bernard (1813–1878) Fr physiol; experimental physiology.	DSB
	— J. Mayer (1814–1878) Ger physics; energy.	DSB
	— H. Geissler (1814–1879) Ger inst maker; glassblower, Hg pumps.	DSB
	— C. Darwin (1809–1882) Eng naturalist; evolution.	DSB
	— T. Schwann (1810–1882) Ger physiol; germ & cell theory.	DSB
	— G. Mendel (1822–1884) Aust botany, plant breeding, pre-genetics.	DSB
	— F. Henle (1809–1885) Ger pathol; germs cause disease.	DSB
	— J. Joule (1818–1889) Eng brewer, physics; conservation of energy.	DSB

CHRONOLOGY OF NUCLEAR MEDICINE — 1890–1894

		Scientific and Technical Background		Ref.
1. Basic —	1890	B. Tchitcherine proposes first "solar" atom design.	[1913]	BSIM
—	1890	E. von Behring discovers antitoxins.	[1883]	CDD
—	1893	W. Wien's formula fits IR wavelength black body.	[1862]	DSB
—	1894	W. Wien deflects canal rays in parabolic curve.	[1886]	DSB
2. Obser —	1891	G. Stoney names "electron" for Faraday unit charge.	[1881]	DSB
—	1892	H. Hertz: cathode rays go thru gold foil, no effect.	[1888]	APC
—	1892	N. Finson says skin pigments protect from sun's UV.	[1877]	DSB
—	1892	W. CROOKES NOTES PHOTO PLATES FOGGED NEAR URANIUM.	[1867]	Bio
—	1894	J.J. Thomson sees X-rays from Crookes tube — disregards it.		PM
—	1894	A. Goodspeed discards a few X-Ray pics as "freaks."	[1877]	Sc
—	1894	C. T. R. Wilson notices cloud formation on mt peak.	[1880]	Bio
3. # Nuc —	1890	P. Schutzenberger considers "isotopes" — drops idea.	[1885]	V98
—	1891	D. Mendeleev foresees more new elements, but not clearly.		Bk
—	1894	Rayleigh & Ramsay discover argon.	[1886]	DSB
—	1894	W. Ramsay adds gases to Periodic Table's 77 elements.	[1869]	HRC
4. # Med —				
		Organizations and Internal Politics		
5. Pols —	1890	Global influenza epidemic are concern of politics.	[1883]	EB
6. Socs —	1892	W. Osler sets format in "Principles and Practice of Med."		Bk
7. Event —	1890	K. Auer produces "Welsbach Mantle" (first use of Th).	[1885]	HRC
—	1890	H. Hollerith uses punch-card tabulator in census.	[1869]	FV
		Instruments, Units of Measurement, and Drugs		
8. Instr —	1891	S. Langley begins experiments in aerodynamics.	[1783]	DSB
—	1892	J. Dewar invents the "thermos flask."	[1643]	DSB
—	1894	CROOKES TUBE IS COMMON INSTR IN SCIENCE LABS.	[1896]	GSR
—	1894	P. Lenard adds an Al window to Crookes' tube.	[1895]	HRC
—	1894	L. Lumiere invents the cinematograph.	[1889]	DSB
—	1894	M. Marconi reads Hertz, begins wireless research.	[1888]	Bio
9. Units —	1893	A. Michelson suggests Cd-red wavelength meter std.	[1881]	Bio
—	1893	J. Mallet says mass of H @ 1 is proper unit At Wt.	[1860]	JCS
—	1893	Electrical Cong (Chicago) suggests Int Amp & Ohm.	[1948]	NBS
—	1894	G. Heinrichs "true" unit At Wt is 1/12 carbon.	[1860]	EB
10. Concp —	1891	W. Judson invents the zipper to replace buttons.	[1919]	EB
—	1891	E. Dubois discovers pithecanthropus erectus in Java.		DSB
—	1892	First automatic telephone switchboard devised.	[1880]	EB
11. Drugs —	1890	T. Curtius produces azoimide from organic source.	[1872]	DSB

Radioiodine, P-32, and Radioactive Therapy

12. I-Res	—	1890	V. Horsley proves thyroid deficiency in myx, cret.	[1873]	BMJ
13. I-Dx	—				
14. I-Rx	—	1891	G. Murray treats myx pt with sheep thyroid extract.	[1850]	BMJ
	—	1894	G. Reinhold treats goiter with sheep thyroid extr.	[1889]	MMW
15. P-Rx	—				
16. Tele	—				
17. Other	—				

Scans and Other Tests of Function in Various Organs

18. Brain	—	1890	I. Pavlov establishes the conditioned reflex.	[1861]	DSB
	—	1894	C. Sherrington finds 1/2 muscle nerves are sensory.	[1837]	DSB
19. Heart	—	1890	E. Starling studies nature of myocard contraction.	[1831]	DSB
	—	1891	F. Trendelenberg studies physiol and path of veins.	[1875]	Bk
	—	1891	S. Riva-Rocci describes a mercury sphygmomanometer.	[1846]	CDD
	—	1893	W. His demonstrates the A-V bundle.	[1843]	Bk
	—	1894	G. Stewart derives formula for rate of blood flow.	[1870]	JPh
20. Liver	—	1891	K. Voit shows mammals convert sugars into glucose.	[1856]	DSB
	—	1894	E. Starling discovers liver's lymphatic drainage.	[1740]	JPh
21. Lung	—				
22. Bone	—				
23. Kidney	—				
24. Gut	—				
25. Blood	—	1892	L. Vaques describes Polycythemia Vera Acuta (PVA).	[1845]	CDD
26. Other	—				

Radiation Hysteria and Health Physics * Obituaries *

27. Hyst	—				
28. React	—	1894	A. Yersin discovers the plague bacillus.	[1876]	DSB
29. Respo	—				

* * *

30. Obits	—	J. Stas (1813–1891) Belg chem; precision chem, atomic wts.	DSB
	—	E. Siemens (1816–1892) Ger elect physics; indust electricity.	EB
	—	H. Helmholtz (1821–1894) Ger physics & physiol; conserv energy.	DSB
	—	H. Hertz (1857–1894) Ger physics; electromagnetic waves.	DSB

DALTON WEIGHS THE ELEMENTS
(Babbage Uses Color Blindness)

At the second annual meeting of the British Association for the Advancement of Science, Oxford 1832, four honorary doctorates were awarded by Oxford: to M. Faraday, David Brewster (polarized light), Robert Brown (nucleus in cells), and John Dalton. It was one of the few honors Dalton would ever accept. His strict Quakerism abhorred the praise of man. But he had been a school teacher all his life and considered the degree a thank-you.

His Atomic Theory made Dalton's fame world wide, and a group led by Charles Babbage felt that he should receive England's highest honor: presentation in person to William IV. To be presented to the king required wearing formal court dress including a sword — anathema to a Quaker. However, Babbage explained to Dalton, it is proper and expected that you wear academic robes.

Years later Babbage was asked how he had overcome the Quaker's horror of wearing the brilliant scarlet doctoral robes of Oxford, an ostentation as severely proscribed as wearing a sword. It was simple, answered Babbage, I dressed him in robes of shades of gray, and the Court was dazzled by Oxford scarlet. Two robes can be worn by the same man at the same time because Babbage was one of the few who had read Dalton's 1798 article in the Memoirs of the Manchester Philosophical and Literary Society; thus, he knew that Dalton was totally color blind.

Dalton Sees an Atomic Theory of Matter

For 200 years people had been arguing Newton's particulate atom. Dalton, not an accomplished chemical technician, did something previously unheard of — he tried to weigh atoms. On 21 October 1803 Dalton read a paper to the Manchester Phil & Lit Society (published 1805): *"An inquiry into the relative weights of the ultimate particles of bodies is a subject, as far as I know, entirely new: I have already been prosecuting this inquiry with remarkable results."*

Dalton had been interested in the atmosphere (he agreed and taught Lavoisier's 2-gas theory) and in rain, and the gases absorbed in water. He took a volume of water, weighed it, then absorbed material in it to saturation and reweighed. He never gave a complete explanation of his technique, but listed a table of twenty elements and their comparative weights:

Hydrogen	1	Strontian	46
Azote	5	Barytes	68
Carbon	5.1	Iron	50
Oxygen	7	Zinc	56
Phosphorus	9	Copper	56
Sulphur	13	Lead	90
Magnesia	20	Silver	190
Lime	24	Gold	190
Soda	28	Platina	190
Potash	42	Mercury	167

Two of his friends disagreed with Dalton on important details of the Atomic Theory: William Wollaston and William Prout; both were highly skilled at chemical manipulation and did not consider Dalton's precision sufficient to match his speculations. Wollaston discarded the Newtonian atom for the point force atom of Bośković. He was an analyst who worked with eyedroppers and drops on a glass slide, but no one ever saw him in his mini-lab. (He was no fake, and as the only man to make platinum malleable he became independently wealthy.)

Wollaston remeasured all 45 known elements and arranged them into a *Table of Equivalent Weights*. His Table was widely used until Crookes changed them to "atomic weights" in 1864 and they became a Periodic Table. [For one thing, however, he is forever cursed. He was responsible for Parliament turning down metric scales and adopting the British Imperial (and hence, U.S.A.) System of Weights & Measures in 1819.]

The second dissident was the young William Prout. Prout was struck by the fact that wildly different substances had the same "weight" (e.g., silver & gold) which he knew was an error in measurement. He also noted that all element weights were whole numbers (or nearly so) — or was this just poor weighing? As a fanatic on precision, he remeasured all the elements he could get in pure form. From his own measurements, that he knew had a degree of inaccuracy, he formulated what we know as The Atomic Theory of Matter.

[See Vig1815 .WP, Prout's whole numbers]

DELAMDRE MEASURES THE WORLD
(The First SI Basic Unit)

As a young man Jean Baptist Delamdre (1749–1822) tutored the children of aristocrats of Paris in languages and history. Thinking he might add mathematics to his lessons he attended the astronomy lectures at the College of France. To make mathematics interesting he talked one student's father into setting up a small astronomy laboratory. Celestial measurements made astronomy calculations more meaningful to his students (and, incidentally, to him).

During one lecture at the College the professor mentioned an astronomical event referred to in an obscure third century BC poem. Delamdre, who had a prodigious memory, corrected the reference by quoting the entire passage in Greek. Then, translating into French, he added some Greek, Latin, and medieval commentary on the poem. He rounded out with some pertinent annotations to the professor's mathematical derivation. The professor, a very smart man, did not get angry. He hired Delamdre on the spot as his assistant; in a few years the language tutor was a collaborator.

Beginning a Decimal Metric System

Six years later (1786) Delamdre was the only astronomer in Paris to observe a transit of Mercury across the sun. All the other astronomers had given up because they had used the professor's predicted time tables which were 3/4 of an hour off. Delamdre, however, persisted in his observations because he had also read Halley's tables which were 3/4 of an hour off in the opposite direction. His report of the actual time of transit pointed out the horribly inaccurate nature of astronomical time.

Astronomers had been using the Huygens meter-second pendulum as a measurement "standard." But what was a meter if the second was 1/86,400th of a variable day? The French Academy of Science decided they must have a "uniform system of measures ... on a natural and invariable basis." On 8 May 1790 Talleyrand proposed to the French Assembly that some such system, possibly the new metric system, be established for all France. His reasons were all political: TAXES.

[No single person invented the metric system. The decimal point had been in use since 1612. Thomas Jefferson had devised a base 10 or metric decimal system for many measures and Congress accepted it for the new U.S. monetary system. Mathematicians and others with six fingers preferred a duodecimal scale, but James Watt's clever interrelation of length, area, volume, and mass on a base 10 decimal scale convinced Talleyrand.]

On 22 Aug 1790 Louis XVI approved the Assembly's decree. The Academy appointed a commission (Borda, Condorcet, Lagrange, Lavoisier, Tillet). It quickly decided that decimal-metric was the only sensible way, and a new system of all units would henceforth be called a "metric system." On 19 March 1791 they rejected the Huygens meter-second pendulum because it linked units of length and time. If either was inaccurate it would affect the other; hence a new principle: every basic unit must be independent of all others.

The First Unit Is Measured

The commission also recommended a new unit of length. They chose the most invariable natural thing they could think of as its unit: one ten-millionth part of a quadrant of a terrestrial meridian. Such a unit would be in the range of a man's reach (English yard) or his stride (Roman pace) which has been the natural span of distance throughout history. But they intended to actually measure a 10° arc on the meridian through Paris from Dunkirk to Barcelona: a task of unheard of panache.

The arc was divided into segments. André Mechain was given a 170,000 toise (old French unit of length: a fathom) segment from Rodez to Barcelona to measure by triangulation. Jean Delamdre was given the 380,000 toise from Rodez to Dunkirk. But — this was two years after Bastille day. The political situation was still unstable.

Mechain was the first to be thrown into jail. The citizens of Essone, his third observation site, knew that the only use for complex surveying equipment with spyglasses was to set up artillery pieces. They stopped this counter-revolution on the spot. Mechain talked his way out of jail with difficulty, but Delamdre had real troubles. By the time he triangulated his way into Paris the government had changed. Delamdre had the wrong passports and was thrown out of town. With intercession of the general committee he got new passports. But the government changed hands again. A new Committee on Public Safety informed him that he had lost his job. (He was lucky, Lavoisier lost his head.) Another change in government saw the work revived. Delamdre was ordered back to work.

By 1799 he completed his survey and began incredible calculations. His instruments had been calibrated, by order of the original metric commission, on the new metric 100° circle. To make the calculations, Delamdre had calculated a new set of log and trigonometric functions for the metric circle. A new commission under still another new government changed rules. They wanted decimal positioning on base 10 for length and mass, but were not metric enough for angles and especially for the clock face.

Delamdre recalculated back to a 360° circle. It took him years because Mechain had died in 1804. Delamdre had to finish Mechain's calculations and prepare the final report. All of the field work was complete and so, at the age of 55, he got married and settled down to writing three volumes on the history, observations, and computations of the new meter.

In 1810 the third volume was finally printed. In a formal ceremony Delamdre presented it to Napoleon, Emperor of still another government. The "meter" (Greek for measure) was defined as one ten millionth of a quadrant of a meridian through Paris. It was the first unit to have a precise definition of a *measured* quality and it was accurate.

[In the 1970s a direct measurement was made from outer space. Delamdre's error was found to be less than 1/3rd of a meter in over 10 kilometers measured.]

Politics Completes the Unit

But the intent of Jefferson, Watt, and Talleyrand was not yet fulfilled. The meter was not yet an "international" unit. On 22 Feb 1821, in a report to the U.S. Senate, John Quincy Adams proposed an international conference on the metric system. Almost a half century later, 1 Sep 1869, a decree of Napoleon III summoned an international conference to produce new and absolutely exact standards of mass and length. Fifteen nations responded and sent delegates to Paris on 8 Aug 1870. The conference disbanded and the delegates got out of France quickly because the Germans were invading France.

But the conferees didn't give up. Two years later, 24 Sep 1872, thirty nations sent delegates to confer. They not only conferred but passed resolutions like mad — 40 resolutions in 18 days. Their most important resolution involved a new alloy: 90% platinum 10% iridium, eventually called "Invar" (invariable) because it didn't distort (much) with temperature change. It resisted chemical action, and took a high polish for precise machining. Replicas could be made of a primary standard for each country to have its own "primary" calibrated against the "Metre des Archives" kept in Paris.

Treaty of the Metric Convention

Thirty-one such meter prototypes were made, but this took seventeen years. Meanwhile the deliberations of the conference had to be formalized. On 20 May 1875, 19 nations met in Paris and 15 (including the U.S.A.) signed the Treaty of the Metric Convention. They also set up the Bureau International des Poids et Mesures (BIPM) to be controlled by an international committee which had one technically knowledgeable member from each of the participating states, but which in turn would be under the direction of a diplomatic body (which in 1889 became the Conférence Général des Poids et Mesures, CGPM). France donated a site at Sévres for the BIPM, declaring it neutral territory.

Thus the "meter" became the first international measure, but only technically. With the Pt-Ir "invar" alloy for making standards, a "kilogram" became a possible unit. It has no "natural" model but is related to the mass of the liter suggested by James Watt to Talleyrand as a unit of volume.

[See Vig1790 .Wat. Watt's meter[3]]

COURTOIS DISCOVERS IODINE
(A Medication a Century too Early)

Bernard Courtois (1777–1838), who discovered iodine, was born across the street from the famous old Dijon Academy in France. His father ran the local saltpeter works and was a "Demonstrateur" for the lectures on chemistry at the Academy. Bernard was, in due time, admitted to the Ecole Polytechnique. He was a brilliant student of chemistry. In 1799 he had reached the age when all Frenchmen pay for the privilege of living in France. He served as a pharmacist in the regional military hospital.

Upon discharge from service he returned to help his father. Within a few years the saltpeter (potassium nitrate) business was failing. Their product was good, and there was a huge demand by the main customer. (Saltpeter is a component of gunpowder.) The French government wanted more but had a fault — they paid little and usually very late. In fact, they might, according to rumor, tax the raw material which was French property.

The raw material was dried seaweed. The seaweed was burned and its ash contained potassium carbonate plus unwanted sulfites. It was leached at the saltpeter works, and, to get rid of sulfites and hyposulfites, Bernard would add sulfuric acid. One day late in 1811 he must have added too much, too fast. To his astonishment beautiful clouds of violet vapor arose to fill the room. The vapors condensed on cold surfaces, but not with droplets of liquid; instead, dark crystals with metallic sheen were formed.

Bernard's chemical training immediately surfaced. He gathered some crystals and fired them to red heat — they did not decompose! The crystals did not form compounds with oxygen or carbon, but they did combine with hydrogen and phosphorus. The new material combined with some metals but without efflorescence, and it was explosive when combined with ammonia. Courtois suspected that he was dealing with a new element, but he realized that his laboratory was too poorly equipped to prove it.

About July 1812 he asked two friends from the Dijon Academy if they would please investigate further and announce the discovery. He would furnish a supply of the crystals.

His friends were happy to oblige and on 29 Nov 1813 they announced the discovery to the Institute de France, giving Bernard Courtois full credit. (N. Clément, one of the friends, made the first publication in Ann de Chimi 88:304, 1813.) Samples of the new element were sent to Gay-Lussac and Humphry Davy. Gay-Lussac named it "iode" from the Greek for violet; Davy called it "iodine."

Iodine had unusual properties, and chemists throughout the world were so interested that Courtois could not prepare it fast enough to supply the demand. His price was sufficient to support the old saltpeter business until, in 1824, an industrial process was devised that brought the price down below subsistence levels. By 1831 Courtois was in abject poverty and the Academy of Sciences awarded him a 6000 franc prize. He continued to eke out a living selling iodine until 1838. But his efforts were not unrewarded because on iodine's 100th anniversary (1911), at a solemn civic ceremony, a plaque was placed on his birthplace. They also named a street for him in Dijon.

Iodine is Medicinal and Ubiquitous

Within a year of its announcement, a physician-chemist in London, William Prout, had made some of his own iodine. He made an obvious connection that only a chemist who was also a physician could make. Burnt sea sponge was a remedy for goiter, iodine came from burnt seaweed: let's try iodine in goiter. He tried it in 1816 and in 1819 it was standard therapy in St. Thomas Hospital. (There was no publication.) A year later J. Coindet made the same observation in Geneva and published it. [Ann Chim Phys 15:49, 1820]

A Parisian chemist noted that free iodine produced a blue color in starch and made it a test in 1914. The German analytic chemist, F. Stromeyer, devised a detection to a sensitivity of 1 part per half-million. By 1825 chemists were finding iodine in spring water, ground water, lava, plants, pigments, fossils, granites. Iodine was truly ubiquitous — but not quite: absence of iodine was noted in 1907.

[See Vig1893 .Doc, Goiter & Iodine]

THE FECES OF A BOA CONSTRICTOR
(Leads to Prout's Whole Number Rule)

In 1815 an exotic-animal exhibition was held on the Strand in London. It was the scientific event of the year. An "animal chemist" named William Prout (we now call it clinical pathology) attended the exhibit and was astounded by what he saw in the boa constrictor's cage — not the snake, but the feces the snake had just deposited. He called the animal caretaker and asked for a sample. Grave robbers were an ongoing scandal, but this was the first feces lover the incredulous caretaker had ever seen. A high-church Anglican, he crossed himself 3 times, muttered a Hail Britannia, swept the entire feces into a small box and gave it to the nut. Prout took the sample and hurried back to his surgery (the British term).

It could not have been unusual, in 1815, for a clinical pathologist to practice medicine from home, because Prout was the first and only existing clinical pathologist. He had graduated MD from Edinburgh on 21 June 1811. He walked the wards of Guy's and St. Thomas's hospitals in London to earn his licentiate from the Royal College of Physicians 22 December 1812. In addition to seeing patients, he analyzed urine and blood using his own methods and equipment. (35 years later an obituary would point out that Prout had *"a taste for extreme exactitude and an unrivaled manual expertness never achieved by John Dalton."* [Med Times 1:15, 1850]) He also gave lectures at his home attended by London's top physicians.

Prout's request for snake feces is easily explained. A year earlier he had been first to obtain pure urea. He prepared it from human urine. He used his Animal Charcoal method (soon standard textbook chemistry). Prout knew what urea looked like — but coming from a snake?

Upon arriving home Prout dissolved the snake feces in muriatic acid and analyzed the undissolved precipitate: it was almost pure (99.16%) uric acid. He went one step further. His friend, the geochemist William Wollaston, had gone beyond Dalton's crude "weights of elements" to build a "Synoptic Scale of Equivalents." (These "equivalent weights" lasted until 1864, when W. Crookes changed the name to "Atomic Weights.") Prout measured the "proportional number" (empirical formula weight) of urea at 37.5. (F. Wöhler used this weight in his urea synthesis that initiated organic chemistry.
[Pogg Ann d Physik 12:88, 1828])

Man's Greatest Intellectual Achievement

Twenty-six years earlier, Lavoisier had counted 33 chemical elements. H. Davy and others had added a few, until by 1815 40–45 elements were recognized. [See How Many? Appendix] Prout measured as many of the elements as he could obtain and checked the weights given by Dalton, Davy, Wollaston and others.

> [In order to understand Prout's hypothesis you must project yourself back into the intellectual milieu of 1815.]

According to the orthodox science of the day, if each of the chemical elements had been separately and independently created by God, the atomic weights could be haphazard and random. If, however, the elements were all derived from the single creation of one primordial *protyle,* then the atomic weights of the elements should follow in orderly succession. This conclusion was theologically sound and hence must be scientifically demonstrable.

Prout showed that all atomic weights were whole numbers — or very nearly so. As a fanatic on *"extreme exactitude,"* Prout argued that if he were able to measure more accurately, all atomic weights would be multiples of *"1,"* the atomic weight of hydrogen. Hydrogen was thus the primordial matter, the *protyle,* from which the universe was made. (105 years later Rutherford listened to Prout and renamed it *proton.*) [Vig1918 .ER5]

In 1815 Prout published his findings anonymously in the Annals of Philosophy. [5:413, 1815] When the hypothesis was highly praised, he quickly acknowledged authorship. The hypothesis was widely accepted among scientists — until:

Prout's Hypothesis Is an Illusion

The atomic weight of oxymuriatic acid (we now tend to call it "chlorine") was not known with accuracy until Jöns Berzelius in 1928 measured and put it halfway between 35 and 36. Berzelius' accuracy was as unassailable as Prout's.

In 1832 The British Association appointed William Prout and John Dalton to a committee, and gave them L-50 to test the whole number hypothesis. They never did report because they became embroiled in a bigger hassle on chemical nomenclature. The question of atomic weights was "settled" by another precision chemist. In 1860 J. Stas, the great Belgian chemist, using equipment far beyond Prout's, said the whole number was *"une pur illusion."*

Prout's hypothesis was dead, until 1888. W. Crookes, a generation beyond Stas and a fanatic on accuracy, surveyed the Rare Earths and felt uneasy about the atomic weight concept *"... Probably our atomic weights merely represent a 'mean' value around which the actual atomic weights vary...."* [CN 1888]

Prout's Hypothesis is Scientific Law

By 1901 H. Strutt (soon to be Lord Rayleigh) voiced a new scientific consensus, *"... we have strong reasons for believing in the truth of Prout's laws...."* In 1905 Otto Hahn began the discovery of a series of "look alike" elements (e.g., RaTh & Th) that could not be explained until 9:32 PM on 23 Nov 1912 in Karlsruhe Germany, when K. Fajans discovered that two different substances could occupy the same place on the periodic table. A year later F. Soddy called them "isotopes." [See Vig1912 .KF1]

In 1913 H. Moseley noted *"... We are led by experiment to the view that ... (the number of charges) is the same as the number of the place occupied by the element in the Periodic system...."* Element Number 1 was hydrogen. After 98 years Prout's hypothesis was no longer a hypothesis.

[See Vig1913 .Mos & Vig1919 .Ast]

Prout Was a 19th Century Leonardo

In 1814 a new element called iodine was discovered in seaweed. Many chemists investigated, but only Prout had the combined chemical-medical knowledge to make a connection between iodine seaweed-goiter-therapy. He made some potassium iodate and swallowed a few small doses to test its safety. He then tried it on a patient with goiter and found it superior to the standard burnt sea sponge because it didn't cause the expected severe stomach cramps. He recommended it to John Elliotson, chief of medicine at St. Thomas, who tried it and made KI a standard medication for goiter. For this reason, Prout is father (or is it grandfather?) of Endocrinology.

In addition to gravimetric analyses of urine specimens with a hydrometer he invented (it soon became the standard), Prout also analyzed for nitrate, sugar, sugar of milk, and diabetic sugar. When Gay-Lussac introduced copper oxide (1816), Prout devised a spirit lamp modification that was more accurate. In 1821 he published a textbook on the gravel, calculus and diseases of the urinary tract. Hence Prout is grand- or great-grandfather of Urology.

In 1823 Prout wrote a book on Gastroenterology, but suddenly withdrew it from the publisher because he made an unbelievable discovery: in the vomitus of patients he detected free hydrochloric acid. After rigorous and elaborate investigation Prout was obliged, in spite of what he had been taught, to conclude that the stomach contained *"muriatic acid and no other."* This great discovery was announced to the Royal Society on 11 December 1823. (10 years before Beaumont's story of Alexis St. Martin.) Hence Prout is the great-grandfather of Digestive Physiology.

Prout had a very active association with committees and commissions of the Royal Society, British Association, and the Royal College of Physicians. He investigated the cause of London's Cholera epidemics with demographic methods. His home-made barometer was for a time the official instrument at the Royal Observatory. He named carbohydrate, protein and fat as the three aliments. He was father of epidemiology, medical statistics, nutritional physiology, instrument design. In his spare time Prout built an organ to play hymns and anthems he composed himself. About 1834, with increasing deafness he withdrew from science to practice medicine. Both the Royal and Chemical Societies ignored his death in 1850, but his scientific eclipse ended in 1919 when Rutherford named the *Proton* and Aston gave every isotope a whole number.

[Best Ref = W.H. Brock, Med Hist 9:101, 1965]

THE LITER ALMOST BECOMES THE KILOGRAM

(The Second SI Basic Unit)

The popular word "weight" implies a mass of substance under the influence of gravity. The first CGPM (Conférence Générale des Poids et Mesures) accepted the kilogram as the unit of weight in 1889. Some scientists protested: the kilogram is not a "weight." The standard mass of water was compared to a platinum prototype "kilogram" on an equal-arm-beam-balance. Gravity acted equally on two bodies and cancelled. Weight = mass × gravity. A kilogram is a unit of "mass."

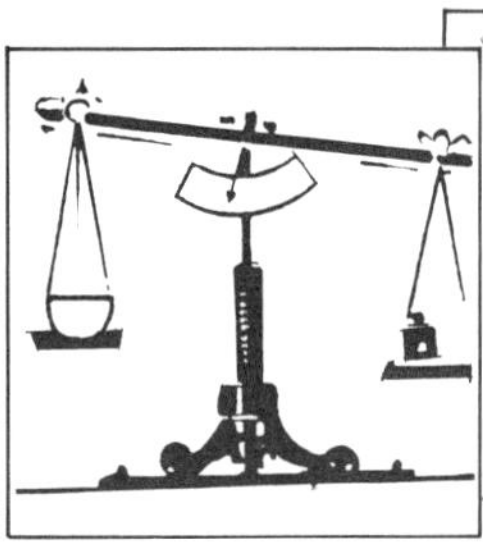

Balance

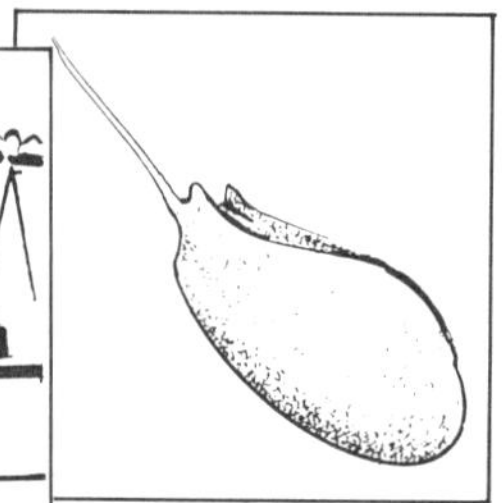

Grain

"Mass" is from the Greek "maza," or barley cake. For many centuries (most of man's existence) the accepted unit of mass was a grain of barley or wheat. The **"grain"** was a handy unit for precious stones or pieces of money (**carat** and **shekel**). Number-of-grains was handy for powerful drugs and for condiments: a **scruple** of poison, or a **dram** of spirits. Eventually, the **troy ounce** shifted from bakery to drug store at 437.5 grains with the **apothecary ounce.** ("Troy" weights come from a medieval trade fair held in *Troyes,* France.) The **avoirdupois** ounce became 480 grains.

The Pound Was Standardized in Rome

For everyday use, food, clothes, common objects lifted by both adults and children, a heavier standard was needed — something that had about the heft of Roman soldiers' "Libra" or battle axe. The only "standardized" weight for centuries, it was carried all over the known world. It weighed about a **"pound,"** or big stone, rather than a **"scruple,"** or little stone. Eventually avoirdupois (means weight) developed around the heft of a **"libra"** called **"pound"** (still "Libra" in South America).

[See Vig1889 .kg]

But farmers sold fruit by the peck and wheat by the bushel (dry capacities, not weights), wine and honey by the skin or jug of liquid. Two skins of wine, or two pecks or barrels, did not necessarily contain the same "amount" and nobody expected this — except C. Talleyrand, a tax collector who outlived the French revolution, hence was a great politician.

Tax Collection and Foundations of Science

Around 1790 Talleyrand had joined the French Ministry of Finance. As tax collector, he was being ripped off by farmers who sold wine in big skins but paid taxes in little skins. Every village had a different system of measures. In an after-dinner conversation in London around 1790 he complained to James Watt, how could he collect taxes? There was no standard for measurement of weight. James Watt suggested one way to make one. [See Vig1790 .Wat]

Make a little metal cup of standard length, width, and depth for each tax collector. Have them fill it with cold water and declare this *THE* legal unit of "weight." A standard unit of length, to be called a "meter" (Greek for measure), was already under discussion in France. Talleyrand, being a politician, referred the matter to a committee of the French Academy of Science. [See Vig1657 .mks] But the Bastille was stormed on 14 July 1792 on the matter of tax collections. For a few years French governments came and went. Standards of *Poid et Mesure* had low priority.

[See Vig1794 .Lav]

John Quincy Adams Says Go International

In 1821 John Quincy Adams (Secretary of State, to be President in 1824) reported to Congress on the state of measures used in the 24 states. They were, he reported, in a confused mess. Bushels, pecks, baskets, barrels, all under the generic "Weights and Measures," varied from town to town.

[Note that "Weight" comes before "Measure." ("Measure" then meant unit of distance.) Actually the coinage precedes "weights" in metrology, but coins were once weights of precious metals. Length or distance had many obvious "standards": hand, foot, etc. There was, and still is, no "natural" standard for "weight," the basis for taxes. Taxes feed politicians, which explains why a prototype *"Kilogram des Archives de France"* was a first unit.]

Adams was the first high government official to propose an international conference on the metric system, but Congress stalled on carrying it out.

The First Prototype Kilogram & Meter

A French committee had tried Watt's suggestion and made a cubic centimeter container. They filled it with water at maximum density (water gets lighter above and below 4°C) and called it a **gramme** (Latin for small unit) of weight. It was too small for everyday use: cups, ladles, cooking pots.

Following metric principles, they multiplied the gramme cup by 10: ten cm long by 10 cm wide by 10 cm deep made 1000 grammes. This mass of cold water, naturally, was a **kilogramme,** but was too sloppy to keep as an official standard. They matched its weight on a beam balance with the most permanent metal they knew, platinum. (At the same time, they made standards for Delamdre's 1810 meter. [See Vig1810 .1SI]) The U.S. Minister, knowing of Adams's interest, bought copies of the standards for the United States.

Our copy of the kilogramme was a right cylinder 39.5 mm in diameter and height. It was certified by the French physicist, M. Arago, to differ by less than 1 mg from the *"Prototype kilogramme des Archive de France."* British, European (especially French) scientists had been trying to intercompare standards of weight and length, but realized that the "language of measurement" was primarily political. The French government assembled 15 nations in Paris in August 1870. They had to disband after 5 meetings because the Germans were marching on the city. They reconvened two years later.

A 238 kg ingot of "alloy of 1874" was rejected at the Second International Conference. A precise definition of a new platinum-iridium "invar" alloy was offered the commission by a British firm of platinum refiners. They made an "invar" (for invariable) alloy satisfactory for standards to BIPM chemists

On 20 May 1875, at a *diplomatic* conference, 17 nations (of the 19 present) signed the *Treaty of the Metric Convention.* The French government ceded a piece of ground in the park of Saint Cloud at Sévres, near Paris, as neutral territory. A laboratory was set up to become the final international authority on standards: the *Bureau International des Poids et Mesures.* [See Vig1889 .CGP]

The Kilogram is Finally The Unit of Mass

In 1887 31 prototype meters and 40 prototype kilogram standards were cast and sent to the BIPM to be compared with the *"Métre des Archives"* and the *"Kilogramme des Archives."* After approval by the International Committee (CIPM), on 26 September 1889, the Conférence Général (CGPM) chose the prototypes closest to the old "Archives" standards. These were declared the *International Meter* and *International Kilogram* and deposited at the BIPM in Sévres. A vault with three locks had keys for 1) Custodian of the Archives of France, 2) President of the CIPM, and 3) Director of the BIPM. This vault must not be opened more than once each year.

Two meter and two kilogram primary standards were assigned to each signatory country. Each set was accompanied by a certificate of comparison with the Archive's primary, two hard glass thermometers and a piece of invar metal cut off from the meter standard. The USA was allotted #21 & #27 meter and #4 & #20 kilogram standards. Received at the White House by President Harrison on 2 January 1890, he ceremoniously deposited them in the Office of Weights and Measures. By approval of the Secretary of the Treasury, on 5 April 1893 the International Meter and Kilogram became the fundamental standards of length and weight (in 1903 changed to mass) in the United States. On 1 July 1901 control was passed to a new National Bureau of Standards.

From 1092 weighings of kilogram #20 in Paris an error of $\pm <0.002$ mg had been accepted. That's 2 parts/million precision, but how accurate? The meter had a natural meridian to copy. All of the busy-work and pageantry of official "International Standards" does not hide the fact that there is no natural mass. The "kilogram" is an arbitrary decision, hence is the only "exact" (by definition) unit we have.

Reference: The full story of standards is much more complex. A very complete reference is: W. Hallock and H.T. Wade; *The Evolution of Weights and Measures and The Metric System.* Macmillan, 1906.

JOULE DISCOVERS ENERGY CONSERVATION

Einstein did not overthrow Newton's laws of motion, nor did he overturn the laws of conservation of mass and energy; he merely put them in their proper place. Above molecular, but below astronomical, sizes, shapes, and speeds the numbers are within a middle range. Conservation of mass was recognized by Lavoisier in 1789. Conservation of energy was announced by J. Meyer in 1842, but was disregarded. The Mechanical Equivalent of Heat had to be demonstrated first, and in many ways. It was an absurd concept in the 1840s; heat was "coloric," an Aristotelian element. James Joule supplied overwhelming evidence that it was energy, but nobody believed him — until a mathematics prodigy put Joule's thoughts into proper form.

Joule Trains Himself in Science

James Joule (1818–1889) was the second son of a wealthy brewer. A spinal injury and poor health as a young man encouraged a life of study. He was enrolled as a pupil of Dalton from whom he learned the necessity for experiment. James' father supplied him with a small laboratory where, unlike Dalton, he developed a passion for precision measurements, primarily of temperature. He was making thermometers that read to 0.005°F. Few scientists believed it — primarily because they couldn't do it.

By 1840 he had worked out an empirical formula for the heat developed by an electric current, but, like Faraday, he was innocent of mathematics and couldn't write it up in acceptable form (acceptable, that is, to science journals). He went on to measure every kind of heat transfer he could imagine: water churned by paddles, water forced through holes, expanding and contracting gases, etc.

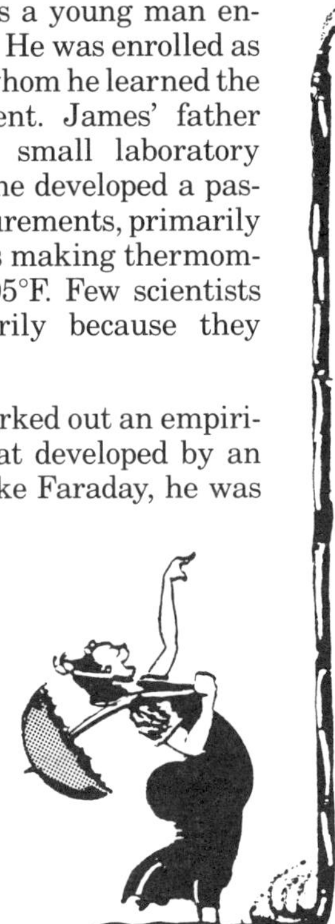

In 1847 he decided to get married. His bride chose a scenic waterfall in England for a honeymoon. Joule went prepared with two thermometers that read to 0.02°F. He measured water temperature at top of the falls with his wife measuring simultaneously at the bottom. There was a difference, it was hotter at the bottom. His conclusion: the falling mass of water was mechanical work, equivalent to the amount of heat generated.

He wrote up 10 years of experiments in a single article. All scientific journals rejected the article as the work of a rank amateur (a brewer at that). He was reduced to presenting his work at a public lecture in Manchester and then paid to have it published in a newspaper where his brother was music critic.

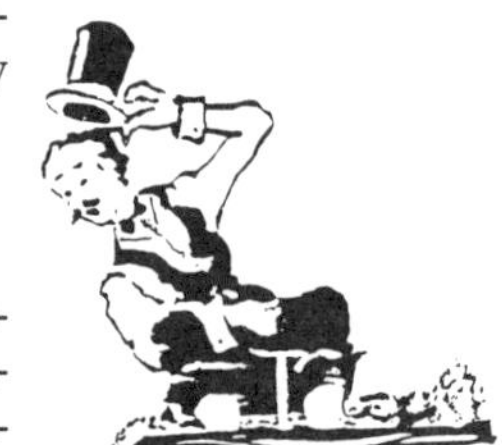

Joule is Recognized as a Scientist

A few months later Joule was allowed to present his talk to a scientific audience that paid no attention — except one 23-year-old mathematical prodigy named William Thomson (later Lord Kelvin). Thomson collaborated with Joule and put the measurements into proper scientific language with a physical explanation of the mathematical formulae. Joule's ideas were then quickly adopted. In 1849 he read a paper before the Royal Society with Faraday as sponsor.

Thomson, using Joule's gas expansion and contraction temperature measurements, calculated backwards to where no thermal motion occurred. This he defined as "absolute zero," −273°C. Because of this concept the basic thermometry unit is called the kelvin. (Celsius is a subsidiary unit indicating degree-of-change in temperature.)

Joule, now recognized as a major though non-academic scientist, went on to demonstrate that a loss of mechanical energy is always accompanied by a gain in thermal energy, or vice versa. All of Joule's experiments involved very small changes in temperature; there was usually nothing obvious to sensation.

But the energy transfer is pervasive: eating a lump of sugar, burning a ton of coal, dropping water over a cliff, lifting your hand, just standing upright involves considerable transfer of energy.

The law of conservation of energy became, and still is, scientific dogma, with only two shakeups in its domination of all science:

1. the discovery of radioactivity by Becquerel in 1896 required some heat exchanges so small that even Joule could not have measured them;
2. in 1906 Einstein made a major revision when he proved that mass and energy were convertible (under certain conditions).

But the law did not stand alone. It complemented Newton's laws of motion, and used the same units, albeit with a modification. Joule, through Kelvin, had revived an ancient Greek speculation that everything material was motion of mass through space in time.

Motion in Space / Time

Motion through space has speed:

$$\mathbf{m/s}$$

If it changes speed it has acceleration:

$$\mathbf{m/s^2}$$

A Mass accelerated for a distance is a force. Its unit was named for the man who discovered the laws of motion:

$$\mathbf{1\ newton = kg \cdot m/s^2}$$

Stretch your arm out to one side with your hand open, palm up. Have some one place an apple in your hand. You feel one newton of force.

Because Joule had shown that energy is nothing more than masses under acceleration, the SI unit of energy is called a joule:

$$\mathbf{1\ joule = kg \cdot m^2/s^2}$$

Watt described horsepower as a measure of energy in joules per second or:

$$\mathbf{1\ watt = kg \cdot m^2/s^3}$$

With the units Watt, Kelvin and Joule used, mensuration was not so simple. The need for a coherent system of units was already becoming obvious by 1889.

[See Vig1889 .CGP; Weights & Measures]

BLOOD VOLUME AS NO-NONSENSE PHYSIOLOGY

M. Gregersen defined "blood volume" as simply the ml of cells and plasma inside the circulatory system — but then he hedged. Does it include the volume inside the liver's sinusoids? Three quarters of these are closed at any one time. How much plasma-extravascular fluid interchange is included? J. Peters said we can't measure circulating plasma accurately. [NEJM 1948]

During the centennial celebration of "Blood Volume," Gregersen summarized about 100 blood volume techniques. [PhR 1959] He concluded that volume measured by technique-X was an accurate measure of whatever technique-X measured. 100 years earlier physiologists did not know enough about blood to be confused.

H. Welcker noted in 1854 that hemoglobin (Hb) is confined to red cells. He withdrew a few ml of an animal's blood as a standard, then canulated a large artery and drained all blood while pouring in saline through a large vein. He minced all muscles and extracted the Hb. The Hb in his standard divided by the sample amount times the dilution factor was the animal's blood volume. [AAF 1854]

How about human bodies? Two years later T. Bischoff used Welcker's method. Two humans, normal except for nasty criminal habits, were about to be beheaded. Bischoff convinced the authorities that their decapitation could serve both law and science. Following Welcker's method he found that 1/13 of their body weight was "circulating blood."

Forty years later a more practical method, but using the same principle, was devised by J. Haldane. [JPh 1899] Hemoglobin exposed to carbon monoxide turns a bright cherry red — a quantifiable tag. Haldane exposed a small aliquot of the patient's blood to CO as his standard. He had the patient take a few breaths of CO and then took a sample of blood. This was the first method to use the "tagging" principle, but, as Starling said, ". . . it is important not to give too large a dose of CO gas." The method never became clinically popular.

[See Vig1942 .BV, Blood Volume]

TO MEASURE LIGHT, FIRST CATCH A WHALE

(The Sixth SI Basic Unit)

The Royal Hydrographer had to be a mathematician, but one who made many measurements. Hydrography — geography of the seas — was an important subject in 18th century France. In 1713 the royal professor of hydrography at the College of Paris died. The professorship did not stay empty for long; the dead mathematician's son, a 15-year-old mathematics prodigy, Pierre Bouguer, was appointed. Within a few years his abilities were such that he was THE French authority on all things nautical.

"Brightness" is an Unmeasurable Unit

In 1721 a French academician proposed a problem that involved relative amount of light from the sun at two altitudes. No answer was possible because there were no units for measuring "amount of light." The problem asks for a measure of "brightness," which we still have not solved. (Brightness is a psychological, not a physical, concept.) This question was not academic play. Hydrographers mapped coastlines from shipboard by estimating distances to shore. Did a distance "appear the same" at noon, at sunset, and in moonlight?

On a moonlight night Bouguer compared an average candle's brightness to that of the light from a full moon. Its brightness was low compared to daylight. He couldn't match direct sunlight with a candle, so he tried a new idea.

On 23 Nov 1725 Pierre Bouguer solved the first step in measuring light. His first measurement marks the foundation of the science of Photometry (physical branch). Pierre made a box with a split screen of translucent paper. Behind each half screen, and shielded from the other, he placed the most common portable source of light in his day: a candle. Each of the candles could be moved closer for a brighter, or more distant from the screen for a dimmer, illumination. He measured the distance from the screen to each candle and found that relative brightness followed the inverse square of its distance to the screen.

When the two halves of Pierre's screen were equally bright he called the distances to each candle a measure of relative "candle-power." However, he was not measuring "brightness." The screen's appearance to his eyes could have seemed darker to an older man. He had really measured a *relative intensity of light* with his candle distances.

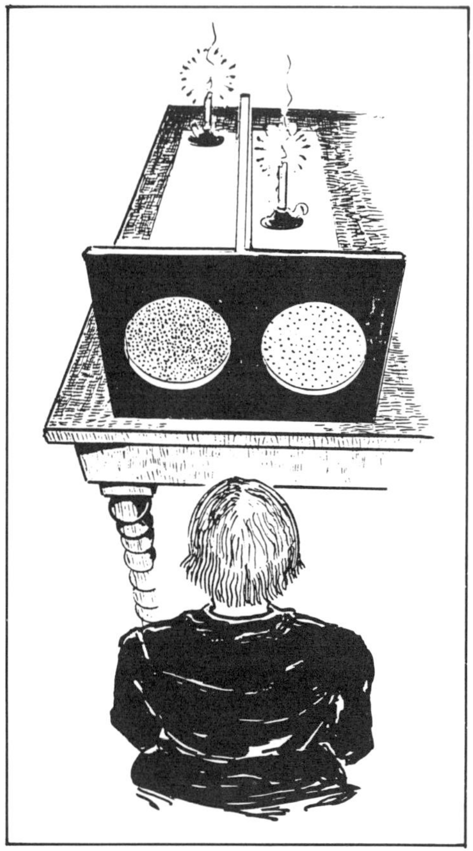

Pierre Bouguer invents candle power in 1735.

From Relative to Absolute Candle Power

For over a hundred years candle power was used to compare pigfat sooty candles with oil lamps, wood fires, and tree pitch. All sources gave off a flickering colored light of low intensity. English scientists formed a Photometry Committee with instructions to find a single reproducible standard source of light to serve as a standard unit of light intensity.

The Photometry Committee in 1860 selected a spermacetti candle as the cleanest, most intense, and whitest light they could find. And it didn't offend the nose. Although it was expensive, spermacetti was a product of a major industry and could never end. Hence, as required for every universal unit's standard, spermacetti candles would always be easily available.

First catch a sperm whale. Remove from its skull a handful of white waxy spermacetti. Now thread 3 strands of 18 strand cotton through the center of a candle maker's mold and cast a 10″ spermacetti candle, 9/10″ on the bottom tapering to an 8/10″ top diameter. Trim the cotton wick to burn 120 grains of wax per hour. This is, by definition, a one *candle power* light source.

A New "Candle" But the Same Candle Power

The standard candle served well for two generations, until in 1909 a more constant, more brilliant, and cleaner source, the electric light bulb, put candles out of date. The U.S., UK, and French committees on standards selected one type of carbon filament electric light bulb as the *International Candle.*

Thirty years later (1939) a new International Committee made a complete break from photometric practice. They recognized the requirements of a new breed of photographic and lighting engineers. They recognized Bouguer's 1725 misinterpretation; a source had to project light onto a surface. Put a small frosted glass sphere around a candle power source (e.g., a light bulb). The glass surface is bright. Put a much larger frosted bulb around the same candle. The total illumination is the same, but fewer light rays reach each unit of glass surface and the light is dimmer.

A constant light source is required in photometry (to be called the *new candle*). Also, the intensity of light projected spherically outward into space is a separate concept (called a *lumen*). Still different is the effect of lumens projected onto a surface (to be called the *lux*).

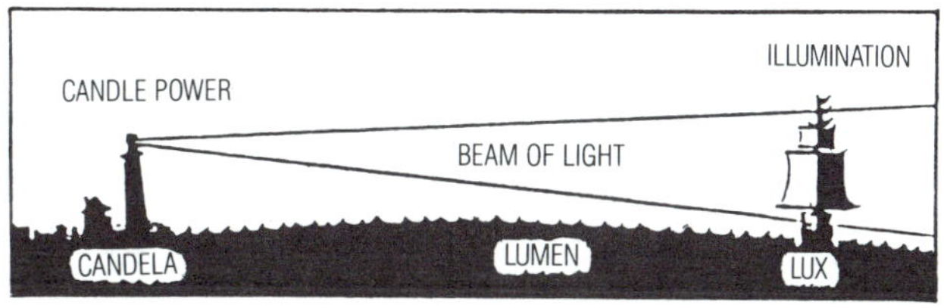

Imagine yourself on a ship a few miles from a lighthouse on a dark night.

The candle in the lighthouse
its intensity is now measured in *candela* (cd) to set it apart from the previous new and old candles
is projected as a beam of light
now measured in *lumens* (lm)
one lm = 1 cd • 1 steradian
(a steradian is a 3-dimension angle.)
to illuminate the surface of the ship
now measured in *lux* (lx)
one lx = 1 cd • sr/m^2

Three Branches of Photometry

Neither the candela, nor the lumen or the lux, measures the "brightness" of light. Brightness still depends upon the efficiency of someone's eyes. If you have 20/20 vision (you see at 20 feet what is normally seen at 20 feet) and I have 10/20 vision (I see at 10 what is normally seen at 20 feet) we have different scales of brightness. In the retina of the eyeball, 4 kinds of light detectors are sensitive to red, green, and blue wave lengths, or to shades of gray. No two persons have exactly the same response to white light. Thus, a subject matter of *physiological* photometry is superimposed on *physical* photometry.

Railroad tracks converge to a point at eye level on the horizon. We all know that this is visual illusion. All of us can be fooled by clever 3-dimensional distortion pictures. Thus *psychological* must be superimposed on a *physiological* which is superimposed on a *physical* photometry. All three add separate units of measurement to cd, lm, and lx.

For the past century physical photometry has been an exact science, but 250 years after Bouguer we still have no unit for "brightness." However, we now measure *absolute* rather than *relative* candle power. But the precise definition of a candela is more complicated than catching a whale was in 1860. [See Vig1967 .cd The Candela]

SPIRITUALISM AND THE ATOMIC WEIGHT OF Tl

which leads Crookes to the Radiometer,
which leads to the Crookes tube (1880)
(also to the electron, neon signs, etc.)
which leads to Roentgen's rays (1895)
(also to vacuum pumps, television, etc.)
which leads to Becquerel's rays (1898)
(also to radium, radon, anti-nukes, etc.)
which leads to Rutherford's decay (1899)
(also to natural $4n + x$ series, RaTh, etc.)
which leads to Fajans' isotopes (1913)
(also a nuclear atom, transmutation, etc.)
which leads to Joliot's isotopes (1934)
(also to cyclotrons, supervoltage, etc.)
which leads to Evan's iodine (1937)
(also to fission, bombs, secrecy, AEC, etc.)
which leads to Seidlin's cure (1946)
(also to regulatory clowns, NRCs, etc.)
which leads to Nuclear Medicine.

On 22 September 1867 27-year-old Phillip, youngest brother of William Crookes, died of yellow fever while on a cable-laying expedition in Havana, Cuba. William, one of eighteen siblings, was deeply affected because he had been partly responsible for getting Phillip onto the voyage. The circumstances of death were confused. Was Phillip, the only electrician aboard, exhausted by overwork? Why had Phillip contracted a fatal disease? (Remember, mosquitos were still 30 years in the future.) Crookes published an attack on the **India Rubber, Gutta Percha, and Telegraph Works Company** expedition's officers. This was no minor news note. Crookes, a well known 38-year-old chemist, was editor and publisher of *Chemical News* (since 1859), the most widely read scientific publication of its time. The commander of the expedition took action for libel against Crookes.

Crookes Hears Voices From the Other Side

For his legal defense Crookes chose to describe conditions aboard ship. He consulted Mr. Varley, a telegraph technician on board. Were conditions on cable expeditions unhealthful? Yellow fever was not a contagious disease. Who contaminated Phillip? If he could only talk to his brother, William sobbed. Mr. Varley, a fellow in the Royal Society, thought that maybe he could. Having just become interested in Spiritualism, Mr. Varley described some of the messages he had received from the other side.

Spiritualism Triggers the Atomic Age

Spiritualism, an import from America, was a current rage in England. In 1848 the Fox home in Hydesville, NY, had been the site of "rappings" accredited to spiritual agencies. Later two Fox sisters moved to Rochester, NY, where they became spiritualist "mediums." Spirits of the dead, they said, could only talk through a "medium" — somebody had to make money out of this. They went into trances for a price and reported on the "other world." A large group of copy cat fakers spread the word, and adopted religious trappings to escape exposure by police.

By 1894 a National Spiritualists Association was incorporated in Washington D.C. with 75,000 members, about 200 churches, 500 ordained ministers, $7.5 million in church property, and their own seminary. The next year Sigmund Freud published "The Interpretation of Dreams," and Psychiatry gave a medical tinge to the spirit world. By 1925 there were over 500 churches and 2000 "mediums" in the U.S.A. They charged high fees. Psychiatry had renounced the spirit world for an even more lucrative scam with sub, super, and split consciousness states. Spiritualism and its sister religion, Psychiatry, make up the major intellectual perversion of the 20th century, but in 1870 its converts were just gaining strength.

Crookes is the Scientific Voice

During the late 1860s the movement spread into England and many top intellectuals were caught up in the enthusiasm: A. Balfour, W. Gladstone, Oliver Lodge, William James, J.J. Thomson, Alfred Tennyson, John Ruskin, Lord Kelvin, R.L. Stevenson. William Crookes used scientific methods to verify the "physical phenomena" behind the "psychic force."

His "psychic force" was no more ethereal than Faraday's "fields of force" and was a lot more practical — if you wanted to talk to your dead brother. Crookes took over the editorship of the *quarterly Journal of Science* to publicize his inquiries into Spiritualism. He came dangerously close to capturing the Royal Society as a vehicle. But Faraday's opinion saved English science: "Many dogs have the power to come to much more logical conclusions."

Crookes Must Reestablish His Reputation

It took a magician, The Great Houdini, to prove spiritualism a fraud.

[I rank Houdini with Faraday as an experimental craftsman because he duplicated every "psychic manifestation."]

Most scientists saw the error, but like reformed sinners they almost read Crookes out of scientific society. Crookes was deeply hurt by the bitterness of his peers. In despondency he turned to scientific scut work — something to saturate his mind. He would measure something so precisely that no scientist could ever raise the slightest objection. He would measure the atomic weight of his 1861 discovery, the element thallium. In his search for precision he inadvertently set off the fuse that began the atomic age.

If William Prout was called an "exacting chemist" and J.S. Stas a "specialist in precision," Crookes became a fanatic:

"The most extraordinary pains have been taken to secure the absolute purity both of the thallium employed and the agents used to act upon it. The glass and other apparatus have been especially constructed for these researches, and the balances and weights have been of an accuracy never before surpassed in any research."

[D'Albe, Biog, Appleton, 1924]

The new balance was enclosed in a glassed-in vacuum. The expandability of the weighing arms, knife edges and beam were measured. The weighing pans were matched to microgram precision. Friction of forceps against weights was obviated with special platinum hooks. The thallium samples to be weighed and all of the reagents used were prepared from multiple re-precipitations, re-filtrations, and re-crystallizations. Crookes used the Tl_2NO_3 method and arrived at an atomic weight of 203.642. Today's accepted value is 204.37. If it can be called an error, he made one error: he used the latest Stas atomic weights of nitrogen and oxygen.

If Crookes had used 1961 N and O values, his atomic weight would have been 204.02. The correct weight (if our stable isotope proportions are correct, which they probably are not) is 204.41. Only two or three of the next generation of scientists could match such precision. And then H. Moseley made such measurements obsolete in 1913. In 1919 F. Aston's mass spectrometer measured, instead, miniscule deviations from the whole number rule.

Crookes Makes His Greatest Discovery

The important point historically is that Crookes sensed even greater error: not in chemical technique — impeccable — but in the physical concepts around "atomic weight." In 20 years (1888) he would make the first speculation on the existence of "meta-elements." (We call them isotopes.) His habits of work made the suspicion possible. He habitually worked in his chemistry lab (probably the best equipped in the world) in the mornings, attended meetings at the Royal and other societies in the afternoons, and returned to his lab in the evenings.

Crookes, therefore, weighed samples on his new balance at two different times. He soon noticed that the excursions of the sensitive balance needle seemed greater in the sunlit room in the morning than in the half-light of evening. For a while he thought he had discovered gravitational X-force; but tests with massive objects on and near his weighing pans said no. Only a variation in light affected the balance. If true, then his platinum balance was too massive to be grossly affected, so he suspended two pith balls from a broom straw and balanced it on the knife edge in his balance's vacuum case. In half-dark he directed a beam of white light at one pith ball — it moved.

He directed different colored lights against the pith ball. The ball was moved more by red light than by other colors. Crookes demonstrated the phenomena to the Royal Society on 11 December 1873. It was successful in that the demonstration provoked controversy.

"I wish to avoid having a theory," said the still controversy-shy Crookes. Such shyness was unnatural for him, but was reinforced by the realization that the experiment was not good. Pithballs balanced on-a-straw-in-a-vacuum was highly unstable. Crookes went home to build something better.

[See Vig1875 .WC2, The Radiometer]

CROOKES INVENTS THE RADIOMETER

(A Toy Shakes the Foundation of Physics)

William Crookes (1832–1919) had suspended pith balls on the ends of a straw balanced on a knife edge in a vacuum. A light shining on one ball caused a slight movement. [See Vig1872 .WC1] He showed this to the Royal Society on 11 Dec 1873. For explanation he considered gravitational forces or heat, but various modified experimental devices cancelled them out. The idea of direct repulsion by light was a possibility.

Crookes' paper, submitted to Philosophical Transactions of the Royal Society, was refereed by James Maxwell, then director of Cavendish Laboratory. Maxwell felt that some of Crookes' "heat repulsion" data disagreed with his newly published *Treatise,* but he recommended publication. Osborne Reynolds, professor of Engineering at Owens College (he invented the *Reynolds number* in fluid dynamics), said not light pressure but the increase in heat motion of the molecules remaining in the evacuated globe caused the pith ball to move.

Crookes had no training in higher mathematics and was unaware that Maxwell had predicted a pressure from light in his 1873 *Treatise on Electricity and Magnetism.* Maxwell also proposed experiments of the type Crookes was about to devise. [Woodruff, Isis, 1966]

Crookes Invents the Radiometer

After trial experiments Crookes arrived at an instrument design that satisfied all the criticisms of his 1873 demonstration. He called in his lab assistant, Charles Gimingham, a young chemist and expert glass blower. Charles not only made instruments, but also made a long series of measurements on these instruments. Crookes wanted four disks of pith, black on one side, white on the other, attached to wire arms suspended on a steel point so as to revolve horizontally. The vanes enclosed in a glass bulb at the highest possible vacuum should be free to rotate.

In the first machine the arms revolved when exposed to bright light. Crookes called the device a "light mill" or, because its rotation was proportional to light intensity, it was a "radiometer." He demonstrated the radiometer to the Royal Society on 22 April 1875. It was a smash hit.

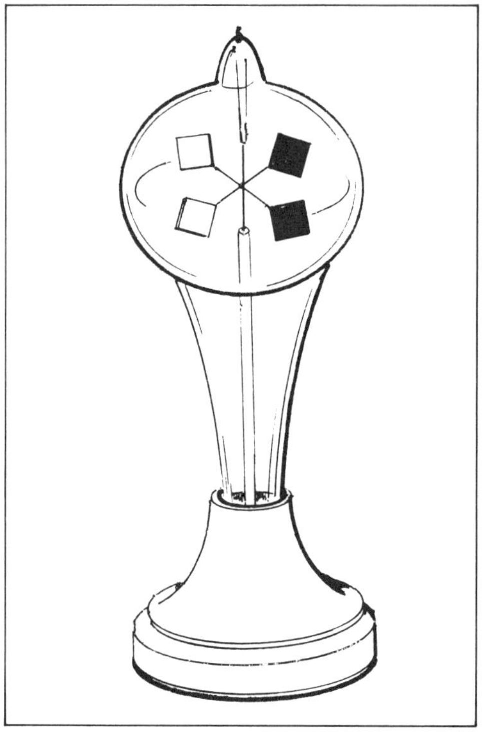

Crookes' Radiometer (1875)

Coggia's comet had made a spectacular appearance in the skies over Europe during the summer of 1874. Scientists observing the position of its tail away from the sun were prepared to accept the concept that light can exert a pressure. Maxwell's 1875 electromagnetic theory was uppermost in physicists' minds. It provides for light to exert a pressure. A light particle falling on a black surface should be absorbed and transfer its momentum to the vane. Falling on a white surface the light particle would reflect, transfer some energy, and the vane should recoil with a momentum equal and opposite to the reflected ray. Thus the white surface doubles the momentum of the black and Crookes' radiometer will rotate clockwise . . .

. . . but it didn't.

It rotated counterclockwise!

For Every Action An Opposite Reaction

Mathematical physicists quivered when they saw the radiometer rotating in the wrong direction. Sir William Thomson (later Lord Kelvin) sat immobile and stared at the radiometer for a half hour and then left without saying a word. Many others went home to build their own, or invited Crookes to demonstrate to their students.

Arthur Schuster was a demonstrator in the new physics laboratory at Owens College in Manchester. He was about to join Maxwell's staff at the Cavendish. In a few years (1881) he would become professor of applied mathematics and then hold the Chair in Physics at Owens. In 1907 he would give up the professorship (he was independently wealthy) in favor of his choice for successor, E. Rutherford. Schuster was the first to investigate the spectra of electric discharges through evacuated Geissler tubes, and suggested that gases "dissociated" to conduct a current. (This became "ionization" to J.J. Thomson.) He was the first to suggest the measurable e/m ratio that helped Thomson discover the electron. Although primarily a mathematical physicist, he forecast the rise of experimental physics.

In 1875 Schuster was just a "demonstrator," an instructor who set up "experimental" demonstrations to illustrate lectures in science. In the midst of the explosive controversy started by Crookes' radiometer, Schuster suggested an alternate to Maxwell's (and Crookes') "pressure of light" explanation. Large numbers of gas molecules left in the glass globe after reaching "high vacuum," impinge on both black and white surfaces of the vanes according to the kinetic theory of gases. When light strikes a black surface it gets hotter, repels the molecules with greater energy, and their recoil rotates vanes counterclockwise.

Osborne Reynolds, Professor of Engineering at Owens, asked Schuster for proof. If the vanes rotate from pressure of light, the globe itself will not be affected. But if the recoil is from molecules within the globe, it must rotate in the opposite direction. If the recoil impulse is so small that it can't be measured, Schuster thought of a way to demonstrate: he would suspend a radiometer on a thread from a high ceiling in a well lit room. The globe could then rotate as freely as the vanes.

The aura and credibility of mathematical physics was hanging by a fine thread at Owens College. In his "Recollections . . ." 62 years later, J.J. Thomson described the anxiety of physicists throughout England on the morning of the experiment:

> *"I can still remember the excitement and anxiety with which I waited for the verdict. And the relief on hearing that the case had rotated in the opposite direction to the vanes."*
>
> [MacMillan, 1937]

Crookes, a Chemist, Shakes the Foundations of Physics

Crookes had severely shaken but had not cracked the foundations of science. Moreover, although he continued to believe in Spiritualism until his death in 1919, he was no longer strident and his reputation as a scientist was never again questioned. Hundreds of publications on the radiometer appeared in the scientific and popular literature in the next few years. Most teachers of science could make a workable radiometer and it soon became (and still is) a staple of instrument makers. But Crookes received many requests for demonstrations. On 7 March 1876 his lab assistant, Charles Gimingham, made a note in Crookes' laboratory notebook:

> *"Making radiometer for exhibition . . . all went well until putting in bulb when all came to grief . . . I have tried hard to finish it, but find it impossible today."*
>
> [D'Albe, Biog, Appleton, 1924]

Later that night Crookes wrote under this entry: *"Cheer up,"* and then sketched in the first rumble of an earthquake that would ultimately crumble the foundations of 19th century physics. He sketched two platinum wires embedded in a glass tube to act as anode and cathode under very high vacuum. It was the prototype of the "Crookes tube" that puzzled Roentgen 19 years later.

[See Vig1879.WC3, Crookes' & Geissler's. . .]

THE CROOKES TUBE

When in 1875 William Crookes asked his laboratory assistant to blow a glass tube with embedded lead-in wires, he was not making a simple request. [See Vig1875 .WC2] To seal metal wires in a glass tube that would have to maintain a vacuum was a special trick in the glassblower's art. To achieve a vacuum, or something close enough to be considered "highly evacuated," had only been achieved recently. Charles Gimingham, Crookes' lab assistant until 1882, had remarkable glass blowing dexterity and achieved many of Crookes' unreasonable instrument designs. With his expertise, Crookes improved the Geissler mercury vacuum pump.

Faraday Looks at Sparks in a Wire Gap

Crookes, from his beginnings as a scientist, considered Michael Faraday an ideal. He tried to emulate the experimental style: a simple experiment would illustrate an explanatory lecture. Much of Faraday's work had been on the passage of electricity through liquids; no glass blowing was involved. He and others had observed colored sparks produced in a gap in wire connecting the two poles of a Leyden jar. In CO_2 atmosphere they were red. In nitrogen, green. In coal gas they were partly green and partly red. He was beginning to investigate currents passing through different gases in the 1830s.

Charles Wheatstone, inventor of the "Morse" telegraph, turned to brush discharges instead of sparks. Following his lead, Faraday studied discharges in gases, but this required containment in glass bottles. A current flowing through the gas caused a glow extending from cathode to anode. The glow was always interrupted near center by a dark region (soon known as "Faraday's Dark Space"). About this time Faraday fell ill. When he returned to work in 1844, his interest was in a new subject, magnetism. But he had stimulated another person to action.

Plücker Becomes a Physicist

Julius Plücker, Professor of Mathematics and Physics at Bonn, turned from pure mathematics to experimental physics in 1846. After correspondence with Faraday he became interested in the passage of electricity through gas, particularly

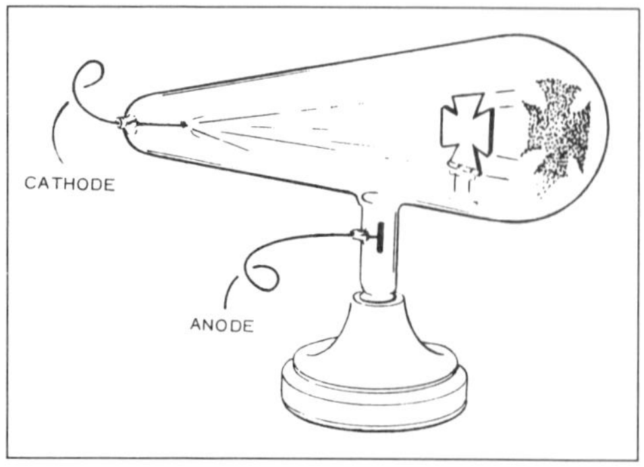

Crookes' "Shadow" Experiment (1877)

through a *pure* gas. Many physicists had followed Faraday on currents through "discharge tubes" (two wires imbedded in glass walls), but the vagaries of colored glow must, Plücker thought, be due to impurities. To get a pure gas he must first evacuate the air from a discharge tube. He sought the aid of Heinrich Geissler, Bonn's instrument maker.

Geissler's Tubes, A Major Physical Event

Geissler was probably the only glass blower ready to "seal" wires in glass, but the vacuum was poor. Around 1855, he improved on Torrecelli's vacuum by inventing a mercury vacuum pump: two glass tubes with thick rubber seals were manually raised and lowered to pump air in or out of a hermetically sealed tube. It took time and patience, but hitherto unknown vacua could be achieved. A very low pressure glass tube with electrodes imbedded at either end soon became known as a Geissler Tube. (And still is. Fill with neon after 1930 and call it a neon sign.) By 1868 Geissler's work had become so widespread that the U. of Bonn awarded him an honorary doctorate.

Geissler gave the first tube with a reasonable vacuum to Plücker. On the first attempt to fill it with "electric fluid" from a Leyden jar, Plücker could not see a thing. Patches of fluorescence obscured the improperly annealed glass. At least Plücker thought it was improper annealing, but Geissler didn't make that kind of mistake. Almost by accident Plücker discovered that the patches could be moved around the glass walls with a simple hand magnet. Something susceptible to a magnetic field was emerging from the cathode and fluorescing on the glass wall. In 1859 he reported his results. By 1864 he had degenerated back to pure math and died in 1868.

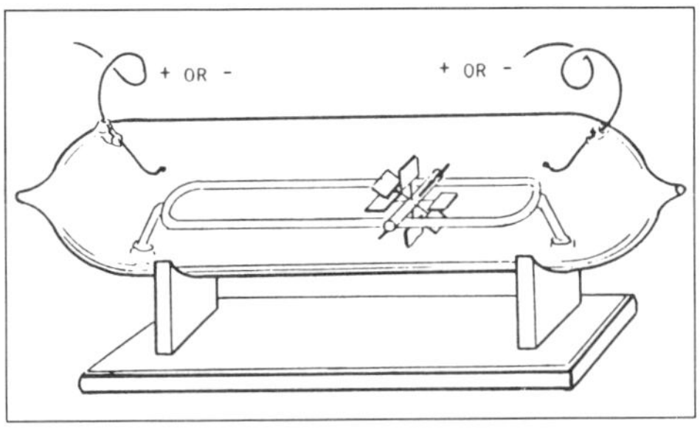

Crookes' "Paddle-Wheel" Experiment (1879)

With Plücker's death, Johann Hittorf, a former student who had seen a possible fault in the 1859 work, could now revive the experiment. (In those days you did not encroach upon The Professor's field.)

Hittorf's Shadow Experiment

In 1869 Hittorf, now professor at the U. of Münster, blew a Geissler tube in an L shape to get the anode out of line-of-flight from the cathode. The glow, he noticed, was then confined to the cathode arm. By accident he found that any solid object in the beam cast a shadow. He sharpened the cathode in his next tube to a fine point to demonstrate the shadow's sharp lines; therefore, whatever emanated from the cathode followed optical laws. It was a wave phenomenon in the luminiferous aether. This was Hittorf's famous shadow experiment of 1869.

Crookes Makes a Better Shadow

A few years later, after his triumph with the radiometer, William Crookes saw an answer to Hittorf's demonstration of wave theory. He had Gimingham blow a glass tube with an arm at 90° to contain the anode and drawn to a dull point at the cathode end. In the pathway of the cathode rays he inserted a mica maltese cross on a hinge. With a flick of the wrist the cross could be stood up or knocked down. Upon activation of the tube a shadow cast by the cross was surrounded by fluorescing glass. After a while the fluorescence began to fade, presumably from fatigue in the glass. The cross was knocked down and the shadowed glass now fluoresced brilliantly while the fatigued glass remained dark. This was Crookes' famous 1879 shadow experiment.

Crookes' improvements over Hittorf were not only in showmanship. He had much stronger batteries and was the first to achieve a vacuum at one millionth the molecules of room air. (Both Edison and Swan gave Crookes credit for the high vacua in their electric light bulbs.) He repeated the early Faraday discharge tube work and found a second stripe in fluorescence; the "Crookes Dark Space" appeared at low vacuum and increased in size until it filled the tube at high vacuum. (The "Hittorf L shaped tube" became widely known as "the Crookes Tube" when used by Roentgen in 1895.) Crookes disagreed that Hittorf had given evidence of the wave nature of cathode emission. To dispute wave theory he built another tube device.

Crookes inserted a pair of glass rails so a paddle-wheel with mica vanes could roll from cathode to anode in the highly evacuated tube. The vanes masked the line-of-sight from cathode to anode. He sent a current into the cathode. The paddle-wheel rolled toward the anode. He reversed the current and the paddle-wheel rolled back. Hence cathode rays had mass.

Eugen Goldstein at Potsdam Observatory disagreed with Crookes. A broad cathode, substituted for Hittorf's point source, showed that the shadow's edge had both umbra and penumbra. He introduced the word "kathodenstrahlen" because these were rays like light. Crookes went a step further. He put two cathodes in one tube and interposed a shield with two fine slits. When cathode A was activated a ribbon of rays caused a fine line of fluorescence on the glass wall. When cathode B was activated, another ribbon of cathode rays fluoresced on the same focus. When both were activated simultaneously, two lines fluoresced. Thus the two ribbons repulsed each other! Light rays could not do this.

Crookes built another tube to remind Germans of Plücker 25 years earlier. A fine ribbon of cathode rays was directed along a plate chalked with phosphorescent powder. The ribbon could be seen from slit to anode. A horseshoe magnet was set astride the tube. The ribbon was deflected upwards. The magnet was reversed and the ribbon deflected downward. By Faraday's rule the cathode ray was negatively charged. In 15 more years J.J. Thomson not only agreed, but measured the size of the "corpuscle" (we say "electron").

YOUR MOST IMPORTANT DECISION
(The CGPM is validated every day)

When you woke up this morning you opened your eyes, looked at the clock, and decided to get up — the most important decision in your life. Not the getting up part; the world could easily have done without you for a few more hours. Your acceding to the measurement of time as shown on the face of the clock was the important decision.

You did not have a vote in deciding that the clock face goes from noon to midnight through 12 numbers, but you agreed to go along with the crowd in measuring "time" (a word you probably can't even define). You accept 60 seconds for every minute and 60 minutes in every hour when you know that 60 seconds of toothache and 60 seconds of pleasure are not the same span.

You Are Subservient to the CGPM

Thus, with your first gasp this morning you have subordinated your biological clock to the deliberations of a Paris bureaucracy called the *Conférence Générale des Poids et Mesures* (CGPM). This international *political* body made the decision on how long it takes for the second hand to go from tick to tock.

When you got out of bed you took ten paces to the bathroom, but we haven't used "paces" to measure distance for a few hundred years. The architect for your house probably used inches to indicate distance, but nobody has actually measured the "inch" in your lifetime. The Conference on Weights and Measures precisely defined a unit of length and called it the "meter" (a Greek word for "measure"). Hence, in 1889 when they got started, their name was really "Conference on Weights and Meters." The word "Weights," translated from the French "poids," is also wrong.

At their Third Conference in 1903, some nit-picking scientist had pointed out that a "weight" was a mass of substance pulled down by the force of gravity. This force changes from place to place. The CGPM had canceled gravity by using a dual arm balance; hence, they had defined "mass" in 1889, not "weight."

Because a unit of measurement is nothing more than a precise, nit-pick proof definition of a word, the Conference had to agree with the nit-picker. In 1903 they admonished all never to use the word "weight" when "mass" was intended. Naturally, as a political body on "Mass and Meters" they continued to call themselves the Conference on Weights and Measures.

Continuity With Past Units is Necessary

When you first turned on the lights this morning you used up some CGPM units of energy. In 1889 electricity was just coming into widespread use; its units had to be added to those of the meter, kilogram, and second. If your light bulb burned out this morning you replaced the old 60 watt with a new 850 lumen bulb. "Watts" are being phased out, to be replaced by an 1860 candle power unit of luminous intensity. Of course the "Candle Power" unit was brought up to date in 1967, but the CGPM retained a continuity by calling it the "candela."

This *continuity* with past units is why the CGPM is a political, not a scientific body. The "second" is still *almost* the same duration of time as the heart beat of primitive man. The "meter" is still *almost* the same length as the Roman Pace. The "kilogram" is still the same gob of metal stashed in a Paris vault in 1889. Scientists may change their units of measurement at the drop of a decimal point, but most people will not change units during their lifetime.

Everything people breath, eat or bump into throughout the day is perceived in the units of measurement they learned in childhood. It is difficult to overcome psychological imprinting. The next generation *might* make the change if scientists in the parent generation prove a new unit desirable, practical, and measurable, and if the political body supports the change. This mixture of politics and science is illustrated by the developments and structure of the Conférence Générale des Poids et Mesures (CGPM).

Historically units of measurement, especially a nation's coinage, are a property of the divine right of kings or the military might of warlords. In 1781 a change occurred.

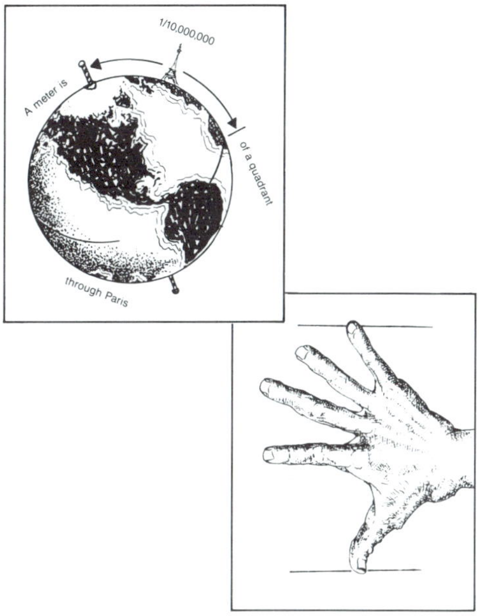

Many units of measurement were originally based on natural phenomena.

"Units" Become True International Units

In 1781 13 sovereign states (at least they considered themselves sovereign states) assembled in a Continental Congress to confederate their politics. Taxes, and British mercantile policy, sparked the revolutionary discontent. The unit of measurement in their economics was the coinage system. Thomas Jefferson, impressed by a new system of counting by 10s, convinced the new Confederation to adopt a "metric" coinage. Thus, in revolutionary fervor, the United States was the first government to adopt a "metric system."

The most important interaction between states was commercial trade. Each state, and often communities within the state, had its own bushel and peck, its own sunrise and sunset; distance was measured by how long it took to get there. But the old British Imperial System was the only system they knew: for pounds & ounces, and yards & inches.

A new "Constitution of the United States" in 1789 provided some relief from confusion. Sec 8, Art 1 reads, "The Congress shall have power to fix the Standards of Weights and Measures . . . ."

In England and Europe an even more complex plethora of units was hindering commercial trade. A new "scientific" (the word had not yet been coined) discipline was beginning to measure things. Metrology, the science of measurement, began on the eve of the French Revolution.

In 1795 the French Academy of Sciences defined the "metre" as a unit of distance based upon a natural phenomenon (the size of the earth). The committee making the decision survived the Revolution (only one member, Lavoisier, had his head chopped off). After 90 frustrating years their successors realized that the metre could be a commercial success only if it were a "universally" adopted unit.

By 1875 the French "scientists" (the word, coined in 1840, can now be used) managed to gather diplomats from 17 nations (the industrial world) in Paris to sign a "Treaty of the Metric Convention" — the first step in a system of units. To add flesh to the definition of units they created a *Bureau International des Poids et Mesures* (BIPM) in Paris. It would be a scientific laboratory to make standards for adoption by the diplomatic body.

In 1889 the treaty signers reconvened in Paris as the *First Conférence Générale des Poids et Measures* (CGPM). This new diplomatic body defined the meter and the kilogram with platinum-iridium prototype standards made by the BIPM. They also defined the "second" as a fraction of the mean solar day, and adopted a centigrade temperature scale.

The General Conference continued to meet about every six years (wars permitting), adopting new units in new fields of science. At their ninth meeting, in 1948, they recognized that the new units were just as *incoherent* as the mess Thomas Jefferson had complained about in 1781. The word *"coherent"* has a special meaning in metrology: no "unit" could be a fraction, hence all begin with "1." The 1889 CGPM began a new chapter and a "system" that lasted until 1960.

(See 14th CGPM 1971)

GEORGE DOCK SEES ENDEMIC GOITERS
(And Finds a Goiter in Lucy's Squirrel)

George Dock completed medical training in Philadelphia in 1890. After a couple of years in Galveston he set up a practice in Ann Arbor, Michigan. He was soon bewildered by the number of goiters he saw in the populace and even in animals. A well-known physician in Baltimore named William Osler had pointed out that goiter was common among the French Canadians along the Detroit River.

Osler's information had come from insane asylums, but Dock's practice was in a vigorous farming community. He made an effort to find goiter among the indigenous Indians, but they had been cheated so often they trusted no white doctor. Dock paid little attention to stories of the commonplace nature of goiter until he saw it in his own practice.

One day early in the spring of 1893 Dr. Dock got a message to stop by the home of a farmer who had a touch of the ague, his little girl had caught the croup, and the missus was feeling a bit peaked. He made a call the next morning. A dab of laudanum took care of the farmer, but in addition to her cough the little girl had a swelling in her neck. The mother said not to pay no mind because it was natural in the family. She had carried a good sized goiter all her life, as the doctor could plainly see. To prove her point, a second daughter came into the room and Lucy too, had a goiter.

"All my children have generous necks," said the mother, *"Lucy, call in Mary and Melinda."* They too had goiters. Then a fifth daughter came in the room. She had a goiter; then the sixth and the seventh. The eldest daughter was working in the barn, but she too had a goiter. Nine women in one family, and all had goiters. *"Obviously,"* said Dr. Dock, *"goiter is a family disease." "Mebbe so,"* said the farmer, *"but it must be catchin' because my horse also has a big neck."*

Dr. Dock couldn't believe this, so they went out to the barn to look at the mare. She had a goiter. In the barn a ewe and her lamb had goiters. By this time Lucy had retrieved her pet squirrel (sex unidentified) to prove that it was part of the family.

Speculation On the Cause of Goiter

George Dock had been taught that goiter was neither hereditary nor catching, but nobody mentioned what it was. Goiter was rare in newly arrived Michiganders. But once they settled down, the youngsters, especially girls around puberty, began to get swollen necks. They didn't resemble the grotesque masses said to be common in Switzerland, but there were so many. Up in Otsego county one fourth of the children reaching puberty had goiter. In Calumet, in one day, Dock saw six goiterous horses.

In Switzerland, living near glaciers or in protracted mists and fogs was suggested, but no glaciers cooled Michigan. The women did not carry heavy loads on their heads, a theory that carried some weight in Europe. The current medical fad was microbes and toxins, but Dock's patients were not sick — they just had big necks.

Dock Scores a Near Miss on the Cause

Dock thought he had a hint: *"... of the cases of goitre I have seen, a very large proportion have used well-water, and almost without exception my correspondents state that the same is true of cases they report. Near Ann Arbor ... one of my patients, a girl of sixteen years, developed goitre a few months after a new well was put in use. Dr N. Taylor, of Ludington, writes that goitre has become much less frequent there since lake-water has been substituted for well-water."*

[TAAP, 10:101, 1895]

The possibility of a contaminant in well water was an astute observation. For him to have considered the absence of iodine as a cause was impossible. As his article went to press, E. Bauman's discovery of iodine in the thyroid was in print but hadn't reached Michigan. And anyway iodine was well known to be geochemically ubiquitous. The *absence of something* was not acceptable pharmacology in 1895. An investigation of inconsistent results from a new therapeutic agent, desiccated sheep thyroids, would put David Marine on the right track in 1907.

[See Vig1907 .Mar]

THESE MEN MADE NUCLEAR SCIENCE A REALITY

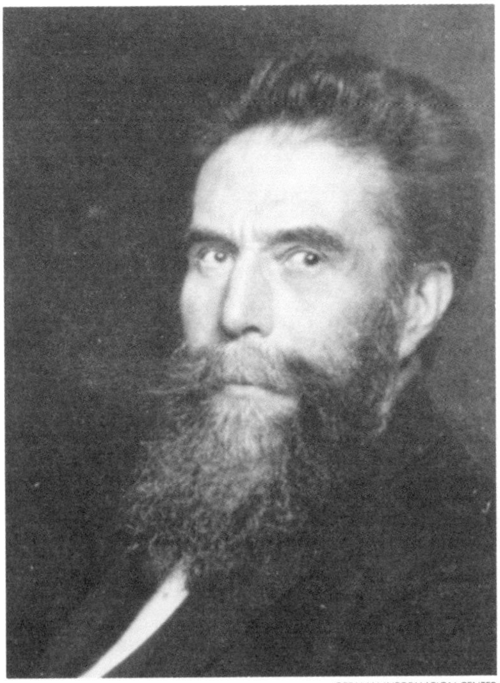

GERMAN INFORMATION CENTER

William Konrad Roentgen, Ph.D., 1845–1923

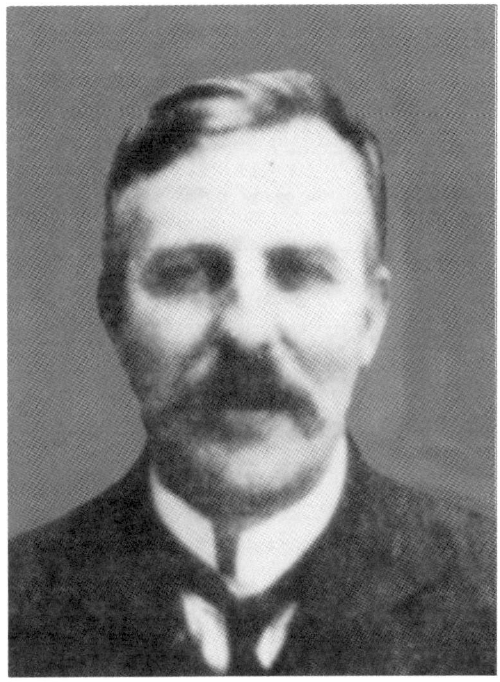

Ernest Rutherford, 1871–1937

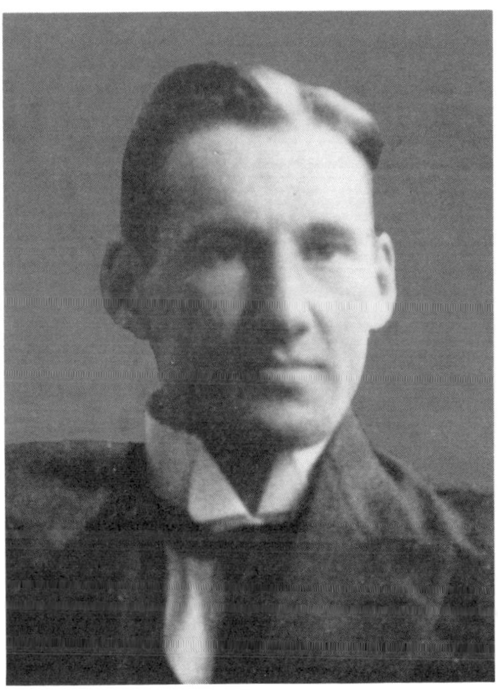

Kasimir Fajans, Dr.Nat.Phil., 1887–1975

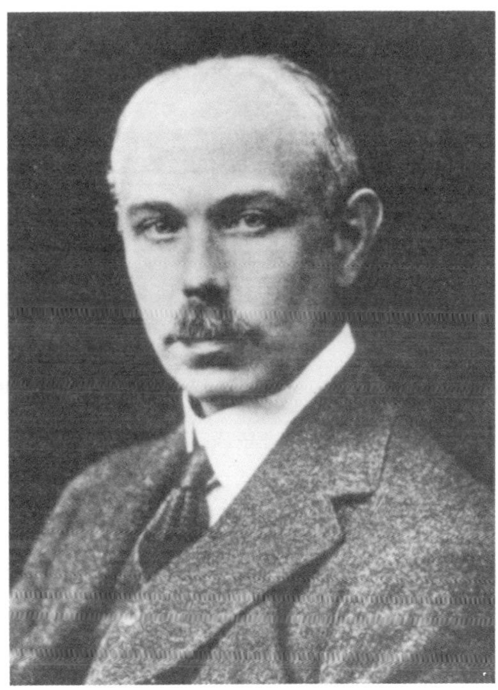

Francis William Aston, 1877–1945

CHRONOLOGY OF NUCLEAR MEDICINE — 1895

			Ref.
	Scientific and Technical Background		
1. Basic	— W. ROENTGEN DISCOVERS X-RAYS ON 8 NOVEMBER IN WÜRZBURG.	[1877]	GSR
	— J.J. THOMSON DISCOVERS X-RAY IONIZATION IN AIR, names it after Faraday's ionization in liquid.	[1825]	Bio
	— G. FitzGerald says motion increases length in same direction.		WoA
2. Obser	— S. Freud publishes "Studien Über Hysterie."	[1850]	Bio
3. # Nuc	— Ramsay & Rayleigh discover He in gas from uranium ores.	[1868]	HRC
	Organizations and Internal Politics		
5. Pols	— Japan defeats China, begins military build-up.	[1941]	AP
7. Event	— G. Marconi invents wireless telegraphy.	[1889]	DSB
	— J.J. Thomson takes Rutherford as first grad student (exp Physics).		Eve
	— K. Gillette invents the safety razor.	[1890]	EB
	Instruments, Units of Measurement, and Drugs		
8. Instr	— J.J. Thomson invents cotton plug ion trap.	[1881]	Bio
	— J. Perrin collects cathode rays in cup inside tube.	[1894]	HRC
	— C.T.R. Wilson builds his first cloud chamber.	[1894]	Bio
	— W. Roentgen covers his Crookes tube with black paper.	[1894]	GSR
	— W. Einthoven invents the electrocardiograph.	[1893]	PAP
	— C. Linde builds a machine to make liquid air.	[1892]	DSB
	— Elster & Geitel invent the photocell.	[1896]	AnP
10. Concp	— A. Lumie're invents a motion picture camera.	[1894]	EB
	— K. Isiolkovski describes rocket propulsion principle.	[1880]	DSB
	Radioiodine, P-32, and Radioactive Therapy		
12. I-Res	— E. Baumann discovers iodine in normal thyroid gland.	[1852]	ZPC
	— G. Dock finds great incidence of goiter in Michigan.	[1657]	TAAP
	Scans and Other Tests of Function in Various Organs		
18. Brain	—		
26. Other	—		
	Radiation Hysteria and Health Physics * Obituaries *		
27. Hyst	— S. Freud starts psychiatric therapy. Psychiatry replaces phrenology as major medical hoax.	[1832]	Bio
28. React	—		
29. Respo	—		

* * *

30. Obits	— K. Ludwig (1816–1895) Ger physiol; exp physiol & instruments.	DSB
	— L. Pasteur (1822–1895) Fr chem; germ theory, pasteurization.	Bio
	— T.H. Huxley (1825–1895) Eng biol; first major supporter of Darwin.	Bio
	— L. Meyer (1830–1895) Fr chem; accepted Avogadro, Periodic Table.	DSB

ROENTGEN DISCOVERS A NEW FORM OF LIGHT

(As Told in 1897 by Silvanus Thompson)

Silvanus P. Thompson, a good friend of Crookes, Kelvin, Lodge, J.J. Thomson, and all English physicists, was working on electrical discharges from the Crookes Tube around 1894. He discovered a discharge early in 1895 that he reported as "hyperphosphorescence." After the 6 Jan 1896 news story revealed Roentgen's discovery, friends of Thompson spread the word that he had published first. Thompson scotched this by publishing a retraction: his work had not recognized the fundamental X-ray discovery. But he became an enthusiastic president of the first (British) Roentgen Society. To learn the story of the discovery he went to Würzburg to visit Roentgen and was able to give as close to a first hand account as ever recorded. On 5 Nov 1897 at St. Martin's Town Hall he told this story:

"November the eighth, 1895, will ever be memorable in the history of Science. On that day a light never seen was first observed. The observer, Prof. William Konrad Röntgen. The place, the Institute of Physics in the University of Würzburg in Bavaria. What he saw was a faint flickering greenish illumination upon a bit of cardboard painted over with fluorescent chemical. The faintly luminous surface was crossed by a line of dark shadow. All this was in a carefully darkened room, from which every known kind of ray had been scrupulously excluded. In that room a Crookes tube, stimulated internally by sparks from an induction coil, had been carefully covered with a shield of black cardboard. It was impervious to every known kind of light. Yet in the darkness, expressly arranged so as to allow the eye to watch for luminous phenomena, nothing was visible until the hitherto unrecognized rays, emanating from the Crookes tube and penetrating the cardboard shield, fell upon the luminescent screen.

"From seeing the line of shadow across the fluorescent screen, tracing it back to the object, and verifying the source to be the Crookes tube, was, to the practiced investigator, but the work of a few minutes. The invisible rays — invisible except on the chemically painted screen — were found to have a penetrative power hitherto unimagined. They penetrated cardboard, wood, and cloth with ease. They would even go through a thick plank, or a book of 2000 pages. But metals such as copper, iron, lead, silver, and gold were less penetrable, the densest practically opaque. The discoverer, interposing his hand between the source of the rays and his bit of luminescent cardboard, saw the bones of his living hand projected in silhouette upon the screen. The great discovery had been made."

Silvanus Thompson's story was published in the first radiographic journal: THE ARCHIVES OF SKIAGRAPHY. This journal lasted for 2 issues when a new "medical" journal took over: ARCHIVES OF THE ROENTGEN RAY.

His wife said that Roentgen seldom emerged from his laboratory in the next six weeks. He had progressed from painted cardboard to fluorescent screen to glass photographic plate. One of the first photos was that of his wife's hand wearing a wedding ring (soon to become the most famous photo in history). On 28 Dec 1895 he emerged with a preliminary manuscript for the WÜRZBURG PHYSICAL MEDICAL SOCIETY. (He would speak to them on 28 Jan 1896.) But he couldn't hold his excitement. He wrote a few friends, enclosing a positive of his wife's hand.

Prof F. Exner, a physicist in Vienna, put the letter in his pocket and went to a dinner party of fellow scientists. For dinner conversation he showed the remarkable photo he had received from Roentgen. One physicist asked to borrow the photo to show to his father-in-law (who published the Wiener Presse). This editor knew a news item when he saw it. A story with photo was in the next morning's paper where it was picked up by the London Times and cabled to the world on 6 January 1896. On 7 January every physicist in the world who owned a Crookes tube was taking his first X-Ray picture.

[See Vig1896 .X-R]

CHRONOLOGY OF NUCLEAR MEDICINE — 1896

Scientific and Technical Background			Ref.
1. Basic	— W. Roentgen's article translated into English.	[1895]	Sc
	— H. Becquerel discovers uranium gives off "X" rays.	[1892]	CRS
	— G. Stokes says X-rays have very short wave length.	[1889]	Eve
	— J. Perrin finds electrified bodies lose charge in X-ray.	[1895]	CRS
	— H. Lorentz says volumes contract to "0" at speed of light.	[1893]	WoA
	— P. Zeeman proves vis light spectrum splits in mag field.	[1873]	DSB
	— Elster & Geitel discover emission from hot filaments.	[1897]	DSB
2. Obser	— C. Henry sees Al transparent to X-rays (used ZnS crystals).	[1892]	CRS
	— S. Thompson reads uranium rays as hyperphosphorescence.	[1895]	PM
	— E. Rutherford detects electromagnetic waves.	[1888]	Bio
	— M. Curie finds more radiation in natural/synthetic chalcolite.		Bio
	— J. Dewar finds X-ray opacity proportional to Atomic Wt.	[1895]	CN
3. # Nuc	— W. Ramsay discovers helium on earth.	[1868]	DSB

Organizations and Internal Politics			
6. Socs	— F. Venable publishes "Development of the Periodic Law."	[1869]	Bk
	— W. Roentgen's first paper published on March 9.	[1895]	GW
	— F. Exner receives copies of Roentgen's first X-rays about	5 Jan.	GSB
	— WIENER PRESSE PUBLISHES ROENTGEN'S LETTER TO A FRIEND.	5 Jan.	GSR
	London press cables discovery of X-rays to world	on 6 Jan.	GSR
	Many physicists with Crookes tubes check news story.		GSR
	Most science and medical journals note X-ray discovery in weeks.		—
	JAMA notes "somatic illumination by electricity"	on 1 Feb.	JAMA
	W. Magie pubs first article on "medical X-Rays"	in March.	AJMS
	Arch of Skiagraphy publishes first of 2 issues	on 2 Apr.	—
	Elihu Thomson pubs first book on Roentgen rays (Van Nos)	Aug.	Bk
	50 books & 1000 papers published on X-Rays in first year.		GSR
6a.	Early X-Rays were made by anybody who had a Crookes tube; some were:		
	— S. Thompson takes first X-Ray picture in England	on 6 Jan.	Bio
	— F. Almy, Grinnell College, takes pics of student's hands,	7 Jan.	AP
	— Davidson College students use Crookes tube, first AM X-Ray	(1926	Rad)
	— M. Pupin takes first diagnostic X-Ray picture in America	? Jan.	Bio
	— Diagnostic X-Rays being made in Vienna.	11 Jan.	GSR
	— F. Exner demonstrates X-Ray of hand to Vienna meeting.	17 Jan.	GSR
	— -. Mosetig-Moerhof shows 2 pics of hands in Vienna.	24 Jan.	WKW
	— S. Rowland says X-Rays are important medical Dx tool.	8 Feb.	BMJ
	— M. Pupin publishes first description of X-ray physics.	12 Feb.	EW
	— J. Burry shows a few clinical X-Rays to surgeons.	29 Feb.	JAMA
	— X-ray machine used in S. Africa by March.	? Mar.	GSR
	— S. Rowland expands on the new photography in medicine.	18 Apr.	BMJ
	— J. Chappuis shows biliary and renal calculi.		BAM
	— E. Davis studies infant in pregnant uterus by X-Ray.		AJMS
	— W. Fuchs starts first private (lay) X-Ray lab in Chicago.		AP
	— A. Goodspeed illustrates X-Ray application to surgery.		AJMS
	— R. Guiteras demonstrates a needle in pts foot.		NYMR
	— W. Keen applies X-Rays to surgical diagnosis.		AJMS
	— C. Leonard, A. Wright, H. Rowland, all show surg X-Rays.		AJMS
7. Event	— Court allows X-Ray of bullet as evidence, first use.	4 Mar.	CDDR
	— Denver court gets first suit on X-ray damage (Rocky Mt News).		AP
	— J. MacIntyre takes first 40 ft roll of cine radiography.		GSR
	— X-Ray of bone projected on dog's brain makes dog hungry.		AP
	— D. Kotogakko discovers X-rays emanating from glow worms.		AnP
	— A. McKissick sees radiation from sugar penetrate 2½" wood.		EW
	— W. Shrader (U of Mo) uses bacteriocidal X-rays on diphtheria, begins an era of "kill bacty hence possibly cure disease."		N
	— J. Trowbridge studies "The New Photography."		NYMR

Instruments, Units of Measurement, and Drugs

8. Instr	— C.Wilson exposes his cloud chamber to X-ray beam.	[1877]	Bio
	— T. Edison invents X-ray fluoroscope (Feb ?), gives public demo.		EW
	— J. Blyer manufactures a new photo-fluoroscope (1 July).		EE
	— S. Thompson works on developing intensifying screens.	[1895]	Na
	— Liverpool hosp is first in UK to install med X-ray instr.	(1906	ArRR)
	— W. Magie explains X-ray apparatus and its use.	[1895]	AJMS
	— O. Schallenberger describes Roentgen ray tubes.	[1894]	AE
	— E. Thomson makes stereoscopic X-Rays, describes method.	[1895]	EE
9. Units	— C. Guillaumi discovers alloy (9Fe – 5Ni) invariable to temp; this "Invar" is used for Pt-Ir second standards.	[1889]	DSB
	— G. Stover describes graduated time exposure skiagraphs.	[1895]	NYMR
10. Concp	— J.J. THOMSON SAYS X-RAYS CAUSE IONIZATION IN AIR.	[1895]	Bio
	— E. Buchner proves fermentation a chem action not "Life-Force," marks the end of mystical "Vitalism" in Science.	[1849]	DSB

Radioiodine, P-32, and Radioactive Therapy

12. I-Res	— E. Baumann says iodine appears to be essential in gland.	[1895]	ZPC
13. I-Dx	— A. Magnus-Levy studies Basal Metabolism Rate (BMR).	[1950]	BKW
16. Tele	— E. Grubbe treats Rose Lee for ca of breast (29 Jan).	(1933	Rad)
	He is a pharmacist-homeopath and is disregarded;	(1949	Bk)
	after getting MD he claims first radiotherapy	on 20 Jan.	Bio
	— D. Voight relieves pain of nasopharynx ca with X-ray.		GSR

Scans and Other Tests of Function in Various Organs

18. Brain	— J. Daniel wants X-Ray of big brain — gets Dean of Vanderbilt, Dean is X-Rayed — 20 days later first epilation. Dean does not appreciate being first in history.		Sc
19. Heart	— E. Starling describes extracard phase cardiac failure.	[1876]	La
	— S. Riva-Rocci invents a blood pressure measuring cuff.	[1891]	DSB
20. Liver	— F. Pick studies adhesive pericarditis with cirrosis.	[1854]	ZKM
	— B. Naunyn "produces" gallstones with infections of GB.	[1894]	BK
24. Gut	— J. Head discusses pain & sensation in visceral disease.	[1886]	B
	— J. Hemmeter shows photograph by X-ray of human stomach.	[1895]	BMSJ
	— H. Boas can diagnose from X-Rays of stomach and gut.	[1895]	DMW
26. Other	— C. Eijkman discovers dietary deficiency (Vit B in chick).	[1881]	DSB
	— L. Popcelski finds nerve stimulation of pancreas juice.	[1926]	ZPh
	— E. Codman shows radiograph of fetal arm.	[1895]	BMSJ

Radiation Hysteria and Health Physics * Obituaries *

27. Hyst	— L. Stevens makes first report of skin reaction to X-rays.	[1897]	BMJ
	— E. Grubbe seeks help for his first X-ray burn on 27 Jan.	[1913]	Bio
	— R. Bowles describes the new sunburn of X-rays (12 Mar).	[1898]	La
	— C. Leonard writes about X-ray dermatitis.	[1898]	AXJ
	— T. Edison & asst note eye smarting after hrs exposure.	[1899]	Na
	— E. Thomson proves damage from X-rays, not electricity.	[1904]	EE
	— J. Daniel reports hair fallout after skull X-Rays.	[1910]	Sc
	— W. Marcuse reports epilation and dermatitis after many X-Rays.		DMW
	— L. Stevens reports that X-rays cause a dermatitis.	[1912]	BMJ
28. React	— Jury awards $10,000 for radiation damage, first law suit.	[1977]	CDDR
	— Niagara Falls opens largest electric plant, hazard ???	[1879]	AP
	— N. Finsen finds shortwave light (UV) is bactericidal.	[1801]	DSB
29. Respo	— NY City Health Dept says X-rays stimulate TBC bacilli. PROBABLY THE FIRST HINT OF RADIATION HORMESIS.	[1901]	AP

* * *

30. Obits	— A. Nobel (1833–1896) Swed indust; leaves will with prizes.		AP

CHRONOLOGY OF NUCLEAR MEDICINE — 1897

Scientific and Technical Background			Ref.
1. Basic	— J.J. THOMSON ANNOUNCES DISCOVERY OF "CORPUSCLE" (ELECTRON),	[1881]	PM
	says photoelectric effect occurs with X-rays.	[1895]	PM
	— Rayleigh's formula for long wavelength black body.	[1893]	DSB
2. Obser	— Elster & Geitel say U gives off hyperphosphorescence.	[1896]	BAP
	— G. Stokes: X-rays = "particulate irreg pulse repetition."	[1896]	DSB
	— C. Barkla relates secondary rays from Ni to atomic wt of Ni.		PM
	— J.J. Thomson notes third kind of ray (later = gamma ray).	[1900]	ArRR
	— R. Wood describes diffraction of a cathode discharge.	[1896]	PR
	— Irene Curie born Sept, 9 months before Po discovered.	[1933]	Bio
	— F. Blaise studies effect of X-rays on bacteria.	[1908]	CRB
3. # Nuc	—		
4. # Med	—		

Organizations and Internal Politics			
5. Pols	— W. Crookes becomes "Sir" at Q. Victoria's diamond jubilee.	[1875]	Bio
6. Socs	— Brit Med Soc announces new Brit Roentgen Soc (BRS).	[1896]	BMJ
	— Arch of Roent Ray takes over Arch of Clin Skiagraphy.	[1920]	ArRR
	— H. Roberts starts an X-Ray journal in St Louis.	[1918]	ArRR
	— B. Dardy starts Les Rayons X in Paris.	[1896]	ArRR
	— J. Gevennel starts an X-Ray journal in Hamburg.	[1896]	ArRR
	— H. Albers-Schönberg founds the largest and longest-lasting radiology J: Fortsch a d Geb d Roentgensthrahlen.	[1896]	FGR
	— W. Hedley makes first survey of medical use of X-ray.	[1951]	ArRR
	— J. Mackenzie-Davidson shows precise X-Ray localization.	[1896]	BMJ
	— 400 persons at inaugural meeting of Roentgen society (UK).		ArRR
	— S. Thompson (first pres BRS) describes Roentgen's discovery.	[1895]	ArRR
7. Event	— Z. von Mateuffel introduces rubber gloves in surgery.	[1907]	ZfC
	— W. Hedley writes first history of Roentgen rays.	[1951]	ArRR
	— J. Gardiner takes first X-Rays of reptiles and molluska.	[1876]	ArRR
	— R. Ross proves disease can be carried by a mosquito.	[1881]	DSB

Instruments, Units of Measurement, and Drugs			
8. Instr	— C.T.R. Wilson notes X-rays are detected in cloud chamber.	[1896]	PCPS
	— F. Braun develops a Cathode Ray Tube (CRT).	[1855]	DSB
	— J. Macintyre gathers X-Ray records for cinematography.	[1896]	ArS
9. Units	— E. Dorn measures first X-ray quantity (air thermometer).	[1881]	WAP
10. Concp	— D. Russell makes first (?) autoradiograms (metal plates).	[1859]	ArRR
11. Drugs	— Blaise & Sambue measure X-ray lethality on bacteria.	[1896]	GSR

Radioiodine, P-32, and Radioactive Therapy

12. I-Res —			
13. I-Dx —			
14. I-Rx —			
15. P-Rx —			
16. Tele —			
17. Other —	H. Gocht said to be first to try X-ray Rx of breast ca.	[1896]	FGR

Scans and Other Tests of Function in Various Organs

18. Brain —	P. Erlich notes IV dyes stain all organs except brain.	[1913]	Bio
19. Heart —	V. Eisenmenger studies congenital heart disease.	[1822]	CDD
—	W. Broadbent studies pericarditis.	[1755]	CDD
—	G. Stewart tries to measure cardiac output.	[1870]	JPh
20. Liver —	A. Buxbaum gets in vivo photo of gallbladder.	[1954]	WMP
—	W. Gilbert photographs biliary calculi with X-rays.	[1650]	CRS
21. Lung —	A. Crane gets skiagraphs of the lungs.	[1963]	PMJ
—	F. Williams describes use of X-Ray in thoracic disease.	[1896]	AJMS
22. Bone —			
23. Kidney—			
24. Gut —	D. Walsh: diarrhea & GI distress follow hi-dose X-ray.	[1958]	BMJ
—	C. Leonard introduces bismuth as opaque emulsion.	[1896]	JAMA
25. Blood —			
26. Other —	F. Clarke localizes foreign body in eye with X-Ray.	[1896]	AXJ
—	H. Hansell uses X-Rays in ophthalmic surgery.	[1896]	AJMS
—	J. Swain views calculi with X-Rays in Bristol.	[1896]	BMCJ

Radiation Hysteria and Health Physics * Obituaries *

27. Hyst —	C. Leonard says X-Rays will not add to phys diagnosis.	[1896]	JAMA
—	C. Leonard: burns are not due to X-rays, but to electricity;	[1898]	JAMA
	proof: cover skin with Al foil — stop most burns!	[1913]	JAMA
—	T. Gilchrist describes a case of X-ray dermatitis.	[1896]	JHHB
—	A. Kibbe: first microscopic exam of X-ray damaged skin.	[1896]	NYMJ
—	N. Scott describes X-ray injuries.	[1896]	AXJ
—	D. Walsh documents first radiation dermatitis patients; first mention of "radiation sickness."	[1896]	ArRR
—	N. Tesla says thin wire gauze protects skin from X-rays.	[1903]	ArRR
—	FB's (Illinois) leg is X-Rayed 3 × 40 min @ 5", gets ulcer, leads to amputation, sues, gets $10,000.	[1896]	AP
28. React —	First Radiation Protection Committee is formed by BRS.	[1942]	ArRR
29. Pespo —			

* * *

30. Obits

CHRONOLOGY OF NUCLEAR MEDICINE — 1898

Scientific and Technical Background

			Ref.
1. Basic	— W. Roentgen publishes his second paper.	[1896]	AnP
	— W. Wien proves canal rays deflected in magnetic field.	[1894]	VPG
	— E. Rutherford moves to Montreal as Prof Exper Physics.	[1895]	Eve
	— E. Rutherford detects °gas from thorium salts.	[1894]	TRSC
2. Obser	— P. Schutzenberger suggests an element's At Wt may vary.	(1929	JCE)
	— H. Rieder observes effect of X-rays on bacteria.	[1897]	MMW
	— R. Wolfender observes effect of X-rays on bacteria.	[1897]	La
3. # Nuc	— M. CURIE DISCOVERS POLONIUM (July) AND RADIUM (Dec).	[1896]	CRS
	— M. Curie says potassium salts are weakly radioactive.	[1936]	CRS
	— G. Schmidt: thorium salts and minerals are radioactive.	[1898]	WAP
	— M. Curie independently notes activity in thorium.	[1896]	Bio
	— W. Ramsay discovers Xe, Kr, Ne; Mendeleev adds new group.	[1894]	DSB
4. # Med	—		

Organizations and Internal Politics

5. Pols	—		
6. Socs	—		
7. Event	— J. Dewar makes liquid H, reaches temp of 14° K.	[1891]	DSB
	— M. Beijerinck discovers Tobac-Mosaic filterable virus.	[1937]	Sc
	— First photograph taken using artificial light.	[1895]	EB

Instruments, Units of Measurement, and Drugs

8. Instr	— J.J. Thomson devises parabolic photo record of "+" rays.	[1894]	Bio
	— W. Crookes tries Os, In, U, Pt, Th anticathode hard rays.	[1896]	ArRR
	— J. Mackenzie-Davidson sets up a stereoscopic system.	[1897]	BMJ
9. Units	—		
10. Concp	— W. Crookes calls low-energy rays "soft," high-energy "hard."		CN
11. Drugs	—		

Radioiodine, P-32, and Radioactive Therapy

12. I-Res —			
13. I-Dx —			
14. I-Rx —	Brit Pharmacopoeia includes extract of sheep thyr gland.	[1890]	CDD
15. P-Rx —			
16. Tele —			
17. Other —			

Scans and Other Tests of Function in Various Organs

18. Brain —	P. Rodet exposes 2 G-pig spines to ? dose, gets paraplegics.		PrM
19. Heart —	M. Levy-Dorn studies the heart with X-Rays.	[1897]	FGR
20. Liver —	J. Adami describes portal cirrhosis.	[1826]	BMJ
—	W. Osler describes cholelithiasis.	[1896]	La
—	P. Manson notes abscess of liver in "tropical disease".	[1894]	Bk
21. Lung —	J. Bergonie notes lung inflammation in exposed G-pigs (dose?).		AEM
22. Bone —			
23. Kidney —			
24. Gut —	W. Cannon feeds bismuth to a cat to observe GI motility.		AJPh
—	F. Williams repeats Cannon's Bi meal in humans.	[1920]	Bk
—	A. Benedict defines the limits of the gastric area.	[1897]	Med
25. Blood —			
26. Other —	G. de Takats describes Acute Pancreatic Necrosis.	[1889]	AnS

Radiation Hysteria and Health Physics * Obituaries *

27. Hyst —	C. Leonard says static elec not X-ray causes bio effect.	[1921]	NYMJ
—	E. THOMSON EXPOSES FINGER TO X-RAY, PROVES BIOLOGICAL EFFECT.		AXJ
—	W. Rollins burns from a vacuum tube not emitting light.	[1896]	ER
28. React —	Brit Roent Soc rad hazard sub-comm gives first report.	[1897]	ArRR
—	Little attention to hazard until death of Hall-Edwards.	[1906]	ArRR
—	G. Atkinson: irradiated algae grow faster than controls.	[1896]	Sc
29. Respo —			

* * *

30. Obits —	J. Newlands (1837–1898) Eng chem; law of octaves periodicity.		DSB

CHRONOLOGY OF NUCLEAR MEDICINE — 1899

			Ref.
	Scientific and Technical Background		
1. Basic	— E. RUTHERFORD DISCOVERS DECAY & INVENTS HALF-LIFE ($I_t = I_o e^{-\lambda t}$).		Eve
	— E. Rutherford discovers a gaseous emanation from thorium.	[1898]	Eve
	— E. Rutherford discovers and names alpha and beta rays.	[1900]	PM
	— Elster & Geitel first announce transmutation, ignored.	[1902]	AnP
	— S. Meyer says beta particle is an electron.	[1897]	PZ
	— P. Curie learns Becquerel's rays cause bio effects.	[1898]	CRS
2. Obser	— H. Becquerel recants: his rays are same as Roentgen's.	[1896]	CRS
	— W. Sutherland first uses the word "neutron" as a particle.	[1920]	DSB
	(N. Feather's history of "neutron" in Contemp Physics,	1960)	
	— 2 French minerol find U ore in Colorado: name carnotite.	[1789]	EB
	— J. Loeb stimulates parthenogenesis in sea urchins.	[1838]	DSB
3. # Nuc	— E. Rutherford announces "active deposits" of radium.	[1898]	Eve
	— A. Debierne discovers actinium (21.8y Ac-227).	[1898]	CRS
	— A. Debierne discovers Ac emanation (3.92s Rn-219).	[1898]	CRS
	— Elster & Geitel find °activity in lead (many doubt it).	[1897]	AnP
	— F. Giesel discovers a new radioactivity (5.0d Bi-210).	[1898]	AnP
4. # Med	—		
	Organizations and Internal Politics		
5. Pols	—		
6. Socs	— The Roentgen Society (London) has 140 + 5 Hon members.	[1897]	ArRR
	— D. Hilbert publishes "Foundations of Geometry."	[1889]	DSB
7. Event	— First use of X-Rays on battlefield in Boer war (portable ???).		ArRR
	Instruments, Units of Measurement, and Drugs		
8. Instr	— C. Townsend discovers the avalanche effect in gases.	[1928]	Eve
	— G. Girdwood devises a stereoskiagraph.	[1898]	AXJ
9. Units	—		
10. Concp	—		
11. Drugs	— E. Rutherford discovers "induced radiation" is a gas.	[1900]	TRSC

	Radioiodine, P-32, and Radioactive Therapy			
12. I-Res	—			
13. I-Dx	—			
14. I-Rx	—			
15. P-Rx	—			
16. Tele	—			
17. Other	— -	Southgate-Leigh describes a therapeutic X-ray effect.	[1896]	AXJ
	Scans and Other Tests of Function in Various Organs			
18. Brain	—	A. Church describes first cerebellar tumor seen on X-Ray.	[1949]	AJR
19. Heart	—	A. Gasmann reports rad effect on blood vessels (animals).	[1896]	FGR
	—	H. Huchard writes cardiol textbk, studies hypertension.	[1895]	Bk
20. Liver	—			
21. Lung	—	H. Rieder displays X-Rays of the chest.	[1897]	MMW
22. Bone	—			
23. Kidney	—			
24. Gut	—	E. Starling describes movements of small intestine.	[1898]	JPh
25. Blood	—	J. Haldane measures human blood vol by CO color change.	[1862]	JPh
26. Other	—	K. Grossmann locates foreign bodies in eye by X-Ray.	[1897]	GSR
	—	W. Price applies X-Rays to dentistry.	[1896]	AXJ
	Radiation Hysteria and Health Physics	* Obituaries *		
27. Hyst	—	F. Williams takes 3000 X-Rays at Boston City Hospital.	[1897]	JAMA
	—	Joachimsthal pitchblende used in uranium dyes to 1900.	[1882]	EB
28. React	—	F. Williams urges greater use of X-Rays in children.	[1897]	JAMA
29. Respo	—			

* * *

30. Obits	—	R. Bunsen (1811–1899) Ger chem; spectroscopy, lab burner.		DSB

CHRONOLOGY OF NUCLEAR MEDICINE — 1900

Scientific and Technical Background

			Ref.
1. Basic —	M. Planck derives formula for all black body rad, but IT REQUIRES ENERGY TRANSFER IN MULTIPLES OF "QUANTA."	[1897]	WoA
—	H. Lorentz equation verified: mass varies with velocity.	[1896]	DSB
—	E. Rutherford measures energy to produce an ion pair.	[1899]	PRS
2. Obser —	P. VILLARD SUGGESTS NON-DEVIABLE RAYS ARE HARDER THAN X.	[1899]	CRS
	(E. Rutherford calls them gamma rays.)	[1904]	Eve
—	K. Hofman thinks lead from pitchblende is radioactive.	[1899]	CB
—	J. Trowbridge says Ra emits rays with no loss of energy.	[1899]	JAMA
—	E. Rutherford's "Half Value Period" is accepted term for $T_{1/2}$.		
3. # Nuc —	F. Dorn discovers radium emanation, called niton (now Rn).	[1899]	ANG
—	W. Crookes discovers uranium X (24.1d Th-234).	[1913]	PRSI
—	5 radioactive substances (elements ?) known in nature.	[1979]	GSA
4. # Med —			

Organizations and Internal Politics

5. Pol —			
6. Socs —	First Int Cong of Med Electrology & Radiology in Paris.	[1925]	AEM
—	Roentgen Soc of US (later Am R Ray soc) meets in StL.	[1899]	JAMA
7. Event —	W. Rollins gives F. Williams (Harvard) 500 mg Ra therapy source.		GSR
—	F. Williams buys additional Ra for new Boston Clinic.	[1898]	Bio
—	N. Tesla promotes alt (ac) over direct (dc) current.	[1879]	DSB
—	Everything painted white, hospitals, bathrooms, kitchens, giving impression of being bacteriologically clean.	[1927]	AP

Instruments, Units of Measurement, and Drugs

8. Instr —	E. Thomson constructs device for stereoscopic X-Rays.	[1907]	ArRR
9. Units —	E. Rutherford uses bolometer to measure X-ray quantity.	[1897]	PRSI
10. Concp —	L. Weigel gives practical tips in using X-rays in med.	[1898]	PMJ
11. Drugs —			

Radioiodine, P-32, and Radioactive Therapy			
12. I-Res —			
13. I-Dx —			
14. I-Rx —	F. Williams does first X-ray therapy of exophthal goiter.	[1903]	Bk
15. P-Rx —			
16. Tele —			
17. Other —			
Scans and Other Tests of Function in Various Organs			
18. Brain —			
19. Heart —	G. Pagano describes the carotid sinus reflex.		Bk
20. Liver —	C. Beck detects calculi in liver and gallbladder.	[1896]	NYMJ
21. Lung —			
22. Bone —			
23. Kidney—			
24. Gut —	Barium mixed with refreshments at Rad Society (Lon) meeting to show involuntary intestinal movements by X-ray.	[1898]	ArRR
—	G. Holzknecht shows Dx of esophageal stenosis.	[1898]	DMW
25. Blood —			
26. Other —	E.Opie sees degenerate Islets of Langerhans in diabetes.	[1889]	CDD
Radiation Hysteria and Health Physics	* Obituaries *		
27. Hyst —	-. Walkoff gives first biol report on effects of radium.	[1896]	PoR
—	F. Giesel applies 200 mg Ra to skin and records results.		(Curie Bio)
—	Joachimsthal mined for radium content of pitchblende.	[1884]	EB
—	S. Freud replaces phrenology with a new "scientific" fraud; from "reading bumps" to "Interpretation of Dreams."	[1832]	Bk
28. React —	K. Wolfenden: lo-dose stimulates seed germination.	[1898]	ArRR
29. Respo —			

* * *

30. Obits —

CHRONOLOGY OF NUCLEAR MEDICINE — 1901

			Ref.
	Scientific and Technical Background		
1. Basic	— ELSTER & GEITEL DISCOVER BACKGROUND RADIATION IN ATMOSPHERE.		V105
	— W. Nernst discovers third law of thermodynamics.	[1900]	DSB
2. Obser	— Becquerel & Crookes argue about uranium regeneration.	[1902]	V96
	— P. Curie verifies Becquerel's Ra skin burn on his arm.	[1900]	DSB
	— K. Hofman says radium is the same as lead.	[1900]	CB
	— J. Perrin says radioactive change may be within the atom.	[1897]	RS
3. # Nuc	— R. Strutt (Rayleigh): Prout's hypothesis can't be chance.	[1887]	PM
	— F. Clarke remeasures many At Wts, supports Prout's idea.	[1887]	CN
	— E. Demarcay discovers europium.	[1898]	DoE
4. # Ned	—		
	Organizations and Internal Politics		
5. Pols	— Third CGPM recognizes and corrects its own mistake.	[1889]	NBS
6. Socs	— Nat Bureau of Standards (NBS) formed in US.	[1889]	NBS
	— F. Williams (Harvard): first textbk in clinical radiology.	[1897]	Bk
7. Event	— First Nobel prizes: W. Roentgen for X-rays.	[1895]	DSB
	E. von Behring for antitoxin.	[1892]	DSB
	— First submarine launched (British Navy).	[1954]	EB
	Instruments, Units of Measurement, and Drugs		
8. Instr	— Editorial: X-Ray equipment essential in every hospital.	[1897]	ArRR
9. Units	— Third CGPM says Kg measures mass, not weight;	[1889]	CGPM
	adopts "liter" (dm^3) as measure of fluid vol.	[1889]	NBS
	— P. Curie says Ra produces 140 cal/g per hour.	[1897]	Bio
10. Concp	— F. Dessauer begins depth dose measurements in water.	[1943]	FGR
11. Drugs	— J. Takamine isolates epinephrine, "adrenal" hormone (?).	[1902]	DSB
	— F. Zeit compares direct with ac currents on bacteria.	[1896]	JAMA
	— E. Aschkinass studies Becquerel ray effects on bacteria.	[1896]	PAP

Radioiodine, P-32, and Radioactive Therapy

12. I-Res —			
13. I-Dx —			
14. I-Rx —			
15. P-Rx —			
16. Tele —			
17. Other —	-. Danlos spreads Ra on metal disk, first Rx device.	[1899]	ADS
—	G. Phaler treats skin ca with remarkable success.	[1896]	AXJ

Scans and Other Tests of Function in Various Organs

18. Brain —	A. Froehlich describes pituitary lesion without acromeg.	[1886]	CDD
19. Heart —	L. Morquio describes congenital heart block.	[1888]	CDD
20. Liver —			
21. Lung —			
22. Bone —			
23. Kidney —			
24. Gut —	W. Bayliss studies small intestinal movements.	[1899]	JPh
25. Blood —			
26. Other —			

Radiation Hysteria and Health Physics * Obituaries *

27. Hyst —	H. Becquerel's Ra sample in vest pocket burns skin.	[1899]	CRS
—	Bar & Boule describe deaths from massive dose to fetus.	[1913]	RFC
—	W. Rollins notes lethal dose (in min exposure) to G-pig.	[1985]	BMJ
—	W. Rollins gives large dose and aborts a pregnant G-pig.	[1951]	BMJ
—	Lady sues Paris radiographer for burn, gets 5000 fr.	[1897]	La
28. React —			
29. Respo —			

* * *

30. Obits —	A. Fick (1829–1901) Ger physics, physiol; blood flow, dilution.	DSB
—	G. FitzGerald (1851–1901) Ir physics; light velocity constant.	DSB

CHRONOLOGY OF NUCLEAR MEDICINE — 1902

Scientific and Technical Background

			Ref.
1. Basic —	R. Abegg explains Kekule's bonds as electron transfer.	[1916]	DSB
—	E. Rutherford says radioactive decay is "Transmutation."	[1899]	JCS
	"NATURAL TRANSMUTATION" BEGINS A NEW ERA IN SCIENCE		
2. Obser —	F. Soddy: "transmutation," in 1902, was ultimate heresy.	(1932	Bk)
—	W. Nernst postulates neutrons and positive electrons.	[1920]	Bk
—	P. Lenard is first to see atom as mostly empty space.	[1911]	DSB
—	P. Lenard: + & − charges are evenly distributed in atom.	[1906]	DSB
—	P. Lenard begins study of photoelectric effect.	[1905]	DSB
—	M. Gardiner sees no evidence X-rays are wave phenomenon.	[1926]	ArRR
—	M. Curie says radium priced at 750,000 francs/gram.	[1824]	Bio
—	O. Heaviside observes a layering of the atmosphere.	[1882]	DSB
—	O. Richardson sees electrons emitted from hot bodies.	[1896]	PCPS
3. # Nuc —	F. Giesel discovers "emanium" (it's Debeirne's actinium).	[1899]	CB
—	W. Markwald separates Joachimsthal pitchblende "isotopes."	[1900]	DSB
—	E. Rutherford discovers thorium X (3.64d Ra-224), unannounced.		V95
—	E. Rutherford discovers active deposit (10.6h Pb-212).	[1898]	Eve
—	E. Rutherford discovers thorium C (1.0h Bi-212).	[1906]	Eve
—	E. Rutherford finds emanations are gases of noble class.	[1900]	Eve
4. # Med —			

Organizations and Internal Politics

5. Pols —			
6. Socs —	ICAW (Int Comm Atomic Weights) founded.	[1889]	ICAW
—	Second Int Cong of Med Electrol and Radiol meets in Berne.	[1900]	AEM
—	MDs form Electro Therap Soc (becomes sect of Roy Soc).	[1905]	GSR
—	F. Ostwald founds a journal on "Philosophy of Science."	[1883]	—
—	F. Williams textbook goes into second edition.	[1901]	Bk
7. Event —	G. Holzknecht's secret "chromoradiometer" makes enemies.	[1900]	GSR
—	A. Frieden notes first cancer caused by radiation (???).	[1901]	FGB

Instruments, Units of Measurement, and Drugs

8. Instr —	L. Benoist's "Radiochromator" for penetration of X-rays.	[1901]	CRS
—	R. Wayer develops a "Skiameter" to measure hardness.	[1901]	FGR
—	G. Holzknecht invents "secret" chromoradiometer.	[1900]	GSR
—	R. Zsigmondy builds an ultramicroscope (scattered light).	[1938]	DSB
—	A. Miethe invents the panchromatic plate.	[1889]	DSB
—	E. Caldwell has apparatus for small field localization.	[1896]	NYMJ
9. Units —	3H (Holzknecht units) = minimal skin reaction.	[1897]	CIER
—	G. Contremoulins suggests a stnd fluorescence intensity unit.		CRS
10. Concp —	Editorial says ca disappears after X-ray Rx of erysip.	[1900]	ArRR
—	W. Reed proves etiology of yellow fever.	[1876]	JH
11. Drugs —	C. Richet discovers anaphylaxis.	[1885]	DSB

Radioiodine, P-32, and Radioactive Therapy

12. I-Res —			
13. I-Dx —			
14. I-Rx —			
15. P-Rx —			
16. Tele —	Editorial says X-ray therapy still looks good after 5 years.		JAMA
—	Editorial: X-ray is only known Rx to cure some cancers.	[1897]	ArRR
17. Other —	W. Pussey: first to try deep X-ray therapy (Hodgkin's dis).	[1897]	JAMA
—	U. Portmann says first deep rad Rx by N. Senn in Chicago.	(1934	Rad)
—	F. Williams says no ca pt fails to benefit from X-ray.	[1897]	JAMA
—	F. Williams thinks rad causes prostatic hypertrophy.	[1900]	Bk
—	M. Sharpe cures skin tumors with fractionated lo-dose.	[1897]	ArRR
—	W. Coley compares effects on various sarcomas.	[1898]	NYMJ
—	W. Johnson promotes X-ray therapy of ca.	[1896]	AmM
—	A. Soiland treats case of breast ca with X-ray.	[1896]	GSR

Scans and Other Tests of Function in Various Organs

18. Brain —	H. Cushing studies the pituitary body.	[1901]	CDD
19. Heart —	J. Mackenzie writes "Studies of the Pulse."	[1899]	Bk
—	A. Carrel sutures small blood vessels end-to-end.	[1906]	DSB
—	W. Bayliss studies blood pressure effect on vessel wall.	[1899]	JPh
20. Liver —			
21. Lung —			
22. Bone —	T. Fletcher studies diet of 26 gout patients in USA.	[1876]	JAMA
23. Kidney —	E. Fenwick uses fluoroscopy during lithectomy.	[1897]	BMJ
—	G. von Illyes directs cathether under fluoroscope.	[1897]	GSR
24. Gut —	E. Starling: secretin influences pancreas — first "hormone."	[1900]	DSB
—	W. Cannon studies gut movements with X-Rays.	[1901]	AJPh
25. Blood —			
26. Other —	W. Bayliss gives mechanism of pancreatic "secretion."	[1896]	JPh

Radiation Hysteria and Health Physics * Obituaries *

27. Hyst —	W. Rollins first "tolerance" dose = "no fog on photoplate in 7 min." (estimated in 1930 to be about 10 to 20 r/day).	[1897]	BMSJ
—	C. Wilson discovers fresh fallen rain is radioactive.	[1901]	ArRR
28. React —	C. Hall-Edwards asks, how can we cure derelicts of surgeons?		ArRR
—	Editorial says value of X-ray Rx on proper pts unknown.	[1901]	ArRR
—	W. Scholtz says X-rays do not effect organs below skin.	[1901]	DMW
—	E. Codman studies all recorded accidental X-ray burns.	[1901]	PMJ
29. Respo —	Editorial: every new Rx agent since 1875 has been oversold, followed by reactionary disappointment.	[1771]	JAMA
—	M. Sharpe: Dermatitis not due to X-ray but to electricity; proof: Al filter in beam stops dermatitis.	[1896]	ArRR

* * *

30. Obits —	R. Virchow (1821–1902) Ger pathol; microscopy, cell theory.		DSB

CHRONOLOGY OF NUCLEAR MEDICINE — 1903

Scientific and Technical Background

			Ref.
1. Basic	— O. LODGE: ACCELER OF ELECTRON PRODUCES ELECTROMAG RAYS.	[1897]	WoA
	— E. Rutherford says Ra alphas show spectrum of helium.	[1895]	Eve
	— H. Nagaoka describes a "saturnian" atom of electrons.	[1890]	PM
	— P. Curie measures heat emitted from radium salts.	[1901]	CRS
	— J.J. Thomson says "X" are electromag waves & can scatter.	[1900]	Bk
	— W. Barkla approximates electrons/atom from scatter.	[1900]	PM
2. Obser	— D. Turner says radium rays may be seen by blind persons.	[1896]	BJN
	— Rayleigh says Prout's idea was too close to be random.	[1901]	PRSL
	— P. Villard's non-deviable rays called "gamma" by Rutherford.	[1900]	JCS
	— H. Albers-Schönberg discusses bioeffect on organs.	[1896]	MMW
	— H. Heineke experiments on bioeffect in animals.	[1896]	MMW
	— G. Bohn studies influence of radium rays on animals.	[1896]	CRS
3. # Nuc	— E. Rutherford DISCOVERS FIRST RADIUM A (3.05m Po-218). RADIUM B (26.8m Pb-214). RADIUM C (19.8m Bi-214).	[1902]	PM
	— H. Geiger discovers "E" rays; actinium A (0.002s Po-215).	[1899]	BDCG
	— A. Debierne says Giesel's emanium is his 1899 actinon.	[1902]	CRS

Organizations and Internal Politics

5. Pols	— Russ Social Dem Party splits into Mensheviks and Bolsheviks.		AP
6. Socs	— Third Int Congress of Electrology and Radiology meets.	[1902]	RITP
	— (H. McCoy describes his first 1903 work with °isotopes	in 1937.	BACS)
	— F. Williams third edition of 1901 textbook of radiology.	[1902]	Bk
	— W. Pusey writes textbook, "Practical Application of . . ."	[1901]	Bk
7. Event	— Editorial, The Times (4/17), first use, radioactive "hot."	[1901]	—
	— W. Crookes: RESEARCH IN SCIENCE HAS ONLY PROVISIONAL VALUE.		CN
	— U. of Aberdeen "Anatomy" has X-ray machine for teaching.	[1901]	ArRR
	— Royal Marsden sets up Radiol & Electrotherapy Dept.	[1951]	ArRR
	— Wright brothers make first airplane flight.	[1783]	EB
	— Nobel Prizes: H. Becquerel, P & M Curie, physics; S. Arrhenius, chemistry.	[1901]	AP

Instruments, Units of Measurement, and Drugs

8. Instr	— W. Crookes invents Zn Sulfide crystal "Spinthariscope."	[1875]	Na
	— B. Walter invents scale to measure "hardness" of X-rays.	[1902]	ArRR
	— Dr. Cotton exhibits cardboard X-Ray 3-D stereoscope.	[1900]	ArRR
	— R. Zsigmondy invents an ultra-microscope.	[1942]	DSB
	— W. Hardy notes light & rad release I in iodo-chloroform.	[1961]	Na
	— Holzknecht's dosimeter secret is I color reaction.	[1902]	
	— G. Holzknecht: "Chromo-radiometer" measures X-ray quantity only, not "quality."	[1902]	RITP
	— W. Einthoven invents string galvanometer, see Heart.		CDD
9. Units	— 12 tone color scale reads in "H-units" (Holzknecht).	[1902]	RITP
	— C. Guillaume notes diff "cc & ml"; CGPM requires "ml."	[1901]	DSB
10. Concp	— F. Dessauer describes need for "depth dose" measurement.	[1901]	MMW
	— G. Schwartz irradiates chicken eggs for Doctoral Thesis.	[1905]	APh
	— W. Rollins says X-rays spread in spherical waves.	[1901]	BMSJ
11. Drugs	— S. Tracy detects radioactivity in waters of health spas.	[1901]	MRNY

Radioiodine, P-32, and Radioactive Therapy			
12. I-Res —			
13. I-Dx —			
14. I-Rx —			
15. P-Rx —			
16. Tele —			
17. Other —	F. Soddy advises breathing Ra or Th emanation for "phthisis."		ArRR
—	Alx Gra Bell suggests implanting Ra glass tubes for Rx.	[1900]	AM
—	E. Grubbe says he treats epitheliomas with success.	[1896]	TARR
—	W. Morton treats uterine fibroid with X-rays.	[1900]	NYMR
—	H. Robarts treats prostatic disease with X-rays.	[1900]	AXJ
—	C. Skinner attempts really deep abdominal therapy.	[1902]	TARR
—	R. Pfeiffee attempts therapy in bacterial diseases.	[1902]	BKW
Scans and Other Tests of Function in Various Organs			
18. Brain —	H. Pancoast displays skiagraph that shows brain lesion.	[1899]	GSR
19. Heart —	W. Einthoven invents string galvanometer, measures elec.	[1872]	DSB
—	W. Einthoven also introduces phonocardiography.	[1902]	Bk
—	E. Hering records auricular fibrillation on kymograph.	[1847]	CDD
—	K. Wenckebach introduces quinidine for Rx.	[1749]	CDD
20. Liver —			
21. Lung —	H. Hulst shows skiagrams of the chest.	[1900]	TARR
22. Bone —	W. Haughton shows structure of bone with X-Rays.	[1941]	ArRR
23. Kidney—	A. Baclére makes stereoscopic study of urinary calculi.	[1902]	LPMc
24. Gut —	K. Lennander writes "Sensibility of Abdominal Cavity."	[1896]	Bk
25. Blood —	E. London is first to note effect of X-rays on blood.	[1905]	BKW
—	O. Stiles shows prevalence & distribution of hookworm.	[1902]	PHR
26. Other —	USPHS describes Rocky Mountain spotted (tick) fever.	[1876]	PHR
Radiation Hysteria and Health Physics	* Obituaries *		
27. Hyst —	Editorial: The Times (4/17) suggests Ra street lighting.	[1900]	—
—	T. Edison uses 1/2" lead shield after asst's arm amputated.	[1898]	EM
—	H. Albers-Schönberg: sterility in rabbit after X-ray,	[1964]	
	aspermia after about 30% erythema dose.	[1946]	MMW
—	H. Heinke irradiates thymus gland in young rabbits.	[1968]	APe
—	F. Soddy says "no toxic action" from breathing Rn or Tn.	[1907]	ArRR
—	A. Frieden notes azoospermia after radium Rx.	[1900]	MMW
—	J. Danysz implants Ra in scalp (mice), sick in 3h, death in 12h.		CRB
—	R. Blondlot describes a new kind of light: "N" rays.	[1904]	JdP
	(This top-rank physicist must be taken seriously.)		
—	Britain sets motorcar speed limit at 20 miles/hour.	[1902]	AP
28. React —			
29. Respo —			

* * *

30. Obits —

CHRONOLOGY OF NUCLEAR MEDICINE — 1904

Scientific and Technical Background

			Ref.
1. Basic	— W. Bragg describes range of alphas in "Bragg peak."	[1899]	PM
	— B. Boltwood finds Rn/U (and Po/U ?) constant in all U ores.		EMJ
	— J.J. Thomson studies interact of electricity and matter.	[1902]	Bk
	— G. Barkla proves X-rays are transverse (light) waves.	[1903]	DSB
	— A. Eve studies coefficient of absorp of X and gammas.	[1902]	PM
	— BERGONIE AND TRIBONDEAU "LAW" SAYS IMMATURE CELLS SENSITIVE.		CRB
2. Obser	— G. Hofmann notes that lead has a "number of °activities."	[1901]	AdP
	— B. Boltwood says "°elements" must find place on Periodic Table.		LRB
	°ACTIVITIES OCCUR IN PARENT-TO-DAUGHTER CHAINS	[1903]	LRB
	— J. Hall-Edwards sees no proof of X-ray caused bio effect.		ArRR
	(Dead 2 years later from exposure to unproved effect.)	[1906]	ArRR
3. # Nuc	— A. Debierne discovers actinium B (36.1m Pb-211).	[1899]	V97
	— S. Meyer discovers radium E (5.0d Bi-210).	[1903]	V97
	— B. Hoffman discovers radiolead (22.3y Pb-210).	[1899]	V97
	— F. Giesel (also T. Golewski) discovers Ac-X (11.4d Ra-223).		V97
	— H. Brooks discovers actinium C (2.13m Bi-211).	[1899]	V97
	— H. Brooks says "active deposits" are radium A, -B, -C.	[1903]	Na
	— E. Rutherford notes "active deposits thorium" A, -B, -C.	[1846]	PM
	— 20 radioactive species have been found in nature.	[1900]	GSA
4. # Med	—		

Organizations and Internal Politics

5. Pols	— Russo-Japanese war begins Japan's rise to industrialism.		EB
6. Socs	— Third Int Cong of Med Electricity & Radiology in Milano.	[1902]	ArRR
	— J of Roent Soc is established, specs in radiol physics.	[1924]	BJR
	— A. Soiland sets up Radiol Dept at U Southern California.	[1903]	USC
	— E. Rutherford's "Radio-activity," first ed, published.	[1900]	Bk
	— H. Heineke publishes monograph on path of rad effects.	[1902]	MMW
	— Holtzknecht & Kienbock plea: recognize radiol as new science.		WKW
	— E. Caldwell pubs textbk, "Roent Ray in Therapeutics . . ."	[1903]	Bk
	— W. Rollins publishes "Notes on X-light."	[1896]	Bk
	— C. Allen (dermatology) pubs "Radiotherapy & Photother."	[1903]	Bk
7. Event	— T. Holland says chest X-Ray has replaced stethescope.	[1816]	ArRR
	— M. Curie graduates PhD from Sorbonne, gets Nobel prize.	[1898]	Bio
	— R. Abbe buys first US Ra from Curie, 150 mg — 300 K units.	[1901]	ASAT
	— E. Rutherford gives his first Bakerian lecture to Roy Soc.	[1919]	Eve

Instruments, Units of Measurement, and Drugs

8. Instr	— W. Crookes' scintill crystal is primary counting device.	[1903]	CN
	— J. Elster devises first practical photoelectric cell.	[1901]	DSB
	— J. Flemming uses thermionic tube to generate radio waves.		DSB
9. Units	— G. Holzknecht: first clin dosimeter, "Chromoradiometer."	[1902]	ArRR
	— J. Hall-Edwards says there is no measure of rad dose.	[1903]	ArRR
	— Sabouraud-Noire pastilles introduce clinical dosimetry.	[1902]	LPM
	— L. Freund invents iodo-chloroform solution color change.	[1903]	WKW
	— C. Guillaume finds 1 kg water fills 1000.028 cc volume,	[1903]	DSB
	HENCE, WE MUST USE ml, NOT cc, FOR LIQUID VOLUME.	[1903]	DSB
	— W. Keen finds 2 mm (?) of German Ra = 1,800,000 Uranies.	[1903]	ASAT
10. Concp	— G. Perthes uses "depth dose" for skin-sparing filtration.	[1901]	FGR
	— L. Freund: iodoform-chloroform turns red upon exposure.	[1903]	WKW
	— G. Perthes studies meaning of tissue X-ray transparency.	[1903]	FGB
11. Drugs	—		

Radioiodine, P-32, and Radioactive Therapy

12. I-Res —			
13. I-Dx —			
14. I-Rx —	R. ABBE CURES FIRST EXOPHTH GOITER PATIENT WITH Ra TUBE.	[1900]	ASAT
—	C. Mayo describes thyroidectomy for exophthalmic goiter.	[1923]	MR
15. P-Rx —			
16. Tele —			
17. Other —	H. Doninici first to use metal tubes filled with radium.	[1901]	GSR
—	A. Hock succeeds Rx of prostatic hypertrophy with X-ray.	[1902]	PMW
—	R. Abbe describes his first use of 300,000 units of French Ra.		ASAT
—	W. Keen treats 22 with German Ra, gets only pain relief.	[1902]	ASAT
—	R. Abbe replies: French Ra better than German Ra.		ASAT
—	H. Brauth has success in treating epilepsy with X-rays.	[1903]	PMJ
—	C. Brown cures (symptomatically) a case of leukemia.	[1901]	JAMA
—	B. Bryant treats 2 case of splenomedullary leukemia.	[1902]	MR
—	G. Dock discusses treatment of leukemia with X-rays.	[1902]	AM
—	11 authors (e.g., L. Grosh) treat leukemia with X-rays.	[1902]	JAMA
—	K.Strassmann uses radium emanation in Rx of skin dis.	[1903]	ADS

Scans and Other Tests of Function in Various Organs

18. Brain —			
19. Heart —	L. Aschoff studies Aschoff nodules, myocarditis.	[1840]	CDD
20. Liver —	M. Seldin finds liver has low sensitivity to X-rays.	[1900]	FGR
21. Lung —	T. Holland says X-Rays must be used for Dx of TBC.	[1898]	ArRR
—	D. King evaluates X-Ray Dx in bronchiectasis.	[1902]	GSR
22. Bone —	P. Hickey studies development of skeleton in children.	[1896]	TARR
23. Kidney—	J. Donath discovers paroxysmal hemoglobinuria.	[1849]	MMW
—	B. Klose outlines renal pelvis on X-Ray with bismuth.	[1900]	DZC
24. Gut —	T. Elliot studies anti-peristalsis in human colon.	[1901]	JPh
—	J. Murphy describes 2000 appendectomies.	[1554]	AJMS
25. Blood —	W. Osler describes chronic cyanotic erythremia (PVA).	[1951]	BMJ
26. Other —	H. Heineke is first to note rad effect on thymus & spleen.	[1903]	MW
—	W. Freudenthal reports larynx irritation after hi-dose.	[1919]	AEM
—	W. Sweet locates foreign bodies with X-rays.	[1901]	TARR

Radiation Hysteria and Health Physics * Obituaries *

27. Hyst —	P. Gilman is first to note hi-dose rad effects on embryos.	[1951]	AJPh
—	G. Baermann produces albuminuria in irrad of G-pigs.	[1951]	MMW
—	R. Milohner: RBC most sensitive of marrow cells (rabbits).	[1903]	BAW
—	G. Holzknecht estimates his life-dose exposure @ 8000H.	[1902]	WKW
—	NY police arrest woman for smoking cigarette in public.	[1964]	AP
28. React —	M. KOERNICKE NOTES LO-DOSE STIM, HI-DOSE DEPRESS PLANTS.	[1900]	BDB
—	R. Wood discredits Blondlot "N" rays before media go mad.	[1903]	SA
29. Respo —			

* * *

30. Obits —	C. Winkler (1838–1904) Ger chem; discovered germanium.	DoE
	E. Demarcay (1852–1904) Fr chem; discovered europium.	DSB

CHRONOLOGY OF NUCLEAR MEDICINE — 1905

Scientific and Technical Background

			Ref.
1. Basic	— A. Einstein publishes special theory of relativity.	[1902]	WoA
	— Bacteria "cause" disease IF "Koch's postulates" occur: THE ONLY ACCEPTABLE "PROOF" OF "CAUSE" IN SCIENCE	[1876]	Bio
	— F. von Lerch: transmutation to more electroneg daughter.	[1913]	JaR
	— H. Nernst says entropy approaches "0" at absolute 0°temp.	[1849]	DSB
	— M. Wind measures wavelength of X-rays @ 1/10,000 vis light.		ArRR
	— C. Barkla tries to polarize roentgen radiation.	[1906]	PRSL
	— B. Walter explains Roentgen's law of absorption.	[1895]	FGB
2. Obser	— B. Boltwood hints at 3 natural decay chains: Ac, U, Th:	[1904]	AJS
	— B. Boltwood 22 world wide U samples show U is parent of Ra.	[1904]	PM
	— B. Boltwood cannot find RaTh in thorianite (see Hahn).	[1905]	LRB
	— W. Duane finds radium emanation ionizes air.	[1896]	CRS
	— F. Soddy gets 1.5×10^{-9}g Ra from 1 kg U after 30 months decay.		Na
	— H. Bordier observe action of X-rays on platino-cyanure.	[1895]	AEM
	— L. Halberstadter observes action of X-rays on ovary.	[1904]	BKW
	— P. Bridgmann fails to achieve a moderate high pressure.	[1915]	DSB
3. # Nuc	— J.J. Thomson discovers: alkali metals (K) emit electrons.	[1906]	PM
	— O. HAHN DISCOVERS RaTh (1.9Y Th-228) HAS Th CHEMISTRY.	[1913]	PM
	— Rutherford and Boltwood cannot believe RaTh exists.	[1903]	LRB
	— T. Godlewski discovers Ac X (11.4d Ra-223), analog of UX.	[1899]	Na
	— E. Rutherford extends radium decay chain, RaA...to...RaF.	[1904]	Na
	— J. Slater separates pure Thorium C (now 1.1h Bi-212).	[1904]	DoE

Organizations and Internal Politics

5. Pols	— First (& last) meet of Int Cong for Study of Rad & Ion (Liege): purpose was to emphasize natural bkgd rad,	[1978]	ArRR
	ask for preservation of pitchblende supplies.	[1898]	ArRR
	— Berlin Roentgen Congress celebrates X-ray's 10th anniversary: Walther (Ger) criticizes lack of dose measure. Kienbock (Ger) says measurement in every pt required. Holthusen (Ger) explains different ways to measure dose. Kowalski (Den) proposes some std unit be adopted. Beclere (Fr), Leonard (Am), Salmonson (Fr), agree with Butcher (Eng) that measurement of dose is primitive.	[1896]	ArRR
6. Socs	— Philadel Roent Ray Soc organized for "good fellowship."	[1900]	AJR
	— Deutsche Roentgen Gesllschaft organized in Berlin; publishes Verhandlungen der Dtch Roent Ges.	[1898]	VDRG
7. Event	— Lise Meitner is second woman to get PhD from U of Vienna.	[1904]	Bio
	— Ernst Mach believes atoms after viewing spinthariscope.	[1903]	DSB
	— B. BOLTWOOD WORKS OUT RADIOACTIVE DATING TECHNIQUE.	[1945]	LRB
	— A. Soiland purchases radium for Los Angeles Rx center.	[1904]	V109
	— First neon signs made (Geissler tubes).	[1855]	EB
	— G. Kunz gets U.S. patent for Ra dial "cold light" paint.	[1977]	FR

Instruments, Units of Measurement, and Drugs

8. Instr	— P. Villard measures penetration with "Radiosclerometer."	[1902]	ArRR
	— J.J. Thomson adapts Wien's parabolas to measure + rays.	[1894]	Bio
	— H. Piffard builds a "safety tube" out of leaded glass.	[1896]	NYMJ

9. Units	— R. Kienbock proposes paper AgBr strips for dosimetry.	[1904]	FGR
	— P. Villard says quantity unit must be in c.g.s. system.	[1903]	ArRR
	— Angstrom unit of length adopted by special comm.	[1889]	Sc
10. Concp	— W. DUANE DISCOVERS THAT IONS FROM MEASURING-CHAMBER WALL DISTORT ION MEASUREMENT.		JdP
	(Duane biog, del Regato.	1978	IJO)
	— F. Dessauer makes first "depth dose" measurements in H_2O.	[1903]	AG
	— A. Einstein says Rieman's geometry better than Euclid's.	[1854]	Bio

Radioiodine, P-32, and Radioactive Therapy

12. I-Res	—		
13. I-Dx	—		
14. I-Rx	—		
16. Tele	— F. Dessauer: first paper on homogenous rad Rx fields.	[1903]	MK
17. Other	— C. Luraschi reports X-ray Rx of enlarged prostate.	[1904]	ArRR
	— W. Coley tries radiotherapy of cancers and sarcoma.	[1902]	AnS
	— F. Williams notes good effects on enlarged prostate.	[1903]	BMSJ

Scans and Other Tests of Function in Various Organs

18. Brain	—		
19. Heart	— N. Korotkov explains auscultation.	[1816]	Bk
	— N. Korotkov measures peripheral diastolic blood pressure.	[1896]	Bk
	— P. Grocco explains value of cardiac percussion method.	[1761]	Bk
	— F. Bleichroder passes ureteric catheter into heart.	(1912	BKW)
20. Liver	— H. Christian describes the fatty liver.	[1978]	JHHB
21. Lung	— K. Quadrons sees inflammation after rad Rx for leukemia.	[1898]	ZIM
22. Bone	—		
23. Kidney	—		
24. Gut	— J. Edkin finds chemical mechanism for gastric secretion.	[1902]	AJDD
	— H. Hulst examines the stomach & intestines with X-Rays.	[1904]	TARR
	— H. Rieder examines stomach and intestines with X-Rays.	[1904]	FGR
25. Blood	— G. Schwarz studies rad effects on rabbit blood cells.	[1903]	WKW
	— G. Schwarz confirms leukocytosis shortly after hi-dose.	[1903]	WKW
26. Other	—		

Radiation Hysteria and Health Physics * Obituaries *

27. Hyst	— M. Franklin says Dx X-ray burns are truly alarming.	[1897]	ArRR
	— L. Halbersen irradiates ovaries (mice), sees no damage.	[1902]	BKW
	— L. Philipp sees azoospermia in 2 pts after rad Rx.	[1824]	FGR
	— T. Brown notes azoospermia in 18 workers after irrad.	[1903]	AJSr
	— San Francisco earthquake kills 700 persons.	[1906]	EB
28. React	— H. Heinke: first descrip of Acute Rad Syndrome (rabbits).	[1959]	MCJ
	— H. Heinke notes leukopenia, spleen, sensitive thymus.	[1903]	MCJ

29. Respo —

* * *

30. Obits —

CHRONOLOGY OF NUCLEAR MEDICINE — 1906

	Scientific and Technical Background		Ref.
1. Basic —	G. Barkla discovers X-rays can be polarized.	[1904]	PRSL
—	H. Nernst discovers the third law of thermodynamics.	[2850]	DSB
—	C. Regaud reports mitosis (sperm) is most rad sensitive.	[1903]	CRB
—	Bergonie & Tribondeau implicate rate of cell division.	[1905]	CRB
2. Obser —	R. Lucas says transmutation to more electroneg daughter.	[1905]	PZ
—	O. Hahn says RaAc (Th-227) chemically like RaTh (Th-228).	[1905]	PM
—	E. Rutherford describes "isobars," same mass, diff chem.	[1918]	Bk
—	J.J. Thomson's H atom has 1 electron and large + mass.	[1902]	Bio
—	G. Barkla describes K & L X-rays (limits of resolution).	[1904]	DSB
3. # Nuc —	B. Boltwood discovers "ionium" (Th-230 as parent of Ra).	[1905]	AJS
—	O. Hahn discovers Th C (later C′ is 3×10^{-7}s Po-212).	[1905]	PM
—	O. Hahn discovers RaAc (18.2d Th-227) between Ac and AcX.	[1905]	Bio
—	N. Campbell discovers that potassium is radioactive.	[1901]	PCPS
4. # Med —			

	Organizations and Internal Politics		
5. Pols —	U.S. Pure Food and Drug Act passed by Congress.	[1985]	FR
6. Socs —	Fourth Int Cong of Med Electr & Radiol meets in Amsterdam.	[1904]	ArRR
—	H. Klickstein reviews P. Curie's science achievements	(in 1947	SA)
—	Am Roent Ray Soc establishes Am Quarterly of Roent.	[1913]	AJR
7. Event —	A. Carrel succeeds in transplanting organs.	[1902]	Bio
—	R. Harrison grows frogs nerve, in vitro tissue culture.	[1938]	DSB
—	Nobel Prize (Chem) goes to Moissan not to Mendeleev.	[1921]	—

	Instruments, Units of Measurement, and Drugs		
8. Instr —	O. Hahn uses Rutherford's home-made tobacco can instr.	[1905]	Bio
—	L. DeForest describes a triode radio wave amplifier.	[1895]	DSB
—	D. Gramegna copies Crookes' 1875 radiometer to measure X-rays.		ArRR
—	G. Pfahler installs a "roentgen filter" to increase keV.	[1903]	TARR
—	M. Tsvett invents chromatography (color writing).	[1926]	SN
9. Units —	H. McCoy devises a °activity standard: 1 g pure uranium.	[1903]	PM
10. Concp —	B. Lepine: production up of some chemicals after irrad.	[1900]	CRB
—	C. von Pirquet coins "allergy" in medical use.		CDD
—	C. Regaud suggests a "latent period" in bioeffects.	[1904]	BANM
11. Drugs —	E. Paschen reviews agents in vaccination therapy.	[1902]	MMW

Radioiodine, P-32, and Radioactive Therapy

12.	I-Res	— G. Dock observes exophthalmic goiter.	[1904]	AM
13.	I-Dx	—		
14.	I-Rx	— C. Pfeiffer reports X-ray Rx of goiter has no effect.	[1904]	BKC
15.	P-Rx	—		
16.	Tele	—		
17.	Other	— J. Ewing studies rad effects in infec lympho sarc (dogs).	[1905]	JMR
		— E. Eitner pleads for increased iodoform dosimetry use.	[1903]	ArRR
		— R. Kienbock pushes quantimetric Ag paper strip dose.	[1905]	ArRR
		— H. Pancost discusses roentgen therapy of blood disease.	[1905]	QAR
		— P. Oudin describes use of radium in gynecology.	[1904]	CRS

Scans and Other Tests of Function in Various Organs

18.	Brain	— C. Sherrington develops a theory of reflex action.	[1894]	DSB
19.	Heart	— A. Fraenkel gives first IV strophanthin for conges fail.	[1903]	CDD
20.	Liver	— R. Werner describes liver changes after radium implants.	[1904]	BKC
		— C. Holland radiographs a case of gallstones.	[1904]	ArRR
21.	Lung	— H. Anders sees a pulmonary abscess spontaneous resolve.	[1901]	IC
		— G. Pfahler discusses Roentgen Dx of the lungs.	[1905]	JAMA
22.	Bone	— G. Rankin describes achondroplasia.	[1902]	BMJ
23.	Kidney	— J. Volker studies pyelography with radiopaque collargol.	[1904]	MMW
24.	Gut	— P. Krause notes severe GI effects after hi-dose to mice.	[1951]	BKW
		— P. Krause effects noted to as low as 0.1 erythema dose.	[1905]	FGR
		— E. Starling reviews physiology of digestion.	[1896]	Bk
		— G. Holzknecht studies many X-Rays of the stomach.	[1905]	BKW
25.	Blood	— G. SCHWARZ: LOW RADIATION DOSE STIMULATES WBC PRODUCTION.	[1905]	WKW
		— G. Schwarz finds hi-radiation dose depresses WBC counts.	[1959]	WKW
		— A. Warthin notes decreased blood cells after rad expos.	[1903]	IC
		— A. Wasserman introd complement fixation test for syph.	[1876]	Bk
26.	Other	— F. Hopkins discovers and names "Deficiency Diseases."	[1896]	JAMA
		— C. Bowen has new tech to localize foreign body in eye.	[1904]	AQR
		— E. Caldwell uses skiagraphy in Dx of accessory sinuses.	[1905]	TARR
		— G. Pfahler measures the pelvic diameters of women.	[1903]	AQR

Radiation Hysteria and Health Physics * Obituaries *

27.	Hyst	— O. Hahn notes first rad contamination in Rutherford lab.	[1942]	Bio
		— P. Krause: rad is lethal when Malpighian bodies killed.	[1905]	FGR
		— D. Recamier reports that hi-dose retards growth of teeth.		AEM
		— W. Wills treats acne successfully with X-ray.	[1903]	ArRR
		— W. Wills says he would like method to measure X-rays.	[1905]	ArRR
28.	React	— C. Regaud notes recovery from azoospermia in low doses.	[1905]	CRS
29.	Respo	—		

* * *

30.	Obits	— S. Langley (1834–1906) Am astron; bolometer.		DSB
		— P. Curie (1859–1906) Fr physics; piezo-elec, radioactivity.		DSB

CHRONOLOGY OF NUCLEAR MEDICINE — 1907

Scientific and Technical Background

			Ref.
1. Basic	— T. Morgan discovers the fruit fly, invents exp genetics.	[1860]	Bio
	— H. Minkowski's physics requires a 4-D Space-Time.	[1916]	WoA
	— C. Barkla measures secondaries and At Wt of nickel.	[1905]	PM
2. Obser	— E. Rutherford questions radon growth from actinium.	[1905]	LRB
	— B. Boltwood says Th & RaTh are chemically similar,	[1903]	AJS
	and ThX and MsTh-1 are also similar.	[1905]	AJS
	— B. Boltwood proves RaG is stable lead.	[1903]	AJS
	— B. Boltwood calculates age of earth's crust from °activity.	[1950]	LRB
	— H. McCoy, after 200 ppts, cannot separate Th from RaTh.	[1903]	JACS
	— O. Hahn cannot separate MsTh-1 from Ra.	[1905]	PZ
	— T. Richards asks "are Atomic Weights really variable"?	[1885]	SC
	— J. Crowther: gases exposed to X-rays emit secondaries.	[1903]	PM
3. # Nuc	— B. Boltwood reports ionium (80,000y Th-230) parent of Ra.	[1906]	Na
	— O. Hahn discovers mesothorium-1 then MsTh-2.	[1905]	BDCG
	— G. Urbain discovers lutetium (Lu #71).	[1906]	DSB
4. # Med	—		

Organizations and Internal Politics

5. Pols	— Sociétté de Radiologie de Paris established.	[1912]	ArRR
6. Socs	— L. Jones writes "Medical Electricity" handbk of Rx tech.	[1906]	BMJ
7. Event	— E. Rutherford arrives at Manchester.	[1886]	Eve
	— R. Kienbock: 1899–1905 erythemas caused by "no dosimeter."	[1897]	ArRR
	— R. Harrison develops tissue culture techniques.	[1906]	DSB

Instruments, Units of Measurement, and Drugs

8. Instr	— E. Rutherford counts alphas with Crookes' ZnS crystal.	[1904]	PRS
	— P. Snook invents an interruptionless transformer for X-rays.		AJR
	— R. Koehler invents X-Ray cinematography for lung motion.	[1896]	ArRR
	— L. Luminére invents 3-color photography.	[1894]	DSB
9. Units	— H. Bordier: Rx beam penetration changes with field size.	[1905]	ArRR
	— G. Graham measures "Uranies" with gold leaf electroscope:	[1906]	GSR
	unit is amount of activity in unit mass of U.	[1906]	ArRR
	— R. Kienbock says X-ray tubes require a biologic unit.	[1904]	ArRR
	— W. Salomonson summarizes 12 units of X-ray "intensity."	[1905]	ArRR
	— G. Schwarz proposes calomel (HgCl) ppt for dosimeter.	[1904]	FGR
	— C. Phillips describes many methods to measure dose, but NO SATISFACTORY UNIT MEASURES "QUANTITY."	[1904]	ArRR
	— H. Guilleminot designs new "quantitometer" for X-rays.	[1904]	CRS
	— M. Kassabian summarizes radiometric dosimetry.	[1906]	QAR
	— C. Phillips attempts limited standardization of measures.	[1906]	QAR
10. Concp	— W.H. Bragg: secondary electrons, not gamma, make most ions.	[1906]	PM
	— G. Graham says alpha rays, not betas, are bactericidal.	[1904]	ArRR
	— G. Graham says beta rays inhibit the growth of bacteria.	[1903]	ArRR
	— P. Ehrlich finds Typan Red a "tag" and an Rx agent.	[1884]	DSB
11. Drugs	— E. Fischer proves proteins are amino acid chains.	[1934]	DSB

Radioiodine, P-32, and Radioactive Therapy

12. I-Res — D. MARINE SAYS IODINE NECESSARY FOR NORMAL THYROID FUNCTION. [1896] JHHB
— D. Marine finds iodine deficiency in goitrous sheep. [1898] AnIM
13. I-Dx —
14. I-Rx — D. Marine says dessic thyroid made from goitrous glands. [1898] AnIM
15. P-Rx —
16. Tele —
17. Other — H. Dominici shields out necrosis causing beta rays. [1904] CFM
— G. Graham reports cures of many diseases with radium. [1902] ArRR
— H. Bordier says deep Rx "illusory," X-rays too shallow. [1902] ArRR
— A. Gray treats bladder malignancy thru sup-pub incision. [1904] QAR
— A. Stengel attempts new and rational Rx of leukemia. [1905] TARR

Scans and Other Tests of Function in Various Organs

18. Brain — I. Pavlov studies conditioned reflexes in dogs. [1906] DSB
19. Heart — A. Keith describes the S-A node. [1893] JAP
— A. Sahli puts sphymobolometry (pulse records) in Phys Dx. [1872] Bk
20. Liver —
21. Lung — L. Cole plans for early Dx of tuberculosis. [1904] TARR
22. Bone — F. Nichols describes "arthritis deformans." [1903] JMR
23. Kidney — A. Warthin notes urea after ARS leukocyte destruction. [1904] AQR
24. Gut — C. Herter describes bacterial infections of intestine. [1904] Bk
— S. Melter studies causes of "peristaltic rush." [1904] AJPh
— R. Chitenden pubs "Physiological Economy in Nutrition." [1906] Bk
— G. Pfahler explores the alimentary tract with X-Rays. [1906] JAMA
25. Blood —
26. Other —

Radiation Hysteria and Health Physics * Obituaries *

27. Hyst — Editorial: Radiotherapists overstate their results. [1902] BMJ
— J. Cinzet sees slow breast develop after animal irrad. [1924] CRB
— R. Kienbock treats "burns" with lunar caustic and ointments. Safe exposure is 18min @ 6", or 72min @ 12". [1902] ArRR
but is highly variable. [1905] ArRR
— G. Graham finds Ra salts vary in popular health spas: Bath, Bad Gastein, Plombieres, are highly radioactive. [1905] ArRR
— C. Bardeen irrad toad sperm, gets abnormal fertilized ova. [1903] JEZ
28. React — C. Leonard pleads to enclose X-ray tube in lead box. [1903] NYMJ
— F. Dessauer suggests leaded aprons, gloves and shields; [1903] MMW
and limit fields of irrad. [1901] MMW
29. Respo — W. Salant studies radium excretion. [1939] AJPh
THIS MAY BE THE FIRST RADIUM METABOLISM ARTICLE

* * *

30. Obits — D. Mendeleev (1824–1907) Rus chem; Periodic Table of Elements. DSB
— W. Thomson (1824–1907) Eng math physics; energy. DSB
— F. Moissan (1852–1907) Fr chem; discovered fluorine. DSB

CHRONOLOGY OF NUCLEAR MEDICINE — 1908

		Scientific and Technical Background		Ref.
1. Basic	—	E. RUTHERFORD PROVES THAT ALPHA PARTICLE IS HELIUM ATOM.	[1903]	PM
	—	E. Rutherford measures unit + charge at 4.65×10^{-10} esu (now 4.77).	[1897]	Eve
	—	J. Dewar finds 1g Ra (equlib) produces 5.32 cc helium/s.	[1903]	Eve
	—	J. Dewar calculates 1g Ra contains 3600 horsepower-hours work.		Eve
	—	R. Kleeman finds 3 types of scattered secondary rays.	[1903]	PM
2. Obser	—	B. Boltwood says U cannot be split into 2 kinds by chem.	[1905]	LRB
	—	B. Boltwood cannot separate ionium from thorium chemically.	[1907]	AJS
	—	B. Boltwood finds ionium parent (2.5×10^5y U-234) 0.057% of U.	[1905]	LRB
	—	W. Markwald finds ionium (Th-230) same chem as thorium.	[1906]	BDCG
	—	W.H. Bragg discusses origin of gamma and X-rays.	[1901]	Na
	—	L. Baekeland invents Bakelite.	[1925]	EB
3. # Nuc	—	O. Hahn discovers 1.6×10^{-4}s Ra C′ (Po-214).	[1906]	Bio
4. # Med	—			
		Organizations and Internal Politics		
5. Pols	—			
6. Socs	—	Fifth Int Cong of Med Elect & Radiol meets in Barcelona.	[1906]	AEM
7. Event	—	W. Ramsey: Li, Ne, Ar formed from Cu and Rn (discredited).	[1898]	LRB
	—	H. Kamerlingh-Onnes makes liquid He (4° K).	[1898]	DSB
	—	Nobel prize: E. Rutherford, chemistry.	[1903]	Bio
		Instruments, Units of Measurement, and Drugs		
8. Instr	—	E. Rutherford finds electric method for counting alphas.	[1904]	PRS
	—	H. GEIGER: FIRST TUBE CATHODE WITH A CENTRAL WIRE ANODE.	[1899]	PM
		News item considers Geiger's counter a hot subject.		EE
	—	P. Villard invents a "Radiosclerometer" (electrometer).	[1905]	AEM
9. Units	—	W. Butcher uses 1 Half-Value-Layer Al as hardness unit.	[1899]	ArRR
	—	W. Butcher defines 1 roent-candle = 1 mg Ra unit of intensity.		ArRR
		1 radion = 1 roent candle at 1 cm.	[1925]	ArRR
		1 radion minute = 1 unit of quantity.	[1905]	ArRR
	—	W. Butcher says Hungarian Sci Soc uses ergs/s for intensity.	[1905]	ArRR
	—	P. VILLARD GIVES FIRST DEFINITION OF "R" = 1 esu/cc_{air}.	[1928]	AEM
	—	Int Electricity Congress adopts the Ampere and Ohm.	[1948]	NBS
10. Concp	—	F. Dessauer uses 2 tubes, dist, filt to get "hard" rays.	[1905]	MMW
	—	S. Gager exposes germ cells to check response.	[1904]	Sc
	—	H. Minkowski formulates a 4-dimensional geometry.	[1905]	DSB
11. Drugs	—	W. DUANE SUGGESTS USE OF A RADIUM-TO-RADON COW SYSTEM.	[1954]	PR
	—	S. Flexner develops serum, Rx of cerebrosp meningitis.	[1903]	JEM
	—	F. Haber synthesizes ammonia.	[1900]	DoE

Radioiodine, P-32, and Radioactive Therapy

12. I-Res	—		
13. I-Dx	—		
14. I-Rx	—		
15. P-Rx	—		
16. Tele	—		
17. Other	— W. Duane suggests radon instead of radium for therapy.	[1900]	BMSG
	— G. Holzknecht notes germs disappear from irrad field.	[1907]	MMW

Scans and Other Tests of Function in Various Organs

18. Brain	—		
19. Heart	— J. Mackenzie studies auricular fibrillation.	[1903]	CDD
	— S. Tawara describes node of Aschoff-Tawara.	[1904]	CDD
	— L. Buerger describes thromboangiitis obliterans syndrom.	[1806]	CDD
20. Liver	— J. McCrae implicates phosphorus in cause of jaundice.	[1906]	JPB
	— H. Oertel describes biliary cirrhosis.	[1898]	ArIM
21. Lung	— W. Pasteur describes massive collapse of lung.	[1904]	La
	— A. Gray evaluates Dx by X-Ray of chest disease.	[1906]	NYMJ
22. Bone	—		
23. Kidney	— G. Macalister describes pathol of paroxys hemogl'uria.	[1904]	QJM
24. Gut	— G. Pirie shows diagnosis of esophageal stricture.	[1905]	ArRR
25. Blood	—		
26. Other	—		

Radiation Hysteria and Health Physics * Obituaries *

27. Hyst	— Arch Roentgen Ray documents first Radiation Hysteria.	[1924]	ArRR
	— L. Wickham says betas are Rx agent, hence do not filter.	[1907]	BAEC
	— W. Harvey exposes rabbit adrenals, gets late hemorrhages.	[1904]	JPB
	— Chlorination of water in Jersey City begins a new hysteria.		AP
	— S. Arrhenius says CO_2 buildup in atmos is a "heat trap."	[1984]	Bk
28. React	— W. Butcher says only a fool burns himself or patients.	[1907]	ArRR
	— C. Gager notes lo-dose stimulates growth of many seeds.	[1906]	BK
	— H. Albers-Schönberg: 10 min in dark before fluoroscopy.	[1896]	ArRR
29. Respo	— Am Roent Ray Soc considers protection of Radiologist.	[1897]	ArRR
	— Royal Med Soc (Lon) considers protection of Radiologist.	[1897]	ArRR

* * *

30. Obits	— H. Becquerel (1852–1908) Fr physics; uranium rays and °activity.		DSB

CHRONOLOGY OF NUCLEAR MEDICINE — 1909

Scientific and Technical Background

			Ref.
1. Basic	— W. Bragg measures wave lengths by diffraction of X-rays.	[1905]	Bio
	— G. Barkla discovers characteristic radiation.	[1906]	PM
	— J. Madsen notes wave length changes when rays scatter.	[1922]	PM
	— J. Madsen defines "quality": ability to penetrate absorbers.	[1905]	PM
2. Obser	— D. Stromholm cannot separate Th X from Ac X chemically.	[1906]	ZAC
	— B. Keetman cannot separate Th-RaTh; Ionium-UX chemically.	[1906]	JaR
	— W. Johannen coins word "Gene" (Gr = give birth to).	[1907]	DSB
	— G. Kaye plots distrib of rays from a focus bulb.	[1907]	PTRS
3. # Nuc	— O. Hahn discovers ThD, later AcC" (4.8m Tl-207) by recoil.	[1908]	Bio
4. # Med	—		

Organizations and Internal Politics

5. Pols	— Women admitted to German universities.	[1903]	EB
	— Rockefeller Sanitary Commission founded (to be Rkflr Fndatn).		EB
6. Socs	— W. Gardiner writes "Origin, History & Devel of X-Ray Tube."		ArRR
7. Event	— L. Bakeland mfgrs "Bakelite" (a "tissue equiv" plastic).	[1925]	GMP
	— T. Morgan begins study of "Genetics."	[1907]	Bio
	— J. Costa describes daily activity in English X-Ray office.		ArRR

Instruments, Units of Measurement, and Drugs

8. Instr	— -. Mugge uses autoradiography for mineral distribution.	[1901]	GMP
	— G. Kaye studies intensities from diff metal cathodes.	[1906]	ArRR
	— P. Eykman extolls roentgen-cinematography.	[1897]	ArRR
9. Units	— C. Phillips: 1mg Ra ionization = unit of radioactivity.	[1906]	ArRR
	— J. Dewar: 1g Ra (equilib) emits 13.6×10^{10} alphas/sec.	[1905]	ArRR
	— J. Watson proposes "Radion #1–#6" based on Benoist hardness, #1 Radion = 30 cm spark-gap, 10 amps @ 1 m for 1 min.	[1908]	ArRR
	— C. Phillips: 1 g Ra stores 3600 horsepower-hrs work.	[1908]	ArRR
	— S. Sorensen suggests neg-log-[H] be a scale for pH.		EB
	— H. Bordier lists 5 ways to measure X-ray "quality": 1. Hurmuzesku's electroscope, 4. Gaiffe's milliammeter, 2. Beclere's Spintermeter, 5. Courtard's Radiometer. 3. Benoist's Radiochromometer,	[1908]	ArRR
	— H. Bordier lists 7 ways to measure X-ray "quantity": 1. Holzknecht's Chromometer, 5. Kienbock's Ag paper strips, 2. Freund's iodoform soln, 6. Guilleminot's Pt-Ba-Cyan, 3. Sabouraud-Noire Pastilles, 7. Contremoulin's Ag deposits. 4. Kohler's tube thermometry,	[1907]	ArRR
	— E. Rutherford finds world Ra measurements vary by >20%.	[1910]	Eve
10. Concp	— RUTHERFORD AND CURIE PROPOSE BRUSSELS CONFERENCE ON RA STD.	[1910]	GMP
	— S. Allen tells how to measure X-rays (spark-gap).	[1905]	ArRR
	— C. Phillips notes stories: irrad of one part changes another.		ArRR
	— C. Nicolle experiments with transmission of typhus.	[1876]	CRS
11. Drugs	— P. Ehrlich makes "salvarsan" (606) for Rx of syphilis.	[1901]	DSB

Radioiodine, P-32, and Radioactive Therapy			
12. I-Res —			
13. I-Dx —			
14. I-Rx —			
15. P-Rx —			
16. Tele —			
17. Other —	L. Wickham devises the first intrauterine Ra applicator.	[1946]	GSR
Scans and Other Tests of Function in Various Organs			
18. Brain —	S. Lange examines the mastoid region on X-Rays.	[1907]	QAR
19. Heart —	M. Pachon develops an oscillometer to study BP.	[1896]	Bk
—	T. Lewis writes monograph on graphic pulse recording.	[1902]	Bk
—	H. Christian reviews viewpoints on chronic myocarditis.	[1908]	JAMA
—	A. Hewlett measures rate of blood flow to arm.	[1927]	Ht
—	C. Rothberger describes premature beats.	[1908]	CDD
20. Liver —	J. Abel: some phthaleins excreted exclusively in bile.	[1959]	JPET
21. Lung —	F. Wohlauer irrad G-pigs to hyperven, no alveolar change.	[1898]	DMW
—	F. Trendelenberg develops surgical embolectomy.	[1888]	Bk
—	E. Beck uses stereoscopic view to Dx tuberculosis.	[1906]	GAR
—	C. Leonard reviews Dx of tuberculosis by X-Ray.	[1906]	QAR
22. Bone —			
23. Kidney—	E. Keyes studies renal pelvis and ureter with X-Rays.	[1907]	TAUA
24. Gut —	C. Phillips says bismuth motility studies are routine.	[1900]	ArRR
—	G. Holzknecht sees normal colon peristalsis with X-Ray.	[1907]	MMW
—	R. Cecil shows pathology of pancreas in 90 diabetics.	[1921]	JEM
—	J. Edkins studies chem mechanism for gastric secretion.	[1905]	JPh
—	F. Reiche demonstrates a gastric ulcer.	[1897]	FGR
—	A. Hurst pubs "Constipation and Allied Disorders."	[1907]	Bk
25. Blood —	E. Aubertin: acute radiation means loss of lymphocytes.	[1906]	ZIM
—	G. Weaver analyzes serum disease.	[1876]	ArIM
26. Other —			
Radiation Hysteria and Health Physics	* Obituaries *		
27. Hyst —	C. Phillips says 1906 radiation hysteria is dying out:	[1908]	ArRR
	X-ray burns are caused by ignorance of operator.	[1905]	ArRR
28. React —			
29. Respo —			

* * *

30. Obits —

THE FIRST X-RAY PICTURE IN AMERICA

During November & December of 1895 the freshman class at Davidson College (NC) had been entertained by the play of colors in a Crookes Tube. A few Junior students assisted the science professor in the demonstration. Upon return from the Christmas vacation in January the professor told them of a wonderful discovery made in Germany on this same type of electrical tube.

On Sunday night, 12 Jan 1896, three skeptical but enterprising Juniors put the discovery to test. They obtained a finger from the dissection laboratory and alternated as look-out guards to prevent academic reprisals, because this was unauthorized homework. Upon activating the Crookes tube they exposed the finger for a few hours. The picture was a huge success and was circulated among the student body like a French post card. The picture was never published and remained secret until a freshman snitch spilled the story in an editorial in Radiology 7:257, 1926.

The First X-Ray in America at Grinnell

A Grinnell College, Iowa, newspaper (Feb 29,1896) reported that Prof F. Almy took some "Kathodic Ray photographs" in the college laboratory. A Rühmkorff coil with many batteries (about 120,000 volts) was attached to a Crookes' tube. At a distance of about 8 to 12 inches over a Cramer Photographic Dry Plate, he exposed a steel key ring with 2 large iron keys for about an hour. A good shadowgraph negative was produced.

"On Friday evening (28 Feb) a third attempt with an exposure time of about 12 minutes was made . . . aluminum wire photographed perfectly . . . The lead of a pencil appears with no trace of the wood . . . A fountain pen in which only the pen can be seen clearly was seen . . . [Some photos] do not seem in harmony with the work of Lenard."

Many other examples of "the first X-Ray" are in many newspapers of the time. The science lab of most colleges had a Crookes tube. The best story described the first fee for a medical X-Ray.

THE FIRST X-RAY FEE IN AMERICA

(From Pupin's Immigrant to Inventor, 1923)

Michael Pupin, Prof of Electromechanics at Columbia U, had earned a Ph.D. (Berlin) on vapor pressure of salt solutions. His research required fancy glassware and he became a friend of Herr Mueller, who had blown the vacuum tubes for Goldstein's work on "canal rays." Mueller stimulated Pupin's interest in electrical discharges in high vacua. Consequently, when Pupin set up the first experimental physics lab in America it was loaded with vacuum tubes. He was better equipped to take X-Ray pictures than Roentgen, but that was not his line of research.

When Roentgen's discovery was first noted in the newspapers he immediately confirmed it by taking a picture, and discarded it. But an incredible demand for X-Ray photography had been whipped up by the newspapers. Pupin was deluged by requests from physicians, none of which he honored — with one exception.

A patient of a surgeon friend accidentally received the full charge of a shot gun in his hand. Upon entreaties from the surgeon Pupin attempted, unsuccessfully, to display the embedded shot. Both patient and Pupin could see the lead pellets on a fluorescent screen Thomas Edison had recently sent to Pupin, but the pain was too great for the patient to sit still for an hour film exposure.

The fluorescent screen was far more sensitive to X-rays than a glass photoplate. Why not, thought Pupin, let the film record fluorescent light from the screen rather than X-rays. *"The combination worked even better than I expected. A beautiful photograph was obtained with the exposure of a few seconds."* The surgeon operated and removed every pellet.

This first intensified X-Ray picture was also the first surgery done with X-Ray guidance. It also yielded the first fee in Radiology. The grateful patient established a fellowship at the Century Club entitling Pupin to two toddies daily for the rest of his life. Thus Radiology became one of the highest paid specialties in Medicine.

BECQUEREL BREAKS THE LAW
(He Discovers a Physical Impossibility)

Monday 20 January 1896: the regular meeting of the French Academy of Sciences featured a demonstration of Roentgen photography by Henri Poincaré. The Roentgen story leaked to the press had been well written; it told how Roentgen took the picture. (Roentgen wouldn't give his first report until three days later.) Most physicists had a Crookes tube available for a quick check. Henri Poincaré had fired up his tube immediately. His verification (before the first paper) was being published that day in Comptes Rendus.

Henri Becquerel, as always, attended the meeting. The distinguished occupant of the Chair of Physics at the Musee d' Histoire Naturell had to respond to the latest scientific sensation in the news. (His father, Edmond, had occupied the Chair, as had his grandfather Antoine, and as son Jean would after he died.)

It was a simple matter for Poincaré to take an "X-ray" picture. Literally hundreds of physicists had demonstrated the tube to thousands of students for years. (But only two had done it in a dark room with a Pt-Ba-cyanide screen close by, and one of these, Silvanus Thompson, made a wrong interpretation.) After Poincaré's demonstration, Becquerel asked a question: *"From where do these remarkable rays originate"?* *"Undoubtedly,"* answered Poincaré, *"from the spot on the glass wall rendered fluorescent by impingement of cathode rays."*

Becquerel hurried back to his lab. He was about to break the most sacred law in science, the mathematically sacrosanct Conservation of Energy. Poincaré had NOT said fluorescence caused "X-rays," but Becquerel understandably misunderstood. His father, Edmond, had been the world authority on light from phosphorescence. His grandfather, Antoine, had received the Copley Medal from England's Royal Society for studies of fluorescent minerals. If anybody was genetically coded to discover radioactivity in uranium it was Henri. As a demonstrateur for his father fifteen years earlier Henri had prepared a double sulfate of uranium and potassium that was remarkably phosphorescent after exposure to sunlight.

[Twelve years later, in an obituary to his old friend, William Crookes described the excitement of 1896 (in a slightly shortened, but direct quotation; PRSL 83:xx, 1910):]

"I (W. Crookes) visited Henri Becquerel's laboratory one memorable morning when experiments were in progress which culminated in the discovery of 'Becquerel rays'. Uranium salts of all kinds were in glass cells inverted on photographic plates enclosed in black paper. Starting with the discovery that sun-excited uranium nitrate gave out rays capable of penetrating opaque paper, he had devised another experiment in which, between the plate and the uranium salt, he interposed a sheet of black paper and a small cross of thin copper. The apparatus, completed on a cloudy day, was put into a dark cupboard and left for an opportunity for insolation. But it was cloudy for several days, until, tired of waiting (or with the unconscious prevision of genius), Becquerel developed the plate. To his astonishment, instead of a blank, the plate had darkened under the uranium as strongly as if the uranium had previously been exposed to sunlight. The image of the copper cross shined out white against the black background. This experiment was the foundation of a long series which have made 'Becquerel Rays' a standard expression in science."

The emission of rays was an emission of energy. Whence comes that energy? Becquerel disproved every external source but found no explanation. His break with "Conservation of Energy" was under severe challenge. He was nibbling away at each criticism (including his own disbelief), when the Curies gave him a pinhead of their first glowing radium in a glass vial. He carried the vial in his vest pocket to show to disbelievers. It gave off light, produced heat, and did not diminish with time. Soon there were no disbelievers; but still no explanation. Becquerel had broken the law of conservation of energy.

Then he noticed a slight burn on his skin underneath the vest pocket.

[See Vig1898 .Ci; Vig1906 .Rn3]

THE CURIES DISCOVER POLONIUM
(Also Radium to Clean Up the Source)

Marie Curie received her licencée in physics in 1893, mathematics in 1894, married Pierre in 1895, and was awfully pregnant in 1897. The idea of getting a doctorate was growing in her as was Irene. Her first baby (and second most important contribution to science) was born on 12 September 1897. She then needed a subject matter for her doctoral thesis.

The curious subject matter discovered by Professor Becquerel almost two years before had not yet been the subject of a thesis (because few people really believed it). More important, radiation was said by J.J. Thomson to cause a small electrical current. Her husband could help her because he had invented a quartz piezo electroscope and was a specialist in very small currents.

Pierre Shifts to Electrical Measurements

Becquerel accepted Marie as doctoral candidate and, about the same time, began to shift to a simple gold leaf electroscope. But this was not for Marie: Pierre set up a very sensitive but precise system. Marie began with a survey to find if anything else was radioactive. On 25 Jan 1898 G.C. Smith announced to the Physical Society of Berlin that thorium was [radio]active (VPG 17:14, 1898) — but he never exploited the discovery. Eleven weeks later, apparently independently, Marie announced the same discovery (CRS 126:1101, 12 Apr 1898) — but she had just begun to work.

Becquerel had already proved that uranium compounds emitted rays in proportion to the percentage of uranium in the compound. It followed that no compound could be more active than pure uranium, which measured 2.3 "activity units."

[In Pierre's passion for electrical precision he adjusted Marie's electroscope to read "1" unit for a lab standard set at a saturated ionization current of 10^{-11} amps.]

Marie surveyed some of Becquerel's uranium ore samples with astounding results:

Johanngeorgens't pitchblende	8.3 units
Joachimsthal pitchblende	7.0 units
Carnotite	6.2 units
Chalcolite	5.2 units

Chalcolite was interesting. As a double phosphate of copper-uranium dioxide it could be made artificially in the lab from measured materials. Marie made some pure chalcolite. It should have read about 1.15 units — it read 0.92! Therefore, the natural chalcolite *must* contain something else with "activity."

Marie Gets a Ton of Pitchblende

The Austrian mines at Joachimsthal had been researched by a thousand geologists in a few hundred years. First mined in 1518 for silver to make "Joachimsthaler" (later "thaler," even later "dollar"), it was a source of bismuth, nickel, zinc blend, and later, uranium. The "something else" that "*must*" be present had to be in very small amounts to escape so much scrutiny, and intensely active to overpower uranium.

The early discoveries of the Curies were not accidents; everybody knew what was entailed. The French Academy contributed a small stipend. Through Becquerel the Austrian government contributed a ton of Joachimsthal tailings. The school contributed an unused shed. Marie, about to become a one-woman ore extraction plant, received more help than any other female doctoral candidate in history (so far).

Pierre had a full time teaching job, but he helped in off hours. His mother had died a few weeks after Marie delivered Irene, but his father (a 19th century equivalent of a pediatrician) moved in with the Curies to help take care of Irene.

A Classical Ore Separation, etc., etc.

Marie didn't have the slightest clue as to a proper chemical procedure. Pitchblende contained every metal known to science, including the still confusing rare earths. She followed a routine fractional precipitation of classical chemistry: dissolve a batch of ore in water, decant, precipitate the solution with HCl, measure the undissolved. Put solution and precipitate under the electroscope. Select the sample with the most active electroscope reading and dissolve it in something else; precipitate and measure, select the most active. Repeat; dissolve, decant, precipitate, measure; repeat . . . repeat . . . repeat . . . occasionally a fractional crystallization was required, or fractional sublimation to break an obstacle, but mostly repeat . . . repeat . . .

Eventually the samples got smaller, then soon the bottles on the shelves were faintly luminescent:

"One of our joys was to go into our workroom at night; we then perceived on all sides the faintly luminous silhouettes of the bottles or capsules containing our products . . . The glowing tubes looked like faint, fairy lights." [P.C. biog by M.C. p. 45, Dover, 1963]

About this time Marie and Pierre began using the word "radioactivity." Now each increase in radioactivity required a spectrogram. In one batch they precipitated sulfides of Bi, Cu, and Pb, and a few others. It was more active than anything they had seen. Marie eliminated Bi, Cu, and Pb. A fast spectrum showed bismuth lines and no other.

Polonium is Discovered First

Bismuth? . . . ridiculous! Marie had removed bismuth. She did a fractional sublimation in a vacuum; at one end of the cooling tube a black substance deposited itself. Upon measurement, an aliquot had 700 times more radioactivity than uranium. On 18 July 1898, on radiation evidence alone, the Curies announced a new element they called "polonium." [Soon RaF, now 138.4d Po-210; CRS 127: 175, 18 July 1898]

Critics said the spectroscope showed bismuth. Then the world's master spectroscopist, William Crookes, silenced the critics: the only fault in the Curie discovery was their poor spectroscopy. In between the characteristic bismuth lines were a number of new lines never seen before. But the Curies didn't have time to stop and repeat.

Radium, Almost Overlooked, Is a Surprise

In dissolving the metallic sulfates in water, the soluble portion had yielded their polonium. The insoluble portion, measured as an afterthought to the excitement caused by polonium, turned out to be even more radioactive. Spectroscopy said it contained sulfates of Ca, Ba, Pb. Marie removed these contaminants one by one until only a small intensely active sample remained. The spectroscope said barium chloride. Fractional crystallization was repeated several times. Ultimately Marie had one portion of inactive barium chloride crystals and a similar batch of crystals-with-a-difference: they glowed *in the light,* and gave off heat.

Pierre took a small aliquot to a gold-leaf electroscope. The scope collapsed before he got there. The sample was cut in half, and then diluted, then diluted again, and again, and finally had to be measured at a distance. Pierre calculated that it was a million times more radioactive than uranium.

The polonium criticism the Curies were still suffering from did not apply. Every separation had shown a barium spectrum with a strong new ultraviolet line. With each additional purification the barium lines sank into the background and a dozen new lines proclaimed a new element. On 26 Dec 1898 the Curies announced the discovery of their second new element. They called it "radium."

Something Must Be Wrong!

A few days later Pierre checked his measurements. If anything the sample was more active than he thought. During the next month it became still more radioactive, but something was going wrong. The electroscope seemed to be itself radioactive. Their papers, glass, metal, everything in the laboratory had become somewhat radioactive. It was unbelievable!

But it was believable. In Montreal at exactly the same time, fall of 1898, Ernest Rutherford was struggling with instrumentation problems in working with the much shorter-lived daughters of thorium. By Christmas time he would demonstrate that a gas "thoron" (now 55.5 sec Rn-220) was emanating from his samples.

"Radon" (now 3.8 day Rn-222) was emanating from the Curie's samples.

[See Vig1898 .ER]

RUTHERFORD DISCOVERS A RADIOACTIVE GAS

($I_t = I_0 e^{-\lambda t}$, $T_{1/2}$, Begins Nuclear Physics)

In 1898, at McGill University in Montreal, a new physics laboratory had just been built. John Cox, a Cambridge mathematician, was professor of physics. He recognized his own lack of flair for a new experimental physics and went back to Cambridge to find an "experimental man." J.J. Thomson, Oliver Lodge, G. Stokes and others recommended J.J.'s first assistant: Ernest Rutherford.

Many years later the man who had been Dean of Law in 1898 reminisced: "*... Cox made a remark to me before Rutherford came which has stuck in my memory. He said that one day he was feeling rather dispirited because there seemed nothing new going on in physics. The main things, he said, had all been found out.*" (Things were about to change abruptly.) [Eve Biog p. 59, 1939] Rutherford accepted in August, and set to work finishing a paper on ionization in air caused by a film of uranium salt.

Back in 1896 Roentgen's discovery had caused J.J. Thomson to interrupt his near final work on the "electron." He sloughed much of the work in discovering that X-rays caused "ionization" in air onto Rutherford, who was continuing with Becquerel's similar rays:

> "*... there are present at least two distinct types of radiation — one that is very readily absorbed, which will be termed for convenience the Alpha radiation, and the other of a more penetrating character, which will be termed the Beta radiation.*" (Eve p. 107) Gamma radiation, though recognized, wasn't named. [See Vig1908 .Vil]

Toward the end of the paper he notes that G.C. Schmidt's new thorium radiation (Jan 1898) was more penetrating than uranium radiation. He did not have time for details; he mailed the paper to Phil Mag on 1 Sep 1898 and packed his bags.

Rutherford Discovers an Element

Upon arrival in Montreal Rutherford set up electrometers and scopes. On 24 October he sent a rush request to the Cavendish for some uranium and thorium preparations. He had just met the new professor of Electrical Engineering, Robert Bowie Owens. The older man (he was 28, Rutherford was only 27) was looking for a likely research subject. Rutherford suggested one.

Rutherford had been checking how thorium emissions differed from uranium emissions. He had set up a thin layer of thorium oxide in a metal dish. A thin wire was stretched a few cm over the dish. The dish was attached to one pole of a battery, the wire to the other to capture some of the ions of emission. When attached to one pole, the wire became intensely radioactive. Attached to the other pole, the wire gathered no radioactivity. Disconnected, the wire gathered a small bit of activity. This wonderful experiment had only one fault: about half the time it didn't work.

Owens Demonstrates a Thorium Gas

When a physicist has a perfect experiment that doesn't work he calls in an instrument repairman. The battery made the experiment electrical — Owens was an electrical engineer. "Find out what's wrong with my battery?" suggested Rutherford. Owens thought the simple straight-forward problem was a fine way to break in a new laboratory.

He spread a uniform layer of thorium oxide on a thin platinum planchet and centered it on a brass plate connected to one quadrant pair of a delicate Thomson electrometer. The other pair went to a wire directly above the oxide. Rutherford had already shown with uranium that the rate of achieving quadrant equilibrium was proportional to current flow, and proportional to ionization in the air, and proportional to alphas emitted. Slips of aluminum foil could be inserted to measure penetration, hence alpha energy. Owens forgot only one thing — Murphy's law.

"It was very early observed that the radiation from thorium oxide was not constant, but varied in a most capricious manner."
(Roy Soc Canad, read 26 May 1899.)

Owen's first measurement read the way Rutherford had predicted. To illustrate his scientific bent he repeated the entire setup. This time while exposing the electrometer a secretary walked past the lab bench with skirts a-swishing.

[Unlike today, an 1898 skirt on a properly built female could swish up a micrometeorologic wind storm.]

Owens emitted a low wolf whistle in appreciation and focused back to the measurement. The experiment did not work properly.

So he repeated, following the academic principle that if you can't do it right the first time, repeat it ten times and report the average. Eventually he began to notice that every time a breeze passed through the laboratory the experiment didn't work.

Owens put the entire setup in an air tight vessel. He pumped a stream of air past the thorium oxide. The rate of current leak registered on the electroscope was reduced by a third. After cutting off the air flow the readings gradually recovered to a steady maximum.

Nothing had ever been wrong with Rutherford's instruments! The thorium oxide was giving off a *gas*. Owens did not know enough chemistry to realize the heresy he had committed. He gave the results to Rutherford with a snide remark on the expulsion of gases and went off on summer vacation.

Rutherford Accepts the Gas Concept

Rutherford was trying to save enough money to go back home (New Zealand) to pick up a bride. He could not afford a vacation, but this gave him time to puzzle out the rapid build-up or washout of activity from thorium oxide. *"Suppose,"* said Rutherford, *"Owens is correct. In addition to ordinary radiation, a large number of radioactive atoms are given out from the mass of active substance."* Such an 'emanation' could pass through considerable thicknesses of paper.

By bubbling the emanation thru water he proved it was not a dust. In an early type cloud chamber he proved it itself emitted radiation. The emanation could pass a plug of cotton in a glass tube. It was unaffected by bubbling through hot or cold sulfuric acids (the old trick for trapping ions). It passed through gold foil and mica and behaved like a gas. But it didn't last long.

[Proof that 'emanation' was a gas had to wait until 1900 because another characteristic, half-life, dominated his thoughts. So many 'emanations' occurred in the next few years that I (MB) will use their 1923 names: thoron, radon, actinon.]

Rutherford Discovers Half-Life

The short and unbelievable life of the new thoron emanation posed a problem in measurement. Rutherford devised an insulated cylindrical can to act as a gas sample container. At the same time it was an integral part of a quadrant electrometer that trapped gas within its poles. A paper of thorium oxide was put into a tube and a slow current of air blown past it into the electrometer.

Rutherford showed that the radiation intensity of the gas *"fell off to one-half its original value in about one minute."* This was the first description of exponential radioactive decay. (Phil Mag 49:1, 1900; submitted 1 Sep 1899.) He then derived the now familiar decay formula: the intensity at any time (I_t) is equal to the intensity at time zero (I_0) multiplied by $e^{-\lambda t}$, where "λ" is the decay constant: thus, $I_t = I_0 e^{-\lambda t}$.

The decay constant "λ," by a stroke of public relations genius, he had already converted from a mathematical symbol to an easily understood "half-value-period." "λ" $= 0.693/T_{1/2}$, the time interval for the intensity to fall to half of its initial value. Thus, the concept of *"half-life"* was introduced in 1899, but the term "half-value-period" or something similar was used well into the 1940s.

["Half-life" was shorthand slang at Berkeley during the 1930s. The first printed use I can find is G. Seaborg's review (Chem Rev 27: 199, 1940). In spite of its misuse for "half-time" by biologists it is a precisely defined word.]

Rutherford considered the concept of half-life decay fundamental to nuclear science. When he was created a Baron in 1931 he put his 1899 decay and recovery curves for thoron (and all other radionuclides) on his coat-of-arms.

[See Vig1900 .C&B]

X-RAYS CAN KILL GERMS
(or Can They?)

The major change between 19th and 20th century lifestyles was caused by proof that a bacterium caused anthrax in sheep. The population quickly became obsessed by bacteria. Soon "all disease was caused by germs." Fortunately, equally well known was the popular wisdom that "sunlight killed all germs."

On 6 January 1896 a WIENER PRESSE news item was cabled by the TIMES from London to all the civilized world: "... Professor Routgen (sic) of the Würzburg University has discovered a light which for the purposes of photography will penetrate wood, cloth, and most organic substances."

If solar radiation is germicidal, are these new X-rays also germicidal? Three weeks later, in the 1 Feb 1896 issue of LANCET, T.G. Lyon of London noted a destructive effect of Roentgen's rays on tuberculosis and diphtheria bacilli. Three weeks still later (17 Feb 1896) he backtracked and reported no effect. However, some physicians disagreed. On 26 April 1896 THE CHICAGO TRIBUNE announced a possible cure of diphtheria by X-ray.

These scientists were not stupid. A reason for the next decade's repeated confirmations and refutations was that NO units of quality or quantity existed. Only one biological effect was certain: people exposed to X-rays tended to get a "sunburn." Even serious overexposure caused only a superficial ulceration; therefore, superficial skin disease might be treated with X-ray. Then, in 1904, based upon investigations in the rat testicle, J. Bergonie & L. Tribondeau found actively dividing cells especially susceptible to radiation.

Radium Becomes a Therapeutic Agent

X-rays directed at fast-growing surface cancers produced real "cures." If you could get radiation to deep cancers they too could be killed. Such depth was possible with radium in tubes.

Many months after Roentgen's discovery, publicity was still in full cry. Henri Becquerel's discovery had not caused much of a splash. Discovery that thorium is radioactive went unnoticed by the public. Polonium's discovery didn't even make page one, and radium's most newsworthy feature was its discovery by a woman. Radium was unobtainable, except to dedicated chemists, and then for decades it was prohibitively expensive. Radium also had a serious fault. Pierre Curie had discovered that radium *induced* radioactivity in everything it came near. Rutherford had proved this untrue, but it took time for the word to spread from Canada. Radium decayed to a short-lived °gas that seemed to plate out on anything, leaving an "active deposit" of radium A; this changed to radium B to C, D, ... ideas on this were changing rapidly.

Radium initially emitted another "gas" called alpha by Rutherford. William Ramsay, in 1903, tried to prove alpha was helium. Rutherford had shown that alpha rays were doubly-charged mass — 4 particles with emission speeds of 9000–12000 miles per second, but they could be stopped by a piece of tissue paper. Gamma rays were inconstant around 1900/5. (Ra & Rn emit a weak gamma, no beta rays; not until well into daughter decay do the gammas become significant.) Gamma rays caused almost no effect compared to alphas.

Bacteria exposed to fresh *unsealed* radium were killed, and no doubt about it (unless the radium was in paper). A fresh *sealed* source of radium might or might not kill bacteria; a month old *sealed* radium source always did. Until the decay scheme was cleared up (c 1910) radiobiology was a chancy science.

Each day 0.0001% of radium atoms became radon, and 16.5% of accumulated radon atoms decayed. Eventually as many radon atoms were decaying as were produced from the radium source. This same equilibrium occurs with each decay from RaA (Po-218) through RaG (Pb-206). After a few months, a sealed radium source is a remarkably consistent source of *supervoltage* radiation. (The word was coined to describe radium gamma rays.)

By 1914 radium's complex decay chain explained the biological discrepancies. Radium, more specifically, radon (unmentioned in newspapers) was about to become a major factor in cancer therapy.

[See Vig1915 .Cow]

"WHITE" MEANT "BACTERIOLOGICALLY CLEAN" IN 1900

Those of us born too late for 1900's turn-of-the-century festivities must rely on pictures to see what we missed — or escaped, depending upon your point of view. The stretch between 1890 and 1910 was a shining peak in the golden age of *science & technology*. A few scientific discoveries had major impacts upon the public's way of life.

> [I use an ampersand to link science with technology because by 1900 they were separate only in academia: if it's taught for glory it's "science"; if it makes money it's "technology."]

The 19th and 20th Centuries

Compare 1890 with 1910 photographs. In 1890 people wore black or grey clothing. Kitchens and bathrooms had dark wainscoting. Fretwork moldings and filigree indicated craftsmanship. Hospitals were dark and, hence, healthful tombs. By 1910 kitchens and bathrooms had lost the wood paneling and were painted white. Doctors wore white labcoats. Nurses wore starched white uniforms. Hospitals used white-lead as the only clean and, hence, healthful pigment. The most visible difference between the 19th and 20th centuries is white paint on flat surfaces.

This transition to "white" was supported by Robert Koch's 1876 proof that anthrax in sheep was caused by bacteria. He thereby founded bacteriology.

> [— but was this "science"? Bacteriology was an academic backwater until country doctor Koch proved it had immediate practical value. Research was strictly mission-oriented. By definition early bacteriology was an exercise in "technology."]

The golden age of science (c1850 to c1940) was split down the middle by the turn of the century. The most obvious difference between the 19th and the 20th centuries was the eruption of white paint on anything supposed to be "clean."

Who Started the Bacteria Hysteria?

R. Koch did not start the anti-bacterial frenzy that marked the turn of the century. He merely proved that the man who did start it was correct. In 1865 J. Lister, English surgeon, learned of Pasteur's cure of bacterial diseases. In 1867 he used carbolic acid hand washing before surgery to stop surgical wound infections. His success led to a "bacteria clean" concept (as opposed to dirt clean). Getting rid of dirt was the first step to bacteria clean and this was easy if white towels were used, then white sheets, then white uniforms, then white walls. Eventually, to be "bacteria clean" everything had to be white. (Don't laugh; Lister knew this was false but it is what people believed.)

Koch discovered the bacterial cause of tuberculosis in 1882. He and his students followed with the cause of glanders, Asiatic cholera and diphtheria in 1884; gonorrhea, strep & staph in '85; pneumonia in '86; Malta fever, tetanus, the plague, botulism, dysentery were proved bacterial in short order. By 1900 many knowledgeable people were saying that ALL disease was caused by "bacteria." To prevent disease, kill bacteria. To kill bacteria, clean up. To assure clean surfaces, paint them white. Thus the 20th century opened in obligatory white.

By 1930 "White" is No Longer Required

Another technology carried over from the 19th century did not require cleanliness and could be painted black. All automobiles were black until, in a frenzy of sales pitchery one of them broke the color barrier. In 1923 Willys-Overland came out with the "Red Bird." The next year General Motors marketed colored Duco Lacquers. The true break, however, came in 1925 when Crane Co advertised colored porcelain bathroom fixtures. The final blow to white came in 1926 when the Cannon Mfg Co advertised (in color of course) colored bath towels.

By the mid 1930s Alexis Carrell committed the ultimate heresy: his surgical team was dressed in light green. "White" held on as a clean color until after World War II, but it no longer meant "bacteriologically clean."

Another hysteria took its place in popular maladjustment. In 1927 Herman Muller noticed that X-rays caused mutations in fruit flies which, to him, were practically human. "Radioactivity clean" replaced "bacteria clean" in phobias.

[See Vig1901 .E&G Background Radiation]

CROOKES & BECQUEREL OPEN THE CENTURY

(They *Almost* Discover Transmutation)

In his youth William Crookes was a pioneer photographer. (He became "Sir" at Victoria's 1897 diamond jubilee.) At the age of nineteen (1851) he read his first scientific paper to the London Chemical Society on a remarkable parallelism between sulfur and selenium. His idea came 18 years before Mendeleev and 6 years before Dumas mentioned periodicity. Incidentally, it was the first and also the last paper Crookes would ever write on pure chemistry.

Photography, then spectroscopy, and finally metrication of any kind became Crookes' passion. His dexterity in the chemistry laboratory led to an interest in Fox Talbot's new photographic discoveries which, at the time, were more chemistry than artistry. He learned the Talbotype process from Talbot himself and soon adapted photo-recording to meteorographic registration at the Radcliffe Observatory. His wonderfully sharp photos of the moon brought him to the attention of Professor Wheatstone (of bridge fame), who was attempting to get solar and lunar spectra. Crookes adapted the photographic method to spectroscopy and built the first spectrometer-camera. He became an authority, and eventually the world arbiter, in spectroscopic analysis.

Crookes Supports Himself as a Publisher

Crookes, with no family money, had to earn a living. He managed at first by editing the Liverpool and then the London Photographic Journals (1856). With three years experience, he purchased the *Chemical Gazette* (founded in 1845). With himself as editor, on 10 Dec 1859 he began issuing the *Chemical News*. For the next sixty years practically everything that went on in science (because Crookes defined "chemistry" as "science") passed under his eyes.

Therefore, Crookes was more than interested when his good friend Henri Becquerel used photography to make a major scientific discovery. [See Vig1896 .Bq] When radium was announced in 1898, Crookes exposed every mineral in his cabinet — an extensive collection — to sensitive film for 48 hours each. Of 16 minerals that gave autoradiograms, each was active in proportion to its uranium or thorium content.

Crookes Makes The First °Standards

Crookes, age 65, was an old fashioned chemist. If the young Curies could separate radioactive elements from pitchblende, maybe he could separate them from uranium, which is where his autoradiograms said they should be. However, with the distrust of a seasoned chemist he would have to do his own purifications from raw ores. He purchased a half-ton of pitchblende, had it worked up systematically by a friend who ran a chemical works. He ran through Marie Curie's months of labor in a few weeks without getting his hands dirty. But each filtrate and precipitate was compared autoradiographically against a uranium salt "tentative standard."

One crystallized uranium nitrate was very active compared to an especially pure metallic uranium sample he had obtained from M. Moissan in France. This sample would become his "permanent standard." He dissolved a few pounds of the very active uranium nitrate in ether and by repeated crystallization got uranium nitrate crystals of great purity. He put these crystals on a photographic plate to test an exact 24 hour exposure density: "Not a trace of image could be seen." He repeated the experiment. Again, he washed the radioactivity out of uranium contrary to Becquerel's assertion. He immediately sent a note off to his old friend, but he had to find that lost activity.

Crookes dissolved a full pound of pure crystallized uranium nitrate in a pound of methylated ether. The portion insoluble in ether contained all the activity (by the photographic method he was using). Further, a fraction dissolved in ammonium carbonate and dilute HCl no longer contained uranium by spectroscopy, but was still radioactive.

"For the sake of lucidity the new body must have a name. Until it is more tractable I will call it provisionally UrX — the unknown substance in uranium."

[Proc Roy Soc 66:409, 1900]

Crookes went through a series of time consuming tests, always diluting the sample, to characterize UrX. Only then did he put it under the spectroscope. Nothing showed up.

Uranium X (UrX later UX) is 24.1 day thorium-234. Gigayear U-238 decays by alpha emission (photographically cold by Crookes' technique) to a photo-hot beta Th-234, through an even hotter Pa-234, to another photo-cold U-234. Buried between two long-lived uraniums, Crookes' UrX was present in very small quantity. Crookes used the spectroscope like we use eyes. He always followed every extraction analysis with multiple spectrograms. But just this once, confused by the extremely sensitive photo technique, he forgot his own rules. If he had spent 15 minutes on a spectrum at the first stage of pure crystalline nitrate when UX is in its most concentrated form, he would have recognized distinctive thorium lines. He had missed by 15 minutes the greatest scientific discovery of the 20th century — transmutation.

Crookes Says Becquerel is Wrong

But Crookes partially made up for his mistake by setting in motion a chain of events that led to Rutherford's discovery. After his first ether separation of uranium nitrate, the note to his old friend Becquerel stated, *"I've washed the radio-activity out of your uranium,"* then told him how to do it.

Becquerel Tells Crookes to "Look Again"

Becquerel opened the envelope and exploded, "Impossible"! He immediately duplicated Crookes experiment and confirmed Crookes — but not quite. By this time Pierre Curie had won Becquerel over to use of the electroscope in addition to the photo film. The precipitate was very weak but not totally inactive. The mother solution contained almost all the activity, as Crookes had written.

[You must realize for the next paragraphs that Crookes was a pack rat. He didn't throw samples away. Becquerel, on the other hand, saved not only his, but his father's, and had quite a few of his grandfather's collections. It was the autoradiogram of one of his grandfather's uranium samples that had prompted the "always radioactive" statement.]

What had he done to make such a mistake four years ago when he proved uranium was permanently radioactive? He reviewed his old work then, 4 months later, went back to the Crookes confirmation samples. Just to be complete he remeasured them. The cold uranium samples were hot, but now the mother solution was cold. He made some new uranium crystals and began all over again from scratch. But first he dashed off a note to Crookes, *"Measure your samples again."*

When Crookes received Becquerel's note he was in the middle of answering a letter from Rutherford giving him instructions on where to buy some pure thorium nitrite. After checking Becquerel's finding, he added a final paragraph:

> 18 Dec 1901: *"... M. Becquerel told me a curious circumstance and asked if I could verify it. He prepared some time ago an inactive uranium nitrate. Now, on repeating his experiments with that identical sample he found it had resumed its radioactivity. I am at work on old compounds of my own to see if I can get similar results."*

Rutherford Takes the Hint from Crookes

Upon receiving the letter from Crookes, Rutherford immediately checked all of his old (weeks) thorium X samples. All of the dead thorium precipitates were now active again. All of the hot thorium X samples were dead cold.

But what is thorium X (now 3.7 day Ra-224)? No one had ever announced the existence of such a substance. *"Hmmmmm ...,"* thought Rutherford. He didn't know it yet, but he was about to resurrect medieval transmutation and begin the 20th century.

[See Vig1902 .ER2 Transmutation]

IS THERE BACKGROUND RADIATION?

(Elster & Geitel Find it in the Garden, and Giesel Introduces °Body Burden)

Johann Elster and Hans Geitel were considered by J.J. Thomson to be the world's most remarkable life-long partnership in physical research — and one of the most productive. Both Elster and Geitel went to Heidelberg in 1875, and transferred to Berlin in 1877. Elster went back to Heidelberg for a doctorate in 1879, but Geitel, with a certificate to teach secondary school, got a job in Herzoglich Gymnasium in Wolfenbüttel, south of Braunsweig, Germany. Elster joined him in teaching science and math in 1881. They were still teaching in 1920.

Elster was a true example of the absent-minded professor. Once when told he had put a 10 pfennig stamp on a letter requiring only 5, he neatly crossed it out and glued a 5 pfennig stamp over the 10. The door of his house had a large and a small doorlet cut in the bottom. When asked why, he said it was because he had both a large and a small dog. Geitel represented Germany at the 1910 Brussels Conference on Radium. He received honorary doctorates from Heidelberg in 1915 and Berlin in 1919. The two lived in the same house for almost 40 years, had a renowned flower garden and raised brilliantly colored butterflies.

Elster & Geitel Anticipate Discoveries

Elster and Geitel collaborated on almost 150 publications in the new field of electricity and the movement of electrons. In 1895 they invented the photocell. In 1897 they discovered negative emission from incandescent filaments to bolster a new "corpuscle" theory by J.J. Thomson. After Becquerel's announcement they proved his rays were not affected by air pressure or temperature.

Elster & Geitel had been highly influenced by Thompson-Rutherford's 1896 announcement that Roentgen's rays ionized the air. Because they were busy measuring small quantities of electricity in air, they invented the electrometer to confirm X-rays; and continued to discover that Becquerel's rays also ionized air. After the Curies announced polonium they set up the efficient method for separating it in commercial quantity. After the December 1898 announcement of radium, they looked further in Joachimsthal tailings and found radioactive lead (before half-life, but it was probably the same as Rutherford's Radium B (Pb-214)).

E & G Anticipate Transmutation

Marie Curie suggested that uranium's emission *"is fluorescence of uranium excited by a very penetrating radiation that fills all space, hence it is radioactive, i.e., activated by radiation."* These words came out of Becquerel's laboratory and could not be taken lightly. Elster & Geitel wondered, where was the evidence for this radiation *"that fills all space."* They set up a program to find it, and meanwhile they restated Marie Curie's speculation:

> *"An atom of radioactive element behaves like an unstable compound that becomes stable upon release of energy. To be sure, this conception would require the acceptance of a gradual transformation of an active substance into an inactive one and also, logically, of the alteration of its elementary properties."* [AnP, 1899]

This statement is the first to announce transmutation, but there was no evidence beyond observing radioactivity which most scientists had not done. (It was left for Rutherford to announce transmutation, *with evidence*, three years later.) However, Elster & Geitel were so concerned about the evidence that they measured "everything." They soon observed a leakage of current from their electroscope. An electroscope is about the simplest instrument available; nothing much can go wrong. There must be residual radioactivity, presumably in air.

E & G Discover Background Radiation

Elster and Geitel strung a wire one meter long and a meter above the earth in their garden; they set it at −2000 volts potential against the earth. Within a few hours the wire itself was appreciably radioactive. Did it come from the sky or earth? They drove a hollow pipe a meter into the earth and withdrew some very radioactive air. [PZ 1903] Over the next decade they measured the radioactivity in rain,

THE FIRST AND ONLY
DEATH FROM BACKGROUND RADIATION

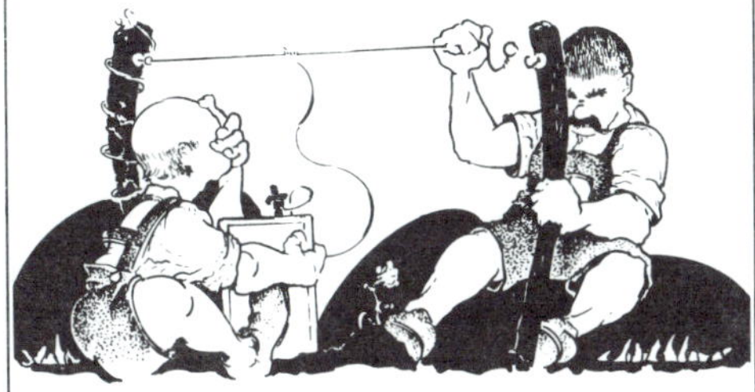

"HANS! YOU HAF ON DER BLÜMCHEN GESTOMPED."

streams, lakes, oceans, plains, valleys, mountains, health spas. They took trips to gather samples, wrote letters to friends for samples. They measured radiation in everything.

While this was going on others joined in. At Cambridge C.T.R. Wilson suggested an extraterrestrial source for background radiation (eventually known as cosmic rays [See Vig1923 .VH]). In 1902 he detected radioactivity in freshly fallen snow around Cambridge. Because so many sources of radioactivity were being reported by so many people in so many places, J.J. Thomson decided to settle the matter by drawing a glass of Cambridge tap water and demonstrating that it, too, was radioactive.

> [But he hadn't solved the problem: 75 years later a Tucson, Arizona, newspaper would "warn" the public by reporting normal radioactive urine samples collected throughout the city as "contaminated." They reported a harmless H-3 spill was "potentially lethal," demanded, and got the death penalty for the company involved.]

Herr Giesel and the Hot Body Problem

Meanwhile, back in Wolfenbüttel, a close friend from Braunschweig (now Brunswick) was measured for radioactivity. Friedrich Giesel (1852–1927) had studied industrial chemistry at the Königliche Gewerbeakademie, Berlin. With an 1876 doctorate from Göttingen, he became chief chemist at Büchler & Co (a quinine factory in Braunschweig). 18 years later, 1898, he read the announcement of radium and began, first as a hobby but later as a business, the production of ultra-pure sources of radium bromide. He used an improved fractional crystallization technique. (The Curies produced a weaker RaCl.) He developed many radioactive luminous compounds, and was the one who advised Crookes to use ZnS to detect scintillations from alpha rays (a technique learned from Elster & Geitel). Rutherford said he was first in nuclear science because he supplied everybody with sources: Rutherford, Hahn, Boltwood, Bragg, Ramsay, Soddy, et al.

In 1904 E & G went to Braunschweig and asked Dr. Giesel to blow into a special electroscope 18 hours after he had left his lab; his exhaled breath had higher radioactivity than anything they had tested. Herr Giesel not only had "background," he was himself a radioactive body. [ArRR, 9:179, 1905] In his opinion, much of the seemingly ubiquitous terrestrial radiation was really the gaseous emanation from radium, thorium, and from Giesel's new "emanium" (that Hahn was about to identify as actinon).

[See Vig1905 .OH1]

Giesel had breathed radon, thoron, and actinon in higher dose (many times Marie Curie's level) than anyone with the possible exception of Otto Hönigschmid. According to Health Physics Gospel he had to die of lung cancer. But his good friend Otto Hahn said he died in 1927 at the age of 75 with a *"radiation induced carcinoma on the left index finger."* It was death "with," not "of," cancer. In 1954 K.Z. Morgan corrected history and had him die properly of lung cancer. "Cause-of-Death" became a "Health Physics," not a "Pathology" opinion. [See Vig1761 .Mor]

Background Radiation is a Known Fact

In 1913 Geitel published a summary of over 10 years of data collection. In the "Handbuch der Radiologie," the largest survey of background radiation (until 1978) showed a wide range of background levels: "Die Radioacktivität der Erde und der Atmosphäre." Unfortunately neither the "roentgen" unit of radiation nor the "curie" unit of activity had yet been accepted. In 1940 my generation learned about background as a local cpm (counts per minute). By 1978 the world of radiation changed with a few but widespread background measurements.

[See Vig1923 .VH & Vig1978 .Bkg]

RUTHERFORD RESURRECTS TRANSMUTATION

1898 saw the discovery of polonium and radium in the Curie laboratory. The Curies had poor equipment and no assistance. About this time André Debierne, chemistry preparateur at the Ecole Polytechnique, began to drop in at the shed to help out. He became a close friend of the family and was soon a full collaborator. The problems associated with radium were too vast for one person. They decided to divide: Pierre on physical aspects, Marie on chemistry (remember, this was still her unfinished thesis problem), André would search for the "other" element they knew had to be in their non-radium residuals. (He discovered actinium within the first year, 1899.)

Pierre Finds "Induced Activity" (False)

A major problem for Pierre was in keeping Marie's electroscope honest. It kept drifting to higher readings. In 1899 Pierre and André put a small necked flask of radium solution inside a large closed beaker. Five clean plates of mica, copper, cardboard, and ebonite were positioned around the flask; one was put behind a thick lead shield. After a day's exposure all the plates were equally radioactive. Debierne tried the same thing with his new actinium, with the same result. They called the phenomenon "induced activity." Uranium and polonium, they found, did not cause "induced activity."

Rutherford Disputes "Induced Activity"

Meanwhile, Rutherford in Montreal had completed his work on the build-up and decay of thoron. He knew (but did not have positive proof yet) that thoron was a gas. At the end of his article he added a note on the galley proof:

"As this paper was passing through the press, the Comptes Rendus of Nov 6, 1899 was received, which contains a paper by Curie . . . on the radiation excited in bodies by radium and polinium (sic) . . . no mention is made of whether there is an 'emanation' from radium and polonium as there is from thorium compounds. Curie concludes . . . excitation by radiation, in the case of thorium such a theory is inadmissible."

[Phil Mag 49:161, Feb 1900]

Within a year F.E. Dorne of Halle had discovered "niton" (our radon, 3.8 day Rn-222) to prove that Rutherford was probably correct. [ANG 1900]

A Brief Transition Period

The two most active radioactivity laboratories paused momentarily in 1900. Pierre was offered the Physics Chair at the University of Geneva with an official slot for Marie. They visited Switzerland, worried a great deal, and almost accepted; but it would interrupt Marie's doctoral thesis. Henri Poincaré got Pierre appointed Asst Prof of Physics, Chemistry and Natural History, at the Sorbonne. (A required course for medical students with a heavy teaching load and no lab space.) Marie obtained a teaching post at the Normal Superior School for Young Girls at Sedres. They kept the radium shed operating as their only laboratory and wasted hours each day commuting from home to lecture room to laboratory. In Marie's biography of Pierre, she describes it as a "painful period."

The pause in Montreal was for a happier reason. Rutherford had finally saved enough money to get married. In the spring of 1900, he returned to New Zealand to marry his fianceé. Upon his return for the autumn semester he met a chemist just graduated from Oxford, who had joined McGill's faculty. The head of the chemistry department had no interest in inorganic or the new so-called radio-chemistry. The new man, Frederick Soddy, was anxious to do experimental work. Rutherford gladly put him onto the chemical characterization of thoron and its active deposits.

Rutherford Discovers Thorium X

In catching up on his reading Rutherford came across Crookes' article on UX. Maybe thorium also had an X. He got Soddy to repeat Crookes' procedure, but on thorium. Sure enough, there was a "thorium X" that decayed to half its value in 4 days (now 3.7 day Ra-224). But they made no announcement of the discovery of Thorium X because they were busy writing a major article on the radioactivity of thorium.

It would be historically interesting to see the first draft of the Rutherford-Soddy article on the Radioactivity of Thorium Compounds. [JChS 81:321, 1902] The published second draft gives the first hint of "transmutation." How, in the first draft, did they explain the concentration of short-lived (55 sec) activity growing out of long-lived (14 Gy) thorium? Rutherford admits it can't be explained when he contradicts himself in mid-paper to prove that thorium X (Ra-224) is different from thorium. You can't find any literature reference to the discovery of thorium X — it just materialized in the middle of a page. But thorium X made the second half of their paper a logical extension of the first half.

Thorium Decay Requires Transmutations

Look at today's Chart of the Nuclides to see what was happening: 14 Gy Th-232 decays by pure alpha emission to 6.7 y Ra-228. A weak beta emission takes the series to 6.1 h actinium-228 (practically unknown in 1902); then back to a 1.9 y Th-228 that is chemically indistinguishable from the original thorium. Th-228 decays back to another radium, 3.7 day Ra-224 which has a very hot (5.7 MeV) alpha emission. Radium-224 is what Rutherford discovered as Thorium X. It decays to 55 sec Rn-220, which was familiar to Rutherford as thorium emanation, or thoron gas. Then follow the thorium "active deposits."

Rutherford didn't see all of this in 1902. All he could see was that permanently radioactive thorium decays to a queer 4-day thorium which decays to a gas which decays to a short-lived active deposit (compared to radium's deposit). An investigation of thorium's "active deposit" was on Rutherford's schedule, but first he had to clear up the Th X decay. Thoron's 1 minute half-value-period was too short for accurate chemistry. Thorium X, fortunately, had a comfortable 4-day period that allowed both radioactive and chemical measurements.

Because there was "no decay" in the original thorium its activity was a kind of natural background. (14 Gigayears did not qualify as decay in 1902.) Thorium X had a slightly irregular decay on day 1. (THIS WAS IMPORTANT, see end of page.)

But, thereafter, it had perfect exponential decay. The build-up during recovery of the de-emanated thorium was the exact inverse:

"There can be no question that Th X and UX are distinct types of matter with definite chemical properties." This said "transmutation" without saying the bad word.

[Trans Chem Soc 81:837, 1902]

Transmutation is Announced

Rutherford's work had been severely impeded by his miniscule supply of thorium. Soddy was attempting chemical analyses on homeopathic samples. In desperation Rutherford wrote a letter to Crookes to find out where to purchase pure thorium compounds. Crookes was answering the question when he received a hurried note from Henri Becquerel.

[This story is told in Vig1900 .C&B]

On 18 December 1901, after checking Becquerel's bombshell on the reactivation of the de-activated uranium, Crookes finished his letter to Rutherford and added the last paragraph: deactivated uranium reactivates itself. Upon opening the letter Rutherford was astounded to read confirmation of his latest article which hadn't even been printed yet, and by no less than Crookes and Becquerel. He immediately checked his old samples: regrowth after deactivation was also true for thorium X. Another article would have to be written and this time he would include the forbidden words:

". . . the radioactive elements must be undergoing spontaneous transformation."

[Phil Mag September 1902]

Spontaneous transformation, akin to the medieval transmutation, was the most important discovery of the 20th century. But it did not cause a public sensation; in fact it was a scientific obscenity — not mentioned in polite conversation. His senior colleagues at McGill had begged Rutherford not to publish the second thorium article because it would bring disgrace on McGill. Further, the argument was flawed. On day 1 after separation from thoria, thorium X DID NOT decay exponentially. The complex multiple chains of decay had to be unraveled before transmutation would be accepted in science. In three years a private in the German army began the unraveling.

[See Vig1905 .OH1 Otto Hahn Begins.]

CROOKES INVENTS SCINTILLATION COUNTING
(and Convinces Mach that Atoms Exist)

Dig deep enough into the microhistory of anything in nuclear science and Crookes' name will pop up. He was a rarity in Victorian science: no academic support, not wealthy, earned his living as a publisher-chemist — and did much basic research. He could be classified, without disrespect, as a toymaker, if you remember that his 1875 radiometer upset every physicist in England. Its progeny led to discovery of Roentgen rays, the electron, and the atomic age. Another toy, the spinthariscope, would eventually take over Nuclear Medicine (in modified form). [See Vig1948 .XTL]

In late June 1903 William Crookes wrote to F. Giesel, a friend at Büchler & Co. in Braunschweig, Germany (they were selling radium at £12,000 an ounce):

> *"... Can you tell me what is the best way to exhibit the luminosity either of a radium compound or the action of radium on a screen, so that it can remain permanent?"* [Biog, Appelton 1924]

Giesel recommended zinc blende (ZnS, an idea fresh from Elster & Geitel). Crookes painted ZnS solution on a glass plate, and then 12 mg of RaBr onto the dried crystal screen. In the dark, Crookes' screen gave off enough light to read by. [See Vig1901 .E&G]

Marie Curie could never have made this discovery. She hoarded every microgram of radium like a miser and followed a rigid bureaucratic lockup each night. Rutherford couldn't have made it. He had none to spare. But Crookes used his Ra supply freely. As the world's best chemist (his opinion) he had made his own and could always make more. A £5–10 expense was minor; faith in his ability as a chemist made recovery and re-purification a minor chore.

By Murphy's law Marie's lab was the most highly contaminated in the world. A.S. Eve had to take electroscopes home at night; he couldn't calibrate in Rutherford's lab. But Crookes' lab, in his home, was spotless — and for good reason: he did not spill things, and saw no reason to measure contamination.

Radium's glow on ZnS was uninstructive. Under a microscope the glow was dense; Crookes wanted to see detail. He cut a short length of brass tubing, sealed one end and painted the inside surface with ZnS. He threaded the other end and screwed in a microscope eye-piece. A needle on a thumbscrew was mounted in front of the screen with its point dipped in radium. As he screwed the point close to the ZnS screen he saw bright sparks of light flashing — *"resembling a swarm of fireflies on a dark night."* He called his new toy a "Spinthariscope" (from the Greek *spintharis* = spark). With the needle covered with foil, diffuse luminosity covered the screen. With the needle naked each spark registered an individual alpha particle hitting a ZnS crystal.

The Toy Becomes an Important Tool

It is said that the great Ernst Mach (intellectual godfather of Viennese logical positivism) was the last scientific holdout on Atomic Theory. He used it as a handy tool but could not "believe," because it violated science's epistemology. When he was shown a spinthariscope he was converted, because alpha particles were now perceptual evidence.

A few years later (1908) both Rutherford and E. Regener in Germany modified the spinthariscope: first count the number of flashes/time, then substitute the screen with an electrical collector to measure total charge. A simple division gives the charge on each alpha. Rutherford and Regener independently arrived at a charge of 9.3 to 9.58×10^{-10} esu on an alpha particle. J.J. Thomson's charge on the electron was 4.65 $\times 10^{-10}$ esu. Hence, alphas had a double charge. With a known charge the mass could be calculated from e/m studies. It was four times the mass of a hydrogen atom. *"... The alpha particle, after it has lost its positive charge, is a helium atom."*

[Proc Roy Soc 1908]

Much nuclear physics prior to World War I was done on Crookes' ZnS scintillation screens. The idea lost popularity to the GM tube and electroscopes until a Russian displayed a distaste for moth balls in 1948. As a result, 20 years still later, the scintillation crystal would take over Nuclear Medicine.

[See Vig1948 .XTL]

BOLTWOOD PREACHES PATTERNS OF DECAY
(and begins the Natural Decay Series)

From his first interest in radioactivity in 1898, Bertram B. Boltwood tried to answer a challenge he flung at Otto Hahn in 1905: *"prove that a long-lived intermediate connects radium to uranium."* Boltwood proved it himself in 1907 by discovering "ionium" (now 80,000 year Th-230). But Hahn almost beat him to it.

[see Vig1906 .B&H]

Boltwood's major scientific contribution, however, was the concept of ordered radioactive decay patterns. Between 1898 and 1904 he was the first to become convinced that the nine radioactive "elements" were not random freak species, but were part of a rigid decay pattern.

Boltwood was a cousin of Ralph Waldo Emerson, but far more important an uncle was professor of mineralogy at Amherst. Boltwood entered Yale's Sheffield Scientific School in 1889. After a doctorate in 1897, two years post-grad in Munich on chemical analysis were followed by a semester at Leipzig in physical chemistry. He then took an instructorship at Yale.

In 1899 one of his students repeated and wrote a thesis on Marie Curie's separation of radium, and barely missed discovering actinium. Debierne's announcement caused Boltwood to check the thesis and make the first confirmation. (Nine years later he had regrets.) [See Vig1906 .B&H]

World-wide Distribution of Radioactivity

In 1900 Boltwood left Yale to form a partnership with Joseph Pratt as Consulting Mining Engineers and Chemists. Pratt was the field man who sent samples from all over the world to Boltwood for analysis. After Rutherford's announcement of transmutation, Boltwood included measures of radioactivity in routine analyses of mineral samples. Soon he had a unique knowledge of the distribution of radio-chemicals around the world. He thought he could support transmutation by showing a constant ratio between the amounts of radium and uranium in world-wide minerals. He assumed, on little evidence, a generic relationship and set out to prove it.

Boltwood soon recognized that the traces of radium he was seeing were easier to detect — and more accurately — by measuring the radon emanation from radium. The inert gas required only mechanical, not chemical separation. Within months he had built a gas tight gold-leaf electroscope, and went a step further: the amount of emanation was proportional to the amount of radium, also to the amount of uranium.

Boltwood consulted Rutherford by mail. Rutherford was delighted with the work and began a voluminous correspondence and much collaboration. In 1906 they said that one gram of unadulterated uranium contained 3.8×10^{-7} gram of radium (now 3.42). But he could not find direct evidence of a genetic uranium-to-radium link. He was first to try to grow radium from uranium and failed miserably. (F. Soddy would succeed in 1919.)

Not only the beginning of each decay series, but also the final decay product could be seen in his geologic survey. Analyses showed that every uranium deposit was accompanied by deposits of lead. The older the deposit the greater the amount of lead. He was not satisfied with his data on the thorium series. The actinium group was not yet recognized as a series.

Growing out of this end product work was an appreciation of long-lived decay in geologic dating. If the rate of formation of a chemically inactive decay product is known, the amount present must indicate its age. Rutherford had speculated on age-of-the-earth in 1902, but geologists still believed in Kelvin's megayear earth. Radioactive geologic dating began in 1907 with Boltwood pushing gigayears.

After 1910 he was made full professor of radiochemistry at Yale. Increased academic and administrative duties, plus a heavy consultation load, ended his research career. In 1918 he became director of the Yale chemical laboratories. While watching many of his ideas bear fruit, he realized, in the 1920s, that he was out of touch with the field he had helped start. He had bouts of depression and in August of 1927 committed suicide.

[See Vig1907 .B&H]

GERMANY REDUCES THE BACKGROUND OF BRAZIL

Although not a chemist, Rutherford had become popularly known as the world authority on thorium because he could detect minute amounts with his radioactive method. Around the turn of the century, before electric lighting became popular, thorium had one major industrial use: making incandescent gas mantles was a highly prosperous business in Germany.

A woven fabric of cotton was dipped in Welsbach's mixture (thorium plus cerium impurity), fired, and then dipped in collodion for structural strength. Gas burned in this mantle gave off an intense white light. The gas and light industry used millions of mantles and needed a large supply of thorium. The German government had found an ample supply.

For years the German government had been sending large cargo ships loaded with trade goods to Brazil: cuckoo clocks from the Schwartzwald, handblown Christmas tree ornaments, colored glass beads and toys for children. Out of compassion for their fellowman they practically gave this merchandise away. All they asked in return was, could they please load some ballast into the ships for a safe return voyage to get more goodies for the poor?

After some years some Brazilians noticed that the ballast was always taken from the same cove. Was this the well known German dedication to systematic routine? But why so much ballast? Why ships always loaded to the gunwales? Some mining engineer had suggested a thorite deposit, so the Brazilian government sent a man to see Rutherford with a sample of the "ballast." Rutherford thought he recognized the sample. Under an electroscope the monazite sand showed quite a high thorium content.

"Can I purchase some of this sand?"
.... *"What's it worth?"*
"About a pound per ton."
.... *"What's it used for?"*

Rutherford pointed to a gas mantle.

The Brazilian reflected on how many gas mantles were purchased in Rio de Janeiro alone. It is recorded that soon after, the bottom fell out of Brazil's market for cuckoo clocks.

[Eve p. 114]

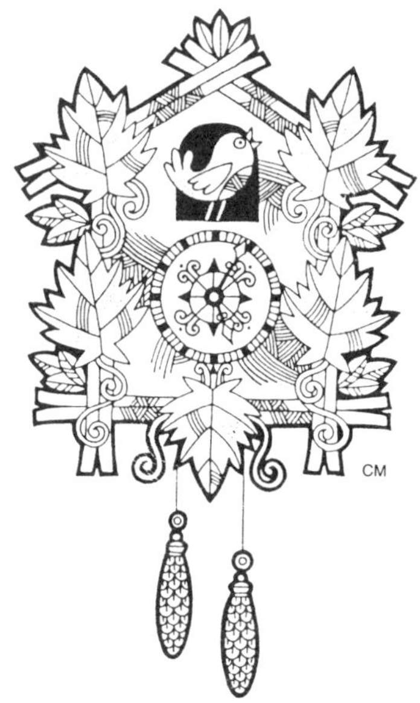

THE LONG GESTATION PERIOD OF "ISOTOPES" (RENAMED NUCLIDES IN 1947)

Date		Author(s)	Event
2 Sep	**1886**	W. Crookes	Audacious speculation on "Meta-elements." (Chem News, London 54:115, 1888)
16 Aug	**1904**	B. Boltwood	Radioelements must find a place on periodic table. (L. Badash, ER & BBB Letters. p. 40, Hopkins)
16 Mar	**1905**	O. Hahn	RaTh and Th have similar chemical properties. (Proc Roy Soc, London A76:115, 1905)
22 Sep	1905	B. Boltwood	RaTh cannot be found in thorionite. (L. Badash, Er & BBB Letters. p. 81, Hopkins)
—	1905	F. von Lerch	Transmutation is to more electronegative daughter. (Jahrb Radioaktiv Elektron 2:470, 1905)
—	**1906**	R. Lucas	Transmutation is to more electronegative daughter. (Phys Z 7:340, 1906)
Late	1906	O. Hahn	RaAc is chemically similar to RaTh. (Phil Mag 13:165, 1907)
26 Mar	**1907**	O. Hahn	$MsTh_1$ cannot be separated from Ra. (Autobiog p. 43; Phys Z 8:277, 1907)
16 Jun	1907	B. Boltwood	RaTh & Th are chemically similar; also ThX & MsTh. (Am J Sci 24:93, 1907)
12 Oct	1907	H. McCoy & W. Ross	RaTh cannot be separated from Th chemically. (J Am Chem Soc 29:1709, 1907)
Jan	**1908**	W. Markwald & B. Keetman	Ionium is chemically similar to Th. (Ber Dtsch Chem Ges 41:49,1908)
28 Feb	1908	B. Boltwood	Ionium cannot be separated from Th chemically. (Am J Sci 25:365, 1908)
Summer	1908	E. Rutherford & H. Geiger	Alpha is double charge, mass 4 atom. (Proc Roy Soc 81:162, 1908)
11 Oct	1908	B. Boltwood	U cannot be chemically split into two substances. (L. Badash, ER & BBB Letters. p. 193, Hopkins)
27 Jul	**1909**	B. Keetman	Th, RaTh, Ionium, UX, are chemically inseparable. (Jahrb Radioaktiv Elektron 6:265, 1909)
	1909	D. Stromholm & T. Svedberg	ThX, AcX, Ra, are chemically inseparable. (Z Anorg Chem 61:338, 1909)
28 Nov	**1910**	W. Markwald	MsTh1, ThX, Ra, are chemically inseparable. (Ber Dtsch Chem Ges 43:3420, 1910)
Jan	**1911**	F. Soddy	Chemical identity can have different atomic wt. (J Chem Soc 99:72, 1911)
May	1911	E. Rutherford	The "nuclear atom" announced. (Phil Mag 21:669, 1911)
	1911	A. van den Broek	First hint of ordinal atomic numbers. (Nature 87:78, 1911)
Late	1911	F. Soddy	There are three disintegration series. (Chem of Radioelements. p. 26, 1911)
Summer	**1912**	N. Bohr	Ordinal number, not atomic weight, is critical. (G. Hevesy, Adventures Rad Research. v. 1, p. 13)
Sep	1912	A. Fleck	UX, AcX(?), same as Th; ThB same as Pb. (Chem News 106:128, 1912)
Oct	1912	A. Russell	Chemical allows position on Periodic Table. (Chem News 107:49, 1912)
Nov	1912	K. Fajans & G. Hevesy	Gossip about recent events in Nuclear Science. (Letter Fajans to Brucer, G. Hevesy Adv Rad Res)
23 Nov	1912	K. Fajans	Attends "Tristan und Isolde," sees displacement laws. (Brucer, Vigs in Nuc Med, #98. Mallinckrodt, 1981)
28 Dec	**1912**	**K. Fajans**	**Inaugural address (Karlsruhe)** states displacement laws. (Med Verein Heidelberg 12:173, Dec 1912)

[See Vig1913 .Iso]

OTTO HAHN BEGINS TO UNRAVEL DECAY

Otto Hahn graduated with a Ph.D. *Magnum Cum Laude* from the U of Marburg in organic chemistry. He then enrolled in the 81st Inf. Regiment in Frankfurt for a required one year voluntary duty. Hahn's rise in the military service was meteoric; within six months he was promoted to private.

Upon completing his military career he was offered the assistantship to his chemistry professor, T. Zincke. It was customary that after two years of preparing lecture demonstrations Zincke would recommend him to a chemical company for a career in industrial chemistry. At the end of his two year stint he was offered an industrial job.

Fortunately for nuclear science a condition restricted the offer. With a brisk international business the company hired only those who had lived in a foreign country and acquired a reasonable skill with its language — it didn't matter which country. Professor Zincke wrote to William Ramsay at University College, London. Would he take a pair of hands for six months? Ramsay answered, yes. In September 1904 Otto Hahn arrived in England with a German/English phrase book in hand.

Sir William Ramsay was away on a trip and Otto had two weeks to visit museums and learn basic English. Upon his return Ramsay found two German postgrad chemists awaiting assignment. Dr. Otto Sackur from Breslau also needed English experience. Sackur was given some minerals and told to check them for radioactivity. This other boy, Hahn, was still having troubles with the language.

Ramsay Assigns an Impossible Task

Ramsay had no trouble understanding Hahn. He not only spoke German, but wrote articles and lectured in English, French, German or Italian and mixed the languages in mixed company. Ramsay, a noteworthy gas chemist, had almost no competence in radioactivity. Frederick Soddy had worked with him the year before and some equipment was still in the lab. But much more important, Ramsay, after his noble gas discoveries, was one of few chemists unintimidated by imponderable amounts of materials.

Ramsay wanted to be the first to determine the atomic weight of radium. "Would you like to work with radium?" Ramsay asked the doltish Otto. "Ich know nichts von radium," answered Hahn in his two week old English. *"Good,"* said Ramsay, *"you can approach the problem without preconceived ideas."*

> [Two years earlier Crookes had said he was the only man in England who knew how to produce radium. Few people in the world knew how — Ramsay was not one. The Curies worked with a ton of ore, Crookes with half a ton, Meyer in Vienna with about five tons. . . .]

Ramsay handed Hahn a bowl containing 100 grams of barium chloride. He said it contained about ten milligrams of radium. He wanted Hahn to follow Marie Curie's procedure, obtain the pure radium (which Marie hadn't done yet), and make a few organic compounds. These organics would crystallize nicely in sufficient bulk to allow an accurate measurement of atomic weight. Hahn accepted the bowl and headed for the library to look up this Marie Curie and, incidentally, how do you measure this radioactivity thing?

Ramsay Has a Quick Priority Job

A few days later Ramsay interrupted his two students with a priority job. He gave them two samples: one was of André Debierne's 1899 "actinium," the other of Friedrich Giesel's 1902 "emanium" that gave off an emanation of short half-value-period. Debierne's original 1899 thorium-contaminated actinium sample had been found to give off an emanation in 1903. But only after Giesel had produced a pure actinium product he called "emanium." A French/German controversy had developed over whether the two were the same. Ramsay suggested the two students compare the radiation from the samples.

Hahn and Sackur wrapped each sample in porous paper, inserted them into cotton filled glass tubes. They blew a puff of air past the papers into a measuring tube inside an electrometer. The electrometer needle jumped but the jumps diminished until at 30 seconds it was quiet. They set a metronome beating at 1.3 sec intervals, and blew in another puff. The two samples had identical half-value-periods — 3.9 sec (now 3.96 sec Rn-219). They collected what Rutherford was calling "active deposit." The two active deposits had the same half-value-periods.

A direct comparison of two samples is not earth-shaking science, but why hadn't somebody already done it? National pride was involved. Only an international charmer like multilingual Ramsay could talk two prima donnas out of priceless samples, and then convince the German that "actinium" had priority over "emanium." (Hahn lived long enough to learn it was neither, it was radon.)

This most valuable training exercise taught Hahn how to measure short-lived activities and the value of the decay rates in analysis. Hahn went back to separating radium from barium.

Hahn Discovers a Disputed Radiothorium

On his early, still highly impure separations of barium chloride, Hahn noted two radioactive decay rates. One was the constant radium, but another kept cropping up in his solutions. He could identify it by its one minute half-value period. It came from a thorium-like fraction. Fractional crystallization led him nowhere. He concentrated it with thorium chemistry to over 100,000 times the activity of thorium (now 1.4×10^{10} year Th-232). It was a highly radioactive thorium so Hahn called it "radiothorium" (RaTh, now 1.91 year Th-228).

[Proc Roy Soc 76A:115, 24 May 1905]

[In two years Hahn would learn why the Curie's fractional crystallization led him astray. Radiothorium grows out of a radium isotope, "mesothorium," but this is the focus of another story. See Vig1907 .BB.]

Hahn Changes His Career to Academia

Ramsay immediately acknowledged the new "element" without further proof (this was improper because international committees would not recognize half-life in the definition of "element" until 1976). He also recognized something far more important. This young chemist had a rare talent for research. He didn't belong in industry doing scut work. You belong at the University of Berlin, he told Hahn. *"But I don't know anybody in Berlin,"* said Hahn. *"Ahh, but I do,"* said Ramsay who knew practically everybody. He sent off a letter telling Emil Fischer what he was missing. During the summer holiday in 1905, Hahn was invited to see the famous Director of Berlin's Chemical Institute. Fischer explained to Hahn that he could not be a privatdozent (a kind of assistant professor) because that had to be in a specialty field, and no such field as *radio*chemistry existed. But he would fix up something.

To shift from industrial to academic chemistry, Hahn realized that he needed more training. He didn't realize that he had already caught up to the handful of chemists laying radiochemical foundations. Ramsay's slight acquaintance came from F. Soddy who came from Rutherford. Hahn decided to start at the top. Ramsay sent off a letter to Rutherford. Rutherford said yes. In September 1905 Hahn departed for Montreal.

Rutherford Prepares for Hahn's Arrival

To Rutherford, Otto Hahn's announcement of radiothorium was a mistake on Ramsay's part. Both F. Soddy and B. Boltwood at Yale had checked the Th to ThX to Tn decay thoroughly. Upon seeing Hahn's article, Boltwood had immediately worked up five grams of thorianite (thereby guaranteeing failure). He used Hahn's procedures but found no radiothorium.

Thorianite contains no radiothorium. Hahn had started with Ramsay's bowl of barium chloride. Thorium-232 decays to radium-228 decays to actinium-228 then back to thorium-228 then to radium 224, which was their thorium X. But this wouldn't be known for another ten years. Boltwood wrote to Rutherford (22 Sep 1905) *"... Hahn's new element is only a compound of thorium X and stupidity."*

He would soon retract this judgment and never again think it of Hahn's work. Rutherford answered, *"... Hahn is coming over to work with me this year. I think he wants to know how to measure things radioactive so as to be able to prove his element. In fact, I think he will 'take physic and throw up his element'."* Rutherford was the first to retract.

[OH autobiog, chap 2] [See Vig1908 .BB]

J.J. THOMSON AND "KANALSTRAHLEN"

(J.J. Sees Ne-22, but Doesn't Believe it)

In late 1905 J.J. Thomson, satisfied with his description of negative particles, looked at the positive half. In 1886 Eugen Goldstein in Berlin reasoned that with negative charges streaming to the anode, positive charges should stream in the other direction — if they had a pathway. He drilled a small hole (he called it a canal) in the cathode of a Crookes tube. As expected he saw a faint bluish glow emanating away from the anode. He put a magnet to it but the glow was not deviated, hence not particulate. He called them "Kanalstrahlen" (canal rays).

Wilhelm Wien, the man who succeeded Roentgen at Würzburg, showed in 1898 that Goldstein had been misled. Canal rays were not small particles easily deflected by a horseshoe magnet. They were heavy particles. Deflection required a powerful magnetic field. Wien set up a system similar to J.J. Thomson's deflector for cathode rays, but with photographic recording. The particles deflected by his magnetic field left streaks on the photo; their separation could be measured. Wien also found that if the gas pressure in his Crookes tube were low enough he could also deflect the rays in an electrostatic field. (The name *Kanalstrahlen* stuck and they continued to be positive *"rays."*) [VPG 17:1, 1892]

The Mass Spectrograph Principle Emerges

If a charged particle crosses a magnetic field it is deflected at a right angle to the field. If it crosses an electrostatic field it is deflected parallel. The amount of deflection must be proportional to the particle's velocity. In Thomson's 1895 cathode ray tube the two fields were crossed, in Wien's canal ray tube the fields were parallel; hence, deflections can be manipulated.

In a Wien tube a positive particle emerges from a hole in the cathode to cross a space between two condenser plates. If the magnetic field is active the particle will be deflected horizontally. If the electrostatic field is active the deflection is vertical. With both fields active the particle strikes the photoplate midway between vertical and horizontal axes. Particles with the same mass and charge but different velocities will make a parabolic streak on the photo. Particles with different masses will make different parabolic streaks.

J.J. Begins Positive Ray Analysis

[So many Thompson/Thomsons were doing physics in England around 1900 that first name initials became necessary. "J.J." soon became the proper name among colleagues and even among students. Even when he was knighted in 1936 he never was called "Sir Joseph," always "Sir J.J."]

Some of Wien's results departed seriously from theory, hence the theory must be wrong. But not for J.J.; to him it meant the experiment was faulty. He looked at Wien's equipment. In his early work on electron beams he had found that errors were caused by too many particles in the field at the same time. Residual pressure in Wien's tube was too high.

In 1905 J.J. began work on a modification of Wien's positive ray tube. With the fields displaced properly in a low pressure tube, the trace on the photoplate should display mass of deflected particles. Thomson knew that positive particles ionized the residual gas in a tube, or could lose part of their charge by acquiring ionization electrons. Interpreting positive ray photos was not easy.

After a few years of calibration, it was possible to read directly in mass numbers, but what was read, atom, molecule, contaminant? In 1910 Francis Aston, a chemist by training, joined the staff as J.J.'s lab assistant. Things began to move a little faster. By 1912 they were working on neon. The first photoplate showed a double parabolic trace, Ne-20 and X-22. J.J. said contaminant. Aston repeated many times. The double trace was always present with neon, never without neon in the tube. On 13 Jan 1913, J.J. told a Royal Institution audience it was Ne-22. The next summer he said "contaminant." Francis Aston, who developed the photoplates, was convinced he could prove it was Ne-22.

[See Vig1913 .Ast]

RADIUM VERSUS RADON

Radium, in 1906, was rare, hence expensive, and dangerous to handle. The danger was to laboratory instruments, not to people. Damage to people did not become important until after World War II. As soon as Health Physicists saw the money in radiation hysteria, the Maximum Permissible Dose came down to background.

None of the early background radiation studies came out of radium-using labs, because their background levels were too high. A.S. Eve tells how he made all his electroscopes at home because Rutherford's lab was so highly contaminated. Marie's lab, on the other hand, was not contaminated for the simple reason that she did not allow health physics type measurements. (People did comment, though, on the high background levels.)

Around 1910 there wasn't sufficient science and industry need for radium to support a mining industry. The big business was in medical therapy. Today we remember the doctor's use of sealed sources of *radium,* but Ra-226 emits alpha rays and an unimpressive splash of gammas during a 1600 year $T_{1/2}$. In sealed sources no alpha rays get through; hence Ra-226 itself is a poor source. However, it decays to a gas, 3.8 day $T_{1/2}$ Rn-222, which in turn decays by alpha emission through daughters (RaA ... RaF) that do have significant high-energy gamma emission. Therefore, radium therapy is really daughters-of-radon therapy.

In much of the early therapy literature and in the popular press the words "emanation," and "radon" (after 1923) were interchangeable with "radium." "Curie therapy" was interchangeable with "Radium Bomb Therapy," but in most cases radon was the actual source.

However, considerable therapy was done with direct injection of radium salts. In 1933 H. Bowing and R. Fricke of Mayo Clinic said that direct injection had been abandoned. (GSR, p. 236) Maybe true in academe, but in the early 1950s the sale of medical doses of liquid radium salts was still an ongoing big business — declining, but still popular.

The Beginnings of Radium Therapy

In April 1901 Henri Becquerel carried a small vial of the Curies' first glowing radium in his vest pocket to show his friends. The skin burn he received prompted Pierre Curie to verify it by exposing his own arm. Pierre saw skin damage that took awfully long to heal. He also saw a possible medical use.

At the suggestion of a friend, Pierre gave a small sample of radium to a Dr. Danlos of St. Lewis Hospital in Paris. After three years Danlos reported that in vivo radium killed animal tissue more easily than it killed bacteria. By 1906 the bactericidal effect of radium was so positive that a Biological Laboratory of Radium was set up in Paris. From this lab many firsts in radium therapy were reported: filtration, source designs, deep therapy, etc.

(GSR p. 211–218)

Robert Abbe, a New York physician, acquired some radium as soon as he could buy it. In March 1905 he inserted a tube of radium into an exophthalmic goiter for 24 hr exposure. The results were astounding. (Six years later he claimed a complete cure. [AnS 1913])

By 1910 tubes, plaques, needles, seeds, salves, ointments, even direct injection of radium salts, had various degrees of success. Little outright failure was reported. Overenthusiasm can be explained by the lack of competition.

A History Lesson for Anti-Radiation Kooks

Most people worried about background radon flux are exploiting radiation hysteria to get a government handout. Honest worriers should consider the lifetime Rn-222 dose from direct Ra-226 injection. Between 1910–1950 hundreds of thousands of patients (no one knows how many) received millicuries (no one knows how much) of radium. We began to live long enough to get cancer, but no epidemic of cancer occurred. More leukemia was diagnosed after 1910, but that's because more doctors saw more people and kept more records. Twice as many of us live twice as long with half as much disease as before radium was discovered. Radium can't be all bad.

[See Vig1981 .Hor]

BOLTWOOD AND HAHN AGREE ONLY ON BEER

When Otto Hahn left England for Montreal, Ramsay gave him two unusual gifts: the original barium sample from which he had extracted radiothorium, and the actinium preparation from which "emanium" was proved identical to actinium. Few laboratories, let alone individuals, had such pregnant sources of alpha rays.

Rutherford had decided to give Hahn a simple but demanding task: measuring the alpha range of thorium. But first Rutherford had to put radiothorium to rest. Hahn arrived in Montreal with a command of English that didn't match his enthusiasm. Rutherford's command of German couldn't hide his disbelief of radiothorium. So Hahn made some — under Rutherford's eyes (but from his own barium chloride source). Rutherford became more excited than Hahn.

Upon hearing of Rutherford's conversion, Bertram Boltwood at Yale yielded, but with a question. If RaTh had a half-value-period of 2 years, as Hahn said, it should be easily detected growing out of thorium salts in a few months; there was no such growth — Hahn's half-value-period must be wrong. It was remeasured in Rutherford's lab — Hahn was correct.

Rutherford suggested a conference.

Boltwood and Hahn Meet in Combat

Boltwood and Hahn met as master and student, arguing fiercely. (Boltwood spoke fluent and idiomatic German.) Hahn suggested the possibility of a long-lived intermediate. *"Prove it,"* challenged Boltwood, who by this time had recognized his equal in chemistry. The conference ended over a glass of beer that made Milwaukee famous. Their only agreement was that Munich beer was better. They parted still arguing fiercely, but no longer as master and student; now they were both students.

Hahn Discovers Two More "Elements"

In 1904 W.H. Bragg (U of Adelaide) had discovered the range limits over thin films of alpha emitting substances. Ionization built up to a peak and then suddenly dropped to zero. This "Bragg peak" was different for each substance. It meant that alpha particles had precise ranges (later, precise energies). Could the range be used to identify the substance? Rutherford gave this problem to Hahn to solve.

[The terminology becomes hopelessly confused and impossible to understand until the 1910 Brussels conference started revisions. I will use modern terminology to describe the events.]

Using Bragg's alpha-range method, Hahn traced some freshly prepared active deposit through its decay. He missed the 0.14 second thorium A. (Geiger & Marsden would pick up Po-216 in 1910.) As expected, Hahn found no alphas in the 10.6 hour thorium B (Pb-212). Totally unexpected, he found two alpha ranges in the 1.0 hour thorium C (Bi-212). One of these had an unbelievable 3×10^{-7} second half-life, It was identified as thorium C′ (Po-212).

On his own time, Hahn was studying Ramsay's second gift, the actinium sample. But by his own, not Rutherford's method. Just as radiothorium came between Th and Th X, he now found a radioactinium between Ac and Ac X. Actinium X (Ra-223) was discovered independently by F. Giesel and T. Godewski. Both had missed the 18.2 day radioactinium (Th-227). Three new "elements" discovered in less than one year — more than anyone had accomplished. Hahn went back to Germany a highly respected full-fledged radiochemist — but his reputation was in a small circle.

Hahn, on His Own, Discovers Two More

Because Hahn was working outside the curriculum, Emil Fischer could give him only an unused basement room called the wood shop. Hahn set up the Rutherford requirement of three electroscopes: one each for alpha, beta, gamma radiation. Charging these was done by the latest high tech method: rubbing a hard rubber stick against a coat sleeve. Hahn considered himself fortunate, and Rutherford had given him a hundred problems. But one challenge wouldn't go away: the long-lived intermediate between uranium and radium. Boltwood had said *"Prove it. I can't — yet."* In the months since their argument Hahn detected a crack in Boltwood's argument. Why was Boltwood's radiothorium (from pure thorium) so much weaker than his (from unpure sources). He needed some thorium to work with.

Berlin's Knofler Chemical firm was the world's largest producer of thorium. He learned that they prepared thorium by a method similar to Boltwood's. [See Vig1904 .ER3] Armed with a letter of introduction from Ramsay, Hahn was offered all the samples he wanted free of charge. He gleefully took a few samples, went back to his lab and was stunned to learn that he couldn't separate his own discovery.

One minor detail caught his eye. For quality control Knofler dated each batch of purified thorium. Hahn noticed that "activity" seemed related to age. Fresh thorium batches were twice as active as those several years old. He went back to Knofler. They had saved samples from the earliest production runs ten years ago. Hahn was again surprised. The oldest samples were almost as active as the freshest. This was the Crookes-Becquerel UX story all over again. [See Vig1900 .C&B] Fresh thorium contained material that decayed out rapidly, but was constantly being replaced. Hahn called the long lived intermediate "mesothorium" (now 6.7 year Ra-228).

Hahn received a second surprise when he compared some freshly separated mesothorium with samples separated a few days earlier. Fresh mesothorium had almost no radioactivity. (Remember the limitations of Hahn's scopes. In 1907 he couldn't detect 50 keV betas from Ra-228.) But a strong beta activity grew out with a half period of six hours (now 6.2 hour Ac-228, 2.1 MeV beta). Hahn called them mesothorium$_1$ and mesothorium$_2$.

Hahn Goes Back to Boltwood's Problem

During his survey of thorium samples Hahn occasionally detected the faintest trace of radon. In aged radium-free purified thorium salts the trace was obvious. Strange — because radium is so easily washed out of thorium preparations. Boltwood's long sought mother substance for radium had to be in a uranium series. Perhaps if he looked at the small thorium fraction of uranium-pitchblende he might find Boltwood's radium parent. Hahn sent a letter to Joachimsthal for samples. But it was too late. The next issue of Nature announced Boltwood's discovery of "ionium." [Na 26 Sep 1907]

Boltwood was working a few months ahead of Hahn on the same type of experiments — but with actinium. Rutherford snorted at actinium and told him to go back and read his own uranium papers. He did just that. They said uranium comes out of pitchblende, so does actinium. Where had he got the idea that no radium was in the actinium fraction? From Debierne's 1898 article. He reread it, but this time with ten years radiochemical hindsight. It was the sloppiest piece of analytic chemistry he had ever seen. He immediately repeated Debierne's work. The first "Debierne fraction" showed a long-lived alpha emitter with a soft gamma. He separated out the actinium and radium. In a short time radon gas could be detected emanating from the new "element." He had finally found the long lived parent of radium in the thorium-bearing portion of an early fractionation in the separation of uranium from pitchblende. He called it "ionium" (now 80,000 year $T_{1/2}$ Th-230).

Why Didn't We Think of Isotopes?

Boltwood had congratulated Hahn on the first mesothorium announcement by promising the beer was on him next year; also he had already sent in a confirmation. In a letter to Rutherford he confessed how he could be so fast (15 May 1907). He had already noticed the dated thorium sample changes that had spurred Hahn and was preparing an announcement. Now, six months later, in the first mail after his announcement of ionium he got a letter from Hahn, "The beer is now on me." Later in discussing it over beer they told each other how close each had come to the other's discovery.

Both Boltwood and Hahn had proved beyond doubt that a few series of rigidly connected decay patterns weaved back and forth among the elements like epicycles in pre-Kepler astronomy. Crookes had practically predicted isotopes that would allow such decay patterns in 1888. 1966 Hahn reminisced: *"Today it seems beyond belief that this knowledge did not suggest the existence of isotopes."* [OH Autobiog p. 50]

In five more years Kasimir Fajans will go to the opera, doze off, and see isotopes.

[See Vig1912 .KF1]

DAVID MARINE PROVES "IODINE DEFICIENCY"

(Lack-of-Iodine Becomes Iodine-Excess)

An inspired association between a paucity of iodine in certain soils and wells in the French Alps had been made by A. Chatin in the 1850s. [CRS 34:14, 1852] How, in the name of Hegelian logic, asked the great Virchow, can *absence*-of-something cause the *presence*-of-anything? It takes special genius to overcome such powerful logic. In 1907 David Marine was prodded by what he considered even more powerful logic — experiment.

Marine was then working in Professor Sollman's clinical lab in Cleveland. As a member of the AMA Council on Pharmacy, Sollman had heard complaints on the extreme variability of a new medication: "desiccated thyroid." He asked Marine to look into it. Marine used Bauman's 1895 iodine content as a scale, and fed desiccated thyroid to dogs. He became impressed by the correlation between thyroid iodine stores and the gland's hyperplasia. Iodine stores, he thought, might be a clue to variability of the pharmaceutical.

He decided to visit a Chicago slaughter house to see how *desiccated thyroid* was made. On his way he stopped off in Michigan to see the raw material: the sheep who supplied the thyroid glands. These sheep were in the same area where Dock had seen goiters 12 years earlier. Marine saw many healthy looking sheep, but they all had fat necks. [See Vig1895 .Doc]

On 23 May 1907 Marine watched workmen in Armour & Company's slaughterhouse collect sheep thyroids. Armour & Co was very cooperative because they worried about the variability of a big money maker. Workmen were instructed to discard all goitrous thyroids. About a third of the glands were discarded. By Marine's standards, from his work on cattle and dog thyroids, at least another third were enlarged, but he would have to run iodines and do histology before he could say for sure. Armour gave him a couple of barrels of glands to take back to Cleveland for assay. Marine did histology and iodine assays and separated the glands into two groups: <1 mg I/g thyroid, and >1 mg I/g thyroid. From these he made two batches of desiccated gland.

Marine Learns How to Prevent Goiter

Desiccated thyroid was fed to dogs for 18 days. Those fed low-iodine content material (from goitrous glands) showed no effect. (Remember, Armour had supplied only "acceptable" glands, goitrous only by Marine's histology.) Those fed high-iodine content material (from normal glands) got diarrhea, weight loss, tachycardia, and showed *thyroid involution*. The histology struck a spark of recognition in Marine. Thyroid involution had been a physiologic response in early studies.

Marine then measured the thyroid's iodine content in a large series of dogs, pigs, cattle, and fish. The degree of hyperplasia varied inversely with iodine content in "normal" animals. The human samples available to him were "surgicals" from Graves disease, "colloid" and "nodular" goiters — too variable in morphology and iodine content to be comparable to his "normal" animals. Therefore he found and measured abnormal animals.

After many experiments Marine reached a conclusion obvious for months: "colloid" goiter was not breakdown or degeneration, it was a physiologic resting stage awaiting the availability of iodine. Goiter was an iodine-deficiency "disease." 40 to 80 micrograms of iodine daily prevented colloid goiter. But *do not* feed too much iodine. Marine stressed the precaution: Coindet had been severely criticized in 1824 for causing toxic nodular goiter; Jod-Basedow's thyroiditis was thought to be caused by abuse of iodine medication. Iodine thyroiditis, though rare, was a clinical entity.

[See Vig1920 .Mar]

In a memorial lecture 35 years after his announcement of iodine prophylaxis for goiter, Marine reminded physicians of a 1929 hysteria: "... *Many kinds of iodine medication, including candies, tablets, and chewing-gum, ran wild; and there occurred a rapid rise in the hospital admission rates of adenomatous goiter with hyperthyroidism.*" [AnIM 41:875, 1954]

Marine's 1954 warning would conveniently be forgotten in the 1980s when it became more profitable to sue for fallout radiation damage.

[See Vig1970 .Iod]

PAUL VILLARD PROPOSES A UNIT OF RADIATION
(Eight Years After Naming the Gamma Rays)

J.J. Thomson had immediately verified the "X-ray" item in the Times (London) on 6 Jan 1896. [See Vig 1895 .X-R] He was on the way to measuring the basic charge on the atom, but allowed a diversion. He enlisted the help of his first graduate student, E. Rutherford, and quickly discovered that the new X-rays "electrified" the air. After naming it "ionization" he went back to his e/m studies, but encouraged the student to study more about this interesting ionization phenomenon.

Rutherford was looking at the ions bounced off sheets of zinc under ultra-violet light when he read about the two Curies' finding materials in uranium more "radioactive" (Marie had just coined the word) than pure uranium. This "radioactivity" was a kind of ionization. He obtained some uranium salts, but soon found thorium salts much more "active" to work with, and, incidentally, cheaper.

In comparing UV light ions with those from a Crookes tube and now from uranium and thorium, he soon learned that two very different types of rays were produced. He called them alpha and beta and intended to add Roentgen and Becquerel's penetrating rays to the list later. As the newly appointed McGill professor of experimental physics, Rutherford had to pack his bags and get to Montreal. He sent his paper on alpha and beta observations to Phil Mag as his first contribution from the new lab. [PM xlvii(5):109, 1899]

In order to characterize the rays, Rutherford had used Plückers deviation in a magnetic field. Beta rays emanating from thorium salts deviated, but alpha rays were non-deviable. (Wrong! Wilhelm Wein had shown that kanalstrahlen were heavy particles and required very strong magnetic fields. He soon learned that alphas are very heavy. [See Vig1906 .JJ])

Some physicists considered the non-deviable rays immaterial waves, but Rutherford concentrated on another difference — their penetrating power. Beta rays showed remarkable penetration of dense matter, up to millimeters. Alpha rays, on the other hand, could not penetrate a thin sheet of paper. Rutherford aimed at characterizing alpha and beta rays; X-rays were pushed aside.

Paul Villard Dissects Non-Deviable Rays

While Rutherford was busy discovering gaseous emanation from thorium, Paul Villard at the Ecole Normale Supérieure in Paris studied the nature of the non-deviable rays from radium. His observations implied two kinds: Rutherford's easily absorbed alphas, and also some rays that penetrated sheets of metal. He borrowed a stronger source of radium from Pierre Curie (a few milligrams), covered it with a 1 cm thick sheet of lead and exposed a photographic plate. Something penetrated the dense metal. Following Rutherford's example he called his "non-deviables" gamma rays. [Compt rend 130:1178, 1930]

He set up an electroscope for more sensitive detection. It was possible, he learned, to detect rays after penetrating 30 cm of iron. They could not be deviated in his strongest magnetic field and they caused considerable ionization in air. He wanted to quantify his measurements, but no unit of "radiation" quantity existed. Marie Curie was using "uranies," a mg of uranium equivalent. The X-ray people had devised a few radiometers for X-rays, but gamma rays were not the same (until Friedrich showed in 1912 that X-rays originated in electron fields, gammas originated in the nucleus).

Villard (1860–1934) was a physical chemist by training and brought a chemical point of view to all of his research on ionizing radiation. He studied the reducing action of cathode rays and X-rays as well. As a physical chemist he thought the unit of quantity should be a measure of ionization that caused changes — the number of electrical charges.

The unit of X-ray quantity is *"that which liberates by ionization one electrostatic unit of electricity per cubic centimeter of air under normal conditions of temperature and pressure."* [Arch d'Elec Med 16:692, 1908]

In 1918 Walter Friedrich would tell his students O. Glasser and H. Behnken to find a way to measure Villard's unit.

[See Vig1928 .R The roentgen]

CHRONOLOGY OF NUCLEAR MEDICINE — 1910

			Ref.
	Scientific and Technical Background		
1. Basic	— J.J. Thomson deflects positive rays in a magnetic field.	[1905]	Bio
2. Obser	— A. Van den Broek: decay of light elements increases At Wt by 2.	[1905]	Na
	— W. Markwald notes MsTH-1, Th X & Ra are chem inseparable.	[1909]	BDCG
	— E. Rutherford can't find + electron in scattered rays.	[1932]	LRB
	— D. Florence relates scattering to angle of incidence.	[1909]	PM
3. # Nuc	— O. Hahn discovers branches Ac C″, TH C″, Ra C′.	[1909]	PZ
	— Geiger finds true ThA (1.78×10^{-3} Po-216); changes names.	[1904]	PZ
	— A. Debierne remeasures the emanation of radium.	[1900]	CRS
4. # Med	—		
	Organizations and Internal Politics		
5. Pols	—		
6. Socs	— Brussels Congress of Radiol & Electricity (13–15 Sep).	[1909]	VPG
	— Sixth Int Cong of Med Electrol & Radiol held in Prague.	[1908]	AEM
	— Whitehead & Russell begin pub: "Principia Mathematica."	[1899]	Bk
7. Event	— M. Curie isolates first metallic Ra, At Wt = 226.4; density 6.	[1904]	CRS
	— T. Morgan finds a white eyed mutant fruit fly.	[1907]	Bk
	— H. Kamerling-Onnes gets down to 0.8° K.	[1908]	DSB
	Instruments, Units of Measurement, and Drugs		
8. Instr	— O. Hahn develops the first beta ray spectrometer.	[1908]	PZ
9. Units	— FIRST INT CONFERENCE ON RADIOLOGY HELD IN BRUSSELS.	[1909]	ArRR
	adopts definition of "Curie" (after Pierre).	[1906]	Na
	adopts terms, Half-Value-Period, "active deposit."	[1902]	VPG
	— Int Ra Stds Comm decides not to make std solutions.	[1940]	GMP
	— E. Mach unit = ion current @0.001 abs elec unit = 3×10^{-13} amp.	[1909]	VPG
	— B. Szillard proposes mega-mega ion unit (forgets walls).	[1905]	DGP
	— E. Speder compares B, BW, WH, W rad "hardness" units:	[1909]	AEM
	compares H, S, B, I, M, X, K rad "intensity" units.	[1909]	AEM
10. Concp	—		
11. Drugs	— A. Debierne devises a Ra-Rn cow system for Curie lab.	[1908]	DSB
	— P. Erlich begins "chemotherapy" (his name), makes salvarsan.	[1935]	DSB
	— J. Loeb says chemical tropisms occur in lower animals.	[1899]	DSB

Radioiodine, P-32, and Radioactive Therapy			
12. I-Res —			
13. I-Dx —			
14. I-Rx —	G. Schwarz cures 90% of 40 Basedow's patients (X-ray).	[1906]	FGR
—	J. Ludin surveys 208 articles on X-ray cures of goiter.	[1906]	CGMC
15. P-Rx —			
16. Tele —			
17. Other —	L. Wickham writes textbook on "Radium Therapy."	[1903]	Bk
Scans and Other Tests of Function in Various Organs			
18. Brain —			
19. Heart —	H. Recklinghausen studies pulse and BP recordings.	[1909]	FM
—	E. Libman: etiology of subacute infectious endocarditis.	[1909]	AJMS
—	W. Obrastzow finds and studies coronary thrombosis.	[1903]	FM
—	H. Vaquez develops theory of R & L ventricular failure.	[1899]	Bk
—	H. Schottmueller studies bacterial endocarditis.	[1904]	CDD
—	W. Straub studies the isolated frog's heart.	[1846]	CDD
20. Liver —	G. Mills notes inflammatory reparable reaction to hi-dose.	[1906]	La
—	G. Pfahler sees gallstones on X-Ray.	[1907]	QJR
21. Lung —	L. Cole describes early tuberculosis.	[1909]	AJMS
22. Bone —			
23. Kidney —	H. Baker measures the capacity of the renal pelvis.	[1902]	SGO
—	W. Braasch lists deformities of renal pelvis.	[1902]	AnS
—	J. Cunningham Dx stricture of urethra by X-Ray.	[1902]	TAGU
—	A. Uhle combines cystoscopy and X-Ray examinations.	[1909]	AnS
24. Gut —	I. Pavlov studies the work of the digestive glands.	[1909]	Bk
25. Blood —			
26. Other —	E. Odie publishes "Diseases of the Pancreas."	[1896]	Bk
Radiation Hysteria and Health Physics	* Obituaries *		
27. Hyst —	Phrenological Journal ceases publication (See 1934).	[1831]	EB
28. React —	H. Guilleminot: lo-dose increases germination of seeds.	[1904]	CRSB
29. Respo —			

* * *

30. Obits —	F. Nightingale (1820–1910) Eng nurse; begins patient care.	EB
—	S. Cannizzaro (1826–1910) It chem; resurrected Avogadro.	DSB
—	R. Koch (1843–1910) Ger bacty; bacteriologic cause of disease.	Bio

CHRONOLOGY OF NUCLEAR MEDICINE — 1911

			Ref.
	Scientific and Technical Background		
1. Basic	— E. RUTHERFORD ANNOUNCES THE NUCLEAR ATOM.	[1902]	PM
	— A. Van den Broek: each element has its own atomic charge.	[1910]	Na
	— K. Fajans discovers branching decay, RaC to RaC'' (Tl-210).	[1910]	PZ
2. Obser	— G. Hevesy asked to separate Ra D from lead (fails).	[1907]	ARR
	— F. Soddy says some new °species are chemically similar.	[1907]	JCS
	— C.T.R. Wilson modifies Cloud Chamber to "see" radiation.	[1896]	V107
	— V. Hess takes an electroscope up in a balloon.	[1925]	V107
	— C. Barkla's measurements lead to nmbr of atom's electrons.	[1908]	PM
3. # Nuc	— H. Geiger's 1903 "E" rays are Actinium A (2×10^{-3}s Po-215).		PM
	— G. Antonoff discovers UY (1.03d Th-231), disputed.	[1913]	PM
	— A. Van den Broek: # of elements must = # of possible charges.	[1910]	PZ
4. # Med	—		
	Organizations and Internal Politics		
5. Pols	— M. Curie awarded second Nobel prize (this time in chem).	[1903]	Bio
6. Socs	—		
7. Event	— R. Millikan devises "falling drop" unit charge exper.	[1908]	DSB
	— Royal Marsden Hosp hires a part time X-ray physicist.	[1935]	ArRR
	Instruments, Units of Measurement, and Drugs		
8. Instr	— F. Groedel describes a cine apparatus for resp motions.	[1909]	FGR
9. Units	— Mache unit (not Mach) used in radon sip & breath Rx.	[1913]	BMJ
	— W. Hampson develops a "radiometer" for short doses.	[1907]	ArRR
10. Concp	— G. Fabre describes how radium stops growth of plants.	[1901]	CRB
11. Drugs	— S. Saubermann notes increased metabolism after IV Rn.	[1908]	La

Radioiodine, P-32, and Radioactive Therapy

12. I-Res —			
13. I-Dx —			
14. I-Rx —	R. Abbe describes 6 year cure of goiter with radium.	[1904]	AnS
15. P-Rx —			
16. Tele —	D. Cheron develops radiotherapy for uterine fibromata.	[1906]	AEM
17. Other —	A. Pinch relates first radon brachytherapy (from Ra cow).	[1908]	BMJ
—	S. Saubermann sums 1000 articles on radon Rx in 12 dis.	[1908]	ArRR
—			

Scans and Other Tests of Function in Various Organs

18. Brain —			
19. Heart —	L. Ehrenberg describes two cases of tumors of the heart.	[1905]	DAKM
20. Liver —			
21. Lung —	H. Dunham: technique for reading stereo chest plates.	[1900]	QAR
—	H. Hulst reviews auscultation vs X-Ray in TBC.	[1909]	QAR
22. Bone —	R. Hammond discusses X-Rays of chronic joint disease.	[1910]	QAR
23. Kidney—	L. Jaches uses opaque dyes to see pelvis and ureters.	[1910]	NYMR
24. Gut —	W. Cannon pubs "Mechanical Factors of Digestion."	[1910]	Bk
—	H. Ashbury confirms Dx of gastric & duodenal ulcers.	[1910]	AQR
—	A. Hurst pubs "Sensitivity of the Alimentary Canal."	[1903]	Bk
—	G. Pfahler sees "adhesions" in the gastric region.	[1910]	JAMA
—	L. Cole lists types of gastric peristalsis.	[1909]	ArRR
25. Blood —	H. Rudberg sees lymphs entering blood after irradiation.	[1906]	BMJ
26. Other —	J. Bergonie shows lower salivary secretion after irrad.	[1984]	AEM
—	W. Manges: how to measure the female pelvis in stereo.	[1906]	QAR

Radiation Hysteria and Health Physics * Obituaries *

27. Hyst —	G. Schwarz shows 3 rad leukemia deaths (chron rad synd).	[1905]	BKW
—	S. Lange introduces thymus irradiation with high doses.	[1905]	QAR
	(S. Lange becomes Pres. Am Roent Soc in 1913.)	[1976]	AJR
28. React —			
29. Respo —			

* * *

30. Obits —	F. Galton (1822–1911) ıg anthropol; eugenics, statistics.	DSB
—	G. Stoney (1826–191´ ır physics; first use of name "electron."	DSB

CHRONOLOGY OF NUCLEAR MEDICINE — 1912

Scientific and Technical Background

			Ref.
1. Basic	— M. von Laue proves X-rays are electromagnetic waves.	[1903]	WoA
	— M. von Laue discovers X-ray diffraction in crystals.	[1909]	WoA
	— K. Fajans determines the radioactive displacement laws. DISCOVERY OF "PLEIADES" (soon called ISOTOPES)	[1913]	V4
	— W. Friedrich clarifies the nature of X vs gamma rays.	[1908]	BAW
	— W.L. Bragg measures the spectrum of mica scattered rays.	[1908]	Na
	— W.L. Bragg derives a law of crystal diffraction angles.	[1908]	PCPS
2. Obser	— W. Bragg sees need for X-ray energy spectrum analysis.	[1909]	WoA
	— G. Hevesy discovers radium D and lead are identical.	[1909]	PZ
	— A. Van den Broek postulates ordinal atomic number system.	[1911]	WoA
	— N. Bohr thinks ordinal atomic numbers must be critical.	[1911]	ARR
	— A. Russell proves Boltwood's "ionium" is thorium.	[1908]	PRS
3. # Nuc	— F. Soddy discovers Actinium C' (0.56s Po-211).	[1909]	CN
	— H. Geiger discovers Uranium II (2.5 × 10^5y U-234).	[1911]	PM
	— A. Fleck: Th B is lead, UX is thorium, but misses on AcX.	[1910]	CN
	— 30 species of °activity exist in nature, but some are disputed.		GSA
4. # Med	—		

Organizations and Internal Politics

5. Pols	— Remains of "Piltdown man" found, Lewes Eng (Hoax! see 1953)		AP
6. Socs	— Seventh & last Int Cong of Med Elec & Radiol held in Lyon.	[1910]	AEM
	— O. Lichenstern pubs "Influenza in the 19th Century."	[1910]	Bk
7. Event	— H. Hoover translates "De Re Metallica."	[1910]	Bk

Instruments, Units of Measurement, and Drugs

8. Instr	— G. Barkla is building a large wall-less ion chamber.	[1905]	ArRR
	— C.T.R. Wilson photographs ion tracks in cloud chamber.	[1911]	PM
	— C.T.R. Wilson adds automatic lights for photos, enlarges chamber.	[1925]	PM
	— H. Geiger's string electrometer measures current leak.	[1895]	PM
	— T. Richards: how submerged float gives fluid density.	[1915]	JACS
9. Units	— Int Ra Std Comm calibrates a 21.99 mg Ra primary std.	[1910]	ArRR
	— W. Marrison builds first quartz-crystal clock (sec/3y).	[1920]	NBS
10. Concp	— T. Christian defines Half-Value-Layer (HVL) as "quality."	[1905]	VDRG
	— F. Billines sees "focal infection" as cause of disease.	[1907]	ArIM
	— P. Debye: theory of "specific heat" of solids.	[1871]	DSB
11. Drugs	— C. Funk coins the name "Vitamine" for vital amine.	[1907]	DSB
	— P. Erlich develops acriflavine as topical antiseptic.	[1908]	DSB

Radioiodine, P-32, and Radioactive Therapy				
12. I-Res	—			
13. I-Dx	—			
14. I-Rx	—			
15. P-Rx	—			
16. Tele	—			
17. Other	—	First implants of Rn tubes at London Ra Institute.	[1908]	ArRR
Scans and Other Tests of Function in Various Organs				
18. Brain	—	V. Kafka injects fluorescein SQ to stain some tissues.	[1904]	ZGNP
	—	H. Cushing pubs "Pituitary Body and its Disorders."	[1886]	Bk
19. Heart	—	E. Starling develops heart-lung preparation in dog.	[1910]	JPh
	—	J. Herrick describes clinical pic of coronary disease.	[1878]	JAMA
	—	F. Bleichroder passes ureteric catheter into heart.	[1905]	BKW
	—	H. Vaquez makes X-Rays an integral part of cardiology.	[1904]	JAMA
	—	G. Stewart writes "The Circulation in Man."	[1897]	Bk
	—	Y. Henderson studies closure of the heart valves.	[1910]	AJPh
20. Liver	—	A. Hess describes icterus neonatorum.	[1908]	AJDC
21. Lung	—	F. Arrillaga describes arteriosclerosis in pulm artery.	[1815]	CDD
	—	L. Hill describes "Caisson Sickness."	[1925]	Bk
22. Bone	—			
23. Kidney	—			
24. Gut	—	C. Regaud describes GI damage from hi-dose rad in dogs.	[1906]	AEM
	—	W. Cannon studies peristaltic reflexes.	[1908]	AJPh
	—	J. Hartwell seeks cause-of-death in intestinal obstruct.	[1909]	JAMA
25. Blood	—	O. Schloss describes etiology, hemorrhag dis of newborn.	[1909]	AJDC
26. Other	—	C. Funk discovers and names some vitamins.	[1906]	DSB
Radiation Hysteria and Health Physics		* Obituaries *		
27. Hyst	—	C. Gauss describes his "roentgenkater "(X-Ray hangover).	[1905]	Str
28. React	—			
29. Respo	—			

* * *

30. Obits	—	J. Lister (1827–1912) Eng surg; developer of surgical sterility.	Bio
	—	L. Boisbandrau (1838–1912) Fr chem; discovered gallium.	DSB

CHRONOLOGY OF NUCLEAR MEDICINE — 1913

Scientific and Technical Background

			Ref.
1. Basic	— After 98 years Prout is proved correct by Moseley.	[1903]	V92
	— N. Bohr revises Rutherford's nuclear atom.	[1911]	PM
	THE TRUE BEGINNING OF NUCLEAR PHYSICS AND CHEMISTRY		
	— E. Rutherford says alpha & beta originate in nucleus.	[1910]	Na
	— E. Rutherford says gammas originate from electrons (wrong).	[1910]	Na
	— W. Bragg confirms Friedrich's origin of X vs gamma rays.	[1912]	PRS
	— A. Van den Broek says charge on nucleus = Atomic Number.	[1911]	Na
	— H. Geiger proves nuclear atom by alpha scattering exp.	[1911]	PM
	— K. Fajans proposes radioactive displacement laws.	[1912]	CZ
2. Obser	— J.J. Thomson's 2 parabolic lines of Ne are called contamination.		Bk
	— N. Bohr says Thomson's parabolic X-3 could be H-3.	[1885]	Eve
	— F. Aston separates Ne-20, Ne-22 by diffusion (questioned).	[1919]	Bk
	— K. Fajans predicts Pb from diff sources have diff At Wt.	[1907]	CZ
	— A. Fleck summarizes 6 chemically similar twin "elements."	[1912]	CN
	— F. Soddy says a few "elements" are chemically identical.	[1912]	CN
	— F. Soddy uses word "isotopes" for first time.	[1912]	CN
	— A. Fleck tells how M. Todd coined "isotope" for Soddy.	(1963	PCSI)
	— 5 scientists say chem identical "elements" have diff At Wt.		V97
	— E. Rutherford: Fajans' UX$_2$ was first proof of isotopes.	[1912]	Lt
	— J. Gray questions wavelength shift in scattering.	[1912]	PM
	— Bragg & Bragg discuss possibilities of a spectrometer.	[1912]	PRS
	— Bragg & Bragg show the crystal structure of diamond.	[1912]	Na
3. # Nuc	— H. Moseley proves Ordinal Atomic Numbers rank 92 elements.		V98
	FIRST ANSWER TO BOYLE'S 1661 QUESTION, "HOW MANY ELEMENTS"?		
	— K. Fajans discovers UX$_2$ called Brevium (1.1m Pa-234).	[1921]	PZ
	— B. Boltwood says actinium D (Pb-207) is stable lead.	[1907]	V97
	— A. Russell assigns RaC" to Pb (wrong), ThD to Pb (correct).	[1912]	CN
4. # Med	—		

Organizations and Internal Politics

5. Pols	— U.S. Bureau of mines estimates 30 g radium are separated.	[1948]	EB
	— J.D. Rockefeller founds Rock Institute with $100 million.	[1909]	AP
6. Socs	— Brit Assoc meets in Birmingham, its most famous session.	[1932]	Na
	— Am J Roent begins publication for Am Roent Ray Society.	[1960]	AJR
	— H. Vaquez sees Roentgenology as a branch of cardiology.	[1909]	CRB
	— German Roent Soc pubs 1 page rad protec (safety) rules.	[1908]	Str
	— J.J. Thomson's "Rays of Positive Electricity" published.	[1964]	Bk
	— G. Hevesy & F. Paneth begin writing on new "°indicators."	[1911]	ZAC
	FIRST PUBLICATIONS ON RADIOISOTOPE TRACERS		
	— Chem Rubber Handbk of Chem and Physics begins publication.		HCP
7. Event	— First radium extraction from carnotite in SW Colorado.	[1899]	GSA
	— K. Fajans explains how the Periodic Table accommodates isotopes.		PZ
	— V. Hess takes Hevesy up in balloon to see "cosmic rays."	[1911]	ARR
	— G. Hevesy does first "°isotope" exp (RaD as Pb tracer).	[1907]	ZAC
	— W. Duane proposes radium cow to Harvard Cancer Commiss.	[1908]	BMSJ
	— First radiology training offered MDs (4 weeks full time).	[1948]	AJR
	— C. Fabry discovers ozone in upper atmosphere.	[1840]	Sc

Instruments, Units of Measurement, and Drugs

8.	Instr	— W. Bragg devises an X-ray spectrometer.	[1912]	BJR
		— W. Coolidge introduces hot cathode, hi-volt, X-ray tube. THE TRUE BEGINNING OF X-RAY THERAPY	[1907]	PR
		— H. Geiger counts betas in charged tube (first step to GM)	[1908]	VDPG
		— H. Geiger develops "point counter," small hole in cathode.	[1908]	VDPG
		— A. Lamb uses submerged float, measures density of fluids.	[1912]	JACS
		— F. Groedel gives technique for roentgenkinematographie.	[1911]	DMW
9.	Units	— NBS gets first 20.28 mg Ra standard (only °std for 21y).	[1912]	NBS
		— Ra Std signed by E. Rutherford, M. Curie, & S. Meyer.	[1910]	GMP
		— H. Mache proposes 0.001 esu of emanation = 3.64×10^{-10} Ci/l.		LPP
		— D. Saubermann says use 1K to 10K Mache units in Rn Rx for pain; the Rn solution must glow faintly in dark.	[1911]	ArRR
		— G. Mackee describes current problems with S-N Pastilles.	[1904]	AmJR
10.	Concp	— G. Holmes proposes a standard Rx dose measure system.	[1909]	AJR
		— M. Bodenstein forms concept of chemical chain reaction.	[1910]	DSB
11.	Drugs	— W. McCollum isolates Vitamin A.	[1907]	DSB
		— R. Willstätter discovers composition of chlorophyll.	[1910]	DSB

Radioiodine, P-32, and Radioactive Therapy

12.	I-Res	— H. Plummer describes the toxic nodular goiter.	[1951]	AJMS
13.	I-Dx	—		
14.	I-Rx	— J. Mannaberg treats Basedow's with X-rays to ovaries.	[1910]	WKW
15.	P-Rx	—		
16.	Tele	—		
17.	Other	— F. Proescher reports first use of IV Ra salts in USA.	[1903]	Bk
		— L. Rowntree sums results of radon Rx in 1038 patients.	[1911]	JAMA

Scans and Other Tests of Function in Various Organs

18.	Brain	— E. Goldmann finds (and names) blood-brain barrier.	[1897]	SA
		— S. Flexner studies poliomyelitis.	[1876]	JAMA
19.	Heart	— Y. Henderson measures factors in arterial volumes.	[1912]	AJPh
20.	Liver	— G. Whipple studies experimental obstructive icterus.	[1909]	JEM
		— N. Brill describes "Gaucher's" splenomegaly.	[1982]	AJMS
21.	Lung	—		
22.	Bone	—		
23.	Kidney	—		
24.	Gut	— A. Hertz describes normal movements of the colon.	[1909]	JPh
25.	Blood	—		
26.	Other	— B. Shick devises diphtheria immunity test.	[1902]	CDD
		— A. Friedlander discusses Dx & Rx of enlarged thymus.	[1911]	AJDC
		— J. Hubbard says scarlet F differs from measles erythema.	[1876]	MR

Radiation Hysteria and Health Physics * Obituaries *

27.	Hyst	— S. Lange's success proves thymus irradiation harmless.	[1911]	AJR
		— A. Solomon does first mammography with X-Rays.	[1953]	AKC
		— A. Fernau first describes hemorrhagic phase of Ac Rad Syn.	[1905]	Str
		— A. Arnstein finds no lung ca in Joachimsthal miners.	(1932	AJC)
28.	React	— O. Loew notes lo-dose U salts stimulate plant growth.	[1910]	CZ
29.	Respo	— U.S. Supreme Court rules X-Ray burn is not negligence.	[1901]	—

* * *

30. Obits —

CHRONOLOGY OF NUCLEAR MEDICINE — 1914

			Ref.
	Scientific and Technical Background		
1. Basic	— O. Hoenigschmidt confirms transmutation by Atomic Wts.	[1900]	Ber
	— M. Siegbahn shows relation, wavelength and absorption.	[1909]	PZ
	— T. Richards proves multiple At Wts/element exist.	[1907]	JACS
2. Obser	— K. Fajans announces Lembert's 2 diff At Wts for Pb.	[1913]	ZE
	— Curie, Hoenigschmidt, Richards, Soddy find multi At Wts for Pb.		DSB
	— H. Moseley says At Numbers, isotopes no longer in doubt.	[1913]	Bio
	— G. Hevesy says isotope not accepted by phys or chemists.	[1919]	PZ
	— K. Nims (1924) says price of Ra is $120,000/g.	[1902]	Rad
3. # Nuc	— O. Hahn discovers UY (1.03d Th-231).	[1912]	PZ
	— Of 70 Rare Earths announced, Moseley's At Numbers allow 16.		V97
4. # Med	—		
	Organizations and Internal Politics		
5. Pols	— Name St. Petersberg changed to Petrograd. [Leningrad in 1924]		EB
6. Socs	— J. Jeans publishes "Radiation and the Quantum Theory."	[1905]	Bk
	— W. Duane teaches physicians diff between X & gamma rays.	[1913]	AJR
7. Event	— Duetsch Bunsen-Gesellschaft toasts Fajans for isotopes.	[1912]	V98
	— E. Rona coins "radioactive label" for isotope use.	[1913]	ZPC
	— Austrian Archduke Ferdinand assassinated, 28 June 1914.	[1939]	AP
	Instruments, Units of Measurement, and Drugs		
8. Instr	— W. Duane invents the parallel plate ionization chamber.	[1912]	AJR
	— W. Coolidge explains hot cathode hi-vacuum X-ray tube.	[1913]	GSR
9. Units	— THE "CURIE UNIT" RADIOACTIVITY STANDARDS ARE ACCEPTED.	[1910]	Eve
	— A. Debierne first uses "millicurie" for med radium dose.	[1916]	CRS
	— W. Duane proposes dose E = esu/cc air; intensity = E sec.	[1908]	AJR
	— B. Szilard proposes mega-mega ion (same as Villard unit).	[1908]	Str
10. Concp	— E. Rosenow sees mouth infection source of systemic dis.	[1912]	JAMA
	— L. Halberstädter exposes trypanosomes to X-rays.	[1909]	BKW
11. Drugs	—		

Radioiodine, P-32, and Radioactive Therapy

12. I-Res — E. Kendall discovers and prepares pure thyroxin. [1907] CDD
13. I-Dx —
14. I-Rx — M. Ludin summarizes Rx of Morbus Basedowii with X-rays. [1910] Chi
15. P-Rx —
16. Tele —
17. Other — C. Regaud uses radon in tubes for experimental therapy; [1912] AEM
is convinced, but can't prove, value of protraction [1926] CRS

Scans and Other Tests of Function in Various Organs

18. Brain — C. McCord views pineal as causing "sexual effects." [1867] JAMA
— W. Manges shows X-Rays of obscure head lesions. [1911] AJR
19. Heart — O. Frank adds a new tech for recording heart sounds. [1907] FM
— T. Lewis describes excitation of auricles. [1907] PTRS
— A. Carrel performs first heart surgery (on dog). [1902] DSB
— D. Gerhardt sums current Vienna ideas on endocarditis. [1910] Bk
— H. Gasser studies effects of exercise on heart rate. [1912] AJPh
20. Liver — A. George demonstrates gallstones with X-Ray. [1913] NEJM
21. Lung — S. Iglauer visualizes (X-Ray) the larnyx and trachea. [1912] JAMA
22. Bone — P. Hickey describes X-Ray techniques for seeing mastoid. [1911] AJR
23. Kidney — F. Volhard studies relation of nephritis & hypertension. [1899] CDD
— F. Barrington describes the physiology of micturition. [1921] QJPh
24. Gut — J. Gunn studies in vivo survival of swine intestine. [1912] QJPh
— J. Case studies visualization of intestinal stasis. [1913] SGO
— J. Case describes (X-Ray) peri- & anti-peristalsis. [1913] NYMR
— A. George describes X-Rays of gut on 1000 patients. [1913] AJR
— F. deQuervain describes (X-Ray) sigmoid diverticula. [1912] DZfC
25. Blood —
26. Other — H. Schmidt notes dry saliv glands after hi-dose irrad. [1965] VDRG
— A. Hess experiments with German measles. [1912] ArIM

Radiation Hysteria and Health Physics * Obituaries *

27. Hyst — D. TIRABOSCHI, RADIOTHERAPIST, DIES OF OVEREXPOSURE TO RAD;
AUTOPSY SHOWS "PROFOUND ESSENTIAL ANEMIA." [1934] ArRR
28. React — C. Holland reports first success in finding lost radium. [1938] ArRR
29. Respo —

* * *

30. Obits — J. Hittorf (1824–1914) Ger physics; Plücker's cathode rays. DSB

CHRONOLOGY OF NUCLEAR MEDICINE — 1915

			Ref.
	Scientific and Technical Background		
1. Basic	— A. Einstein develops General Theory of Relativity.	[1905]	WoA
	— A. Einstein says light rays are affected by gravity.	[1910]	WoA
	— P. Bridgmann achieves a pressure of 20,000 atmospheres.	[1905]	DSB
2. Obser	— F. Soddy proves U is parent of Ra by growth experiment.	[1908]	Bk
	— G. Hevesy: isotopes have slight diff rates of exchange.	[1939]	Bk
3. # Nuc	—		
4. # Med	—		
	Organizations and Internal Politics		
5. Pols	— Western Roentgen Soc formed, publishes J of Radiology.	[1920]	Rad
6. Socs	— T. Morgan's "Mechanism of Mendelian Heredity" published.	[1907]	Bk
	— G. Cantor writes ". . . Theory of Transfinite Numbers."	[1854]	DSB
7. Event	— J. Kendall isolates a dysentary bacillus.	[1905]	CDD
	— E. von Schweiler hails Elster & Geitel discov of bkgnd.	[1901]	Nw
	— W.H. & W.L. Bragg (father and son) awarded Nobel prize.	[1911]	DSB
	Instruments, Units of Measurement, and Drugs		
8. Instr	— L. Adams uses refractive index to measure H_2O density.	[1913]	JACS
	— F. Dessauer ciné X-Rays described in Scientific American.	[1911]	SA
9. Units	— R. Furstenau uses Se resistor for intensity meter.	[1914]	PZ
10. Concp	— C. Evans measures gas metabolism of the heart.	[1907]	JPh
	— J. Case describes the post-op GI X-Ray.	[1913]	JAMA
	— S. Russ debates hard vs soft rays in Rx uses.	[1909]	BJR
11. Drugs	— W. DUANE DESIGNS FIRST RADIUM COW, EXPLAINS ITS ECONOMY.	[1913]	BMSJ
	— W. Duane collects Rn in glass tubes for implant Rx.	[1928]	BMSJ
	— A. Debierne milks Curie's Ra; puts Rn into tubes for Rx.	[1914]	CRS
	— R. Cooke discovers active immunization for hay fever.	[1912]	LI

Radioiodine, P-32, and Radioactive Therapy

12. I-Res	— E. Kendall discovers and crystallizes thyroxine.	[1914]	TAAP
13. I-Dx	—		
14. I-Rx	— G. Pfahler says X-ray is choice exoph goiter therapy.	[1910]	AJR
15. P-Rx	—		
16. Tele	—		
17. Other	— W. Morton says IV radium has great healing powers.	[1926]	MRNY
	— 26 authors (e.g., J. Rosenbloom) document IV Ra cures.	[1911]	AJMS
	— S. Russ pubs early txtbk on Ra Rx — before Rn cows.	[1914]	Bk
	— H. Kelly treats ca of cervix with radium.	[1914]	JAMA

Scans and Other Tests of Function in Various Organs

18. Brain	—		
	— W. Dandy finds nothing from extirpation of pineal gland.	[1914]	JEM
19. Heart	— H. Mautner notes venous discharge of lung, liver sluices.	[1912]	WMW
	— T. Janeway discusses what's learned from blood pressure.	[1910]	JHHB
	— T. Lewis describes excitement of the ventricles.	[1914]	PTRS
	— H. Wessler: role of X-Ray in DDx of obscure heart dis.	[1911]	AJR
20. Liver	— S. Okada studies the chemical reactions of bile.	[1913]	JPh
21. Lung	—		
22. Bone	— E. Locke sees secondary hypertrophic osteoarthropathy.	[1903]	ArIM
23. Kidney	—		
24. Gut	— W. Alvarez begins his study of gut peristalsis.	[1909]	AJPh
	— A. Barclay sees (X-Ray) a peptic ulcer of esophagus.	[1911]	PRSM
	— R. Carman describes (X-Ray) GI ulcers.	[1914]	AJR
	— C. Grandy discusses X-Ray of diaphragmatic hernias.	[1913]	JAMA
25. Blood	— L. Rowntree introduces vital red for plasma volume.	[1899]	ArIM
26. Other	— C. Waters explain X-Ray technique nasal sinuses.	[1911]	AJR
	— G. Rost studies radiation bioeffect of X-rays on skin.	[1905]	Str

Radiation Hysteria and Health Physics * Obituaries *

27. Hyst	— S. SOCHOCKY INVENTS A New RADIUM LUMINOUS PAINT.	[1928]	(1962 JAMA)
	— Epidemic of tetanus in trenches reported.	[1912]	AP
	— M. Sanger jailed for writing first book on birth control.	[1904]	AP
28. React	— J. Murphy notes post-rad resistance in tumor regrafts.	[1906]	JEM
	— Brit Roent Soc suggests safety standards.	[1908]	ArRR
29. Respo	—		

* * *

30. Obits	— P. Ehrlich (1852–1915) Ger bacty; first chemotherapy.	DSB
	— H. Moseley (1887–1915) Eng physics; atomic numbers.	Blo

CHRONOLOGY OF NUCLEAR MEDICINE — 1916

			Ref.
	Scientific and Technical Background		Ref.
1. Basic —	A. Einstein describes a 4-D space-time interdependence.	[1907]	Bio
—	G. Lewis says that chemical bonds are shared electrons.	[1902]	DSB
2. Obser —	E. Gleditsch measures Ra $T_{1/2}$ at 1642-1674y (now 1600y).	[1899]	AJS
—	A. Eddington studies physical properties of stars.	[1905]	DSB
3. # Nuc —			
	Organizations and Internal Politics		
5. Pols —			
6. Socs —	Am Radium Soc formed, publishes with Am Roent Ray Soc.	[1900]	AJR
—	A. Carlson pubs "Control of Hunger in Health & Disease."	[1911]	Bk
7. Event —	Whole blood for transfusion is refrigerated (first time).	[1906]	JAMA
	Instruments, Units of Measurement, and Drugs		
8. Instr —	J. Shearer says kilovolt scales are bad, use spark-gap.	[1909]	AmJR
—	P. Langevin constructs ultrasonics for sub detection.	[1911]	DOS
—	H. Threlkold-Edwards teaches intensifying screen's use.	[1904]	AJR
9. Units —	Britain introduces "summertime" daylight-saving time.	[1948]	AP
10. Concp —	A. da Silvo Mello studies thorium salts in animals.	[1896]	ZKM
—	J. McNee describes louse-borne "trench fever."	[1903]	BMJ
11. Drugs —			

	Radioiodine, P-32, and Radioactive Therapy			
12. I-Res	— D. MARINE FINDS I-127 CLEARED FROM BLOOD BY THYROID.	[1907]	JPET
	— E. DuBois describes clinical calorimetry.	[1915]	AnIM
13. I-Dx	—		
14. I-Rx	—		
15. P-Rx	—		
16. Tele	—		
17. Other	— -. Ionescu does sympathectomy for painful angina pect.	[1914]	CDD
	Scans and Other Tests of Function in Various Organs		
18. Brain	— G. Horrax studies the pineal gland.	[1915]	ArIM
	— E. Skinner shows X-Rays of intracranial aerocele.	[1915]	AJR
19. Heart	— C. Iongsev introduces sympathectomy for angina pectoris.	[1912]	CDD
	— T. Lewis pubs "Clinical Disorders of the Heart Beat."	[1914]	Bk
	— C. Wiggers studies movement of mitral cusps in cycle.	[1915]	AJPh
	— A. Crane discusses roentgenography of the heart.	[1915]	AJR.
20. Liver	— J. Case gives statistics on pos & neg Dx of gallstones.	[1910]	AJR
21. Lung	— H. Dunham details X-Ray Dx of pulmonary TBC.	[1911]	AJR
	— G. Holmes describes resp moves of stomach & diaphragm.	[1915]	AJR
	— A. Moore shows diagnostic X-Rays of bronchiectasis.	[1906]	AJR
22. Bone	— H. Van Allen does accurate pelvimetry with X-Rays.	[1904]	AJR
23. Kidney	— J. Burns finds new agent for X-Ray pyelography-thorium.	[1928]	BJHH
	— A. Granger uses oxygen in X-Ray cysto- & pyelo-graphy.	[1911]	AJr
	— C. Holland describes uric acid calculi in X-Rays.	[1911]	AJR
24. Gut	— E. Sharpey-Schafer says no pancreatic juice in diabetes.	[1900]	CDD
	— H. Glasser studies drug response in small intestine motions.	[1914]	JPET
	— R. Carman finds X-Ray best Dx of duodenal ulcer.	[1915]	AJR
25. Blood	—		
26. Other	— B. Darling sees oral sepsis as a "focal-infection."	[1915]	AJR
	— P. Eisen sees mouth as source of "focal-infection."	[1915]	AJR
	— R. Ottolengui interprets dental X-Rays.	[1899]	AJR
	Radiation Hysteria and Health Physics * Obituaries *		
27. Hyst	— G. Holzknecht's irrad of G-pig "puberty gland" supports rejuv.		WKW
	— M. Sanger opens first birth control clinic.	[1915]	AP
28. React	— F. Pilz: lo-dose stimulates, hi-dose depresses pea growth.	[1913]	JChS
29. Respo	—		

* * *

30. Obits	— E. Mach (1838–1916) Aus physics; philos of science, space/time.	DSB
	— F. Dorn (1845–1916) Ger physics; discovered niton (radon).	DSB
	— S. Thompson (1851–1916) Eng physics; first X-Rays in England.	DSB
	— W. Ramsey (1852–1916) Eng chem; discovered inert gases.	DSB

CHRONOLOGY OF NUCLEAR MEDICINE — 1917

			Ref.
Scientific and Technical Background			
1. Basic	— L. de Broglie shows wavelength — absorption relationship.	[1914]	CRS
	— D. Webster shows X-ray spectrum of platinum.	[1913]	PR
2. Obser	— F. SODDY DISCOVERS "ISOBARS": "ELEMENTS" WITH EQUAL MASS BUT DIFFERENT CHEMISTRY.	[1918]	PRS
3. # Nuc	— O. Hahn discovers UX1 (32 500y Pa-231), credits Fajans.	[1913]	PZ
4. # Med	—		
Organizations and Internal Politics			
5. Pols	—		
6. Socs	—		
7. Event	— K. Fajans becomes Prof of Physical Chem at U of Munich.	[1914]	PI
	— W. Duane becomes first Prof of Biophysics (Harvard).	(1978	IJO)
Instruments, Units of Measurement, and Drugs			
8. Instr	—		
9. Units	— S. Russ suggests "Rad" unit (lethal mouse dose).	[1907]	V104
	— W. Duane shows how to calculate dose of radon.	[1914]	BMSJ
10. Concp	— R. Cecil Rx of arthritis with foreign protein inject.	[1912]	ArIM
	— H. Dunham explains pathology of X-Ray findings in TBC.	[1910]	AJR
	— A. George explains path of X-Rays findings in gbladder.	[1910]	AJR
11. Drugs	— W. Duane sets up first radium cow for medical radon.	[1915]	BMSJ
	— W. Park studies duration of antitoxin (diphth) immunity.	[1876]	APe

	Radioiodine, P-32, and Radioactive Therapy			
12. I-Res	—			
13. I-Dx	—			
14. I-Rx	—			
15. P-Rx	—			
16. Tele	—			
17. Other	— H. Janeway adopts Duane's 1908 "buried emanation Rx."	[1915]	AJR	
	— H. Janeway writes textbk on radium Rx of cancer (pre-Radon).	[1914]	Bk	
	— G. Failla teaches physics of radium Rx of cancer.	[1917]	Bk	
	— W. Duane reports on first 1080 pts treated with radon.	[1915]	BMSJ	
	— R. Frank gives 4000 mg h Ra before surg for cervical ca. (mg h Ra = milligram-hours of Ra exposure, used until 1940s)	[1914]	JCR	
	— W. von Jauregg treats syphilis with malaria injection.	[1915]	EB	
	Scans and Other Tests of Function in Various Organs			
18. Brain	— G. Johnston studies X-Rays of pituitary region.	[1912]	AJR	
	— F. Law describes X-Ray anat of sinuses & mastoid.	[1915]	AJR	
19. Heart	— C. Wiggers displays the time relations of heart sounds.	[1916]	AJPh	
	— C. Bolton discusses the pathology of "dropsy."	[1916]	BMJ	
	— R. Mopris: X-Ray vs percussion in Dx pericardial fluid.	[1896]	JAMA	
20. Liver	— J. Case describes X-Ray cholilithiasis Dx to surgeons.	[1916]	AnS	
21. Lung	— W. Boardman describes the X-Ray in pneumoconiosis.	[1904]	AJR	
	— A. Lanza studies X-Rays, 150 miners consumption pts.	[1916]	PHR	
22. Bone	— P. Hickey shows value of lateral views of spine.	[1916]	AJR	
	— J. Honeij describes bone changes in leprosy.	[1911]	AJR	
23. Kidney	—			
24. Gut	— K. Franz reports GI death after hi-dose Rx attempt.	[1912]	BKW	
	— W. Bayliss pubs "Physiology of Food & Economy in Diet."	[1907]	Bk	
	— I. LeWald shows X-Rays of 19 pts with stomach syphilis.	[1909]	AJR	
	— G. Mills studies relation: body build to visceral form.	[1907]	AJR	
25. Blood	—			
26. Other	— B. Bloch notes skin coloring in Addison's disease.	[1849]	DAKM	
	— C. Waters discusses polyps in maxillary sinuses.	[1915]	AJR	
	Radiation Hysteria and Health Physics	* Obituaries *		
27. Hyst	— S. Sochocky begins luminous dial painting in USA	(in Aub 1952 Med)		
28. React	— W. Davey: lo-dose lengthens life, hi-dose kills Tribolium.	[1916]	JEZ	
	— S. Freud's "Intro to Psychoanalysis" replaces Phrenology.	[1900]	Bk	
	— Four women jailed for picketing White House for suffrage.		AP	
29. Respo	—			

* * *

30. Obits —

CHRONOLOGY OF NUCLEAR MEDICINE — 1918

			Ref.
	Scientific and Technical Background		
1. Basic	— C. Ulrey measures energy of continuous X-ray spectrum.	[1906]	Pr
	— C. Ulrey measures ionization spectrum of W, Mo, Cr.	[1909]	PR
2. Obser	— A. Stewart's "Isobars" have constant At Wt (A).	[1906]	PM
	— E. Owen gives formula for X-ray absorption by At Weight.	[1917]	PRS
3. # Nuc	— O. Hahn names proto-actinium (3.28×10^4y Pa-231).	[1917]	Bio
	Organizations and Internal Politics		
5. Pols	— US Nat Bur of Standards begins X-ray testing and stds.	[1901]	AJR
	— NBS studies Pb-glass and Pb-rubber in X-ray protect.	[1907]	NBS
6. Socs	— Western Rad Soc begins publication of J of Radiology.	[1915]	JR
	— AMA sets up Med Research Brd to study aviation med.	[1786]	JAMA
	— F. Gay writes "Typhoid Fever."	[1907]	Bk
7. Event	— G. Kaye details changeover: glass plates to X-Ray film.	[1889]	Bk
	— RAF (Eng) gives excess "dial" Ra to Med Res Council.	[1915]	MRC
	— M. Planck awarded Nobel prize for quantum theory.	[1900]	DSB
	Instruments, Units of Measurement, and Drugs		
8. Instr	— A. Dempster builds first mass spectrometer (U Chicago).	[1919]	PR
	— W. Coolidge shows improved hot cathode in GE Review.	[1914]	AJR
9. Units	— H. Shapley determines dimensions of the Milky Way.	[1907]	EB
	— W. Friedrich assigns Glasser & Behnken to Villard's "e."	[1908]	Bk
	— S. RUSS ADOPTS "THRESHOLD ERYTHEMA DOSE" AT MEMORIAL (NY).	[1917]	ARE
	— F. Dessauer describes foundations for measuring dose.	[1917]	AG
10. Concp	— W. Friedrich gives physical & biol foundation for dose.	[1908]	Str
11. Drugs	— R. Tunnycliff studies immune reactions (Diplococci).	[1914]	JID
	— D. Cutler cultivates Entamoeba Histolitica.	[1901]	JPB

Radioiodine, P-32, and Radioactive Therapy

12. I-Res	— 30% of Michigan army draftees disqualified by goiter.	[1916]	V91
13. I-Dx	—		
14. I-Rx	—		
15. P-Rx	—		
16. Tele	—		
17. Other	— F. Dessauer gets homogenous dose with 2 beams of X-rays.	[1908]	AG
	— R. Cecil inocculates 12,519 men against pneumonia.	[1916]	JEM
	— B. Krönig & W. Friedrich: text "Phys & Bio Found of R Therapy."		Bk

Scans and Other Tests of Function in Various Organs

18. Brain	— G. Holmes shows X-Ray of intracranial aerocele.	[1916]	AJR
19. Heart	— E. Starling describes the "law of the heart."	[1912]	Bk
	— H. Christian reviews chronic myocarditis since 1909.	[1909]	JAMA
20. Liver	— B. Crawford implicates nitro & amido compounds in jaundice.	[1912]	BMJ
21. Lung	— H. Brooks describes 80 cases of emphysema.	[1912]	ArIM
	— A. Crane shows X-Rays of pulmonary metastases.	[1917]	AJR
	— G. Holmes shows multiple abscesses, spontaneous cure.	[1917]	AJR
	— C. Jackson puts opaque substance into bronchial tree.	[1916]	AJR
	— A. McMahon diagnoses primary ca of lung by X-Ray.	[1908]	JAMA
	— H. Pancoast studies dust inhalation with X-Rays.	[1917]	AJR
22. Bone	— F. Baetjer details DDx of bone tumors.	[1916]	AJr
	— T. Groover demonstrates technique for spine X-Rays.	[1917]	AJR
23. Kidney	— W. Manges sees value in pyeloscopy.	[1916]	AJR
24. Gut	— W. Lane describes surgery for chronic intestinal stasis.	[1916]	Bk
	— W. Alvarez finds irritability gradient in small gut.	[1916]	AJPh
	— J. Case studies X-Rays of colon diverticula.	[1915]	AJR
	— G. Holmes shows X-Rays of pedunculated stomach tumors.	[1917]	AJR
25. Blood	—		
26. Other	— J. Case tells history of X-Ray foreign body localization.	[1914]	AJR

Radiation Hysteria and Health Physics * Obituaries *

27. Hyst	— World wide influenza epidemic terminates World War I.	[1915]	EB
	— E. Steinach rejuvenates mid-aged people by gonad irrad.	[1916]	AP
28. React	— E. Rosa: first NBS project is leaded glass and rubber.	[1907]	AJR
	— J. Geiger describes 1914 German measles epidemic.	[1914]	JAMA
29. Respo	—		

* * *

30. Obits	— G. Cantor (1845–1918) Ger math; infinite series & infinity.		DSB
	— E. Caldwell (1870–1918) Am radiol; early X-Ray apparatus.		AJR

CHRONOLOGY OF NUCLEAR MEDICINE — 1919

		Scientific and Technical Background		Ref.
1.	Basic	— E. Rutherford bombards N (gas) with alphas to produce O + prot.		PM
		THE FIRST "ARTIFICIAL" TRANSMUTATION.	[1902]	
		— Rutherford atom requires "neutrons" (on 1933 hindsight).	[1902]	Eve
2.	Obser	— F. Aston proves "Whole Number Rule," verifies 1815 Prout.	[1913]	PM
		— Observation of solar eclipse is first to verify Einstein.	[1905]	Na
		— L. de Broglie does spectroscopy of x-rays.	[1917]	CRS
3.	# Nuc	— F. Aston's first mass spectrum proves his Ne-22 correct.	[1913]	Na
		— F. Aston says O & C are standard "simples" (no isotopes).	[1931]	Na
4.	# Med	—		

		Organizations and Internal Politics		
5.	Pols	— First meet, League of Nations. B. Mussolini founds "Fasci."		EB
6.	Socs	— T. Morgan publishes "Physical Basis for Heredity."	[1915]	Bk
		— A. Sommerfield publishes "Atombau u Spektrallinien."	[1917]	WoA
		— E. Lippman writes history of alchemy.	[1915]	DoE
		— W. Manges describes Camp Greenleaf (WW I) X-Ray school.		AJR
		— J. Barcat pubs history of H. Dominici (brachytherapy).	[1907]	ARE
7.	Event	— E. Rutherford gives (his) second Bakerian Lecture to Roy Soc;	[1914]	Eve
		predicts the existence of the "neutron."	[1932]	Eve

		Instruments, Units of Measurement, and Drugs		
8.	Instr	— F. Aston modifies Thomson's device (to a mass spectrometer).	[1918]	Na
		— A. Kovarik counts gamma rays with a pre-GM type tube.	[1913]	PR
9.	Units	— C. Regaud uses "millicuries-destroyed/hour" for dose unit.	[1914]	CRS
10.	Concp	— G. Warner: muscle/skin screen soft, hard rays differently.	[1914]	SGO
		— N. Alter notes histology post-rad of cervical ca.	[1906]	JMR
11.	Drugs	—		

		Radioiodine, P-32, and Radioactive Therapy		
12. I-Res	—	G. Murray tells 74y life hist of first pt on thy extract.	[1891]	BMJ
13. I-Dx	—			
14. I-Rx	—			
15. P-Rx	—			
16. Tele	—			
17. Other	—	S. Woleach details therapy of influenza.	[1912]	JHHB
	—	F. Allen treats diabetes mellitus with diet.	[1902]	Bk
		Scans and Other Tests of Function in Various Organs		
18. Brain	—	W. Dandy injects air into cerebral ventricles.	[1918]	AJR
19. Heart	—	A. Spitzer's new theory of Congenital Heart Disease.	[1901]	CDD
	—	C. Wiggers: mechanism to limit ventricular suction.	[1917]	ArIM
	—	T. Lewis describes "soldier's heart" and effort syndrome.	[1914]	Bk
20. Liver	—	J. Holmes describes congen obliteration of bile duct.	[1897]	JHHB
	—	N. Davis implicates cholesterol in jaundice.	[1918]	ArIM
21. Lung	—	R. Boggs describes X-Rays of lungs in influenza.	[1916]	AJR
	—	W. Bowman visualizes coccidioidal granuloma.	[1916]	AJR
	—	G. Pfahler describes malignant disease of lung.	[1918]	AJR
	—	J. Selby describes X-Rays of hemorrhagic pneumonitis.	[1918]	AJR
	—	H. Wessler studies 100 pts X-Rays of bronchiectasis.	[1916]	AJR
22. Bone	—	F. Baetjer studies X-Ray Dx of osteomyelitis.	[1918]	AJR
	—	W. Evans sees multiple myeloma in bone.	[1918]	AJR
	—	H. Mauls shows bone & joint X-Rays in 20 yaws patients.	[1916]	AJR
	—	A. Moore studies metastatic malignancy to bone.	[1903]	AJR
23. Kidney	—			
24. Gut	—	W. Alvarez says gut gradient underlies peristalsis.	[1918]	JAMA
	—	G. Holmes shows pedunculated malig gastric tumors.	[1918]	AJR
	—	B. Orndorff studies pneumoperitoneum with X-Ray.	[1914]	AJR
25. Blood	—			
26. Other	—	M. Hubeny evaluates prostatic calculi.	[1917]	AJR
		Radiation Hysteria and Health Physics * Obituaries *		
27. Hyst	—	O. Halm's irritation (larynx) due to X-ray not infection.	[1904]	ZfC
	—	G. Holzknecht prefers fluoroscopy in busy practice,	[1904]	Bk
		develops skin ca, loses parts of hands.	[1907]	(1931 FGR)
28. React	—	S. Dudley studies toxicity of arsenic enema.	[1918]	JH
29. Respo	—			

* * *

30. Obits	—	W. Crookes (1832–1919) Eng chem, physics; radiometer, Chem News.	Bio
	—	E. Haeckel (1834–1919) Eng naturalist: coins word "ecology."	DSB
	—	Third Rayleigh (J. Strutt) (1842–1919) Eng physics; inert gases.	DSB
	—	W. Osler (1849–1919) Can physician; clinical descrip of disease.	Bio
	—	E. Fischer (1852–1919) Ger chem; estabs chem of sugars.	DSB
	—	J. Davidson (1857–1919) Scot radiol; first Scot to use X-rays.	AJR
	—	H. Dominici (1867–1919) Fr Ra therapist; first to inject Ra IV.	ARE

CHRONOLOGY OF NUCLEAR MEDICINE — 1920

		Scientific and Technical Background		Ref.
1.	Basic —	E. Rutherford names neutral H atom the "Proton."	[1902]	Bio
	—	W. Harkins independently proposes, names the "Neutron."	[1907]	JACS
2.	Obser —	H. Hull describes absorption and scattering of X-rays.	[1906]	JR
3.	# Nuc —	F. ASTON FINDS STABLE ISOTOPES OF Ar, He, H, N, Kr, B, F, Si, Br, S, P, As, Xe.	[1919]	Bk
4.	# Med —			
		Organizations and Internal Politics		
5.	Pols —	Eighteenth amendment (US constitution) goes into effect. (See 1933)		AP
6.	Socs —	Physicists associated with but not members of RSNA.	[1911]	Rad
	—	Rad Soc of N America (RSNA) begins pub of Radiology.	[1914]	Rad
7.	Event —	M. Curie in US asks to see Niag Fall, G. Canyon, & W. Duane.	(1978	IJO)
	—	World population estimated at 1.81 billion.	[1918]	EB
	—	USA population counted at 117.8 million.	[1918]	EB
		Instruments, Units of Measurement, and Drugs		
8.	Instr —	F. ASTON INVENTS MASS SPECTROMETER (FROM THOMSON 1910).	[1919]	Na
9.	Units —	W. Friedrich measures Ra & X-rays with electrostat "e."	[1908]	MMW
	—	L. Seitz proposes precise Df of "Erythema" dose unit.	[1907]	Bk
10.	Concp —	A. Erskine teaches: measure, calculate, use isodose chart.	[1905]	Rad
11.	Drugs —	G. Failla proposes a Duane radium cow for Memorial hosp.	[1915]	AJR
	—	V. Hess builds a small scale radium cow for hospitals.	[1915]	V108
	—	L. Hektoen studies effect of radiation on antibody prod.	[1918]	JCD

Radioiodine, P-32, and Radioactive Therapy

12.	I-Res	—		
13.	I-Dx	— F. Benedict invents a Basal Metab Rate (BMR) clin inst.	[1950]	BMSJ
14.	I-Rx	— D. MARINE SAYS 40–80 μg IODINE/DAY WILL PREVENT GOITER.	[1913]	ArIM
15.	P-Rx	—		
16.	Tele	—		
17.	Other	— L. Seitz says best Rx is largest dose in shortest time.	[1914]	ZGL

Scans and Other Tests of Function in Various Organs

18.	Brain	— H. Cushing develops sub specialty in brain surgery.	[1914]	JAMA
19.	Heart	— H. Pardee describes coronary T wave on ECG.	[1903]	JAMA
		— L. Gallvardin writes monograph on blood pressure.	[1899]	JAMA
		— C. Callander analyzes 447 cases of A-V fistula.	[1918]	AnS
		— T. Lewis writes "Mechanisms of Graphic Represent of Ht Beat."	[1916]	Bk
		— G. Holmes sees pericarditis on X-Ray.	[1897]	AJR
		— M. Hubeny reports pt with patent ductus arteriosus.	[1919]	AJR
		— J. Van Zwaluwenburg pleas for fluoroscopic heart exam.	[1908]	AJR
		— W. Chamberlain studies heart motion with roentgenCiné	[1915]	AJR
20.	Liver	— C. Bailey implicates aesphenamine (syphilis) in jaundice.	[1919]	ArIM
		— W. Stadie describes acute yellow atrophy.	[1919]	ArIM
21.	Lung	— I. Walker reviews fibrous bronchitis.	[1912]	AJMS
		— C. Jackson: localization of non-opaque foreign bodies.	[1918]	AJR
22.	Bone	— C. Williamson describes 116 cases of gout.	[1902]	JAMA
23.	Kidney	— R. Stephon: increased kid function after erythema dose.	[1907]	Str
		— D. Cameron uses iodides in soln as pyelography agents.	[1916]	ArS
24.	Gut	— P. Hanuk sees psychic factor in gastric secretion.	[1909]	AJPh
		— J. Farrell studies motion of isolated gastric pouch.	[1909]	AJPh
		— W. Belden sees a hiatus hernia.	[1905]	AJR
		— L. Cole discusses DDx (X-Ray) diverticula of duodenum.	[1918]	AJR
		— A. George confirms X-Ray value in colon diverticulae.	[1918]	AJR
25.	Blood	— P. Lamson notes Ht error (diff in small, large vessels).	[1915]	JPET
26.	Other	— H. Dachtler shows alveolar infection on dental films.	[1916]	AJR
		— I. Rubin determines fallopian tube patency with O_2.	[1919]	JAMA
		— H. Young injects ejaculatory ducts with thorium.	[1918]	AJR

Radiation Hysteria and Health Physics * Obituaries *

27.	Hyst	— E. Aschenheim first to note rad damage during gestation.	[1955]	AK
		— L. Nurnberger finds uterus very resistant to radiation.	[1906]	Str
		— J. Mortland first to note rad death of Ra dial painter.	[1915]	ARE
		— M. Uhlig finds no lung ca in Joachimsthal miners.	[1913]	(1932 AJC)
		— H. Rorschach invents "inkblot" test, is taken seriously.	[1912]	EB
28.	React	— Am Roent Ray Soc sets up protection comm.	(First report in 1922)	AJR
29.	Respo	—		

* * *

30. Obits — Johann Elster (1854–1920) Ger physics; background radiation. DSB

CHRONOLOGY OF NUCLEAR MEDICINE — 1921

Scientific and Technical Background				Ref.
1. Basic	—	O. Hahn finds first nuclear isomer, UZ (6.75h Pa-234).	[1936]	Bio
	—	T. Morgan postulates chromosome theory.	[1919]	Bio
2. Obser	—	E. Rutherford begins concept of 4 natural decay series.	[1905]	Na
3. # Nuc	—	F. Aston sees isotopes of Li, Ni, Na, K, RB, Cs, (none in Be).	[1920]	Bk
4. # Med	—			
Organizations and Internal Politics				
5. Pols	—	KDKA (Pittsburgh) transmits first commercial radiocast.	[1906]	EB
	—	F. Soddy gets Nobel prize for Fajans' isotopes.	[1912]	AP
6. Socs	—	H. Assmann pubs German textbook on Dx Roentgenology.	[1901]	Bk
	—	R. Carman pubs txtbk on roentgenography of GI tract.	[1901]	Bk
7. Event	—	G. Hevesy successfully separates isotopes of one element.	[1912]	ARR
	—	F. d'Herelle discovers bacteriophage.	[1917]	EB
	—	A. Einstein awarded Nobel Prize for 1905 photoelectric.	[1905]	AP
Instruments, Units of Measurement, and Drugs				
8. Instr	—			
9. Units	—	G. Failla calibrates "threshold erythema" in calories.	[1920]	Rad
	—	I. Solomon proposes a unit "R," ions by 1 gram Ra @ 2cm.	[1920]	Str
	—	K. Hansen quantifies UV biol dose by wavelength.	[1918]	Str
10. Concp	—	W. Coolidge: "absorption" means "out of beam" not dose.	[1917]	JR
	—	J. Mavor eliminates drosophila X chromosome with X-ray.	[1919]	Sc
11. Drugs	—	C. Chase lists American literature on Ra before 1906.	[1906]	AJR
	—	M. Sullivan studies saliva & urine in pellagra.	[1910]	JBC

Radioiodine, P-32, and Radioactive Therapy

12. I-Res	— E. Judd describes laryngeal function in thyroid disease.	[1918]	AnS
13. I-Dx	—		
14. I-Rx	— F. Hutten sees no histol effect after goiter X-ray Rx.	[1910]	MMW
15. P-Rx	—		
16. Tele	— A. Soiland considers 200 kVp "super" voltage therapy.	[1912]	JAMA
17. Other	— A. Lacassagne says alpha and beta must be filtered out.	[1914]	JRE
	— F. Dessauer states his "laws" of radiation therapy: 1. Diff cells show diff sensitivity to same X-rays; 2. Homogenous fields require same quant & quality of rad; 3. Effects are function of dose (quant & quality).	[1918]	AmJR
	— F. DESSAUER ADVOCATES HIGHER VOLTAGE FOR RX.	[1915]	FGR

Scans and Other Tests of Function in Various Organs

18. Brain	— J. Langley publishes "The Autonomic Nervous System."	[1916]	Bk
	— A. Merrill Dx brain tumors with pneumoventriculogaphy.	[1919]	AJR
	— J. Murphy notes intracranial calcifications.	[1918]	AJR
19. Heart	— T. Jonnesco treats angina by cutting sympathetic nerves.	[1916]	Bk
	— R. Lutembacher studies arrhythmias and congenital heart dis.	[1904]	CDD
	— R. Tigerstedt writes textbk on physiol of circulation.	[1918]	Bk
	— O. Loewi finds a vagal substance in the frog's heart.	[1910]	PAP
20. Liver	— E. Graham adds I to phenolphth — X-Ray gall bladder dye.	[1917]	GSR
	— P. Rous studies activity of gall bladder in bile stasis.	[1913]	JEM
21. Lung	— H. Korns describes Rx of eventration of diaphragm.	[1912]	ArIM
	— D. Jarvis notes dust inhalation in granite industry.	[1917]	AJR
	— H. Lynah injects bismuth mixture through bronchoscope.	[1918]	AJR
22. Bone	— B. Widmann reports X-Rays of multiple osteochondroma.	[1918]	AJR
23. Kidney	— F. Barrington studies control of micturition.	[1920]	B
24. Gut	— F. Banting discovers insulin.	[1916]	CDD
	— A. Akerlund displays the duodenal bulb in detail.	[1916]	AR
	— J. Meakins finds histamine in small intestine.	[1918]	JPET
	— A. Hastings sees changes in blood after pyloric obstruc.	[1918]	JBC
25. Blood	— J. Erlanger reviews blood volume measurement to date.	[1920]	PhR
26. Other	— R. Newell does pelvimetry with X-Ray measurements.	[1916]	AJR

Radiation Hysteria and Health Physics * Obituaries *

27. Hyst	— C. Regaud describes GI phase Acute Rad Syndrome in dogs.	[1917]	AEM
	— E. Keller sees denuded GI tract in Acute Rad Syndrome.	[1913]	AEM
28. React	— BRIT RAD PROTECT COMM REPORTS ON SHIELDING FROM RAD.	[1918]	BJR
29. Respo	—		

* * *

30. Obits —

CHRONOLOGY OF NUCLEAR MEDICINE — 1922

Scientific and Technical Background				Ref.
1. Basic	—	W. Pauli proposes the neutrino.	[1920]	WoA
	—	C. Ellis proves that gammas originate in nucleus.	[1913]	Eve
	—	"Compton scattering" announced as hypothesis to APS.	[1905]	AJP
	—	F. Aston restates Whole Number Rule, confirms 1815 Prout.	[1919]	WoA
2. Obser	—	K. Davis: total world radium is 175 grams @ $70,000/g.	[1914]	Rad
	—	US Bureau of mines totals 120g Ra produced in US, 554 produced in rest of world.	[1918]	GSR
	—	C. Regaud sees no diff in biol action of X-rays and Ra.	[1915]	CRB
	—	P. Blackett improves the Wilson cloud chamber.	[1912]	PM
3. # Nuc	—	F. Aston finds stable isotopes of Sn, Xe, Fe, Al, Sb.	[1921]	Bk
4. # Med	—			
Organizations and Internal Politics				
5. Pols	—	Stock market boom begins that will end in 1929.	[1929]	AP
6. Socs	—	Int Soc Radiol decides on Int Congress every 4 years.	[1925]	ICR
	—	Bibliography: Uses of radium 1898 to 1922, by US Radium Corp.		Bk
7. Event	—	N. Bohr awarded Nobel prize in chemistry.	[1921]	AP
Instruments, Units of Measurement, and Drugs				
8. Instr	—			
9. Units	—	W. Duane proposes "e"/sec measured in Paral Plt Chamber.	[1920]	AJR
	—	A. Erskine counts number of Dx expos in erythema dose.	[1920]	AJR
	—	H. Holthusen: "Roentgen Value" is R-units/m at 30 cm.	[1920]	FGP
	—	E. Quimby: Ra applicators, effect of size on skin dose.	[1919]	AJR
	—	C. Regaud discusses time factor for dose in epithel ca.	[1921]	CRB
10. Concp	—	F. DESSAUER SUGGESTS TARGET THEORY AS "HITS ON CELLS."	[1921]	ZfP
	—	J. Ewing: rad Rx is "The first rational Rx of ca devised."		Bk
	—	W. Lazarus agrees with Ewing's statement.	[1911]	MRC
	—	W. Woglom studies tumor radiation-resistance.	[1904]	JCR
11. Drugs	—	H. Evans discovers vitamin E, for anti-sterility ???	[1913]	EB

	Radioiodine, P-32, and Radioactive Therapy		
12. I-Res	— R. Cecil tries clinical calorimetry in arthritis.	[1917]	ArIM
13. I-Dx	—		
14. I-Rx	— G. Pfahler treats thyroid ca with X-rays.	[1915]	AJR
15. P-Rx	—		
16. Tele	— S. Russ reports first Med Res Council Ra Pack complete.	[1918]	MRC
17. Other	— G. Robinson describes therapeutic use of digitalis.	[1918]	Bk
	Scans and Other Tests of Function in Various Organs		
18. Brain	— J. Carlson finds normal visceral sensory nerves.	[1921]	ArIM
	— C. Martin injects air in spine to see intracran passes.	[1919]	ARS
19. Heart	— C. Wiggers discusses physiology of heart sounds.	[1919]	ArIM
	— C. Bardeen estimates cardiac volume on X-Rays.	[1921]	AJR
20. Liver	— S. Rosenthal: bld clearance of PCP tests liver function.	[1909]	JAMA
	— G. Whipple studies origin of constituents of bile.	[1921]	PhR
21. Lung	— H. Wintz reports induration of lung after breast irrad.	[1909]	VDRG
22. Bone	— W. Bowman describes spondolithiasis.	[1903]	AJR
23. Kidney	— T. Paris measure the specific gravity of urine.	[1921]	ArIM
24. Gut	— F. Banting isolates "Isletin" (MacLeod dubs it Insulin).	[1916]	JLCM
	— Banting and Best give insulin to diabetic patients.	[1921]	CDD
	— J. Thomas studies nervous control of pyloric sphincter.	[1921]	JLCM
	— C. King sees an intestinal mucosal motor mechanism.	[1921]	AJPh
	— A. Barclay discusses the normal stomach.	[1921]	La
	— H. Starr measure the pH of saliva.	[1921]	JBC
25. Blood	— C. LEWIN: LEUK & LYMPHOCYTES ARE IMMUNITY AGENTS.	[1960]	MK
	— A. Carrel emphasizes importance of white blood cells.	[1903]	JAMA
26. Other	— J. Ewing describes fibrosis action of radiation on ca.	[1934]	AJR
	— D. Campbell demonstrates nasolachrymal ducts on X-Ray.	[1917]	AJR
	— W. Evans shows X-Rays of stillborn & newborn.	[1912]	AJR

	Radiation Hysteria and Health Physics * Obituaries *		
27. Hyst	— H. SCHINZ: 80% ERYTHEMA DOSE PRODUCES PERMANENT ASPERMIA.	[1906]	SMW
	— T. Morgan discovers the fruit fly.	[1919]	Bio
28. React	— L. Halberstadter: lo-dose stimulates, hi-dose harms wheat.	[1917]	FGR
	— A. Hamilton says mad hatters have chronic Hg toxicity.	[1919]	JIHT

* * *

30. Obits	— A.G. Bell (1847 1922) Am inventor; telephone, first brachytherapy.		Bio

CHRONOLOGY OF NUCLEAR MEDICINE — 1923

	Scientific and Technical Background		Ref.
1. Basic	— A. COMPTON DISCOVERS GAMMA-ELECTRON SCATTER INTERACTION.	[1922]	PR
	— L. de Broglie says wave can be a particle & vice versa.	[1912]	WoA
2. Obser	— A. Russell predicts a 4n + 1 series, U-237 to Bi-209.	[1921]	PM
	— C. Nims says not ca but support cells killed by rad.	[1923]	PM
	— A. Eycleshymer prints cross-section Anatomy (Appelton).	[1605]	Bk
	— P. Debye applies quantum theory to X-rays.	[1922]	PZ
3. # Nuc	— O. Hahn finally realizes two uraniums, UI & UII, exist.	[1917]	Ber
	— F. Aston finds isotopes of Ge, Cu, Sc, Ti, V, Cr, Mn, Co, Ga, Sr, Y, Ag.	[1922]	Bk
	— G. Hevesy discovers Hafnium (Hf).	[1921]	ARR
4. # Med	—		

	Organizations and Internal Politics		
5. Pols	— USSR adopts Gregorian calendar; To make the change: add 10 days to Julian date from Oct 5 1572 to Feb 28 1700, add 11 days to Julian date from Mar 1 1700 to Feb 28 1800, add 12 days to Julian date from Mar 1 1800 to Feb 28 1900, add 13 days to Julian date from Mar 1 1900 to Feb 28 2100.		
	— Oct 4, 1582, Gregorian calendar adopted by Catholic states: Italy, France, Spain, Portugal, Luxembourg, Germany; * 1587, Belgium, Switzerland, Netherlands, & Hungary follow change; * 1700, Denmark & Germany, Switzerland, & Netherlands protestant states; * 1752, Britain & its colonies (including America); * 1753, Sweden; * 1806, France changes in 1793 but returns in 1806; * 1873, Japan; – 1875, Egypt; – 1917, Turkey; * 1912, China to new zero but to Gregorian zero in 1949; * 1923, Greece; * 1924 USSR. FOR FIRST TIME IN HISTORY ALL CIVILIZATION IS ON ONE CALENDAR.		
6. Socs	— Am Col Radiology founded as honorary society.	[1916]	AJR
	— A. Soiland: >1000 AMA members are practicing radiology.	[1920]	JAMA
	— Radiology becomes official publication of RSNA.	[1920]	Rad
	— M. Curie's biography of "Pierre Curie" published.	[1906]	Bk
	— E. Andrade publishes "Structure of the Atom."	[1922]	Bk
7. Event	— G. Hevesy: first °tracer exp. in living tissue (horse bean).	[1914]	BJ
	— Willys-Overland Auto mfgr advertises "Red Bird" automobile; breaks the "color barrier" on bactericidal white.	[1900]	AP

	Instruments, Units of Measurement, and Drugs		
8. Instr	— G. Hevesy makes an ionization chamber for counting samples;		BJ
	counter has 1.4 cm^2 mica window for betas.	[1921]	BJ
	— T. Svedberg invents the ultracentrifuge.	[1919]	DSB
	— W. Coolidge: a water-cooled high volt X-therapy tube.	[1914]	AJR
	— W. Duane measures dose with ionization chambers.	[1922]	AJR
9. Units	— W. Witherbee gives dose formula for std X-Ray positions.	[1920]	Bk
	— W. Duane says X-ray tubes for Rx vary >40% in intensity.	[1922]	AJR
	— A. Erskine measures Dessauer depth dose charts in water.	[1901]	Rad
	— A. Bachem writes "Principles of X-ray and Radium Dose."	[1901]	Bk
	— O. Glasser reexamines gamma ray (radium) dosimetry.	[1922]	AJR
	— H. Behnken formulates Villard's "dose" in precise terms.	[1908]	FGR

10. Concp	— F. Dessauer: both "point heat" & "single hit" bio action.	[1922]	Bio
	— J. Arkwright explains etiology of typhus fever.	[1913]	BJEP
11. Drugs	— J. Howland implicates "Vit-D like" subst in rickets.	[1919]	Med

Radioiodine, P-32, and Radioactive Therapy

12. I-Res	—		
13. I-Dx	—		
14. I-Rx	— J. Bower implants Ra in dog thyroids, no toxic reaction.	[1921]	AJR
	— H. Plummer pretreats Graves surgery patients with I-127.	[1920]	JAMA
	— J. Means tries rad Rx on thyroid patients, 33% cures.	[1915]	AIM
15. P-Rx	—		
16. Tele	—		
17. Other	— W. Duane measures therapy doses with ion chamber.	[1908]	AJR

Scans and Other Tests of Function in Various Organs

18. Brain	— J. Camp studies normal anatomy of sella turcica.	[1909]	Rad
19. Heart	— C. Wiggers pubs "Circulation in Health and Disease."	[1922]	Bk
	— T. Lewis discusses effects of aortic regurgitation.	[1920]	Ht
20. Liver	— G. Delprat notes Rose Bengal bld clearances in liv dis.	[1922]	AIM
	— J. Borak irradiates livers of 7 pts, sees no rad sick.	[1910]	MK
	— P. Nevda: much rad sick in hepatic insufficiency pts.	[1910]	WMW
	— W. Alvarez describes suppurative cholangitis.	[1897]	JAMA
21. Lung	— T. Grover reports abnormal shadows after erythema dose.	[1922]	AJR
	— C. Lungsgaard describes physiology of cyanosis.	[1912]	Med
22. Bone	— J. Race determines role of uric acid in gout.	[1920]	PRSM
	— S. Moore observes osteitis deformans.	[1922]	AJR
23. Kidney	— E. Marshall shows PSP is excreted by convoluted tubules.	[1920]	JHHB
24. Gut	— A. Kuntz studies rhythmic contractions of stomach.	[1922]	PSEB
	— A. Akerlund visualizes diverticulae of stomach.	[1920]	NYMR
25. Blood	— H. Curshman writes "Hyperglobulie" (PVA).	[1904]	MKI
26. Other	— H. Holfelder sees no change in adrenals, 80% eryt dose.	[1920]	Str
	— W. Kennedy locates obstructions in Fallopian tube.	[1921]	AJOG

Radiation Hysteria and Health Physics * Obituaries *

27. Hyst	— California legislates non-MD X-Ray labs; Gov vetos it.	[1899]	AP
	— A. Gurwitch discovers "Mitogenetic" rays (false in 17y).	[1903]	Bk
	— E. Coué in US to preach self deception psychology fraud.	[1900]	AP
28. React	— Roy Soc Med requires bld tests & holidays for X-ray tecs.	[1928]	Rad
	— R. Adams gets patent on Ra spray to stimulate plants.	[1922]	USPat
	— B. Barcroft studies bioeffects of hi-dose activities.	[1911]	PTRS
	— J. Geiger analyzes 7419 food poisonings in USA.	[1919]	JAMA
29. Respo	—		

* * *

30. Obits	— W. Roentgen (1845–1923) Ger physics; X-rays.	GSR
	— F. Hans Geitel (1858–1923) Ger physics; background radiation.	DSB
	— J. Dewar (1865–1923) Scot physics; thermos flask.	DSB

CHRONOLOGY OF NUCLEAR MEDICINE — 1924

Scientific and Technical Background

			Ref.
1. Basic	— H. Barboor designs "falling drop" fluid density measure.	[1911]	BJ
	— J. Robertson diagrams complete electromag spectrum, includes wavelengths from 10 cm electric to 0.01 Å.	[1918]	Bk
	— W. Duane verifies Compton scatter & concedes to Compton.	[1923]	Bio
	— L. de Broglie postulates wave theory of matter.	[1923]	WoA
2. Obser	— K. Davis says "millicurie – microcurie" in general use.	[1914]	Rad
	— A. Compton explains "scattering concept" to radiologists.	[1923]	Rad
	— 500 tons of Colorado ore yields 500 lbs RaBrCl (1g Ra).	[1922]	Rad
	— K. Nims tells hist of Ra production; price is $70,000/g.	[1914]	Rad
	— C. Regaud studies bio-effect of radiation in tissues.	[1922]	AJR
3. # Nuc	— F. Aston shows isotopes of Ba, La, Pr, Nd, Zr, Ce, Cd, Te, Bi.	[1923]	Bk
4. # Med	—		

Organizations and Internal Politics

5. Pols	— St. Petersburg changed to Petrograd then to Leningrad.	[1914]	AP
6. Socs	— Am College Radiology incorporated for social issues.	[1923]	JAMA
7. Event	— G. Hevesy uses "half-life" (but in later translation).	[1899]	CRS
	— G. HEVESY USES FIRST °ISOTOPE IN ANIMALS (RaE IN RABBITS).	[1923]	CRS
	— L. Aschoff describes a reticuloendothelial system (RES).	[1920]	Bk
	— A. Barclay predicts machine-automated Dx and Rx.	[1842]	Rad
	— E. Rutherford tells story of early Nuclear Physics.	[1909]	JFI
	— General Motors introduce Duco lacquer color paints.	[1923]	AP

Instruments, Units of Measurement, and Drugs

8. Instr	— F. Kurie says gold leaf electroscope is reigning instr.	[1937]	ONR
	— H. Behnken uses "thimble chamber" to match parall plate.	[1922]	FGR
	— V. Zworikin patents the Iconoscope (TV tube).	[1906]	DSB
9. Units	— O. Glasser modifies Friedrich's "e" for Ra and X-rays.	[1920]	FGR
	— O. Glasser uses Seeman spectrometer on Dx X-ray machine.	[1918]	Rad
	— German erythema is red skin, French is second degree burn (1F = 3G).	[1922]	AJR
	— I. Kaplan compares German and French threshold erythema.	[1920]	AJR
	— O. Jungling proposes "death of bean sprouts" as dosimeter.	[1907]	WMJ
	— G. Holzknecht wants direct measurements of surface dose.	[1922]	Rad
10. Concp	— O. Glasser relates X-ray energy spect & photofilm dens.	[1902]	Rad
	— D. Webster can calibrate energy distrib of X-ray instrs.	[1921]	Rad
	— A. Lacassagne: micro-autoradiographs, Po in rabbit kidney.	[1909]	CRS
	— J. Crowther: bio-dose is energy transfer, hits on cells.	[1922]	PRSL
11. Drugs	— V. Hess devises a simple 50 mg Ra commercial cow system.	[1920]	PM
	— I. Christiansen studies deposition of °Pb (RaD).	[1907]	CRS
	— H. Ness makes Vitamin D with UV light.	[1913]	JBC
	— Chemical insecticides are said to be first used.	[1962]	EB

Radioiodine, P-32, and Radioactive Therapy

12. I-Res	—	W. Dameshek describes the heart in hyperthyroidism.	[1922]	BMSJ
13. I-Dx	—			
14. I-Rx	—	J. Altland (Mich) uses 0.02% I salt (goiterless in 10y).	[1923]	JMS
15. P-Rx	—			
16. Tele	—			
17. Other	—	H. Doub discusses X-ray Dx & therapy of thymomata.	[1913]	Rad

Scans and Other Tests of Function in Various Organs

18. Brain	—			
19. Heart	—	E. Schwizer: histol change in heart after hi-dose irrad.	[1906]	Str
	—	K. Davis produces lesions after hi-dose in dogs and rabbits.	[1923]	Rad
	—	A. Krogh writes monograph on physiology of capillaries.	[1921]	Bk
	—	J. Moenckeberg pubs German textbook on arteriosclerosis.	[1912]	Bk
20. Liver	—	F. Mann reviews the function of the gall bladder.	[1923]	PhR
	—	J. McNee outlines the causes of jaundice.	[1913]	BMJ
	—	L. Aschoff publishes "Origin of Gall Stones."	[1913]	Bk
21. Lung	—	M. Ritvo describes X-Ray of massive lung collapse.	[1923]	AJR
22. Bone	—	P. Magnuson: why no X-Ray finding in "low back pain?"	[1915]	AJR
23. Kidney	—	G. Dick: skin test for scarlet fever susceptibility.	[1916]	JAMA
24. Gut	—	L. Dragstedt begins research on gastric ulcer.	[1920]	AS
	—	W. Sperry measures the lipids in feces.	[1906]	JBC
	—	J. Gamble notes dehydration following pyloric obstruct.	[1922]	JCI
	—	W. Alvarez reviews intestinal autointoxication.	[1923]	PhR
25. Blood	—	G. Minot treats Chr Myelogenous Leuk with ext radiation.	[1920]	JAMA
	—	G. Minot treats Chr Lymphogenous Leuk with ext radiation.	[1920]	BMSJ
26. Other	—	S. Harris says hyperinsulinism is a disease.	[1919]	JAMA
	—	W. Stone describes X-Rays in multiple myelomata.	[1903]	AJR

Radiation Hysteria and Health Physics * Obituaries *

27. Hyst	—	T. Blum reports dial painters "Radium Jaw" in J Am Dental Assoc.		
	—	R. Carman counts 83 papers on rad protect since 1919. (Crisis?)		RAD
	—	E. Muhlmann sees retarded breast growth in irrad girls.	[1907]	Str
28. React	—	NYC amends sanitary code to include X-ray precautions.	[1923]	Rad
29. Respo	—			

* * *

30. Obits	—	J. Loeb (1859–1924) Ger-Am physiol; physiol of fertilization.		DSB
	—	W. Bayliss (1860–1924) Eng physiol; hormones, peristalsis.		DSB

CHRONOLOGY OF NUCLEAR MEDICINE — 1925

	Scientific and Technical Background		Ref.
1. Basic	— M. Born converts Heisenberg notation into matrix algebra form.		Bk
	FIRST USE OF NON-COMMUTATIVE ALGEBRA IN PHYSICS	[1880]	Bk
	— A. Millikan names the "Cosmic rays" of Hess.	[1913]	DSB
	— W. Pauli tells "exclusion principle," 2 electrons/shell.	[1916]	WoA
	— G. Uhlenberg postulates electron spin.	[1924]	WoA
	— N. Vavilov postulates "gene" centers in chromosomes.	[1921]	DSB
2. Obser	— L. Meitner notes electrons after gamma emission (Auger).	[1922]	ZfP
3. # Nuc	— W. Noddack discovers last stable element #75 rhenium.	[1913]	CN
	— W. Noddack discovers #43 and calls it Masurium. (Error).	[1937]	CN
4. # Med	—		

	Organizations and Internal Politics		
5. Pols	— A. Hitler reorganizes Nazi party, pubs "Mein Kampf."	[1919]	AP
6. Socs	— First (post war) International Congress of Radiology (ICR).	[1922]	BJR
	— First ICR establishes ICRU (Int Comm Rad Units & Measur).	[1912]	ICR
	— Radiology accepted as sixteenth section at AMA conventions.	[1847]	JAMA
7. Event	— O. Glasser told new plastic "Bakelite" is tissue equiv.	[1909]	AJR
	— Crane Co offers colored porcelain bathroom fixtures.	[1924]	AP

	Instruments, Units of Measurement, and Drugs		
8. Instr	— H. Geiger invents coincidence count to confirm Compton.	[1919]	Sc
	— P. Blacket adds a coincidence counter to cloud chamber.	[1922]	WoA
	— V. Bush builds a machine to solve diff equations.	[1833]	SA
	— H. Fricke studies ionization in small chambers.	[1924]	FGR
9. Units	— ICR cannot accept new "r" (Glasser-Behnken variation).	[1924]	Rad
	— R. Glocker defines Unit Skin Dose (USD) as <erythema.	[1924]	Str
	— T. Angus' biol UV radiation dose is bacteria kill rate.	[1925]	PRS
	— E. Ernst measures (ion chamber) Ra tube output before Rx.	[1918]	Rad
	— W. Lahm finds erythema dose different in X-ray and Ra.	[1924]	Str
10. Concp	— S. Scott recommends whole trunk rad Rx instead of local.	[1902]	BMJ
	— E. Jeffreys first (?) suggests age of earth in billions.	[1907]	DSB
	— L. Arntzen studies bioeffect of filtered vs unfiltered.	[1924]	AR
11. Drugs	— J. Sumner discovers urease and enzymes are proteins.	[1930]	DSB
	— F. Wood proposes that immunity is involved in cancer.	[1922]	JAMA
	— U. Portman advocates rad therapy for breast cancer.	[1902]	Rad
	— B. Lee compares pre- and post-op radiation in breast ca.	[1902]	AnS

Radioiodine, P-32, and Radioactive Therapy

12.	I-Res	—		
13.	I-Dx	—		
14.	I-Rx	—		
15.	P-Rx	—		
16.	Tele	— K. Stenstrom uses multiple focused fields to spare skin.	[1924]	AR
17.	Other	— S. Pinzman says 2000 breast ca rad Rx since 1911 in Lon hosp.		Rad
		— S. Lomholt measures °Bi uptake in syphilis Rx (rabbits).	[1924]	BMJ

Scans and Other Tests of Function in Various Organs

18.	Brain	— P. Baily tries X-ray Rx of surgically exposed tumors.	[1924]	AJR
19.	Heart	— N. Anitschoff studies arteriosclerosis and myocarditis.	(1944	BHM)
		— T. Lewis discusses reactive hyperemia.	[1923]	Ht
		— T. Lewis pubs "Graphic Registration of the Heart Beat."	[1915]	Bk
		— J. McWilliams reviews blood pressure in normal men.	[1939]	PhR
20.	Liver	— A. Rich reviews the formation of bile pigments.	[1924]	PhR
21.	Lung	— J. Bancroft writes "The Respiratory Functions of Blood."	[1921]	Bk
22.	Bone	—		
23.	Kidney	— G. Holmes sees recovery after removal of adrenal tumor.	[1917]	QJM
24.	Gut	— A. Ivy finds new humoral agent in gastric secretion.	[1920]	AJPh
		— T. Healy sums X-rays of 53 diaphragmatic hernia pts.	[1933]	AJR
25.	Blood	— P. Weil: "pernicious" (aplastic) anemia after Thorotrast.	[1916]	BSMP
26.	Other	— F. Knistoiez exposes isolated pancreas, gets less juice.	[1926]	CRS

Radiation Hysteria and Health Physics * Obituaries *

27.	Hyst	— German X-ray Protection Comm says .01 erythema is safe.	[1924]	Str
		— ICRU establishes first "safe" dose at 0.1 erythema/year.	[1904]	ICRU
		— State of Tenn forbids sex education in schools.	[1924]	AP
		— H. Ludwig feeds mice irrad food: bad result unconfirmed.	[1985]	Str
		— S. Voronoff combines animal-human rejuvenation research.	[1918]	EB
		— H. Martland notes dangers in radioactive substances.	[1916]	JAMA
28.	React	— E. Schneider irradiates yeast, gets increased growth.	[1922]	Str
		— A. Mutscheller has formula to estimate X-ray tube dose.	[1924]	AJR
29.	Respo	— SCOPES "MONKEY TRIAL" FREES SCIENCE FROM CHRISTIAN DOGMA.		AP

* * *

30.	Obits	— A. von Wasserman (1866–1925) Ger bacty; serum tests for infec.		DSB

THE CURIE UNIT IS DEFINED

By 1910 radioactivity nomenclature was a mess. Becquerel's U (Uranium) decayed through Crookes' UX, Boltwood's Ionium (with evidence for an intermediate UX_{II}) to Ra; then to niton or emanation (but not emanium) and through radium A to B, two C's to Radiolead through an E to F (polonium) to a G that Boltwood thought was really lead. Ernest Rutherford had started "active deposits" back in 1899 with a simple A-B-C terminology, but the system had gone mad with exceptions.

Further, every substance had a different "strength," but everybody also had a different meaning for "strength." Marie Curie began using a "uranies" unit which was related to the activity in a gram of uranium. Bertram Boltwood used an electroscope with time-to-collapse as a unit.

The Brussels Conference Finds a Unit

Everyone in the radioactive business agreed that a unit of amount was essential. In 1910 Ernest Rutherford (England) and his friend Stephan Meyer (Vienna Radium Institute) set up an international committee to define a new unit of radioactivity. It was made up of Rutherford and Meyer (because they originated the idea). Frederick Soddy helped represent England (because his father-in-law financed the organizational meetings). Otto Hönigschmid later represented Austria (because he operated the worlds largest, >4g, Ra source at the Vienna Institute). Marie Curie and André Debierne sat in for France (André was the first chemist to join Pierre and Marie in separating radium). Otto Hahn and Hans Geitel represented Germany (Geitel was chemist for the largest commercial supplier of precision-measured Ra sources). Bertram Boltwood sat for America and A.S. Eve for Canada (Bertram had been the first American radiochemist, and Arthur Eve succeeded Rutherford at McGill).

[A Belgium chemist, Ernest Solvay, picked up the tab, which was why the meeting was held in Brussels. He had made a fortune on a method for $NaCO_4$ production, and wanted to pay back something to science. After the success of this meeting, he financed an International Physical Institute that paid about 20 invited scientists to come to Brussels for the famous Solvay Conferences.]

The committee represented almost every major radium research laboratory, but anybody who used radium could attend. The whole congress would democratically pass on the issues. Physicians wanted a unit of dose (which is beyond physics), but would settle for a unit of activity. Few persons understood °decay (most were on the committee); hence, agreement on a definition of a "unit of radioactivity" was easily reached: *the amount of radium emanation in equilibrium with one gram of radium.*

A standard for such a definition, however, would have to be more specific. Rutherford and the other experts realized that the true measure of radioactivity was not grams of a chemical element, it was the *rate-of-disintegration* of a gram. (Ra expense required working in milligrams or milli-units.) They specified that radium be sealed in Thuringian glass tubes. After sealing a precisely weighed amount of radium, they would wait until the daughters had built up and reached equilibrium. Counting the gamma rays emitted per second in a known geometry gave an estimate of the disintegrations per second (dps) of a gram of radium.

Rate-of-Decay of Radium is Unknown

The curie unit applied only to sealed radium sources. As medical radon became popular after 1915 it too was measured in millicuries. In 1930 a new International Radium Standard Commission stretched the definition to include any daughters of radium. By 1934 Fermi's neutron sources and cyclotron drivers were making a few, then hundreds, then thousands of different "radioisotopes" that bore no relation to radium, but were measured in curie units. In the Atomic Bomb Project scientists recognized that disintegrations per second (dps), no matter what the source, was the real unit of radioactivity.

Attempts to measure the dps of Ra gave results from 3.40×10^{10} to 3.72×10^{10} dps; the best estimates were around 3.67×10^{10} dps. To convert man-made °isotopes to curies of radium-equivalent with an unreliable factor was bothersome. In 1948 an NBS group tried to introduce the "Rutherford," which would be a flat 10^6 dps. It didn't catch on.

To keep the historical meaning but allow greater precision, the curie unit was redefined in 1959 (by the ICRU) as exactly 3.7×10^{10} dps of any nuclide.

> [This makes good sense because we have known for a hundred years that a randomly decaying mass can have no exact dps. A committee decision is easier than a measurement, and may be exact.]

The New Unit Honors Pierre Curie

Remember, in 1898 when radium was discovered, Marie was not yet recognized as a scientist. Until she got her degree (and the Nobel Prize) in 1903, she was a graduate student. Her equipment was made by Pierre. Supervision of her graduate work and hence its credibility was not from her professor, Becquerel, but from Pierre, who already had a reputation in piezo-electricity. The new unit would be named the "curie" in honor of the late Pierre. Marie, a committee member, agreed. She would prepare an international standard of about 20 mg. Stephan Meyer would ask chemist O. Hönigschmid, of Vienna, to prepare a number of secondary standards. After calibration against Marie's primary, these could be purchased by any country's Bureau of Standards. (Marie had only her original small sample of radium; the Vienna Institute had 4 grams.)

But agreement on a standard source and how to measure it was a different matter. Several hundred experts on the use of radium (most were medical uses) attended this first radium congress. Each had prepared his own absolutely correct, without a shadow of doubt, absolute standard (and none had followed the committee's definition).

Motions, in a gabble of languages, for alterations of the committee's definition were made from the floor. Then amendments to the alterations were made in several different languages. Then amendments in German to the alterations in French to the motions in Italian to table the Swedish suggestions for English revisions followed in dizzying succession. The confused chairman (who spoke only three languages) fled the meeting in panic. A substitute chairman's attempt to stem the tide of catcalls, boos, and further amendments brought the meeting to a screaming chaos.

And then — Wilhelm Hallwachs, professor at Technische Hochschule, Dresden, ascended the platform. With a powerful voice and an imperial presence he waved aside the temporary chairman and proclaimed in a tone of finality the consensus of the house: the committee's decision is accepted as written. Those in favor raise your hands. No one dared to count. There was no NO vote. Thus the "curie" was democratically introduced.

> [The curie would be modified periodically during the next half century, but never again has an International Unit been put to popular vote.]

In 1960 the Conférence Générale des Poids et Mesures, the mother authority for all units, instigated the coherent Systéme International d'Unités (SI). A "unit" must be exactly what it says: one, singular, not one-half and not 3.7 × anything. By 1975 they got around to the curie; 3.7×10^{10} dps is incoherent, henceforth, the unit will be 1 dps. But a new unit requires a new name; obviously, it would be "Rutherford" because he was first to use "dps" decay, but . . . .

All successful international conferences have three ingredients: politics, the subject matter, and politics. To substitute an English name for a revered French name would have been stupid. They went instead a step behind Rutherford to Becquerel. Of course Becquerel for years did not believe in Rutherford's disintegrating atoms (Pierre Curie eventually convinced him), but he had discovered radioactivity.

Henceforth, 1 becquerel = 1 dps

Madame Curie's standard would, of course, be maintained at Sévres with the standard meter and kilogram. But there was a reason for Hönigschmid's backup standards. Marie Curie looked frail and sickly to the Committee members. Could she be trusted with such a demanding task? Her frailness was heightened by the deferential way Paul Langevin, her ever-present companion, handled her.

[See Vig1911 .Lan. Marie's honor]

RUTHERFORD "SEES" THE ATOM
(But There is a Flaw Beyond His Math)

"One day (in 1911) Rutherford, obviously in the best of spirits, came into my room and told me that he now knew what the atom looked like and how to explain the large deflections of the alpha particles. On the very same day I (Hans Geiger) began an experiment to test the relation expected by Rutherford between the number of scattered particles and the angle of scattering."

[Eve, p. 198]

In one experiment Geiger collimated alpha particles from a radium source. He fired them at a thin gold leaf and measured their angle of scatter. Rutherford was impressed by the very few that returned at about 180°. There must be a massive central charge to repulse alphas. He had a model built to prove it.

An electromagnet was fastened to a table, N pole facing up. Suspended over, almost touching it, on a 30 foot length of thin wire, was another electromagnet, N pole facing down. The poles repelled each other and if the long pendulum was swung, it would swerve away from the central charge on a comet-like hyperbola. Occasionally it approached and was repelled on the same straight line.

9 Feb 1911, in a letter to W.H. Bragg, then at Leeds, Rutherford gives his thoughts on the nature of the atom. He had been following Geiger's alpha scattering results. The laws of large angle scattering, it seemed, were different from small angle scattering laws. In order to explain this scattering Rutherford pictured the atom as a positive charge surrounded by negative electrons uniformly distributed in a sphere.

For a few months Rutherford had been playing with the idea that the central mass of the atom had a negative charge. But how then could the electrons be held in the atom? He changed his concept to that of an atom with a central positive charge. The alpha particle with a double positive charge had to be repelled by a central positive charge. Rutherford asked post-grad student C. Darwin to look into the mathematics of the business.

Darwin Sees the Birth of a Nuclear Atom

Charles Galton Darwin (1887–1962) was named for his grandfather and Francis Galton, his half first cousin twice removed. He became one of Rutherford's team of post-graduates at Manchester. Primarily a mathematician, he became a theoretical physicist. One notable job was his putting Moseley's mass of measurements into the "staircase" form that revised the Periodic Table. Before then he was working with Rutherford, trying to make sense out of Geiger's alpha scattering.

[See Vig1913 .Mos]

Many years later (1938) C.G. Darwin reminisced: *"I count it as one of the great occurrences of my life that I was actually present half-an-hour after the nucleus was born.*

It was a Sunday supper at [Rutherford's] Manchester house and I remember his saying to us . . . that he had been looking into big scattering of alpha particles and that there must be enormous forces in the atom to do it. Then he said that it would require something like a hundred electrons in the case of the gold atom." [Eve, p. 199]

The "central positive charge" was soon called the "nucleus." It had all the mass of the atom, but no size worth mentioning. (Electrons are miniscule.) The number of units of positive charge was about half the atomic weight. (Moseley would clear up this question in 1913.) Electrons were, presumably, evenly spotted throughout the atom.

Rutherford was not a mathematician. He handled exponentials with familiarity (not common in 1904 physics), but he preferred to let experts work the details. In his pendulum magnet experiment Rutherford remembered a theorem in conic sections. The orbits of his pendulum were hyperbolic with measurable angles of eccentricity.

This atom had one obvious flaw. Electrons floating about would be attracted to the central positive charge. Something out of the ordinary must characterize atomic electrons. Niels Bohr was about to arrive in Manchester to flesh out the Rutherford nucleus with a fixed set of electrons.

[See Vig1913 .Mos]

THE FIRST TRACER EXPERIMENT WAS IN THE SCIENCE OF HOME ECONOMICS

George Hevesy's early education was in Budapest. For advanced work he went to Berlin, then to the Technische Hochshule in Freiburg for a 1908 doctorate in chemistry. His thesis posed a question: why such poor yields of sodium from electrolysis of molten sodium hydroxide? He did not answer the question, but learned how a scientist approaches a question that does not have an answer: go, in person, to an expert — but don't necessarily believe what he says!

R. Willstatter in Zurich had developed a new energy transfer measurement called chromatography. Hevesy went to Zurich and became one of the assistants. Einstein had just become associate professor of theoretical physics; Hevesy was one of about twenty who attended his inaugural lecture on determination of the ratio of charge and mass of the electron. The subject was at the base of Hevesy's molten sodium salt question.

In Berlin Fritz Haber had developed another approach to energy transfer, catalytic synthesis. Hevesy became one of Haber's assistants, but not in catalysis. "Go back to your thesis question," Haber advised: was the oxidation of molten zinc accompanied by emission of electrons? No one in Haber's institute knew the techniques for measuring conductivity of electricity in gases. Hevesy proposed and Haber readily agreed that Hevesy should transfer to Rutherford's laboratory to acquire knowledge in this new field. In the first days of 1911 Hevesy left for England.

Hevesy Goes Back to School

Upon arrival in Manchester Hevesy found he was not a complete stranger. An old friend from Zurich, Kasimir Fajans, was also about to take the first step that Rutherford required of all visiting students. An introductory radioactivity course with laboratory exercises was given by Hans Geiger. The radioactivity Rutherford would allow beginning students to handle was thoron emanation (now Rn-220). It had an easily demonstrated one minute half-value-period (not "half-life" for at least another 25 years). Its active deposit slipped through five decays to stable lead in an 11 hour half-value-period.

> [Even the worst student accident could not contaminate the lab for long. The precaution did not imply danger to people. (Radiation hysteria, an American invention, starts in 1948.) But even minor contamination can drive instruments wild. Rutherford had contaminated his Montreal lab (due to understandable ignorance). It was not going to happen in Manchester.]

Hevesy's First Experiment in Radioactivity

As was customary, visiting students obtained room and board in one of the homes close to the Owens College laboratory. Although Hevesy was well satisfied with the meals served by his landlady, he had a long experience in boarding houses and knew what to expect. The remains of the Sunday meat pie would be served in disguise later in the week — tastily, of course, but still leftovers. There had never been a way to prove conclusively what every boarder knew. While thinking of Geiger's last laboratory exercise he had an inspired thought:

> *"The coming Sunday in an unguarded moment I added some active deposit to the freshly prepared pie and on the following Wednesday, with the aid of an electroscope, I demonstrated to the landlady the presence of the active deposit in the soufflé."* [ARR]

Thus, the first radioactive tracer experiment, strictly speaking, was born in the science of Home Economics. However, this experiment was not the essence of Hevesy's 1913 discovery. Obviously, if you mix a distinctive tracer substance with something, you may or may not be able to trace it in chemically disguised form. Hevesy's great contribution was that a °isotope was *chemically identical* to its stable sibling atoms. It could be traced by radioactivity no matter what chemical torture was applied. Such knowledge was acquired only after a few more years of education.

[See Vig1912 .KF1; Vig1913 .GH2]

PAUL LANGEVIN PROTECTS MARIE'S HONOR

Paul Langevin, an old friend of fellow student Rutherford at the Cavendish Lab, became a student of Pierre Curie and eventually succeeded him as professor of physics. Considered one of France's top mathematical physicists, he was contemporary with Einstein on the equivalence of mass and energy. Paul also taught mathematics at Sévres where Marie Curie taught chemistry. Paul (age 39) often went to the older woman for advice. (Marie, 5 years widowed, was 43.) At the first Brussels International Conference on the Radium Unit (1910), Paul's concern for Marie was noticeable.

Marie had always been dowdy, and always wore black. In later years when her younger daughter Eve persuaded her to buy new clothes, they were still black. Following the Brussels Conference for a brief period her costume changed. She appeared at a party dressed in white. "Marie," conjectured a friend, "must be in love, she appears radiant." (This was true in more than an aesthetic sense. She had been breathing huge doses of radon for 11 years. Gold leaf electroscopes collapsed when she entered a room.)

Marie Applies for the French Academy

About this time a vacancy occurred in the French Academy of Sciences; she decided to present her name. After all, she was France's most famous scientist. (At least she had more honorary degrees and honorary memberships in foreign scientific societies than any two other Frenchmen.) An application for such membership followed rigid rules. A formal visit to each member was required. Marie dutifully complied with the ritual. In her mind a membership might be a small blow for Poland's independence. (She was a vivid Polish activist.)

However, such an unprecedented application (*"A WOMAN IN THE ACADEMY?"*) turned the normally underreported election into a newspaper féte. Where, they asked, would she wear the academician's ceremonial sword? M. Amagat, a minor physicist who had beaten Pierre Curie to election eight years earlier, thundered to the press, *"A woman NEVER."* Poincaré, Roux, and Picard fought just as hard for her admission, but Marie lost by one vote.

Then Came the Scandal

A newspaper reporter looking for something to enliven the rarefied academic atmosphere of Academy selections, got hold of a packet of Marie's love letters to Paul Langevin. (It just happened that Paul was already married. His wife had given the letters to the reporter.) These were definitely not rarefied atmosphere, in fact they were torrid, and the Parisian public was given daily doses. Overnight Marie became *"a beautiful seductress"* (as she was when she got out of that lab coat). *"In such matters, always instigated by the older woman, Marie had enticed that poor young boy . . . ."* (He was only 39.) She was *"the foreign woman," "a Russian"* (although she hated the Russians as only a pre-WWI Pole could). *"A Jewess"* (she had supported Dreyfuss a few years back, so that proved it). *"A German"* (after all, she quoted Heine in her letters). She *"was a Pole"* (which was very, very true).

Then the newspapers got out their end-of-the-world headline type for Paul.

Marie's Honor is Restored

Gustave Téry, an old schoolmate of Paul, was the reporter. Dismissed as a teacher of philosophy because of his political activities, he published a weekly anti-Jewish scandal sheet: L'Oeuvre. He got from a very angry Mrs. Langevin the letters Marie had sent to Paul. In his stories, copied by other papers, he labeled Marie *"the vestal virgin of radium."* But, in somewhat mixed metaphor, he said Paul maintained her *"as a concubine in conjugal domicile."* Only one reasonable action was open to Paul: he must protect Marie's honor. Paul challenged Téry to a duel.

The principals met in the privacy of the Paris Bicycle Stadium on 25 November 1911, at 10:50 A.M. (The classical sunrise was inconvenient for one of the seconds.) Under a black bowler hat the waxed mustache of Langevin faced the waxed mustache of Téry under his black bowler hat at 25 meters. (Any shorter distance, the seconds had agreed, would be dangerous.) Langevin's seconds, dressed in black morning coats, faced Téry's seconds, dressed in black jackets and felt trilbys. At precisely 11:00 A.M. in black cape and top hat, the code-of-honor's referee, P. Painleve (a mathematician, soon to become prime minister), gave the order to fire.

.... Off to one side a small huddle of black robed doctors gripped their black bags at the ready. Perched high on the walls of the securely locked bicycle stadium a long line of newspaper reporters, all dressed in formal black, leaned forward in anticipation. (They had gained admission by a ladder routinely furnished by the management for such occasions.) The only sound came from the middle of the stadium where a flock of pigeons pecked peacefully at the grass ....

Téry, rigid with pistol pointed at the ground, stared at Langevin. Langevin, rigid with pistol half raised, stared at Téry. The pigeons continued to peck in undisturbed tranquility ....

The top-hatted seconds circled the cycle-track to confer with the trilby hatted seconds. All moved to confer with the black robed doctors. No one was sure of the procedure; the code duello made no provision for a total absence of shots. The top-hatted referee, with the consent of his peers, then walked slowly to each contestant, carefully removed the pistols from their hands and fired the shots into the air simultaneously.

Marie's honor was restored

The "Curie" Becomes a Unit of Measurement

Madame was disconsolate. (She missed almost a full day at the laboratory.) In her depression she briefly contemplated suicide. Incommunicado, she retreated to a peaceful haven on the English coast, taking with her some minor calculations that needed revision.

[In reading her actions it is apparent that Marie understood that she had just been paid the highest compliment the French press could bestow on a woman. Marie's "depression" at the height of the scandal had not prevented performance of the most exacting of all chemical tasks. Early in 1912 she became seriously ill with a kidney complaint; a surgical correction was required. She demanded that surgery be put off until after March so that she could attend the radium standard intercalibration. The Vienna radium standards would be calibrated against her (the Paris) 21 mg International Primary Standard. She had prepared the Paris standard during the heat of the scandal and it compared well against Hönigschmid's three backups.]

In December of 1911 the Nobel Prize committee topped off the scandal by awarding Marie her second Nobel award, this time in chemistry (the 1903 award had been in physics). Never had the award gone to the same person twice, and in two different sciences, and to a woman. Overnight the French press reversed itself. The foreign Femme Fatale became *"the perfect representative of our race's genius"* and the Heine-quoting seductress became *"a national glory."*

The "curie" unit and the radium standard would last, officially, for 74 years. It had serious faults, but its world-wide credibility was largely due to Stephan Meyer's sensitivity. Marie was not trusted in science by her scientific peers. Hönigschmid's three Vienna Standards were compared with greatest deference to Marie's "Paris Primary Standard." The Experts all knew why the Vienna standards were made. After calibration the primary had to be pried away from Marie who wanted to keep it *"for sentimental reasons."* B. Boltwood, the American representative, considered Marie *"a plain darn fool."* Rutherford thought she was *"a difficult person to deal with; she has the advantages and at the same time the disadvantages of being a woman."*

[Marie has long been canonized in the hagiology of science. Many people believe this story is Parisian newspaper talk. However, 22 years later when Irene called Marie at midnight to witness the discovery of artificial radioisotopes, both Paul and Marie responded.] [See Vig1933 .F-I]

KASIMIR FAJANS DISCOVERS ISOTOPES
(But F. Soddy Gives Them a Name)

John Dalton's definition of "element" in 1803 did not permit "isotopes," but with a slightly modified second postulate he didn't prohibit them. Mendeleev's Periodic Table did not have a place for isotopes but, as Crookes had shown in 1886, could accommodate them on a statistical basis. Since 1905 O. Hahn and a titer of chemists after him had been finding look-alike elements that could not be separated.

[See Vig1905 .Ges]

At the turn of the century (1900) only six °elements were known. [An "°" before a word reads "radioactive."] By 1911 there were 31, and 4 more were about to be announced. Rutherford's laboratory was busy around the clock. In addition to regular staff, Fajans had spent an academic year (1910–11) working with Moseley. Bohr came up from the Cavendish to finish his year in England. Hevesy had extended his stay beyond a year.

At the end of his Manchester visit, on his way to Vienna, Hevesy stopped off to visit Kasimir Fajans to bring him up-to-date on scientific gossip: A. Fleck was egging F. Soddy to a commitment on the chemical identity of some radioactive "elements"; A. Russell was proving "identity" spectroscopically. Bohr felt that beta rays came directly from the nucleus of Rutherford's nuclear atom. Moseley was proving that an element's ordinal number fitted a progressive series. A Dutch lawyer, van den Broek, had made such a speculation and Bohr was taking it seriously. Alphas, in Bohr's new theory, emerged from the nucleus and changed its mass. Beta emission, however, resulted in an insignificant change in mass. Fajans told Hevesy that Bohr's beta particle ideas fit into his problem.

How Fajans Became a "Radiochemist"

Kasimir Fajans (Fi'-ance) got his doctorate in 1909 from Heidelberg on the physics and chemistry borderline. The subject matter of the 1908 Rutherford-Geiger paper on alpha particle scattering had caught his fancy; his reading on the subject made him the local "expert." During his next year's postgraduate work in organic chemistry at Zurich, one of his duties was to teach undergraduates the esoteric "radioactivity." This stimulated his evolving interest in physical chemistry, and he requested permission to spend the 1910–11 academic year with E. Rutherford at Manchester.

Fifty years later he reminisced:

"Hans Geiger was Rutherford's research assistant and became my nearest advisor for two reasons. He conducted an introductory course in radioactive methods at which I participated together with George von Hevesy .... Since I started to learn English only several weeks before coming to Manchester, Geiger, of German origin, acted as interpreter between Rutherford and me. Geiger's and my research interests became especially close when he concluded that short-lived ThA and AcA must exist and they were isolated and their half-life measured in an investigation which H.G.J. Moseley and I performed near the end of my stay in Manchester." [K.F. Aug 1963, letter in MB's files.]

Fajans thus learned that elements in rapid transition must be searched for. A theory, even incomplete, helps you know where to look. The 1905 von Lerch rule said that every °transformation went to a more electronegative daughter. Soddy's 1911 transmutation series left unacceptable gaps in the Periodic Table.

After Manchester, Fajans had accepted an academic position at the Technische Hochschule in Karlsruhe. His inaugural dissertation to the faculty was scheduled for December 1912, on Radioactive Transformations. Alpha particle mass 4 transforms were obvious, but beta emission involved some queer displacements. Hevesy's visit in November brought news of Bohr's betas coming from the nucleus.

Kasimir Fajans Goes to the Opera

While preparing his dissertation, on 23 November 1912, Mrs. Fajans insisted upon attending a performance of Tristan und Isolde at the state opera. Well into the second act only Tristan remained awake, and in his half-doze Fajans' mind wandered down the Periodic Table from uranium to "thorium-like" to uranium to "thorium-ionium" to "mesoradium" to radiothorium to "radium-like." The orchestra went into a sudden crescendo with cymbals announcing the return of Isolde's husband. Fajans awoke with a start. Of course! It was obvious . . . there had to be more than one kind of uranium. With atomic number in place of weight there were plenty of numbers for uraniums, thoriums, radiums, emanations, even multiple numbers for lead.

Fajans called these multiple occupants of the same slot on the Periodic Table "Pleiades," but the name would not stick. His dissertation was published in December 1912. [Med Verein Heidelberg 12:173, 1912] Two papers explaining the "Displacement laws" were published. [Phys Zeitschr, 4 & 15 Feb 1913] But Fajans realized that "rules" were not "laws" until verified by experiment. He searched for gaps in the Periodic Table for which he could: first, predict on theory, and second, verify experimentally, the presence of an unknown "element." He found one — it had a pattern similar to the AcA he had helped find in Manchester.

Fajans Predicts and Discovers an Element

Uranium I (now U-238) decayed by alpha emission to Uranium X (Th-234), which decayed by betas to Uranium II. Fajans' displacement rule said the gap between UX and UII required a forbidden double beta emission. The missing element should be a Group V, eka-tantalum that should plate out on lead. It must be short-lived or Geiger-Nuttal would have detected it when they discovered UII.

With one of his first graduate students, Otto Göhring, Fajans carried out a series of ingenious experiments. In March 1912 they announced the discovery of Uranium X_2 (1.175 min Pa-234m). This discovery was of a new element and Fajans and Göhring had every right to name it "Brevium" but, just as with "Pleiades," their name would not stick.

Five years later (1918) Otto Hahn and Lise Meitner discovered the long sought parent of actinium and *renamed* it protoactinium. (Renamed because it already had the name *brevium.*) Later shortened to protactinium (now Pa-231), the new brevium isomer had a half-life of 34,000 years. Hahn fully recognized Fajans' priority, but explained that the International Atomic Commission could not bring itself to link "brevium" with 34,000 years.

"Pleiades" is Changed to "Isotopes"

Fifty-two years later, after reading proofs of my Vignette giving him major credit for the concept of isotopes, Fajans admonished me (MB):

"I am anxious not to receive too much credit, although in general Soddy is now getting too much. This is partly due to the fact that the term 'isotope' is better than the one I proposed, 'pleiad'. However, this does not mean that Soddy understood the subject better than I and not even that he was a better philologist than I. I lecture and write in Polish, Russian, German, French, and English, but I did not have either Latin or Greek in high school." [KF to MB, 5 Apr 1966]

The philology referred to by Fajans was first revealed in A. Fleck's obituary tribute after Soddy's death in 1956:

". . . *from* [Soddy's work on displacement rules] *came the introduction of the word 'isotope'. It was suggested by Margaret Todd [a medically qualified Glasgow friend of the family], arising from a discussion that Soddy had at a dinner party. . ."*

[Fleck A, Nature 178:892, 1956]

How Many Kinds of Lead?

Fajans had two graduate students. One, Otto Göhring, stayed home to help discover "brevium" to prove the displacement laws. The other, Max Lembert, was given a technically more difficult task. In September 1912 he was sent to work with T.W. Richards at Harvard. Richards was the master of the special art of precision weighings, and Lembert carried with him samples of lead chosen by Fajans because they probably were of uranium origin. Fajans had realized that "isotopes" made 3 atomic weights for lead necessary. If true, Lembert would prove it. By 21 March 1914 he had a copy of the Richards-Lembert report to read to the Deutsch Bunsen-Gesellschaft. In 1963 Hugh Taylor reminisced on the meeting:

". . . The values for two samples from uranium minerals chosen by Fajans were near 206.58 as compared to 207.15 for ordinary lead . . . The officers of Bunsen-Gesellschaft decided that, at the annual dinner, the special toast should be for Fajans. . . ."

[Ann Rev Phys Chem 14:6, 1963]

Isotopes were now a part of chemistry, but most physicists were NOT converted.

[See Vig1919 .Ast]

ISOTOPES ARE USED BEFORE THEIR DISCOVERY

(G. Hevesy, F. Paneth, and E. Rona)

In 1911 Rutherford, always complaining about a lack of °activity, had a very large source of radium D (Pb-210) in the basement of his Manchester lab. The only thing wrong was that it was imbedded in a few hundred kilograms of Joachimsthal pitchblende — a gift from the Austrian government.

Hevesy Is Assigned a Lifetime Task

It was customary for Rutherford to assign a research job to each "student" after he had completed Geiger's introductory course in handling °activity. The task he gave Hevesy would occupy the rest of Hevesy's life.

One day Rutherford met Hevesy (enrolled as a physical chemist) in the lab basement. *"If you are worth your salt,"* he told George Hevesy, *"you separate radium D from all that nuisance of lead."* During the next year Hevesy tried all sorts of chemical methods. Once he almost succeeded, but soon found it was Ra E (Bi-210) that he had separated. The evidence was overwhelming to him that both bismuth and lead had radioactive "forms" inseparable from ordinary Bi and Pb. A handful of chemists were convinced that radium, thorium, uranium, actinium, had "lookalikes" for which we hadn't found the stable forms.

> [As late as 1930 Hevesy was still searching tellurium and bismuth minerals for a stable polonium. He decided that bismuth was the upper end of stability. In 1935 O. Hahn was still searching for a stable radium.]

Stephan Meyer's Radium Institute in Vienna had separated the most radium. If anybody could separate RaD from Pb they could. Hevesy decided to visit over Christmas holidays. Kasimir Fajans had recently left Manchester for a professorship at Karlsruhe; Hevesy would stop by on his way to Vienna. He didn't know it, but in Karlsruhe he would drop a spark that ignited Fajans' discovery of the isotopic nature of the heavy radioactive elements.

[See Vig1912 .KF1]

With Paneth, "Pleiades" Become Indicators

After bringing Fajans up to date on Manchester gossip, Hevesy continued on to the Vienna Radium Institute. He learned that Fritz Paneth, one of the chemistry assistants, had been given the same job by Stephan Meyer that Hevesy got from Rutherford: separate RaD from Pb. He had covered the same ground as Hevesy, same techniques, same time, and with the same results. Shortly after Christmas holidays Hevesy and Paneth decided that inseparability might be an advantage. By early spring they published 3 papers explaining the use of RaD as an "indicator" to show the movement of one lead salt solution through another. [Stz Ak Wisch Wien, 1913]

They were the first to accept the new Fajans "pleiades." They had already used RaD as chemically "identical" to Pb. By December F. Soddy introduced a brand new term, "isotopes." It was so descriptive that everybody, including Fajans, immediately adopted it. [See Vig1912 .KF1]

For Elizabeth Rona, Isotopes are "Labels"

Radium D (Pb-210) was an isotope. Hence it was chemically "identical" to lead, but not quite. With Elizabeth Rona, Hevesy discovered an important modification of complete chemical identity.

Elizabeth Rona (Ph.D. Budapest 1912) had gone to Karlsruhe for post-doctorate training with Kasimir Fajans. She had just returned to Budapest's Chemical Institute thoroughly grounded in "radioactivity." On an annual visit home (1913) Hevesy was surprised to find a highly trained radiochemist. Impressed by her measurement of the diffusion constant of radon in water, he explained how he and Paneth had measured diffusion of radiolead in stable lead solutions with substances now called "isotopes." He suggested they attempt to answer a perplexing problem:

- Diffusion rate is a function of atomic mass.
- Isotopes differ in atomic mass.
- Can we measure diffusion-velocity differences between isotopes?

Hevesy and Rona mixed some lead and thorium B (Pb-212). Another batch was a mixture of lead and thorium C (Bi-212). They measured the velocity of dissolution from thick layers and from molecular-thin layers. They could not detect differences in rates. The presence of lead ions seemed to slow down thorium B (Pb-212) but not thorium C (Bi-212). Hevesy insisted there must be, by theory, a difference; Rona said, by experiment, there isn't.

A Very Important Footnote

Put into modern terminology, they felt the mass difference between Pb-208 and Pb-212 was too small to detect. They put the first caveat on "identical" chemical behavior of isotopes into a footnote in their 1915 article:

> *"[Chemical identity] does not apply strictly to diffusion processes . . . only those atoms which are both isotopic with and of the same mass as those under study are really ideal "indicators."* [Z Phys Chem 89:1915]

> [Technically, only an isomer can be an ideal *indicator*. Elizabeth Rona had already substituted the term "radioactive *label*" in the 1915 article because "indicator" had another meaning in chemistry. "Tag" appears in 1917, and Hevesy uses "tracer" in 1923. "Isomers" would not be discovered until 1921 and were named in 1936.]

The Hevesy-Rona footnote was not a footnote in Aston's mind when he exploited the difference in his Mass Spectrograph four years later. The great mass difference between isotopes was really recognized 18 years later when Urey used it to separate heavy water. [See Vig1931 .HW] It was not a footnote 28 years later when it became necessary to separate U-235 from U-238. The few lines of type in 1915 were the fattest and most productive footnote in history.

"Isotopes" Are Accepted Among Chemists

Back in Vienna with Paneth, Hevesy proved that RaE (now Bi-210) displaced bismuth and ThB (now Pb-212) displaced lead. These displacements were unseeable and imponderable, a kind of theoretical proof that followed Nernst's theory of mass action — unconvincing except to theoretically inclined chemists. Hevesy wanted to convince many chemists. With the large radium sources of the Vienna Institute (>4 g) Hevesy and Paneth were able to obtain a visible layer of $RaD \bullet O_2$ (now 22 year $T_{1/2}$ Pb-210 oxide) on a platinum wire. This first visualization of a "daughter" isotope was convincing even to the most skeptical chemists.

A few people had seen radium, many had seen its salts, and radium is now a daughter isotope: but not in 1913. Radium was considered to be a primary "element" in 1913, not a granddaughter of uranium. Rutherford and Soddy had seen the effervescent thoron emanation in liquid air back in Montreal in 1902. But this demonstration was long before isotopes were a question. Now (1913), in the midst of a general skepticism among chemists, Hevesy and Paneth had accumulated enough of 22 year $T_{1/2}$ RaD to be a visible something that could be weighed. Fajans' discovery in 1912, Soddy's naming them in 1913, the long trail of "identical elements" starting with Otto Hahn's RaTh & Th in 1905, all were speculative chemical theory. But all chemists had to believe in isotopes when Hevesy and Paneth showed them a platinum wire covered with RaD oxide. [ARR p. 88]

"Isotopes" Are Accepted Among Physicists

The chemists now "believed," but not the physicists. J.J. Thomson, considered by many to be No. 1 in physics, had already shown a double parabola in his positive ray image of neon. He didn't believe it. His chemically trained assistant, F. Aston, proved it was an isotope by diffusion. Nobody believed him. Six years later (1919) he would invent the mass spectrograph and prove that Thomson had been the first to see isotopes. With the first run of mass spectroscopy all physicists had to believe in isotopes. [See Vig1919 .Ast]

George Hevesy was a young, somewhat offbeat perhaps, but still a classical physical chemist. Chemistry to him was the study of the atomic interactions of 80–85 or so stable elements. A few of these elements had an unstable radioactive form. This °active form could quantitatively "label" the stable form, and thus act as an indicator of its chemical interactions. Radioactive lead tags stable lead, and °active bismuth tags stable bismuth. That's as far as it went, and Hevesy, at the time, considered isotopes a minor contribution to science, mostly in inorganic chemistry.

Fritz Paneth, however, would stretch the concept of "labeling" a giant step beyond inorganic chemistry.

[See Vig1917 .FPO, Paneth Goes Organic.]

1913 — THE YEAR OF DECISION FOR "ISOTOPES" — 1914 (RENAMED NUCLIDES IN 1947)

(Documents leading to the discovery and acceptance of isotopes.)

Date	Author(s)	Event
JANUARY 1913		
10 Jan 1913	K. Fajans	Lead must have three stable end points (isotopes). (Karlsruhe Chem Ztg 37:151, 1913)
17 Jan 1913	J.J. Thomson	No room for element-22 on Periodic Table. (Aston, Roy Inst Lec, Mass-Spectra, p. 30, 1933)
22 Jan 1913	A. Fleck	9 beta emitters assigned to 5 elements. (J Chem Soc 103:381, 1913)
31 Jan 1913	A. Russell	RaC" is Pb (wrong); ThD is Pb (right). (Chem News 107:49, 1913)
FEBRUARY 1913		
4 Feb 1913	K. Fajans	First publication of displacement laws. (Chem Ber 46:422, 1913)
7 Feb 1913	A. Fleck	RaC" is Tl (right), ThD, AcD, are Tl (wrong). (Chem News 107:68, 1913)
15 Feb 1913	K. Fajans	Displacement laws assign elements to "pleiad" (isotope). (Phys Zeits 14:136, 1913)
28 Feb 1913	F. Soddy	Displacement laws; quotes Fajans. Lead must have three stable end-points (isotopes). (Chem News 107:97, 1913)
MARCH 1913		
11 Mar 1913	K. Fajans & O. Göring	Discovery of UX_2, experimental proof of disp. law. (Naturwiss 1:339, 1913)
APRIL 1913		
2 Apr 1913	E. Rutherford	Fajans' proof has priority over Soddy's hypothesis. (Letter to K. Fajans, 2 Apr 1913, Brucer file.)
Apr 1913	H. Geiger & E. Marsden	Proof of Rutherford's atomic nucleus. (Phil Mag 25:604, 1913)
Apr 1913	J J. Thomson	Sees 2 neon parabola lines (first isotope proof). (Lecture, Proc Roy Soc A89:1, 1913)
24 Apr 1913	F. Paneth & G. Hevesy	No separation of RaD from Pb is possible. (Sits Akad d Wiss Wien 122:993,1913)
27 Apr 1913	G. Hevesy & F. Paneth	First use of RaD as "indicator" for Pb. (Zeit Anorg Chem 82:323, 1913)
MAY 1913		
10 May 1913	H. Geiger	New beta counter invented (pre-GM tube). (Letter in Eve's Rutherford, p. 222, 1939)
15 May 1913	A. Fleck	Final article on beta-emitter transpositions. (J Chem Soc 103:381, 1913)
May 1913	G. Hevesy	2 neons allows 2 leads; J.J. does not agree. (Letter to J.J., Adven Rad Res p. 16, 1962)
JULY 1913		
July 1913	N. Bohr	First statement of Rutherford-Bohr atom. (Phil Mag 26:1, 1913)
20 July 1913	A. van den Broek	Ordinal numbers, not atomic weight, are critical. (Nature 92:372, 1913)

1913 — THE YEAR OF DECISION FOR "ISOTOPES" — 1914
(RENAMED NUCLIDES IN 1947)

(Documents leading to the discovery and acceptance of isotopes.)

Date	Author(s)	Event
	British Association meeting in Birmingham	**Aug/Sep 1913**
Aug/Sep 1913	F. Aston	Neon-22 separated from 20, unconvincing. (Brit Assoc Report, Aston p. 5, 1913)
Aug/Sep 1913	F. Soddy & A. Fleck	Identical substances can have different Atomic Wt. (Brit Assoc Report, Nature 92:331, 1913)
Aug/Sep 1913	J.J. Thomson	H-3 is a polymerized hydrogen. (Hevesy in Eve's Rutherford, p. 224, 1939)
Aug/Sep 1913	N. Bohr	H-3 could be a different weight hydrogen. (Hevesy in Eve's Rutherford, p. 224,1939)
SEPTEMBER 1913		
Sep 1913	K. Fajans	Max Lembert sent to T. Richards, Harvard. (In Anders, J Chem Educ 41:522, 1964)
Sep 1913	N. Bohr	Electrons determine chemistry, nucleus structure determines radioactivity. Beta particles emitted from nucleus. (Phil Mag 26:476, 857, 1913)
NOVEMBER 1913		
Late 1913	J.J. Thomson	Neon-22 is an element. (Positive Rays of Electricity, 1913)
Nov 1913	A. Fleck	Story of the name "isotopes," coined by M. Todd. (Soddy obit, Nature 27 Oct 1950)
DECEMBER 1913		
Dec 1913	H.G.J. Moseley	Proof of ordinal number series in Periodic Table. (Phil Mag 26:1024, 1913)
4 Dec 1913	F. Soddy	First use of word "isotopes." (Nature 92:399, 1913)
		1914
Mar 1914	M. Curie	Different atomic weight for different Pb samples. (Compt Rend Paris 158:1676, 1914)
Mar 1914	O. Hönigschmid	Different atomic weight for different Pb samples. (Compt Rend Paris 158:1796, 1914)
Apr 1914	F. Soddy	Different atomic weight for different Pb samples. (in Taylor, An Rev Phys Chem 13:5, 1962)
21 May 1914	K. Fajans	Report on different atomic weights of leads. (Bunsen-Des, Leipsig, Zeit Elechem 20:319, 1914)
Jun 1914	T. Richards & M. Lembert	Different atomic weight for different Pb samples. (J. Am Chem Soc 36:1329, 1914)
28 Jun 1914	**Archduke Ferdinand Assassinated. World War I begins.**	

[See Vig1905 .Ger; Vig1911 .GH1; Vig1912 .KF1]

MOSELEY'S STAIRCASE SAYS 92 ELEMENTS
(And Confirms Prout's 1815 Hypothesis)

Henry G.J. Moseley was a properly educated Eton boy who, naturally, went to Oxford. Rather than classics, he took the final science honors exams before graduating from Trinity. The questions involved determination of the mass of atoms. His examiners believed their textbooks — Moseley didn't. Moseley received only second class honors. Whatever the 1910 textbooks said, in just 3 years Moseley would prove them wrong.

In spite of his failure (he considered it failure) Moseley decided to stay in physics. Although he lived with his widowed mother across the road from Oxford, it was no place to study science. J.J. Thomson at Cambridge had come out of Manchester's Owens College. Manchester was where "atomic weights" had started with John Dalton 100 years before. Also a famous mathematician, Arthur Schuster, and the controversial Ernest Rutherford might be good teachers.

Moseley Accepted By Rutherford

Moseley took the train to Manchester to apply in person for a job in the lab. Rutherford must have liked his answers to physics questions because within a week he accepted Moseley as lecturer (and of course lab assistant which everybody was in Rutherford's laboratory). Moseley began on the job in October 1910 just in time to meet Kasimir Fajans, a "student" just arrived from Zurich. Three months later another "student," George Hevesy, arrived from Berlin. Other "students" were from Minnesota, New York, Australia, New Zealand, and London.

New staff or visiting student, it didn't matter; all took Hans Geiger's intensive hands-on laboratory course in handling radioactivity. They were soon converted into experts in electroscopes (each student made his own) and Geiger's latest counting tube (prototypes of the famous 1928 GM tube). As soon as students passed Geiger's muster, Rutherford assigned a problem. He told Moseley and Fajans that emanation from actinium (now Rn-219) seemed to emit 2 alphas which Rutherford had disproved in other decays. How many alphas/disintegration?

Moseley and Fajans, under Geiger's supervision, made a great team. Moseley could help Fajans with his English, as Fajans (who already lectured in Polish, French, German, and Russian) introduced Moseley to science outside medieval Oxford. Further, as recently married Fajans later reminisced, he would count the samples during the day and Moseley, a bachelor, would count them at night.

They soon found reason for a confusing actinium decay. Debierne's actinium 1A (Ac A) was actually Ac B. To time a short half-value-period, Moseley had devised an ingenious rotating disk under two electroscopes. Fajans developed a method to capture the recoiling Ac atom from the rotating disk after it made its first alpha emission. By adjusting the speed of rotation they could measure Ac A (now 0.0018 s Po-215) before it messed up the emission of Ac B (now 36.1 m Pb-211). Geiger announced the new Ac A. In the same issue Moseley and Fajans published their first paper: "Radioactive Products of Short Life." (Phil Mag, July 1911)

Rutherford thanked his two "students" in the only way he thought appropriate. He assigned them a more difficult task: Ra B, C, D emitted betas. How many betas/disintegration? Fajans prepared ultra pure samples for Moseley to count but got stuck on Ra C. It emitted an alpha and a beta. Impossible! (It would take time to solve this one.) [See Vig1911 .KF1] Meanwhile Moseley breezed through his part and answered: one beta/disintegration.

Moseley Finds a Difficult Problem

A German physicist, Max von Laue, had discovered that the atomic spacing in a crystal could be used as a diffraction grating for X-rays. His first picture was shown at Rutherford's regular Friday colloquium (24 May 1912). Moseley was intensely interested. When Geiger shot alpha particles through sheets of atoms they were affected only by the massive nuclei. When smaller betas were projectiles an entirely different picture, but still nuclear, occurred. What would happen when infinitely small X-rays were shot through a stable field of electrons? Niels Bohr, then at Rutherford's lab, gave the electrons equal billing with the nucleus in the structure of the atom.

He discussed the problem with Charles Dalton Darwin, a childhood friend also new at Manchester. Mathematician Darwin could follow Bohr's obtuse reasoning, but was all thumbs in the lab. Moseley suggested a partnership on an experiment involving the nature of X-rays. Rutherford, rusty on X-rays, balked, then gave approval — electrons, after all, were part of the atom.

Moseley built an instrument similar to a device built by W.H. Bragg at Leeds. A thin pencil of X-rays was beamed to a glancing deflection on a crystal. The angles and intensities of beams, both reflected and refracted, were measured. In 1906 C.G. Barkla at Liverpool had shown that both "continuous" X-rays and those "characteristic" of an element were emitted. (He called the characteristic sharp peak intensities 'K' and a lower energy 'L' radiation.) Moseley's device balked on its first run. Rutherford sent him to Leeds for help.

The Braggs, a father and son team in physics, were old friends of Rutherford. W.H. Bragg, the father, was first to measure "Bragg's peak" ionization to specify alpha energies while still in Australia. [See Vig1907 .B&H] They had recently returned to professorships at Leeds and heard of von Laue's discovery at the July 1912 250th Royal Society Anniversary in London. W.L. Bragg, the son, immediately saw a method for mapping a 3-dimensional arrangement of atoms in crystals. W.H. Bragg saw a fundamental problem: X-rays, like light, were propagated as particles, but von Laue showed a wave interference. X-rays glancing off a crystal might be broken into a spectrum. The Braggs hurried home to set up an instrument.

Moseley arrived in Leeds and the Braggs gave help freely. Far more experienced as investigators, the Braggs had already seen and solved Moseley's problem. Moseley had been too precise a craftsman. He had collimated his detector so fine that in scanning over the continuous spectrum he had missed the characteristics. The angles of reflection were so narrow that a wider window was needed to find them. Then you could focus and correct. Each reflecting crystal had its own critical angle.

Moseley's Staircase of Atomic Numbers

Moseley returned to Manchester and corrected his machine. Within weeks he had taken more measurements than the Braggs, and Darwin was beginning to make mathematical sense out of them. Darwin could calculate the wave lengths of angular emissions. He shared his findings with the Braggs. On 7 April 1913 the Braggs published, and gave credit to unpublished work by Moseley-Darwin. They noted a fine detail: *"The frequencies of the X rays and, therefore, according to Max Planck, the corresponding quantum energies are in arithmetical progression."*

[Proc Roy Soc]

In July 1913 Moseley and Darwin published a confirmation of the Braggs, but kept that short note in mind. Niels Bohr was back for a few days to confer on his three nuclear atom papers for Phil Mag. Hevesy, Darwin, and Moseley questioned Bohr at length; Hevesy on 'Pleiades' (not 'isotopes' for another 5 months), Darwin on the physical meaning of mathematics, Moseley on why Bohr used that Dutch lawyer's (van den Broek) suggestion that nuclear charge was a multiple of hydrogen's charge. For a working hypothesis, said Bohr, we need to see the X-ray spectra of many elements. Moseley had already decided to do just that. He could test van den Broek's (or was it Prout's 1815?) hypothesis.

Moseley chose 11 elements, Ca to Zn because they were continuous on the periodic table, and threw in Al and brass at each end. The wave lengths of their spectra showed a pattern. He plotted atomic number against Darwin's W (reciprocal square root of wave length); the elements arranged themselves in their exact "staircase" order.

Moseley published his "staircase diagram" in the December 1913 Phil Mag. In the preceding (Nov) issue Bohr announced the nuclear atom. In the 1 Dec 1913 issue of Nature, Soddy used the word "isotopes," which was theoretical nonsense without Moseley's proof that van den Broek had been correct. Nobody thought to mention that William Prout, after 98 years, was finally confirmed.

But Henry Moseley had another idea.

[See Vig1914 .Mos]

MOSELEY'S TRIUMPHS AND DEATH

Henry G.J. Moseley had shown in the December 1913 issue of Philosophical Magazine (London) that "elements" were best characterized by their nuclear charge. The second part of the paper was in the May 1914 Phil Mag, and showed that the charge on any element was some multiple of the charge on the hydrogen nucleus. This statement was an updated version of what William Prout had said in 1815. It gave evidence that 92 elements existed — the first such estimate ever possible.

That is, of course, provided you believed in a nuclear atom. Few people did. Rutherford never referred to his 1911 Phil Mag paper. It violated the laws of acceleration. It would have died, except Niels Bohr tied the electrons to Max Planck's quantum — which Rutherford couldn't see. The quantum was a third order abstraction: a limitation on a ratio of quantities. Before he could accept Bohr's modification of his nuclear atom Rutherford had to see experimental proof. In the second part of Moseley's Phil Mag article (May 1914), hydrogen atoms and alpha particles marched up the Periodic Table in rigid numerical order. Only a nuclear atom with matching parts could accommodate Moseley's "staircase."

Back in 1911, when Moseley had answered Rutherford's question, *how-many-betas-per-disintegration,* so fast, Kasimir Fajans became stuck on his half of the problem. But his answer was also required for acceptance of the nuclear atom.

Fajans Finds the Pathway to Isotopes

In preparing samples for Moseley, Fajans found Hahn correct in saying that Ra C gave off a beta, then an alpha (RaC′), to get to Ra D. But when measured on Moseley's rotating disk to see extremely fast conversions, in a small portion (now 0.2%) an alpha comes off first followed by a 1.3 minute beta (called Ra C″, now Tl-210). Thus there are two possible routes to radium D. Fajans called this kind of decay pattern "branching."

Fajans finished work on 26 April 1911. His academic year with Rutherford was up. He was due to report to Karlsruhe on 1 June. In Germany new professors do not arrive late. Fajans could not yet see that two beta emissions are required to bring an alpha emission back to the same place on the Periodic Table. Beta emissions could not cause such a change because betas do not come from a nucleus — at least in 1911 they didn't. On a visit from George Hevesy in November he heard that Bohr now thought differently. [See Vig1912 .KF1]

Moseley Moves Back to Oxford

By the end of 1913 Moseley was awarded a fellowship to continue his experiments, but back at Oxford. (This was a minor triumph, because it came through the same group that almost flunked him three years earlier.) He felt that a thorough display of the entire Periodic Table was required to convince most physicists of the atom's true nature.

Moseley built a new apparatus with the final spectrum displayed on photographic film. Inside an enlarged Crookes tube he arranged for multiple targets on a tiny truck on wheels. The beam could be focused, without breaking the vacuum seal, on multiple targets. Chemical preparation was unnecessary; any lump of substance could be a target. In January 1914 he wrote to Fajans for help in getting calibration samples. William Crookes supplied him with some of the Rare Earths.

Early in spring 1914 the great Rare Earth chemist, G. Urbain from Paris, visited Oxford personally to verify some rumors (probably by Hevesy). He couldn't speak a word of English, but William Ramsay did the translating. Urbain gave Moseley an ore sample containing his own mixture of miniscule amounts of Rare Earths, including his recently discovered but unconfirmed celtium (#61). Moseley mounted the samples in his tube with a couple of reference standards. He took a few pictures, then excused himself to make a few calculations.

Two days later they met again and Moseley handed Professor Urbain a piece of paper with the answer: Er (#68), Tm (#69), Yb (#70), Lu (#71), no trace of #61. Urbain stared at the paper in utter disbelief. Later he confided in a letter to Rutherford, "*. . . Moseley confirms in a few days the conclusions of my efforts of 20 years.*"

[Eve, 1939, p. 198]

For a Few Months Moseley is Famous

Urbain and Ramsay quickly spread the word on the significance of atomic numbers. Moseley was becoming famous even before the second half of his paper was published. When published in March it showed the elements from Al (#13) through Au (#79) in precise sequence. Three elements were missing, #42 (Tc), #61 (Pm), and #75 (Re). Welsbach's thulium had 2 lines (TmI & TmII were then considered two elements). Six or seven of the Rare Earth names were mixed up (terminology still unsettled). Moseley concluded that every element has an integer "N" (we now say "Z") identified with the positive charge on the nucleus.

Early in June 1914 Moseley left England to attend the British Association meetings in Melbourne, Australia. While still at sea the Archduke Ferdinand was assassinated. Germany declared war on a few countries. England declared war back. On 7 Aug 1914 Kitchener called for 100,000 volunteers.

Everybody Joins the Army

Upon his return home, Moseley found Oxford empty. Rutherford's lab at Manchester was in complete dissolution. Even his glassblower, an articulate German patriot, had been interned. J. Chadwick, helping Geiger get set up in Berlin, was interned by the Germans. H. Geiger joined the German artillery. C. Darwin joined the Royal Engineers. G. Thomson and F. Aston (J.J.'s son and assistant) went into the Royal Aircraft Factory. W.L. Bragg went to the Horse Artillery but later transferred to a new sound-ranging technique.

> [While at the front trying to sound-range big guns, he was recalled for a few days to join his father in receiving the Nobel Prize.]

George Hevesy was stopped in Holland on his way to Oxford to help Moseley with the Rare Earth mess. He was sent to the Carpathians as technical supervisor of an electrolytic copper works. (He found time to set up a small laboratory.)

Moseley was 26 years old, unmarried, and an Eton graduate (where, as everybody knew, the wars of England are won). He immediately enlisted. Rutherford screamed in protest, but to no avail. He tried to at least get him transferred to a scientific post, but it was too late. Second Lieutenant H. Moseley of the Royal Engineers received orders to sail for the Dardenelles. On 10 August 1914, on a hill on Sazli Beit in a Gallipoli goat track, Lt. Moseley was trying to extricate his 26 man communications team from a major foul-up in this campaign, noted for being in itself a major foul-up. A Turkish soldier did his duty and put a bullet through Moseley's head — a routine casualty along with 19,000 others, give or take a battalion or two.

Obituaries

When the news reached Chicago, R.A. Milliken assessed the cost: *"Had the European war had no other result than the snuffing out of this young life, that alone would make it one of the most hideous and irreparable crimes in history."* Even the enemy (technically) received the news with shock. K. Fajans published a moving obituary in Naturwissenschaften. Rutherford complained bitterly in a letter to Nature: *"It is a national tragedy that our military organization was so inelastic as to be unable ... to use ... scientific men except as combatants on the firing line."*

[Jaffe, Biog, Doubleday 1971]

The official British assessment of Moseley's worth was expressed in a letter to Moseley's mother: *"In him the brigade has lost a remarkably capable signaling officer."*

Kitchener's Gallipoli campaign and much of its foul-up had been the work of The First Sea Lord Winston Churchill. In the next war Churchill selected F.A. Lindemann as his scientific advisor. Practically the only opposition to Moseley's work came in a nasty note in the 1 June 1914 Nature. F.A. Lindemann said the work was only a copy of Rutherford's views. Twenty-five years later this same Lindemann (now Lord Cherwell) would fight a bureaucratic battle against the utter waste of time and money on development of an infant science called "radar."

Lindeman's greatest contribution to science was his nasty refusal to accept Francis Aston's separation of neon isotopes at the 1913 British Association. Aston, rankled over the criticism, was forced to devise a mass spectrometer that nobody could refute. [See Vig1919 .Ast]

WILLIAM DUANE AND THE RADIUM-RADON COW

(I use the 1923 word "radon"; Duane used "emanation," but it can be confused with other "emanations.")

William Ramsay, the acknowledged world expert on handling small amounts of gas, was probably the first to attempt to set up a simple collection system for radon in 1903. Fresh from his discovery of the noble gases, he wanted to study the chemistry of radon; he cared little and knew nothing about its °activity. He had hired F. Soddy from Rutherford's group at McGill to take care of the radioactivity details. He used the same liquid air system he used with the noble gases.

Around 1906 André Debierne, who had just taken the late Pierre Curie's place in the Curie Lab in Paris, set up a chemical radon separation system. It was done to preserve Madame Curie's small radium supply. Helping him was one of four post-doctorate students: William Duane.

> [When preparations were being made in 1921 for Marie Curie's triumphant fund raising publicity tour of the U.S. (her phrase), she was asked what she wanted to see in America. Her answer, *"Niagara Falls, Grand Canyon, and William Duane."*]

Duane was one of the few allowed to handle Marie's precious radium supply. He prepared radon sources for some of the earliest biological and medical work in Paris. Duane was impressed by a lack of need for expensive 1600 y radium, once 3.8 d radon was available. Most experiments at the Curie Lab were done with sealed sources. Ra and Rn sources could not be distinguished, except by their half lives. Around 1908 he asked, *"Why waste precious radium on medical work when only radon daughters are used?"*

Harvard Begins the Changeover to Radon

In 1899 a gift to Harvard Medical School began a special interest in "cancer." It surfaced in 1909 as the Harvard Cancer Commission, dedicated to *"multi-disciplinary"* approaches (a euphemism for fishing expeditions). A grant then allowed the Commission to build Huntington Memorial Hospital, dedicated to cancer research. Surgery was notoriously unsuccessful, chemotherapy ranked with ever popular faith healing, but X-rays were having some success.

Ever since 1901, when Alexander Graham Bell (of Harvard's Otology Dept.) had recommended putting radium in a needle and pushing the needle into a tumor, radium therapy had been astonishingly successful (compared to zilch for surgery). By about 1911 radium therapy was a stable medical business, if at "shocking prices" it could be called business. Radium was horribly expensive, and Harvard owned only 350 milligrams. Then a sarcastic remark by a Harvard Professor of Physics came to their attention, *"It's stupid to pay for radium when you're throwing radon away."* The Commission asked Professor Duane to explain.

Why Use Up Expensive Radium?

Duane explained: 1600 y radium decays to 3.8 d radon which decays to radium A, B, C, which last for minutes and eventually goes through D, E, F, in years to G, which is stable lead. Radium emits only alpha rays that can't get through tissue paper, let alone skin. The gamma rays come from radon, an inert gas that can be collected and stored in containers of any size or shape. Use needle, tube, or seed shaped containers for the strong gamma ray emission of RaA, B, C, or let them sit for a few weeks and use the less intense gammas from RaD, E, F.

Duane explained some other options: Collect the gas in a large container. Insert any medical applicator. Expose for a few hours and the radon daughters will deposit onto it. (Exposure time will be equivalent to the dose the physician wants to use.) Or expose grains of salt dissolved in liquid for IV injection. These devices are not "substitutes-for-radium," they are the actual substance used in radium therapy. The expensive radium meanwhile sits back in the lab making more radon. Because the procedure can go on for thousands of years, isn't it foolish to spend the principal when its interest yield is so high?

Duane was asked and accepted the job of making "emanation" (renamed radon in 1923). He designed the first medical "emanation extraction plant" for Huntington Memorial Hospital in Boston. It would use Harvard's 350 mg of radium element (soon increased to 920 mg). The design was a complex train of glass flasks, bulbs, and tubes that extracted 4.5 Ci of radon each month.

By 1917 over 500 patients/year were being treated (mostly cancer patients). The glass radon tubes (2 to 50 mCi/tube) were applied at various distances over the skin through various filtrations for weeks or months. The results were astonishingly good. [Remember, in 1917 there was no other therapy.]

Failla Designs the First °Cow in Terror

Henry Janeway, one of the first oncologists at Memorial in New York, wanted to duplicate the Boston success. His young physicist associate, Gioacchino Failla, was terrified at the thought of many technicians, even some physicians, playing with a wild gas-producing cow. A little radon contamination would be sufficient to put his precision radiation measurement lab out of business.

> [Late in the 1950s I accused Failla of being the first to call a °generator a "cow." His answer was that radon was called "radium milk" in Europe: if milk, it must come from a cow.]

Failla designed an "automatic radon collection apparatus" so self-contained and simple that any reasonably careful technician needed only to follow standard operating procedures. Although initially expensive (it contained 3.56 Ci of 1920 Ra), it produced up to 17 curies of radon each month.

> [At its 50th anniversary in the mid-1970s Failla's radon cow had produced over 10 kCi of radon without serious incident — the cheapest cancer cure (that occasionally worked) in New York. However, torturing patients with chemotherapy was then in vogue, and the event went unnoticed by the cancer money trust.]

The Radium Cow Goes World Wide

Failla's radium cow was a large scale, but local, manufacturing plant. The "cure" of cancer with radon had a world wide popularity. A simpler device more adaptable to the needs of smaller hospitals was designed by Victor Hess of Vienna. He simplified Failla's modification of Duane's radium cow. As little as 100 mg of radium could produce a millicurie of radon on each milking. During the late 1920s Hess's apparatus became the basis for a popular commercial design (U.S. Radium Corp).

[See Vig1923 .Bal]

The Ubiquitous Radium Cow

Another modification of Failla's plant was the large scale radon extraction plant installed in Rome. Enrico Fermi remembered the Rome cow when the neutron discovery was announced in 1932. He could not get an accelerator, but he knew where he could get 5.4 MeV alphas, up to 800 mCi worth, from Rome's radium cow. His neutron yield was about 1 neutron/4000 alphas bombarding Be atoms, hence 1 Ci radon in Be yields about 10 neutron/second. (This calculation is the origin of the 1940s statement that one cyclotron is worth a kilogram of radium.) When Fermi mixed radon with beryllium in 6mm $\times$ 15mm glass tubes he produced 1000 neutrons/mCi sec — one of the largest scale-ups in technical history. His group was well along in the study of neutron behavior when 3 radioisotopes were announced; thus, he was ready to immediately expand the list to 14, one of which was P-32.

When George Hevesy read Fermi's report, the sentence on P-32 was what he had been looking for for many years: a biologically natural radioactive tag. He knew that Copenhagen's Finsen Hospital of Radium Studies had a large source of radium sulfide in solution, from which they produced radon. He dug a well in the basement of the Bohr Institute. Up to 500 mCi of radon was mixed with beryllium powder in a 10 liter flask of cold sulfide. After it sat in the well for 2 weeks he could separate about a microcurie of P-32. [See Vig1936 .GHP]

Robley Evans, in April 1937, made some I-128 with radon from Duane's 1915 radium cow. Upon being asked if he could make iodine, Evans remembered a sentence in Fermi's 1934 report: iodine could be made radioactive. He gathered the discarded radon needles from Huntington Hospital, mixed their remnant activity with beryllium, and exposed some iodine. Within a month he proudly displayed a few nanocuries of I-128 and began Nuclear Medicine. [See Vig1936 .I]

Scratch almost any subject in nuclear science deep enough and you will find a radium cow. It was developed by William Duane to protect Marie Carie's radium.

[See Vig1927 .Blu Blumgart uses Rn]

PANETH GOES ORGANIC WITH RADIOACTIVITY

(and Hevesy misses a discovery)

In 1917 Fritz Paneth went beyond George Hevesy. He discovered that polonium, then a largely unknown rare element, formed a volatile hydride. This fact by itself was minor; all Po homologues, S, Se, Te, form hydrides, but the method he followed was significant.

Paneth had passed a nitrogen stream over polonium in dilute HCl. The gas, fed into an emanation electroscope, had picked up °activity (radioactivity). A "control" experiment was done with bismuth — known to not form a volatile hydride. The stream of nitrogen was passed over bismuth that had been tagged with ThC (now Bi-212) in dilute HCl. It was known that no transfer of °activity would occur (Bi did not form hydride). When Paneth tried it °activity *was* transferred. Were the textbooks wrong?

Paneth put a glass tube between the ThC (Bi-212) sample and the electroscope. He heated the glass tube to decompose any hydride; this time no °activity reached the electroscope. He prepared a lead sample tagged with °lead. (Lead forms a hydride.) To check this discovery he prepared a lead tetramethyl sample (known to be volatile). When heating the glass tube a lead mirror plated out on the glass wall; non-radioactive methyl had split off to become a free methyl radical. He added another glass tube (one with a pre-formed lead mirror). After the free methyl radical was formed at the first Pb mirror, it was carried to the second Pb mirror which promptly disappeared.

Hevesy later described this first break of radioisotopes from the confines of inorganic chemistry:

"Paneth deduced from this and similar observations the existence of a free methyl radical of very short life. In a hydrogen stream half the methyl disappeared within 0.006 seconds . . . It was the ingenious experimental arrangement of Paneth which alone enabled free methyl, the first free radical, to be discovered." (IAEA Bull. 7:17, Jan 1965)

[See Vig1923 .GH3 °isotopes in Biochem]

Hevesy Believes the Experts; Hence, He Fails to Discover Heavy Water

During World War I George Hevesy couldn't leave Hungary. But shortly after (1919) Niels Bohr invited him, as a physical chemist, to join the Institute for Theoretical Physics in Copenhagen.

In the spring of 1920 a few of the Copenhagen group attempted to exploit the remarkable separations of stable isotopes by Francis Aston at Cambridge. Aston, in his first report, described separating only a few atoms of a few elements. But, by theory, the whole number rule told where to look for other stable isotopes. The potential interactions of the stable isotopes cried out for investigation.

Hevesy was a part of the Copenhagen group but ranked, academically, as a junior member. It might be possible, the group thought, to separate a ponderable quantity of, for example, a stable isotope of mercury. (Hg has 7 stable isotopes, but they didn't even suspect this.) They attempted to capture the faster evaporating distillate of mercury on glass surfaces cooled in liquid air. A lighter and a heavier fraction of Hg was achieved. By a similar distillation of HCl they also succeeded in separating a lighter and heavier fraction of HCl. Nothing much was done with the materials because they realized the extreme dilution of their separations.

Hevesy wanted to extend the work to pure water as a check on the slight differences in the HCl separations. Also he remembered his 1912 discussions with Aston, Bohr, Rutherford and others on triple weight hydrogen. However, older, more respectable, and highly authoritative Danish co-workers disagreed. Only one form of hydrogen and one form of oxygen exists. (Two Germans had searched for other forms by diffusion through porous membranes — and failed.)

While this decision was being made, Aston, back in Cambridge, was getting evidence for the existence of H-2, but of course they didn't know this. Ten years later Harold Urey would discover heavy water using a variant of Hevesy's method. Hevesy soon made up for his mistake by taking radioisotopes into biochemistry.

RUTHERFORD DISCOVERS TRANSMUTATION, AGAIN

(This time ER, not nature, does it)

Ernest Marsden, one of Rutherford's senior research associates at Manchester, did most of the didactic review in the *Introduction to Radioactivity Physics* required of all visiting "students." (Hans Geiger did the lab teaching.) One of his first jobs had been to find out, with Geiger, how many alpha particles were scattered directly backwards after collision with a nuclear atom. It had led to the "nuclear atom." [See Vig1911 .ER4]

Just before World War I broke out, Marsden went to Wellington, New Zealand as Professor of physics. His last study for Rutherford had been to find out if hydrogen nuclei would scintillate on a ZnS screen similar to alphas. Marsden bombarded hydrogen gas with an alpha source and saw many scintillations. Massive alphas struck lighter hydrogen nuclei and drove a few far beyond the greatest possible alpha range. Then he packed his bags and sailed for Wellington.

A Lonely Rutherford Transmutes Atoms

In wartime confusion Marsden's experiment was not dismantled. For the next few years Rutherford's lab was practically deserted. In loneliness he played with Marsden's apparatus, enjoying the flashing sparks. He noticed a minor detail. The number of scintillations increased when the alphas were going through dry air. For fun he substituted pure oxygen, then pure nitrogen, . . . but something happened.

Artificial Transmutation is "Proved"

(It was never really questioned)

From a few years of work with alpha scattering experiments, Rutherford knew that oxygen and nitrogen atoms impelled forward by high speed alphas must be completely stopped by 9 cm of gas. But some particles were going far beyond 9 cm. Laboratory doodling stopped — Rutherford had to find out what was happening.

Rutherford proved that the long-range scintillations could not be due to water vapor or dust. They were affected by the pressure of the gas. From absorption measurements he proved they were from accelerated gas atoms. "*. . . The long-range atoms from nitrogen closely resemble hydrogen atoms.*" [PM 37:581, 1919] These rays came from an atmosphere that contained no hydrogen. "*. . . considering the enormous intensity of forces brought into play . . . The results suggest that if projectiles of greater energy were available for experiments, we might expect to break down the nucleus structure. . .*"

In April 1919 Rutherford wrote up the first artificial transmutation. It was his last paper from Manchester. J.J. Thomson, elected Master of Trinity, did not feel he could do two jobs well. On 2 April 1919 Rutherford was elected fourth Cavendish professor to succeed Maxwell, Lord Rayleigh, and J.J. Thomson.

The Proton is Named to Honor Prout

In June 1919 Rutherford gave the Friday evening lecture at the Royal Institution on knocking hydrogen atoms out of nitrogen. One critic pointed out that the more epochal a discovery the more closely it should be examined. But no alternates were seen. The new Cavendish director had his first job; set up a simple instrument to investigate transmutation. After all, the instrument he used at Manchester was Marsden's design for another problem.

It was about this time that Rutherford began using the name "proton." He introduced it at the 1920 British Association meeting at Cardiff. F. Aston was showing Moseley's Staircase moving up in multiple steps. (Now, everybody called them isotopes.) Rutherford had already approved Aston's forthcoming paper that would convert Prout's 1815 Hypothesis to a "Whole Number Rule." Rutherford wanted people to remember William Prout who, as much or more than John Dalton, had started the atomic business with his "protyle." The name electron was well established, and proton was a better match than "positive electron." The mass of a proton was too high for it to be a "positive electron." (P.A.M. Dirac will predict a real +electron in 1928 and it will be found in cosmic rays by C. Anderson in 1932.)

But the ordinal number and atomic weight did not add up sensibly. Something was still missing from the nuclear atom.

[See Vig1920 .ER6, The Neutron]

THE FIRST MAN TO "SEE" ISOTOPES
(Aston proves Prout, in 1815, was right)

Francis W. Aston, a chemist by training, came to the Cavendish lab in 1910 as J.J. Thomson's laboratory assistant. J.J. was working on the parabolic positive ray detector. J.J. considered the positive ray device a potential chemical analyzer, and that's why he chose a chemist for assistant. They were building a library of calibration standards when they ran across a double-line spectrum. The chemical was neon, hence Ne-20 plus •X-22. Aston leaned toward Ne-22, J.J. said "contaminant."

[Aston, Mass Spectra, 1933]

In many repeat exposures Aston showed that a double line occurred always with neon in the tube, and only with neon. In a lecture to the Royal Institution on 13 Jan 1913, J.J. called it an atom of weight 22. (Fajans' articles were not published until February.) Chemists laughed, and said, look again at the Periodic Table! By spring J.J. recanted. Aston tried differential absorption of neon in charcoal cooled in liquid air; the parabolic streaks were unchanged. He tried diffusion of neon through the fine pores of clay tobacco pipes; the results were only "highly suggestive."

At the 1886 Birmingham meeting of the British Association William Crookes had speculated on "isotopes" (he said meta-elements). Twenty-seven years later, at a second meeting in Birmingham, Aston presented what he always considered the first proof that substances existed with the same chemical and spectrographic properties, but different atomic weights. Only one person agreed — George Hevesy, but he was already using "isotopes" of Pb.

A year later (1914) England was at war. G.P. Thomson was the son and collaborator of J.J. Ten of J.J.'s students became Nobel laureates. Thirty years after J.J. got his Nobel prize for proving that electrons were particles, not waves, George got his for proving electrons were waves. Fifty years later George Thomson reminisced on the uncertainties: [J.J. Biog, 1964]

"*... By mid-1915 I* (GPT) *was living with some other scientific people who had been collected by ... the Royal Aircraft Factory. ... Among our group were Aston and F.A. Lindemann.* [He would, as Lord Cherwell, become Winston Churchill's science advisor in the next war.] *Lindemann had recently come back from working in Berlin under Nernst and was full of quantum theory, then still something of a novelty. He and Aston discussed the neon results. Lindemann was skeptical and I remember long discussions on many nights. Lindemann favored either NeH_2 or CO_2, as the source of the 22-parabola. ... Lindemann had a case, and being a much better theoretician than Aston he always won the argument. But Aston had faith and was unbeatable; next morning he 'was of the same opinion still'. However there was no ill feeling, and when the war ended they wrote a joint paper on separation of isotopes.*"

[J.J. Biog, Nelson 1964]

Aston Proves Isotopes Beyond Doubt

Aston returned to the Cavendish lab after the war and immediately repeated his clay pipe diffusion of neon. After thousands of passages he achieved only half of his 1913 separation. He must go back to a method that never failed, Thomson's parabolic trace. But instead of trying to improve J.J.'s device, he designed an entirely new concept.

An element in gaseous form was stored in a glass bulb in front of a cathode. The positive charges were collimated through two narrow parallel slits, then spread out in a velocity spectrum. A portion of this spectrum was then deflected in a powerful magnetic field. Rays of similar velocity but precisely the same mass would come to focus on a photographic plate. Such a focusing eliminated the velocity effect critical in J.J.'s design.

Aston was able to work only with elements that could be maintained in gaseous state (corrected in a couple of years). He was a fussy experimentalist. Aston trusted nobody but himself to do anything. He needed a constant potential of 1000 volts and decided to use accumulators. He blew 500 glass jars, with all lead plates formed and soldered with his own hands. His fussiness paid off.

The first mass spectrum of neon, published in the Nov 1919 Phil Mag, showed remarkable separation of Ne-22 from Ne-20, "*... with an accuracy of one-tenth percent...*" [NATURE 105:617, 1920]

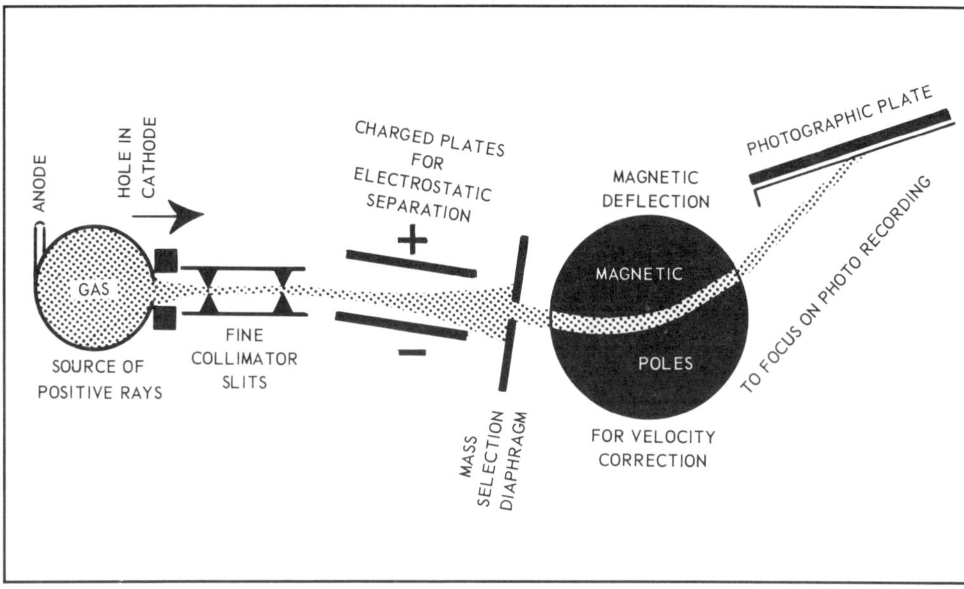

Diagram of Aston's original mass spectrograph.
[Aston F.W.; Nature 105:617, 1920]

The "Whole Number Rule" is Established

Within weeks the stable isotopes of chlorine and mercury were displayed. The stable Ne was for his 1913 humiliation. The two chlorines explained Berzelius' denial of William Prout in 1824. The six (later seven) stable isotopes of mercury illustrated the complexity of "elements." Aston knew he was finally establishing a "Whole Number Rule" as seen by Prout in 1815. (Moseley's 1913 proof was not yet universally accepted.)

Once Aston solved the problem of feeding elements into his mass spectrograph, he ran through the Periodic Table:

Mar 1920 — A, Kr, He, N
Jul 1920 — B, F, Si, Br, Sr, As
Dec 1920 — I, Xe, Mg (By A.J. Dempster)
Feb 1921 — Li (Others now in field)
Apr 1921 — Na, K, Rb, Cs
Jun 1921 — Ni
Nov 1922 — Be, Ca, Zn

In 1923 seventeen more elements were analyzed and some of the less abundant were being found. In 1925 and in 1927 new instruments increased accuracy from 1 part in 1000 to 1 in 10,000. By 1932 only 18 elements (11 Rare Earths) remained unanalyzed. But the Whole Number Rule was not as precise as once thought.

At the end of his 1920 article Aston added *"... with the exception of hydrogen...."* Hydrogen measured out at 1.008 on an oxygen = 16 scale. There was no H-2 to account for the deviation. (Deuterium was way beyond Aston's sensitivity. He even missed Ne-21 which is 175 times more abundant than H-2.) Within a year Aston and G.P. Thomson showed that Li-6 and Li-7 exceeded whole numbers by a small fraction. Then Fe-56 was a little short. The whole-number-deviation, called the "packing fraction," became a regular irregularity: maximum in H, minimum in Fe, and slowly increasing to Pb. Its "binding force" significance would not become apparent until the mid 1930s.

H-2 had not been seen, yet in the late 1920s there was compelling theoretical reason for it. Maybe it would be visible on spectroscopy after diffusion. It was tried and failed. Then in 1931 H. Urey at Columbia had a better idea.

[See Vig1931 .HW, Heavy Water.]

STEFAN MEYER'S VIENNA RADIUM INSTITUTE

(Rutherford Pays Back a Long Term Debt)

Rutherford moved to Manchester in 1907 and found everything agreeable, except maybe the climate and, of course, the great shortage of radioactive material. (Manchester had about 20 mg of pure radium bromide.) He decided to apply to the Kaiserliche Akademie der Wissenschaften of Vienna for a loan of some of the radium preparations in their charge. His request for about a half gram was well received — Rutherford was the world authority on all things radioactive. (At least one of his Montreal students was now working in Vienna.) He was also a new boy in England. The Akademie was a government office that spoke only to governments. To accept radium, William Ramsay at University College, London, was as close to a government body as possible.

The Vienna Akademie Makes Rutherford Rich

The Akademie at Vienna made arrangements for 350 mg of RaBr to go to Ramsay in London, with equal shares to Rutherford. Naturally there was conflict. Ramsay knew little about radioactivity and could imagine only his type of chemical research. He wanted to combine the 350 mg with his personal 150 mg to make a large cow that could be milked every 4 days. The emanation could be sent to Manchester and arrive only 18 hours old, which was good enough for physical experiments.

Such an arrangement was not satisfactory to Rutherford, but the problem was solved by Stefan Meyer, director of the Radium Institute of Vienna (where the radium sources were actually made). Stefan Meyer saw that giving Ramsay control had been a mistake and corrected it in January 1908: Stefan made a personal loan to Rutherford of another 300 mg of radium bromide for his exclusive use. Radioactively speaking, Rutherford was now a rich man.

The Vienna Akademie Falls on Hard Times

In 1910–1914 Meyer and Rutherford were the driving forces behind standardization of radium and the curie unit of activity. Hönigschmid, Meyer's chief chemist, made three international radium standards to back up Marie Curie's one.

[See Vig1910 .Ci]

During the war all communication ceased. In January 1920 Meyer heard of Rutherford's discovery of artificial transmutation and sent him copies of the scientific papers published from the Vienna Institute during the war years. Rutherford resumed their previous correspondence by sending him news of Meyer's friends in England. Meyer answered with news that his old staff had scattered. Hönigschmid was now professor at Munich, as was Fajans. Paneth was professor at Hamburg. Hevesy was in Budapest, but was expected in Vienna soon. Some of Rutherford's students were in Vienna, refugees from the Russians. The Czechs had taken over Joachimsthal and the Austrians expelled; the official language in Joachimsthal was now Czech, although nobody spoke or understood it and communication was quite difficult. The worst problem, however, was inflation.

During the violent inflation in Austria after World War I, Stefan Meyer's Vienna Radium Institute was having great trouble just keeping open. Practically everybody involved with pitchblende, radium, or any radioactivity owed a debt to Stefan Meyer's Vienna group. The 1908 personal loan from Stefan Meyer to Rutherford was well remembered. If England could repay this loan (repayment was never requested) Rutherford thought he might help tide Meyer's Institute over a period of depression and extreme difficulty.

Rutherford Pays Back a "Loan"

First Rutherford sent Meyer several hundred pounds granted by the Royal Society to pay for the 7 mg radium standard Meyer had "loaned" Rutherford before the war (it had been a gift). He asked Meyer about the price of radium so that he could pay for the 1907 supplies. This letter was greeted in Vienna with "vivid joy." The price of radium in America was about $92,000/g. The price in Czechoslovakia was grossly inflated, almost $150,000/g. By 7 Feb 1928 Rutherford informed Meyer that Cambridge University would pay the Vienna Akademie £3,000 for the radium loaned to Rutherford in January 1908. This money kept Meyer's group alive.

[Eve, Rutherford Biog, MacMillan, 1939]

A BALLOON RIDE PAYS OFF IN COSMIC RAYS

(V. Hess Sees Extraterrestrial Radiation)

During his 1913 stay in Vienna while working with Fritz Paneth, George Hevesy was introduced to Victor Hess, a young physicist. [Vig1912 .KF1] Hess was a balloon enthusiast and invited Paneth and Hevesy to take a short flight with him. Because all three worked with radiation they could take electroscope measurements while Hess operated the balloon. He wanted to show how the inverse square law was violated close to a source. (It works only with point sources and detectors, or when the distance between source and detector is many times greater than the diameter of either). However, the decrease should form some mathematical pattern for an infinitely large source.

Hess could not derive a formula, hence on the balloon ride they would measure the decrease while he handled the balloon. Only one thing went wrong: the electroscope readings did not show a decrease in °activity; as the balloon rose an increased activity was unmistakable.

Terrestrial versus Extraterrestrial?

Back in 1900 C.T.R. Wilson suggested an extraterrestrial origin for some background radiation and a few physicists (but with inadequate equipment) tried to prove it. One put an electroscope on the frozen surface of Lake Ontario (the water would shield out the earth.): little change. Measurements made behind thick shields of iron and lead saw minimized, but not abolished, radiation. A 1909 review of the subject [ArRR] concluded that all of the radiations were of terrestrial origin,

A French physicist took an electroscope up Eiffel Tower — no change. A. Gockel, a Swiss physicist, was more realistic; on balloon ascents he saw increased radiation at 5 km. Victor Hess eventually went up to 9 km and saw a substantial increase in radiation. He called this radiation "Höhenstrahlung." They furnished an explanation for the thick layers of metal needed to shield electrocopes on the surface of the earth. Any radiation that could penetrate a 30 km thick blanket of atmosphere must have an unheard of energy.

Höhenstrahlung Become Cosmic Rays

Following World War I, American physicists became interested in the Hess "Höhenstrahlung." Most considered the phenomenon a result of cloud buildup or thunderstorm activity. In 1922 R.A. Millikan, who had *measured* the charge of an electron on a droplet of oil, disagreed. He sent electroscopes up to 19 km in unmanned sounding balloons. He put lead-lined electroscopes on Pike's Peak. But he could not get convincing proof that the rays were of "cosmic" origin.

Lake Arrowhead and Lake Muir in California have similar terrestrial and atmospheric surroundings, except for about 2.2 km altitude. Millikan made electroscope readings at various depths in both. He found the ionization identical in the two lakes, if you corrected for the 2.2 km additional layer of atmosphere over Lake Muir; hence in 1925 he called them cosmic rays (meaning, incidently, "electromagnetic rays").

Are the Rays Really Particulate?

A.H. Compton (pupil of Rutherford), who had discovered the scattering effect of X-rays and named the "photon," turned to the world-wide measurement of cosmic rays in the early 1930s. He documented the variations due to latitude. Millikan had missed this, but later confirmed it. The latitude variation was best explained by the effect of the earth's magnetic field sweeping *charged particles* toward the poles. Millikan could not accept this. After interactions the secondaries could be particulate, but primaries are photons.

During 1930's depression *Cosmic Rays* became a science staple in Sunday Supplement journalism. They were electromagnetic birth cries of stars, according to Nobel Laureate Millikan who had discovered them. If, however, you believed Nobel Laureate Compton, who discovered cosmic rays, they were particles of matter that looked like rays.

[Neither man ever claimed discovery. They both knew Victor Hess and gave him credit. But the Sunday Supplement dog fight was maintained for years as a significant factor in financial support of science during lean years.]

The Cosmic and Solar Rays

After World War II the nature of the Hess Höhenstrahlung became clarified. The sun (and other stars) emits a relatively constant solar wind plus occasional flares. 93% of these winds are hydrogen nuclei, 6% helium and a smattering of heavier elements. Not many of these reach the earth because they are stopped by 25–35 km of atmosphere (78% N, 21% O, a whisper of rare gases). The atmosphere is thin on top, but fairly thick at the bottom. A cosmic ray must get past many trillions of atoms to hit the earth's surface; a couple make it to each square meter of earth each year. Their energies are measured up to tera-electron-volts.

Collisions at GeV, and TeV, are atom smashing energies. Either or both particles may break into smaller pieces of matter: neutrons, protons, or pions. These pions are unstable fragments of protons. Within nanoseconds pions decay to gamma rays or ± electrons. Each of these secondaries at slightly reduced energy is itself a projectile that will collide with another nitrogen in the stratosphere, producing yet more secondaries. Thus an exponentially multiplied cascade of subatomic particles descends through the atmosphere at ever decreasing energies.

A collision is not the most common interaction; a particle is more likely to merely push a nitrogen atom to one side, thereby losing a little energy. Any particle pushed off course will emit radiation. These braking emissions (bremsstrahlung in German) are the same as X-rays — except for point of origin.

Effect of the Earth's Magnetic Field

Beginning with very high energy particles at the top of the atmosphere, this cascade of interactions results in a thick mash of photons, electrons, with some protons and neutrons. At the surface the energies are generally in the keV to >MeV level. The cascade occurs through a 30 kilometer thick atmosphere in a global magnetic field. As expected, the charged particles are swept toward the poles of the earth. At the earth's surface, cosmic ray secondaries are least at the equator and doubled at 80°–90° latitude. (New York City is at 40° N.)

Induced Radioactivities

The energy levels, particularly in the upper reaches of atmosphere, are sufficient to transmute nuclei. Neutrons interacting with N atoms produce C-14. Because of its 5730 year half-life, C-14 production is significant. It is incorporated as normal carbon into all living things and can serve as an archeological dating marker. Also produced are:

Beta emitters		Beta + gamma emitters	
silicon-32	(650 y)	sodium-22	(26 y)
argon-39	(269 y)	beryllium-7	(53 d)
hydrogen-3	(12.5y)	argon-37	(35 d)
sulfur-35	(87 d)	sodium-24	(14 h)
phosphorus-33	(25 d)		
phosphorus-32	(14 d)		

How Much Cosmic Radiation?

The human body occupies roughly a cubic meter of space, usually near the surface of the earth, for about 60 or 70 years. The number of cosmic ray-produced secondaries that pass through this space is too large to be meaningful — many million per second. However, most cosmic rays pass through the body without any effect. Radiations can affect atoms in the body by excitation or ionization. Excitation cannot be measured in the living body, but number-of-ion-pairs can be. The basis for the 1928 roentgen unit is number-of-ion-pairs. A couple of million ion-pairs equal one roentgen, or a couple of thousand per milliroentgen. By just occupying space near the surface of the earth you are exposed to 26–30 mR per year.

26 to 30 mR/year is in pre-1975 roentgen units. Since 1985 we have converted to SI units: 1 old roentgen = 2.58 new SI roentgens, which are in coulombs of charge/kg. Hence, your cubic meter of space is exposed to 7 or 8 milli C/kg each year. This amount is about a quarter of the total exposure most people get from all natural sources.

A couple of other ubiquitous sources account for most of the inevitable radiation that everybody receives. These sources are exhalations of the earth and the composition of living bodies.

[See Vig1924 .°K; Vig1978. Background]

HEVESY INVADES BIOLOGY
(°Isotopes Are Applied to Living Plants)

George Hevesy was called to Niels Bohr's Institute for Theoretical Physics in 1919. But he could not be confined to one lab, or one branch of science, for long. Within a few years he happened to meet a plant physiologist from a small laboratory at the Agricultural School in Copenhagen. The botanist was growing Horse Bean plants *(Vicia faba)* in a culture solution. The amounts of H, O, C, and N absorbed by each plant could be measured. The neat rows of almost identical plant seedlings growing in culture solution set off a knee-jerk reaction in Hevesy: what would happen if radioactive lead were put into the solution?

Within a few days Hevesy returned to the lab with the proper equipment. With the botanist's help a small amount of ThB (Pb-212) in lead nitrate was added to the culture solution. After a period of growth the roots, stems, fruit and leaves were removed, ashed, and measured under the electroscope.

A pattern of absorption revealed the movement of lead atoms through the plant. Hevesy changed the $PbNO_3$ concentrations, then the ThB/Pb ratios. Something more important than simple metabolic movement was revealing itself "*. . . the active Pb atoms are almost completely displaced from their places in the root by inactive atoms. . . .*" [Biochem J 17:439, 1923]

The experiment was far more important than being "the first biological use of radioactive isotopes." Hevesy had discovered the concept of metabolic "turn-over." For years he did not understand the significance of his discovery. His knowledge of biology in the 1920s was not only limited, but he had biases carried over from physical chemistry that were simply not true in biology. However, to him (and this was a rare trait in Bohr's Institute) the experiment, not the theory, was the final truth. The great Danish physiologist, August Krogh, would soon teach Hevesy that the animal body is not a large test tube. Like all physical scientists Hevesy first had to get into the cause and cure of cancer.

[See Vig1924 .GH4]

HEVESY STUDIES °ISOTOPES IN ANIMALS
(In His First Brush With Cancer Cures)

World War I feelings did not fade quickly. Hevesy was anxious to get back to England to update his expertise in radioactivity. In 1921 Rutherford said it was still too early. Hevesy understood and instead reverted to an old idea he had discussed with Moseley just before the war began: the disputed place at #72 on the Periodic Table.

Instead of using the classical chemical search methods he used Moseley's X-ray spectroscopy. In January 1923 he and Dirk Coster announced the discovery of hafnium, element No. 72 (the ancient name for Copenhagen where the discovery occurred). Rutherford, now president of the British Association, took the hafnium discovery as an opportunity to invite Hevesy to address its summer meeting in Liverpool.

A Cancer Cure Gets a Kneejerk Response

At the Liverpool meeting Hevesy heard gynecologist Blair Bell discuss "successful" cancer chemotherapy with colloidal lead compounds. As with most cancer cures, it worked well on every MD's first few patients but not for the first scientist to try it. The words "lead compounds" struck a kneejerk response in Hevesy: lead meant RaD (Pb-210).

Upon returning to Copenhagen he approached the University's biochemist, J.A. Christiansen, about a study of lead moving about in the body. A friend of Christiansen, the dermatologist Sven Lomholt, was interested in the proposal.

> [A dermatologist? Look back to 1923! Syphilis was then a dermatological disease. Bismuth had just become popular in syphilis therapy. RaE was a fine bismuth label.]

Hevesy extracted 5 day RaE (now Bi-210) from 22 year RaD (now Pb-210). He incorporated it into an oil suspension similar to the quinine-bismuth-iodide used in syphilis therapy.

The oil was injected into 9 rabbits. Urine and fecal samples were collected daily. At 15 days the rabbit's organs were ashed and measured under the electroscope. On 7 April 1924 the results were presented to the French Academy in Paris. (Compt Rend 178:1324, 1924) Bismuth is excreted mainly via urine; its distribution in the body is similar to that previously determined by Lomholt for stable mercury.

Hevesy had originally intended only a study of lead, and the same experiment was being run with RaD (now Pb-210). The reason for reporting the bismuth (RaE) results first was that RaD has a soft beta emission (61 keV) difficult to measure with an electroscope. Hence, they stored all their samples for a few months and then measured the hot (1.16 MeV) betas from its daughter RaE.

The radioactive lead distribution in both rabbits and guinea pigs showed high liver concentration, hence fecal excretion. Much more important was Hevesy's training in biological science: *"We have recovered [only] 90 percent of the lead injected."* (Arch Exp Path Pharm 149:336, 1930) Hevesy, the precise physical chemist, had learned that animals are not oversized furry test tubes.

The Cancer Cure Leads to Dynamic Studies

In 1927 Hevesy accepted a professorship at Freiburg. Blair Bell's cancer therapy with colloidal lead still rankled in his head. He explained to Freiburg's pathologist, Ludwig Aschoff, how lead could signal its location in cancers. Aschoff understood the value of dyes as labels in microscopy and was impressed. He assigned his chief chemist, Rudolph Schoenheimer, to the task.

Schoenheimer was introduced to the use of °isotopes, but lead had by this time served its function in cancer money raising and was no longer a cure. Lead was not a normal body constituent and Schoenheimer's interest faded — until the 1932 discovery of heavy water. Hydrogen is a normal body constituent and Schoenheimer immediately began his innovative work on the *Dynamic State of Body Constituents* (published in 1942); a logical extension of Hevesy's discovery of Pb movement in plants. Atoms in living bodies don't stay put.

[See Vig1923 .GH3]

THESE MEN MADE NUCLEAR SCIENCE PRACTICAL

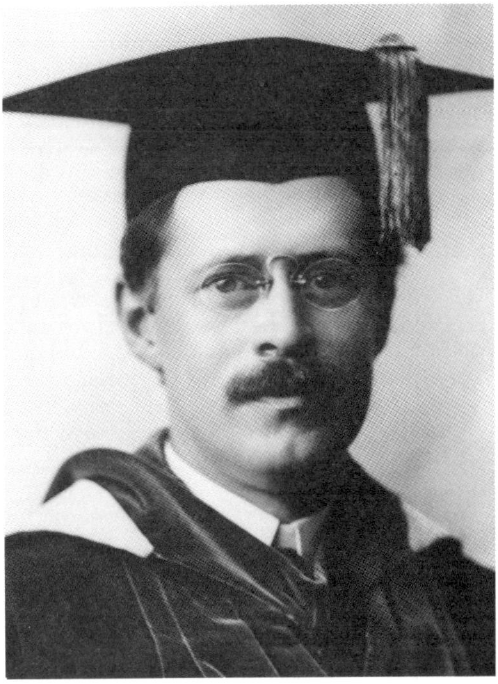

William Duane, Ph.D., 1872–1935

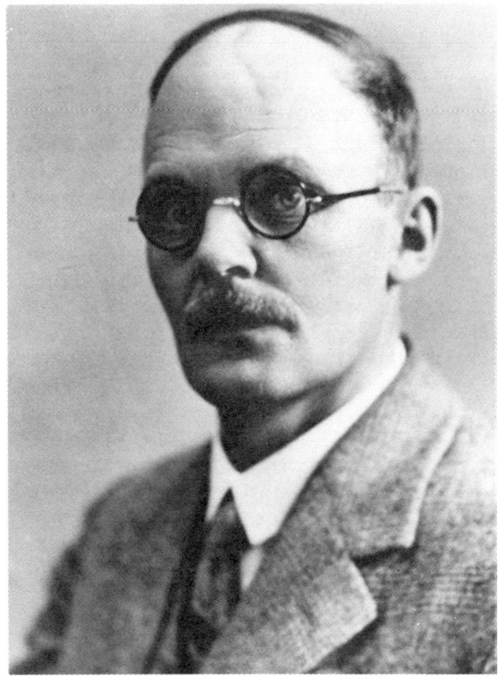

DEUTSCHES MUSEUM, MÜNCHEN

Hans Wilhelm Geiger, Ph.D., 1882–1945

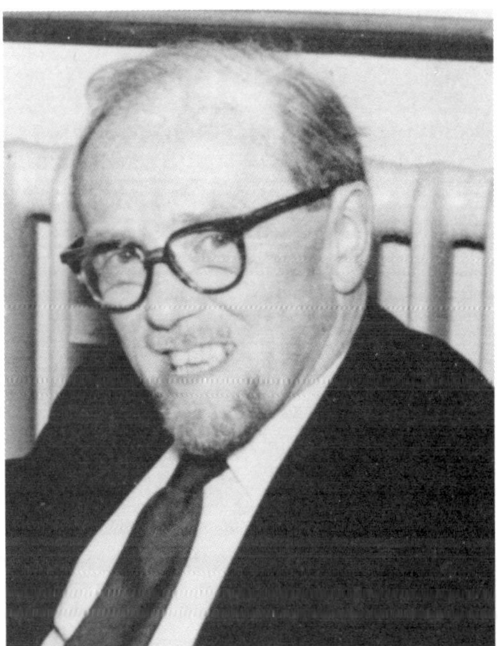

William Valentine Mayneord, Ph.D., 1902–1988

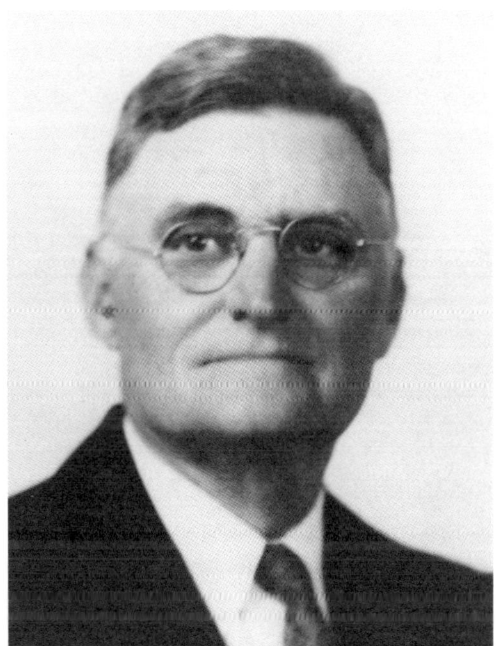

UNIVERSITY HOSPITALS OF CLEVELAND ARCHIVES

David Marine, M.D., 1880–1976

POTASSIUM, HENCE HUMANS, IS RADIOACTIVE

(An Element Essential to Life is °Active)

Through Elster & Geitel's studies, radioactivity was known to be widespread, but only from elements at the top of the Periodic Table. [Vig1901 .E&G] By 1905 hints of an even more prevalent °activity became known. J.J. Thomson mentioned °K in 1905, but potassium was proved radioactive by N.R. Campbell, an experimental physicist under J.J. Thomson at Cambridge. [PCPS 1905–08] The word got around fast. Max Levin wrote to Rutherford from Göttingen about the *"strange fact that potassium is radioactive."*

[Eve, p. 147, 1939]

Potassium was considered permanently radioactive until a billion year half-life was measured by T. Gráf in 1948 (now 1.28×10^9 y). K-40 was one of the first °isotopes known (c1950) to have a combined decay mode: 89% decays by B^- to Ca-40, 11% by e capture to Ar-40. In 1962 a faint trace of B^+ in the decay was detected.

Which Isotope is Radioactive?

George Hevesy was critical of his own use of toxic heavy metals in biology. In 1924, while adapting °bismuth to a biotracer, he recalled a radioactive substance that was natural in biology. Most living organisms, he reasoned, contained potassium, hence its °activity must be biologically acceptable.

Aston had just found 2 isotopes of potassium, K-39 and K-41. [Vig1919 .Ast] Hevesy thought that if he could separate the two he would have a strong biologically "natural" tracer. He used a method successful in separating Hg isotopes. A few kilograms of metallic K were distilled into light and heavy fractions. A difference in counts/min should reveal the °isotope. Hevesy used a new radiation counter built for him by Hans Geiger at his Kiel Institute. (In 1928 it became known as the Geiger-Müller Tube.) The atomic weights of the samples were determined by Hönigschmid in Munich. From these data radioactive potassium was found to be the K-41 isotope.

On a visit to Harvard, Hevesy described his reasoning to G.P. Baxter, successor to T.W. Williams' noted "Atomic Weight" laboratory. K-41 was almost 7% of potassium. Was natural potassium that intensely °active? Baxter, a schoolmate of Hönigschmid under Williams, said Hönigschmid had finally made a mistake. He ran the weights on Hevesy's samples. The radioactive isotope was K-40, with a natural abundance of about 0.02%. This fits the intensity of natural potassium far more realistically.

Other Sources of Background Radiation

The major radioactivity of the human or any other living body is C-14. It is being manufactured continuously in the upper atmosphere by cosmic ray produced neutrons. However, because of its very low energy beta, C-14's contribution to body background *dose* is trivial.

Radium, its gaseous daughter radon, and its 8 daughters with half-lives up to 22.3 years, are usually considered a "body burden" rather than a natural background. Everybody inhales and eats some from natural sources, but the amount is so highly variable that it is considered a "contaminant." The sources contributing to body burden may be a water well with low radon content in one county and 100 times higher in the next, or water from a health spa 1000 times more or from a school yard well in Finland 100,000 times higher. Radium is a daughter of uranium (proved by B. Boltwood in 1907). Hence, uranium and thorium are prime sources of human radiation, but they are not as intimate as potassium.

Natural Body Background

If you are anywhere near the size and shape of a reference man (in the 1950s he originated as the 70 kg "Standard Man") you have 140 g of potassium in your body. 0.012% or 1.68 grams is K-40. The specific activity of K-40 is low because of its 10^6 year half-life, so you contain 12 μCi or 444 kBq of K-40. Most of these 444 disintegrations per second (dps) you absorb yourself, but 11% decays with a 1.48 MeV gamma emission. Hence, you spray about 50 gamma rays per second in all directions. Most of these supervoltage gamma rays go through people without effect, but if you spend days (or nights) close to someone, you add a mrad/year to your partners background. But, in a crowd of people, you are swimming in a sea of gamma rays.

[See Vig1926 .Bkg]

MAX BORN SEES A DIFFERENT PICTURE
(Non-Commutative is Common Sense Algebra)

Soon after physicists got back to work after World War I, they realized that when Bohr's 1913 atomic structure theory was extended to anything more complicated than hydrogen it would not work. Max Born's first paper mentioning "Quantum Mechanics" in 1924 was not quite consistent. In papers with his assistants at Göttingen, W. Pauli in 1922 and W. Heisenberg in 1923, the calculated spectral lines of helium did not agree with measurements. The frequencies of electron vibration were proportional to energy differences in two stationary states, not to an orbit as Bohr had used in 1913.

To find the laws for the "transition quantity" between the higher and lower stationary state was the problem of a new quantum mechanics. It was the substance of daily meetings of Born's staff in theoretical physics at Göttingen in 1925.

Heisenberg Reinvents a Forgotten Math

Heisenberg pursued an idea of his own for a few months. In early July 1925 he brought in a paper and asked Born to check it for possible publication. Heisenberg took off to give a lecture at the Cavendish Laboratory. After a few days Born read the manuscript and was fascinated. Heisenberg had developed a calculus of transition energies in which all quantities are eliminated that are not directly observable and, at least in principle, measurable. Born sent the paper off to Zeitschrift für Physik.

But Born was bothered by the queer manipulation of symbols in the paper. Suddenly on 10 July he saw why. Heisenberg had reinvented matrix algebra. Never used, or even taught in math studies, Born remembered it from student days 20 years earlier. With a pupil, P. Jordan, Born rewrote Heisenberg's idea in matrix notation. Heisenberg hit the books, as did most other physicists, to learn matrix algebra. Matrices have the singular property of being non-commutative. Only in elementary arithmetic does $2+3 = 3+2$. In real life there is a proper and irreversible order to events: a glass must be filled *before* milk can be spilled from it. Max Born, in 1925, put common sense back into physics.

Uranium Cannot Be Radioactive

Ever since Rutherford split a few nitrogen atoms with alpha particles, physicists wanted a higher flux (number crossing a square cm per second) of higher "voltages." In medical usage higher voltage (potential difference between anode and cathode) meant greater permeability through tissue. For nuclear disruptions physicists needed greater penetration through the potential barrier surrounding the nucleus (which wasn't yet fully appreciated). For energy acquired by a charged particle falling through a potential of one volt, the electron volt (eV) was the common unit, usually in denominations of keV.

A prime reason for a hi-energy, hi-flux requirement was to investigate nuclear disruptions in the heavier elements. A good example occurred with uranium. Doubly charged alphas leaving a massive uranium nucleus must, by Coulomb's law, be repulsed to an enormous energy — but it wasn't. Uranium alpha emissions are "only" (relatively speaking) 4 to 5 MeV. Theoretically no alpha particle could ever leave the uranium nucleus.

A Particle is Really a Wave

Erwin Schroedinger, a Viennese physicist at the U of Zurich, was a most conservative mathematical theoretician. He tended toward rigid logic and was devoted to Newtonian mechanics. It is in the nature of science that he should initiate a most radical departure from Newtonian common sense.

In 1920 Schroedinger was a recognized master of the physics of vibrations in continuous media: light waves in the aether, vibrating strings, oscillating bodies; nothing granular or particulate was involved. Bohr's adoption of discontinuous quanta to achieve stationary states in the atom made him unhappy.

In any vibrating system, certain math functions may be treated as though they were integers: amplitudes or periods of oscillation, index of refraction. Bohr's quantized states might be one of those discontinuous aspects of a continuous wave function. When de Broglie discovered the wave nature of particles in 1925, Schroedinger derived a series of equations to clarify DeBroglie's observations. He didn't have the slightest idea of his equation's physical meaning — totally unnecessary that it have any.

A Wave is Really a Cloud of Probability

Max Born was a theoretical physicist at Göttingen in 1925 when he converted W. Heisenberg's incoherent mass of data into mathematically acceptable matrix algebra. For the first time in science, non-commutative algebra and common sense were substituted for the limited intelligence of commutative logics. Everybody beyond moron status knows that if you pull the trigger and then put a bullet in a gun the result is entirely different from when you put a bullet in a gun and then pull the trigger. In kindergarten arithmetic we were taught that $(2+3)$ is the same as $(3+2)$, a commutative numerical algebra that is not true in the real world. Appreciation of non-commutative reality marks the change to 20th century science.

Born was a good friend but intellectual opponent of Schroedinger. He said that there was physical meaning in the wave equations. Schroedinger like DeBroglie, said Max Born, believes in the physical reality of waves. Look at a buzzing violin string. It might be just a piece of cat gut, but to a musician its vibration, the waves, are a real sound. Sheet music might show 12 discreet notes; these are mathematical symbols. The real sound is a continuum. Similarly, electrons at rest — which they never are — must be symbols. Vibrating electrons are not particles, they are vibrational clouds extending in all directions in space.

But the cloud, insisted Born, is not the wave of oscillation or it would retain its structure. The real cloud dissipates as it is propagated in all directions, and eventually the wave can no longer scatter as a particle. The wave therefore is not a physical vibration, rather it is a mathematical expression of the probability of finding a particle in a particular place at a particular time.

Theoreticians Admit That Uranium Might Possibly be Radioactive

According to Born, an electron at rest is a fictitious mathematical symbol; a "real" vibrating electron is both particle and wave at the same time. *"Maxel,"* wrote Schroedinger, *"you know I am very fond of you, and nothing can change that, but I must once and for all give you a big scolding . . ."* [WoA, Chap 64]

Einstein had a different analogy to explain the new common sense in relativity. Bohr was evolving a complementarity. From this new common sense a very practical development was in process. In 1928 George Gamow, a Russian math-physicist who had just spent a year with Bohr, found an answer to why the alpha particle was emitted from uranium at such low energy. He pictured the nucleus as a deep well surrounded by a high coulomb barrier of repulsive force. The alpha inside the nucleus has properties of both particle and wave. When the particle approaches the coulomb wall it is bounced back into the nuclear well.

Its wave property, a Max Born cloud of probability, is not constrained by a potential barrier and the cloud spreads out far beyond the wall. As the alpha particle oscillates inside the nuclear well, there is a finite probability that the particle properties will coexist with the wave properties at any point in time. If the point occurs precisely when the wave is outside the wall, the alpha will be repulsed not back into but away from the nucleus at a low inherent MeV.

The reciprocal of this probability is the lifetime of this nucleus. It is measured as a half-life of many similar radioactive atoms.

> [Don't try to picture this on paper because this is a 4-dimensional space-time event. The only 2-D picture is in Schroedinger's algebraic equations. Don't fret about transcendental tunnels in the barrier. If you can't see physical structure in the equations, you probably never did believe in the tooth fairy.]

Gamow could see physical structure in the equations; he solved them for an alpha particle leaving the uranium nucleus and his calculations agreed with observation.

John Cockcroft, in Cavendish Lab, read Gamow's paper. Why couldn't, he thought, this work in the opposite direction: getting an alpha into a nucleus?

[See Vig1932 .C-W; Vig1939 .MB2]

THE EMBRYONIC DEVELOPMENT OF NUCLEAR MEDICINE 1926 through 1953

FROM Hermann Blumgart's harvesting used radon needles to measure the velocity of blood with a radioactive blood "tag" (he didn't know about Hevesy's studies)...

FROM the Joliot-Curie's accidental discovery of artificially produced radioisotopes (it was a meticulously planned experiment to find something entirely different)...

FROM G. Hevesy duplicating E. Fermi's P-32 production for animal studies of a "normal" metabolic element (all of his previous work had been with very heavy metals)...

FROM Robley Evans harvesting used radon needles to make E. Fermi's almost completely unknown radioiodine...

FROM John Lawrence boldly (wimps said recklessly) trying to cure a leukemia patient with P-32...

TO Sam Seidlin actually curing a patient of metastatic thyroid cancer.

In the midst of a heated anti-Atom Bomb debate, the concept that °isotopes were useful, and possibly a boon to humanity, had grown in headlines. Nobody knew better than Seidlin that a functioning thyroid metastasis was rare, but the newspapers made °Iodine a CANCER CURE and the public forced Congress to act. Congress gave the new AEC a second command: Cure Cancer. (The first command had been: Make Bombs.)

Thus began 28 years of financial support to Unclear Medicine. (The mispronunciation was often true. In 1947 T. Kohman cleared up the "Isotope-tone-bar-mer" confusion by coining the generic term "nuclear," it was hard for some people to pronounce.) During this period the Chronology of Nuclear Medicine (CNM) is dominated by radioisotope therapy, but a single diagnostic procedure, "scanning," changed the emphasis. Nuclear Medicine flowered after P.R. Bell introduced a gamma ray spectrometer that made scanning reasonably accurate:

CNM1926 Cause-&-effect is probablistic.
CNM1927 °Blood velocity is measured.
CNM1928 The "Roentgen" is adopted.
CNM1929 "Dose" is Rad absorption.
CNM1930 A 4-inch "cyclotron" is made.
CNM1931 Radium measured in "r" units.
CNM1932 The neutron is discovered.
CNM1933 "Dynamic State" introduced.
CNM1934 Artificial °isotopes discovered.
CNM1935 P-32 used in rat physiology.
CNM1936 °Iodine suggested for thyroids.
CNM1937 First P-32 Rx to leukemia pt.
CNM1938 "Turnover" concept introduced.
CNM1939 Nuclear fission discovered.
CNM1940 C-14 is discovered.
CNM1941 Sr-89 "cures" bone ca mets.
CNM1942 First reactor goes critical.
CNM1943 °Isotopes reactor starts.
CNM1944 Particle size sets clearance.
CNM1945 Atomic Bombs used in anger.
CNM1946 °Iodine cure of thyroid ca mets.
CNM1947 Name changed to "Nuclear".
CNM1948 NaI(Tl) crystal introduced.
CNM1949 First scanner introduced.
CNM1950 First °drug (°IHSA) introduced.
CNM1951 1000Ci Co-60 teleRx announced.
CNM1952 No adverse reactions to °I Rx.
CNM1953 Medical spectrometer installed.

CHRONOLOGY OF NUCLEAR MEDICINE — 1926

	Scientific and Technical Background		Ref.
1. Basic	— M. BORN'S PROBABLISTIC WAVE THEORY MODIFIES "CAUSE & EFFECT."		ZP
	— E. Schroedinger describes standing wave electron orbits.	[1924]	WoA
2. Obser	— O. Glasser: dose must be measured, cannot be calculated.	[1924]	Rad
	— H. Muller damages fruit fly chromosomes with X-rays.	[1923]	Bio
	— J. Ewing studies morphology of tissue reaction to rad.	[1923]	AJR
	— T. Strangeways finds X-rays prevent cell division.	[1925]	PRS
3. # Nuc	—		
4. # Med	—		
	Organizations and Internal Politics		
5. Pols	— USA population at 115 million.	[1920]	AP
6. Socs	— T. Morgan publishes "The Theory of the Gene."	[1925]	Bio
	— Hevesy & Paneth, "Manual of Radioactivity" published.	[1924]	Bk
	— M. Curie pubs biography, "Pierre Curie" (Macmillan).	[1906]	Bk
7. Event	— G. Hevesy starts Schoenheimer study of dynamic metab.	[1933]	ARR
	— Cannon Mfg Co introduces colored towels for bathroom.	[1925]	AP
	Instruments, Units of Measurement, and Drugs		
8. Instr	— R. Willstatter introduces 1906 chromatography.	[1924]	SN
	— W. Röver calibrates a selenium cell "intensity-meter."	[1925]	Str
	— H. Wintz describes a photometer for use with X-Rays.	[1925]	Str
	— H. Franke modifies his roentgen-cinematography.	[1924]	FGR
9. Units	— H. Fricke attempts (first ?) to measure Dx exposure.	[1925]	FGR
	— G. Failla studies the biological radiation unit problem.	[1921]	AJR
	— R. Glocker urges: standardize a "human size" ion chamber.	[1952]	Str
	— R. Glocker questions effect of wavelength on small chamber.	[1924]	Str
	— O. Glasser compares instr for measuring erythema dose.	[1920]	Str
	— E. Pohle says American Erythema Dose = 1200–1400 "R."	[1920]	Rad
	German Erythema dose = 500–600 "R."	[1925]	Rad
	— W. Giauque gets to within 0.001° of 0° Kelvin.	[1908]	SN
10. Concp	— O. Glasser finds that surface dose varies with field size.		AJR
	— O. Glasser describes backscatter problem in skin dose.	[1924]	AJR
	— H. Coutard begins protracted, fractionated, lo-intensity Rx.	(1934	La)
	— M. Tsuzuki begins first large Acute Rad Syndrome study.	[1921]	AJR
	— M. Tsuzuki gives rabbits cLD_{50} low energy (c80 kev) X-ray.	[1985]	
	— M. Tsuzuki: L-node and spleen lymphocytes give diff reaction.	[1921]	AJR
	— H. Straudinger develops macromolecular chemistry.		EB
11. Drugs	— G. Failla installs 3.35 g radium cow system at Memorial.	[1924]	AJR
	— R. Schoenheimer studies distribution of °Pb.	[1924]	ARR
	— B. Jansen isolates VB_{12} in pure form.	[1955]	CDD

Radioiodine, P-32, and Radioactive Therapy

12.	I-Res	— C. Harrington discovers 4 iodine atoms in T4 molecule.	[1914]	BJ
13.	I-Dx	—		
14.	I-Rx	—		
15.	P-Rx	—		
16.	Tele	— W. Mattick draws depth dose charts for radium pack.	[1923]	Rad
17.	Other	— W. Bell recommends IV colloidal Pb for malig neoplasia.	[1928]	La
		— I. Rubin cures sterility/amenorrhea with X-ray to ovary.	[1918]	AJOG
		— C. Burnham notes Rx of Hodgkin's with 4 gram-hours Ra.	[1922]	JAMA
		— C. Reed gives history of visible light (helio)therapy.	[1774]	Rad
		— G. Failla develops filtered radon implants, gold seeds.	[1919]	AJR

Scans and Other Tests of Function in Various Organs

18.	Brain	— F. Miller reviews physiology of cerebellum.	[1925]	PhR
19.	Heart	— D. Scherf studies the diseases of auricular myocardium.	(1944	BHM)
		— I. Daly studies cardiovascular responses to stress.	[1925]	AJPh
		— W. Chamberlain does roentgen-cinematography of heart.	[1924]	Rad
20.	Liver	— L. Whitaker describes mechanism of gall bladder.	[1924]	AJPh
		— J. Case explains value of cholecystography.	[1921]	AJR
		— G. Higgins explains mechanism of gall bladder emptying.	[1924]	AJPh
		— F. Mann explains formation of bilirubin.	[1924]	AJPh
21.	Lung	— A. Desjardins sees, names "radiation pleuropneumonitis."	[1923]	AJR
		— P. Butler shows X-Rays of metastatic lung disease.	[1921]	Rad
		— H. Grady shows bronchial tree with lipiodol.	[1925]	AJR
22.	Bone	— C. Blacket describes tuberculosis of joints.	[1917]	AJR
		— R. Karshner describes osteoporosis by X-Ray.	[1919]	AJR
23.	Kidney	— F. Hartman irrad dog's kidneys, gets acute nephritis.	[1920]	AJMS
24.	Gut	— G. Falley does fundusectomy to prevent jejunal ulcer.	[1924]	PSEB
		— L. Brown describes X-Rays in intestinal tuberculosis.	[1918]	Bk
		— R. Carman describes X-Rays of ulcerative colitis.	[1924]	AJR
25.	Blood	— G. Minot arrests pern anemia with dietary liver.	[1826]	TAAP
26.	Other	— B. Orndorf irrad tail of pancreas, gets increased juice.	[1922]	AJR
		— A. Ivy discusses the current physiology of pancreas.	[1902]	AJPh

Radiation Hysteria and Health Physics * Obituaries *

27.	Hyst	— H. Fricke says upper limit of safety is 700 r (air).	[1925]	FGR
		— E. Quimby calibrates film badges with photodensitometer.	[1984]	Rad
		— J. Fibiger gets Nobel prize for cure of cancer.	[1921]	Sc
		— Radiologists snub embittered Muller and X-rayed flies.	[1955]	Bk
		— -. Rostoski autopsies first lung cancer from Schneeberg;	[1920]	
		establishes lung tumors in Joachimsthal U miners	(1926	AJC)
		— F. Flynn questions industry safety of °active materials.	[1925]	JAMA
		— Radium Ore Co. sells 155,400 bottles radon drink/year.	[1924]	AP
		— A. Anikin notes effects of mitogenetic rays from nerves.	[1923]	RA
28.	React	— A. Czepa proves Ludwig's irradiated food hazard false.	[1925]	Str
		— M. Tsuzuki studies first dose-controlled Acute Rad Synd.	[1921]	AJR
		— J. Aub discusses and documents Pb poisoning.	[1922]	Bk
29.	Respo	—		

* * *

30. Obits —

CHRONOLOGY OF NUCLEAR MEDICINE — 1927

Scientific and Technical Background

			Ref.
1. Basic	— P. Auger describes the "Auger electron" interaction.	[1925]	WoA
	— W. Heisenberg quantifies wavelength vs spectrum theory.	[1925]	WoA
2. Obser	— H. MULLER DISCOVERS X-RAY MUTATIONS IN FRUIT FLIES.	[1926]	Sc
	— S. Gager notes gene mutations before Muller's paper.	[1908]	PNAS
	— J. Thibaud uses a grating to confirm Compton spectra.	[1923]	GSR
	— C. Packard says same bioeffect at different wavelengths.	[1924]	JCR
3. # Nuc	—		
4. # Med	—		

Organizations and Internal Politics

5. Pols	— Seventh CGPM defines newton, joule, watt, coulomb (elec stds).	[1925]	NBS
	— F. Kellogg (USA) proposes peace pact to stop wars.	[1928]	EB
6. Socs	— S. Meyer compiles a bibliography of tracer studies.	[1924]	Bk
	— F. Paneth reviews the tracers in physical chemistry.	[1913]	Bk
	— I. Pavlov publishes "Conditioned Reflexes."	[1890]	DSB
	— J. Clark publishes "Radium in Gynecology" (Lippincott).	[1915]	Bk
7. Event	— "White lead" ends 25 years of dominance as the only color considered "bacteria clean" in American products.	[1926]	AP
	— H. Blumgart collects Duane's old radon tubes for source.	[1917]	JCI

Instruments, Units of Measurement, and Drugs

8. Instr	— H. Fricke introduces ferro-sulfate color dosimeter.	[1907]	AJR
	— W. Duane measures "absolute r" on parallel-plate chamber.	[1922]	AJR
	— H. Behnken visits Glasser to cross calibrate "r" meter.	[1925]	AJR
	— D. Skobeltyn adds lead plates, mag field to cloud chamb.	[1925]	WoA
	— A. Bowers builds new metal X-ray tubes for Dx and Rx.	[1918]	BJR
9. Units	— A. Bachem says: poor definition of vague "Erythema Dose";		
	measures Erythema Dose on every med student in hosp,	[1926]	Rad
	derives: ED = foc-skin-dist × K / spark gap^2 × mamps.	[1925]	Rad
	— O. Glasser proves that Bachem's formula doesn't work.		Rad
	— O. Glasser says wall effect makes German unit too high.	[1925]	Str
	— H. Behnken discusses standardization of the roentgen.	[1923]	GSR
	— H. Kuester shows relation between erythema dose and "r."	[1930]	Rad
	— K. Hauser notes UV erythema dose varies with wavelength.	[1920]	Str
	— H. Holthusen relates half-value-layer to kilovoltage.	[1916]	Str
	— H. Holthusen proposes injury-to-ascaris-eggs as dosimeter.	[1925]	Str
	— I. Solomon pleads, standardize ionization chambers.	[1926]	JRE
10. Concp	— A. Baclére: arbiter must decide Glasser-Behnken units.	[1909]	JRE
	— C. Regaud is convinced of value of fractionated doses.	[1919]	CRB
11. Drugs	— J. Goldberg implicates Vit B_2 in pellagra.	[1914]	PhR
	— T. Davis discusses early history of phosphorus.	[1670]	JCE

	Radioiodine, P-32, and Radioactive Therapy		
12. I-Res	— C. Harrington suggests T4 is conjugation of two T2s.	[1944]	BJ
	— C. Wegelin: no lymph-infiltrate in Swiss endemic goiter.	[1825]	ICS
13. I-Dx	—		
14. I-Rx	— J. Muir says direct Ra-implants in goiter have 80% cures.	[1923]	Rad
	— U. Portman describes ext beam Rx in 210 malignancies.	[1923]	JAMA
15. P-Rx	—		
17. Other	— H. Ullman finds PbColloid toxic (but antitumor effect).	[1926]	Rad
	— E. Allen tells history of rise and fall of Ra therapy.	[1914]	JAMA
	Scans and Other Tests of Function in Various Organs		
18. Brain	— H. Hering studies the carotid sinus reflex.	(1944	BHM)
19. Heart	— H. Blumgart measures blood velocity with IV Rn-226.	[1927-32]	JCI
	THE FIRST NUCLEAR MEDICINE PROCEDURE	[1936]	
	— H. Frédéricq studies myocardial physiology.	[1924]	Bk
	— L. Brauer designs surgical repair of adhesive pericardium.	(1944	BHM)
	— E. Starling measures energy output of heart.	[1926]	JPh
20. Liver	— C. Schmidt reviews extrahepatic functions of bile.	[1925]	PhR
	— F. Mann studies effect of complete removal of liver.	[1926]	Med
21. Lung	— P. Drinker invents and develops an "iron lung."	[1922]	Sc
22. Bone	— M. Bernstein shows X-Rays of epiphyseolysis.	[1926]	Rad
	— R. Bromer gives X-Ray DDx of infectious osteomyelitis.	[1925]	AJR
	— E. Jenkinson discusses X-Ray Dx of bone tumors.	[1917]	Rad
23. Kidney	— G. Domagic observes chron glom nephritis in irrad pts.	[1926]	MMK
24. Gut	— V. Savich sees secretion after intestinal nerve stimul.	[1924]	CRB
	— J. Evans shows a congenital diaphragmatic hernia.	[1922]	AJR
25. Blood	— E. Ehrenberg estimates bld vol with 10.6h ThB (Pb-212).	[1921]	KW
	— W. Mattick studies bioeffect of radiation on blood.	[1922]	JCR
26. Other	— M. Greenwood describes status-thymo-lymphaticus.	[1913]	JH
	— P. Wilder finds ca of islet cells in hyperinsulinism.	[1924]	JAMA
	Radiation Hysteria and Health Physics * Obituaries *		
27. Hyst	— E. Pohle measures Dx X-ray output for Erythema Dose.	[1920]	
	— E. Pohle: Erythema Dose will give safe Dx exposure limits.	[1926]	Rad
	— H. Chantraine lists tables of skin exposure limits, and	[1925]	
	sets 300 r as a safe exposure limit.	[1926]	FGR
	— M. Baumann finds a sarcoma in pt given thorium dioxide.	[1916]	Str
	— G. Frank compares mitogenetic with ultraviolet rays.	[1923]	RA
28. React	— R. Sayers reviews effects of very abnormal temperatures.	[1923]	PHSB
	— J. Haldane reviews CO as a nerve poison.	[1923]	BJ
	— O. Wuth has a therapy for bromine poisoning.	[1923]	JAMA
29. Respo	—		

* * *

30. Obits	— S. Arrhenius (1859–1927) Swis chem; ionic disassociation.	DSB
	— E. Starling (1859–1927) Eng physiol; secretin, law of heart.	DSB
	— B. Boltwood (1870–1927) Am chem; ionium, first rad chemist.	DSB

CHRONOLOGY OF NUCLEAR MEDICINE — 1928

	Scientific and Technical Background		Ref.
1. Basic	— M. Born changes Schroedinger waves to probability cloud.	[1926]	Bio
	— W. Heisenberg arrives at "uncertainty principle": position-AND-momentum of electron unmeasurable.	[1927]	WoA
	— P. Dirac postulates pair production @ high energies.	[1932]	WoA
	— P. Dirac refines the wave equations.	[1926]	WoA
	— R. Millikan: atoms share electrons in molecular orbits.	[1916]	SN
2. Obser	— A. Compton introduces G. Lewis' term "photon" (e-m rays).	[1900]	Bk
	— R. Wideroe accelerates K^+ ions thru tubes in alternate current. THE BEGINNING OF ACCELERATOR PHYSICS.	[1953]	AfE
	— J. Buchholz gets X-ray defects in F_1 generation chromosomes.		GSR
	— J. Patterson sees somatic cell X-ray changes (fruit fly).	[1927]	Sc
	— L. Stadler sees X-ray changes in chromosomes of barley.	[1927]	Sc
	— P. Vintemberger finds variations in mitosis sensitivity.	[1927]	CRB
3. # Nuc	—		

	Organizations and Internal Politics		
5. Pols	— Kellogg-Briand peace pact pledges 65 states to no war.	[1927]	EB
6. Socs	— "r" accepted by RSNA, NBS, Second ICR, Int X-RAY Comm. THE ONLY MEASURABLE UNIT OF RADIATION	[1908]	Rad
	— ICRP formed by ICRU and Second ICR; adopts British stds.	[1921]	ICRU
	— F. Paneth's "Radio-elements as Indicators" published.	[1926]	Bk
	— F. Paneth founds "Radiochemistry" as a separate science.	[1913]	Bio
	— J. Weatherwax publishes "Physics of Radiology" (Hoeber).	[1922]	Bk
7. Event	— Editorial gives standards for measurement & protection.	[1924]	AJR
	— L. Taylor is chm Advisory Comm on X-Ray and Rad Protect.	[1920]	AJR
	— L. Taylor is Am rep on Int X-ray and Radium Protect Com.	[1925]	ICR

	Instruments, Units of Measurement, and Drugs		
8. Instr	— O. Glasser's Bakelite solves "r" measurement problem.	[1925]	AJR
	— H. GEIGER ANNOUNCES THE BETA AVALANCHE GM COUNTER,	[1919]	PZ
	uses the wall of his tube as the cathode.	[1905]	PZ
	— H. & G. Klemperer announce proportional counter principle.	[1918]	PZ
	— H. Geiger extends GM to alpha, beta, proportional counts.	[1908]	GMP
	— W. Müller (of GM fame) immigrates to Australia, lost to history.		PL
	— A. Bouwers revises X-ray apparat to "complete" rad safe.	[1927]	AR
	— V. Zworykin devises a very fast scanning CRT.	[1924]	SN
9. Units	— The Roentgen unit "r" is same as Villard's 1908 unit.	[1908]	V101
	— W. Duane's parallel plate ion chamber made to define "r."	[1925]	AJR
	— W. Duane measures an "effective" wave length.	[1924]	AJR
	— O. Glasser and H. Behnken "r" calibrations in agreement.	[1927]	Rad
	— A. Barclay's "unit skin dose" measures skin "tolerance." FIRST ATTEMPT TO ESTABLISH A MEASURED HUMAN SAFE DOSE	[1925]	BJR
	— G. Kaye finds Erythema Dose "r" is energy-dependent.	[1927]	Bk
	— R. Braun tabulates dose required for X-Ray exams.	[1923]	FGR
	— F. Dessauer gives theory of Depth Dose Charts.	[1901]	HGS
	— E. Quimby measures intensity around radon needles.	[1922]	Rad
10. Concp	— The "r" is Villard's 1908 definition modified with Duane's 1914 wall effect correction.	[1914]	V104
	— E. Quimby says beam size corrupts inverse square law.	[1926]	Rad
11. Drugs	— W. Duane helps install Ra cow in NY Memorial Hosp.	[1926]	AJR
	— G. Failla substitutes "gold seeds" for Duane's glass.	[1915]	AJR
	— A. Flemming discovers and disregards penicillin.	[1940]	CDD
	— E. Joslin's insulin Rx of diabetes still includes diet.	[1919]	Bk

		Radioiodine, P-32, and Radioactive Therapy		
12.	I-Res	— F. DeQuervain measures iodine bld levels in goiter pts.	[1926]	E
		— D. Marine says iodine prophylaxis abuse causes nodules.	[1924]	V91
		— A. Sturm: no diff in urine I-127 before & after T-ectomy.	[1932]	DAKM
13.	I-Dx	— E. Rose says BMR (basal metabol rate) is most common test.	[1920]	AJR
16.	Tele	— G. Failla puts 4 gram radium pack into operation.	[1926]	AJR
		— G. Pfahler gives theory of high-dose therapy in cancer.	[1925]	Rad
17.	Other	— A. Soiland cannot confirm Bell's PbColloid ca therapy.	[1927]	Rad
		Scans and Other Tests of Function in Various Organs		
18.	Brain	—		
19.	Heart	— W. Hamilton uses dyes and A/V sampling for blood flows.	[1915]	AJPh
		— W. Hamilton adapts Stewart's 1894 outputs to clinical measures.	[1954]	Cir
		— C. Wiggers writes textbk on physiology of circulation.	[1921]	Bk
		— I. Roth describes "Clinical Arrhythmias."	[1925]	Bk
		— F. Hodges measures cardiac output with X-Rays.	[1870]	Rad
		— G. Brown writes "Thromboangitis Obliterans."	[1938]	Bk
20.	Liver	— W. Karuse: effect of foods on gall bladder emptying.	[1927]	AJPh
		— E. Graham pubs "Dis of Gall Bladder and Bile Ducts."	[1927]	Bk
		— A. Ivy studies mechanism of gall bladder contraction.	[1926]	AJPh
		— B. Kirklin discusses effic and limits of cholecystogram.	[1917]	BMSJ
21.	Lung	— W. Belden discusses X-Rays of the mediastinum.	[1926]	AJR
		— F. O'Brien gives meaning of elevation of diaphragm.	[1926]	Rad
22.	Bone	— S. Barrows reviews roentgen analysis of bone diseases.	[1927]	Rad
		— S. Brown describes the X-Ray study of the neck.	[1926]	AJR
		— L. Friedman shows bone changes that accompany icterus.	[1926]	AJR
		— J. Geyman discusses osteochondritis dissecans.	[1926]	Rad
		— A. Shands shows congenital absence of various bones.	[1927]	AJR
23.	Kidney	—		
24.	Gut	— J. Farrell finds gastric mucosa responsive to stimulus.	[1926]	AJPh
		— H. Cooper studies cause-of-death in intestinal obstruct.	[1926]	AS
		— B. Bernstein shows X-Rays of diverticulum of stomach.	[1927]	AJR
25.	Blood	— R. Ehrenberg injects 10.6h Pb-212 for °dilution Bld Vol.	[1927]	KW
		— L. Henderson publishes "Blood," chemistry & physiology.	[1923]	Bk
		— A. Rich describes splenic lesion in sickle cell anemia.	[1923]	JHHB
		— G. Harrot describes Dx and Rx of polycythemia.	[1923]	Med
		Radiation Hysteria and Health Physics * Obituaries *		
27.	Hyst	— T. BLUHNBAUM INTRODUCES Th-232 (THOROTRAST) AS CONTRAST AGENT.		FGR
		— E. Saupe says upper safe limit exposure is 100 r (air).	[1927]	FGR
		— A. Barclay puts daily limit at 0.00028 erythema dose.	[1927]	AJR
		— British MPD stnd is 0.1 erythema dose/y (c 50–100 r/y).	[1927]	BJR
		— S. Veronoff "rejuvenates life" with testicle implants.	[1918]	AP
		— C. Terrs publishes "The Opium Problem."	[1923]	Bk
28.	React	— A. Barclay recommends bld tests, holidays for rad techs.	[1923]	BJR
		— G. Laurence evaluates rad hazard "by nose" (ozone odor = hot).		CNT
		— R. Braun uses 100 r as upper limit for Dx exposure.	[1927]	FGR
		— R. Jaffe discusses pathology of electric shock.	[1923]	APa
		AMA reviews 425 outbreaks of food poisoning in USA.	[1922]	JAMA
		* * *		
30.	Obits	— H. Lorentz (1853–1928) Dut math physics; relativistic scale.		DSB
		— T. Richards (1868–1928) Am chem; precision chem, atomic wts.		DoE
		— W. Wien (1869–1928) Ger physics; deflection of kanalstrahlen.		DSB
		— S. Sochocky (1882–1928) Ra paint; dies of aplastic anemia.	(1962	JAMA)

CHRONOLOGY OF NUCLEAR MEDICINE — 1929

			Ref.
	Scientific and Technical Background		
1. Basic	— O. Klein-Y. Nishina formula on absorption is derived.	[1918]	ZfP
	— A. Einstein proposes a Unified Field Theory.	[1905]	WoA
2. Obser	— E. Rutherford reviews 4n + 3 series, Pa-231 to Pb-207.	[1923]	Eve
	— A. Russell deduces, 4 families of natural decay required.	[1923]	PM
	— K. Lars-Horowitz: ThB-$Pb(NO_3)_2$ penetrates into cells.	[1912]	Na
	— A. Somerfeld explains production of continuous spectrum.	[1927]	PNAS
	— R. Canti lists biologic effects of radium irradiation.	[1928]	AR
3. # Nuc	— F. Aston shows 2 rare isotopes of oxygen.	[1919]	Bk
	— W. Giauque discovers, oxygen has 3 isotopes: O-16, 17, 18;	[1926]	
	hence, oxygen cannot be the At Wt standard.	[1961]	SN
4. # Med	—		
	Organizations and Internal Politics		
5. Pols	— NCRP (NatComRadProtec) formed by ARRS, RSNA, AMA, AAXM, NBS.	[1928]	NBS
	— F. Kellogg gets Nobel prize for stopping all wars.	[1928]	AP
	— Oct 28, "black friday" stock mkt collapse begins depression.		AP
6. Socs	—		
7. Event	— G. Hevesy adds RaD to rock for first °iso-dilut analysis.	[1924]	ARR
	— H. Berger makes first ElectroEncephaloGram (EEG).	[1903]	Bio
	Instruments, Units of Measurement, and Drugs		
8. Instr	— A. Stahel compares Ra & X-ray in new micro-ion chamber.	[1899]	Str
	— H. Schlundt measures 5 μg Ra-226 in human (ion chamber).	[1928]	AJR
	— W. Bleakney designs mass spectrometer to see 0.01% N-15.	[1920]	PR
	— W. Boethe sets 2 GM tubes in line for coincidence count.	[1925]	WoA
	— E. Berliner invents the microphone sound pickup.	[1924]	EB
	— V. Gottheiner describes roentgenkineatographie apparat.	[1926]	GSR
9. Units	— F. Wood says death-of-Drosophila-eggs is biol dosimeter,	[1927]	Rad
	but is only biol calibration of a "physical dose."	[1927]	Rad
	— W. Mayneord: effective atomic no. for tissue depth dose.	[1926]	BJR
	— 1919–1929 Str & FGR publish 59 X-ray dose articles.	[1981]	Str
	— G. Failla says new "r" is not a unit of "dose," it is a unit of quantity of X-radiation.	[1918]	Rad
	— G. Failla says THERE IS NO UNIT OF BIOLOGICAL DOSE.	[1907]	Rad
	— E. Quimby measures skin erythema for gamma and X-rays.	[1925]	AJR
	— W. Morrison introduces a precise quartz-crystal clock.	[1707]	SN
	— A. Leichte considers the time factor in dosimetry.	[1947]	Str
10. Concp	— H. Schlundt measures expired air Rn at picogram level.	[1901]	AJR
	— G. Failla begins bio-dosimetry with energy dependence warning.		Rad
	— L. GRAY SAYS "ABSORPTION" NOT "EXPOSURE" IS PROPER DOSE UNIT.		PRSI
	— W. Mayneord explains physical absorption dose problems to MDs.		BJR
	— W. Mayneord calculates depth dose for X-ray beams.	[1905]	BJR
	— E. Hubble uses "red shift" to measure distance.	[1928]	DSB
11. Drugs	— C. Dam discovers Vit K (for Koagulation).	[1939]	DSB
	— E. Doisy prepares first female sex hormone (estrone).	[1939]	DSB
	— A. Fleming notes effect of penicillin on bacteria.	[1940]	DSB
	— M. Oka introduces Thorotrast to visualize the spleen.	[1928]	FGR
	— A. St George autopsies body 5 years after Thorotrast.	[1925]	APa

	Radioiodine, P-32, and Radioactive Therapy		
12. I-Res —			
13. I-Dx —			
14. I-Rx —			
15. P-Rx —			
16. Tele —	A. Heublein does total body irrad at Memorial NY Hosp.	[1961]	Rad
17. Other —	G. Bucky describes Grenz ray (mostly dermatol) therapy.	[1928]	Bk
—	S. Cade reviews the Radium Treatment of Cancer (Wood).	[1927]	Bk
—	B. Schreiner sums 374 cases Rx cervix ca with radium.	[1927]	RR
—	J. Juul does experimental studies of X-ray Rx of ca.	[1927]	AR
	Scans and Other Tests of Function in Various Organs		
18. Brain —	H. Blumgart: cat's cerebral circ time (RaC) is 6 sec.	[1927]	ANP
—	H. Berger begins clinical electroencephalography (EEG).	[1903]	Bio
—	A. Kapppers pubs "The Evolution of the Nervous System."	[1926]	Bk
—	J. Camp describes X-Rays of intracranial disease.	[1923]	Rad
19. Heart —	W. Forsman passes ureteric catheter into heart.	[1913]	KW
—	A. Master notes stress test with tables of normals.	[1924]	AJMS
—	F. Wilius publishes "Clinical Electrocardiography."	[1916]	Bk
—	T. Lewis studies spasmodic "Raynaud's disease."	[1928]	H
—	P. Stumpf shows cinematography of the heart & stomach.	[1926]	MMW
20. Liver —	P. Radt uses Thorotrast to visualize liver and spleen.	[1928]	KW
21. Lung —	O. Bowen shows acute massive collapse with atelectasis.	[1906]	AJR
—	W. Hudson shows X-ray cine pictures of tracheobronchi.	[1926]	BJR
—	H. Ashbury describes recurrent massive collapse of lung.	[1926]	AJR
—	D. Bowen describes acute massive collapse (atelectasis).	[1926]	AJR
—	A. Hartung pushes use of iodized oil for X-Rays.	[1926]	AJR
22. Bone —	L. Garland describes osteitis and related distrophies.	[1928]	AJR
—	K. Kornblum shows bone changes in Raynaud's disease.	[1928]	AJR
23. Kidney —	E. Muller studies urea excretion in normal subjects.	[1923]	JCI
—	E. Rosenow discusses intravenous pyelography.	[1927]	KW
24. Gut —	J. Case shows X-Rays of colon diverticula.	[1915]	AJR
—	F. Hodges describes mucus colitis.	[1928]	Rad
25. Blood —			
26. Other —	J. McCaughan studies cause-of-death in pancreatic drain.	[1927]	MCP
—	N. Kleitman reviews the physiology of sleep.	[1926]	PhR
—	R. Fraser uses lipiodol to see paranasal sinuses.	[1921]	Rad
	Radiation Hysteria and Health Physics * Obituaries *		
27. Hyst —	J. Lowy autopsies 2 lung ca on Joachimsthal miners.	[1932]	MK
—	No lung ca found in 323 (all) Joachimsthal miners, but, 2/3 of retired "pensioners" have lung ca.	[1926]	AJC
—	Press hypes, League of Nat investigates Joachimsthal.	[1932]	AP
28. React —	AMA will not accept radium drinks because no evidence of value, NOT because any danger has been demonstrated.	[1926]	JAMA
29. Respo —			

* * *

30. Obits —	K. Auer von Welsbach (1858–1929) Aust chem; thorium mantle, R.E.	DSB
—	J. Goldberger (1874–1929) Am physician; pellagra.	CDD

CHRONOLOGY OF NUCLEAR MEDICINE — 1930

Scientific and Technical Background			Ref.
1. Basic	— J. Beardon reasserts temp does not affect absorption.	[1929]	PR
	— P. Dirac suggests a + charged electron: the positron.	[1897]	WoA
	— P. Debye determines molec structure by X-ray diffract.	[1910]	DSB
	— Boethe & Becker detect neutron — don't recognize it.	[1932]	WoA
2. Obser	— G. Laurence's Canada pitchblende ends Congo Ra monopoly.	[1924]	CNT
	— D. Sloan's first Wideroe tubes set up as cyclotron backup.	[1936]	PNAS
	— C. Tombaugh discovers Pluto.	[1941]	EB
	— C. Packard relates cell division rate to sensitivity.	[1906]	JCR
3. # Nuc	— F. Aston shows stable isotopes of Cr, Mo, W.	[1929]	Bk
	— I. Joliot-Curie develops hi-intensity Po alpha sources.	[1887]	V108
	— A. Grosse finds three isotopes of protactinium.	[1918]	JACS
4. # Med	—		

Organizations and Internal Politics			
5. Pols	— C. Regaud organizes a war against cancer.	[1922]	R&R
	— USA population is 122 million.	[1921]	AP
6. Socs	— Rutherford, Chad & Ellis pub "Rad From °substances" (Macmillan).		Bk
7. Event	— L. Rovner tells of GM tube's domination of all counting.	[1932]	Sc
	— D. Sloan accelerates to 1 MeV X-rays. First supervoltage?	[1936]	PR

Instruments, Units of Measurement, and Drugs			
8. Instr	— E. LAWRENCE INVENTS PRINCIPLE AND A 4" CYCLOTRON.	[1928]	Sc
	— C. Lauritsen (& B. Cassen) develops a million volt tube.	[1949]	PR
	— R. Van de Graaff develops an electrostatic generator.	[1896]	WoA
	— A. Busch builds a 2.4 mVp X-ray device for Rx.	[1913]	Nw
	— R. Millikan builds automatic, mag field, multi lead-plate cloud chamber to photograph cosmic rays.	[1927]	WoA
9. Units	— O. Glasser finds r unit differs at different energies.	[1924]	Rad
	— O. Glasser cannot confirm Lahm's Ra/X-ray dose ratios.	[1925]	Rad
	— O. Glasser cannot confirm Stahel's micro-ioniz records.	[1929]	Rad
	— O. Glasser compares effects of geometry & size of 5 chambers.	[1909]	Rad
	— E. Lorenz outlines history of dosimetry to date.	[1929]	Rad
	— J. Barnes pleads for giving exposures in r units.	[1928]	Rad
	— R. Sievert studies the gamma ray intensity of radium.	[1928]	AR
10. Concp	— O. Glasser: Threshold Erythema doesn't relate to r unit.	[1928]	Rad
	— M. Glaser uses iodized rapeseed oil for body cavities.	[1929]	AJR
	— C. Johnson says stereoroentgenometry is for measurements.	[1900]	AS
11. Drugs	— J. Northrup proves that pepsin is a protein.	[1925]	SN
	— A. Allen describes English Ra-Rn cow, emanation plant.	[1928]	JCR

Radioiodine, P-32, and Radioactive Therapy

12. I-Res —			
13. I-Dx —			
14. I-Rx	— E. Astwood says surgery is only practical thyroid Rx.	[1927]	JAMA
15. P-Rx —			
16. Tele	— A. Erskine shows increased depth dose with high energy.	[1917]	Rad
	— A. Soiland preaches highest energy supervoltage.	[1914]	Rad
	— H. Martin calculates tissue dose in beam therapy.	[1928]	AJR
17. Other	— G. Hevesy finds °Pb, °Th, haven't, but °Bi has uptake in ca.	[1927]	ARR
	— B. Bell suggests Pb colloidal agent for cancer therapy.	[1928]	AEPP
	— J. Bloodgood separates surg from radiation first tumors.	[1929]	Rad
	— W. Healy discusses therapy of ca of cervix.	[1928]	Rad

Scans and Other Tests of Function in Various Organs

18. Brain	— J. Camp discusses intracranial calcifications.	[1929]	AJR
	— G. Pfahler describes the roentgenographic base of skull.	[1929]	Rad
19. Heart	— F. Wilson describes bundle branch block on ECG leads.	(1944	BHM)
	— C. Wolferth describes auricles sound and pulse.	[1923]	AnIM
	— M. Hochrein hears sounds of mitral sten & aortic insuf.	[1912]	KW
	— W. Fray shows X-Rays of adult coarctation of aorta.	[1923]	AJR
	— G. O'Kane sets up standardized Left Oblique position.	[1974]	AJR
20. Liver	— BSP & RB contend as "best"; neither good in jaundice.	[1923]	V33
	— M. Oka introduces a new method for visualizing spleen.	[1960]	FGR
21. Lung	— J. Farrell shows chest X-Rays of the new born infant.	[1983]	AJR
	— J. Sagel describes a mediastinal pleural effusion.	[1968]	AJR
22. Bone	— R. Bromer discusses the X-Ray Dx of rickets.	[1924]	AJR
	— P. Bucy lists primary hemangiomas of bone.	[1926]	AJR
	— W. Chamberlain discusses sacroiliac and symphysis pubis.	[1921]	AJR
	— A. Gray lists deforming bone diseases of adolescence.	[1926]	AJR
	— R. Stone shows an ecchinococcic involvement in bone.	[1929]	Rad
23. Kidney	— L. Jaches describes intravenous urography.	[1911]	JAMA
	— von Lichtenberg describes intravenous pyelography.	[1911]	Rad
24. Gut	— J. Northrup crystalizes pepsin and trypsin.	[1925]	DSB
	— T. Kosaka shows fat inhibition of gastric secretion.	[1925]	PSEB
	— L. Dragstedt: effect of total loss of gastric secretion.	[1926]	AJPh
	— H. Florey describes secretion of mucus by colon.	[1929]	BJEP
	— J. Farrell shows X-Ray Dx of ca of esophagus.	[1920]	Rad
25. Blood —			
26. Other	— L. Dragstedt: effect of total loss of pancreatic juice.	[1926]	PSEB
	— S. Donaldson sums 1045 pts with hyperplasia of thymus.	[1913]	AJR
	— H. Doub reviews roentgen Dx and Rx of thymomata.	[1913]	Rad
	— C. Hasley does ciné X-Rays of thymus in infants.	[1926]	JMMS

Radiation Hysteria and Health Physics * Obituaries *

27. Hyst	— THOROTRAST CONSIDERED A GOOD LIVER VISUALIZING AGENT.	[1928]	V33
	— J. Barnes measures Dx film dose at 1–10 r/exposure.	[1928]	Rad
	— 1474 women have been Ra dial painters in US. (AEC est.)	[1915]	AEC
	— "Technocracy" is the current fad for discussion.	[1929]	AP
28. React	— J. Barnes endorses safe dose limit of 100 r; hence number of films allowed per pt (e.g., 320 AP chest)	[1929]	Rad
	— E. Vogt shows lead line sign of plumbism in child bone.		
29. Respo —			

* * *

30. Obits —

CHRONOLOGY OF NUCLEAR MEDICINE — 1931

Scientific and Technical Background			Ref.
1. Basic	— H. Urey evaps liquid H, sees faint H-2 spectral line.	[1920]	JCE
	— W. Pauli postulates particle (called neutrino by Fermi).	[1922]	GSA
	— K. Godel finds some logical statements neither provable nor unprovable. Certainty is impossible in mathematics.	[1926]	SA
	— Joliot-Curies detect neutron (but don't recognize it).	[1919]	WoA
2. Obser	— H. Johnson says stable isotopes in 4n + 0, 1, 2, 3 series.	[1905]	JACS
	— Cockroft & Walton complete their proton accelerator.	[1930]	WoA
	— P. Bridgeman achieves pressures up to 100K atmospheres.	[1929]	DSB
	— J. Lansky observes radio interference from Milky Way.	[1915]	DSB
	— F. Hanson notes lethal mutations following rad exposure.	[1928]	AnR
	— H. Langendorff notes diff sensitivities during mitosis.	[1927]	Str
3. # Nuc	— F. Aston finds stable isotopes of Os, Ru, Re, Tl (U?).	[1930]	Bk
4. # Med	—		

Organizations and Internal Politics			
5. Pols	— ICRP recommends none, adopts NBS Hndbk #15 provisional.	[1928]	ICRU
	— ICRU adopts HVL in Cu or Al to scale "quality" of rad.	[1927]	ICRU
	— FDA established by Congress to administer food laws;	[1885]	FR
	replaces Bureau of Chemistry.	[1906]	FR
	— A. Hollander: "mitogenetic rays" most important problem.	[1940]	QRB
6. Socs	— F. Bainbridge publishes "Physiology of Exercise."	[1927]	Bk
	— F. Martin writes history of X-Ray plates and films.	[1916]	AJR
7. Event	— P. Bridgmann achieves pressure of 20,000 atmos.	[1955]	Bio

Instruments, Units of Measurement, and Drugs			
8. Instr	— E. Lawrence achieves 80 keV protons on 4" cyclotron.	[1930]	Bk
	— M. Livingston achieves 1 MeV protons on 11" cyclotron.	[1930]	PR
	— D. Sloan's linear electron accel tubes achieve >1MeV.	[1930]	PR
	— R. Van de Graaff builds an electrostat generator.	[1930]	GSA
	— B. Rajewsky uses quartz w/UV sens wall for soft X-rays.	[1908]	PZ
	— H. Rein describes thermoströmuhr to study blood circul.	(1944	BHM)
	— W. Coolidge describes how to operate high voltage tubes	[1913]	GSR
	— H. Imboden sums development of modern apparatus.	[1930]	AJR
9. Units	— V. Mayneord uses the r unit to measure Ra (technical OK).	[1928]	BJR
	— ICRU refines definition of "r"; "intensity" is r/sec.	[1928]	ICRU
	— E. Shower measures ear's differential pitch sensitivity.	[1800]	JAAS
10. Concp	— G. FAILLA EXPLAINS CONCEPT OF RBE (RELATIVE BIOL EFFECT).	[1929]	Rad
	— R. Seivert stresses time factors in bioeffect of rad.	[1930]	AR
	— R. Janker discusses all roentgenkinematographie.	[1928]	FGR
11. Drugs	— P. Karrer synthesizes a carotenoid — Vit A.	[1929]	DSB

	Radioiodine, P-32, and Radioactive Therapy		
12. I-Res	— A. Ivy sees high opossum thyroid bld flow (500 ml/dg/m).	[1928]	Rad
	— B. Turner studies I blood levels in various diseases.	[1928]	JBC
13. I-Dx	— AMA committee completes classification of goiters.	[1911]	JAMA
15. P-Rx	—		
16. Tele	—		
17. Other	— A. Hublein develops total body rad therapy.	[1921]	Rad
	— G. Forsell suggests many new Ra brachytherapy devices.	[1917]	JR
	— H. Bowing gives technique for Ra treatment ca cervix.	[1927]	MM
	Scans and Other Tests of Function in Various Organs		
18. Brain	— K. Lange notes IV fluorescein on skin under UV light.	[1946]	DGIM
19. Heart	— H. Rein sees coronary application of "Thermoströmuhr."	[1916]	Bk
	— P. White writes American textbook on Heart Disease.	[1928]	Bk
	— E. Edens writes German textbook on Heart Disease.	[1928]	Bk
20. Liver	— H. Leuth confirms existence of the sphincter of Odie.	[1929]	AJPh
	— E. Barrow discusses bilirubinemia.	[1926]	Med
	— L. Levyn uses a fat meal plus a gallbladder stimulant.	[1928]	AJR
	— L. Whitaker uses an oral agent for cholecystography.	[1928]	NEJM
21. Lung	— E. Friedman shows interlobar and mediastinal effusions.	[1928]	Rad
22. Bone	— H. Anderson describes lesions of the clavicle.	[1928]	Rad
	— W. Belden displays the fifth lumbar vertebra on X-Ray.	[1928]	Rad
	— W. Chamberlain shows bone & joint changes in leprosy.	[1929]	Rad
	— M. Kahn studies the bones of the hands and feet.	[1974]	Rad
	— R. Kegel describes tumors of the lower jaw.	[1930]	Rad
23. Kidney	— T. Addis describes "Renal Lesion in Bright's Disease."	[1827]	Bk
	— A. von Lichtenberg gives principles of IV urography.	[1930]	JU
24. Gut	— R. Jackson says diet methionine can replace cysteine.	(1939	Sc)
	— A. Vineberg gets gastric secretion by vagal stimulus.	[1930]	AJP
	— M. Dahm shows the esophagus on roentgenkinematograms.	[1926]	FGR
	— J. Aurelius shows a "peptic" ulcer of esophagus.	[1926]	AJR
	— J. Bargen describes clin aspects of chron ulcer colitis.	[1926]	Rad
25. Blood	— W. Coley describes Ewing's endothelioma or sarcoma.	[1922]	Rad
26. Other	— H. Margulis classifies tumors of the thymus.	[1927]	AJC
	— R. Beeler uses opaque oils to see maxillary sinus.	[1929]	AJR
	— J. Camp shows osseus changes in hyperparathyroidism.	[1982]	Rad
	— H. Walton: intrauterine cephalometry and pelvimetry.	[1920]	AJR
	Radiation Hysteria and Health Physics * Obituaries *		
27. Hyst	— League of Nations declares tolerance dose is 0.25 r/d.	[1929]	SN
	— H. Martland diagnoses malignancy in radium dial workers;	[1910]	AJC
	says 2400 girls were radium dial painters.	[1925]	AJC
	— H. Schlundt considers IV Ra-226 a therapeutic agent.	[1924]	AJR
	— S. Kadrnka shows many liver-spleen X-Rays by Thorotrast.	[1930]	FGR
	— J. Sparkes discusses pulmonary asbestosis.	[1985]	Rad
28. React	— H. Smyth reviews toxicity of benzene compounds.	[1919]	JIH
29. Respo	— H. Lavery invents "Psychograph" to measure phrenology data; rents to psychologists for $2000, $35/month.	[1900]	AP

* * *

30. Obits	— T. Edison (1847–1931) Am invent; electricity.	Bio
	— E. Goldstein (1850–1931) Ger physics; kanalstrahlen.	DSB
	— A. Michelson (1852–1931) Am physics; speed of light.	Bio
	— G. Holzknecht (1872–1931) Ger radiol; first lead shielding.	WKW

CHRONOLOGY OF NUCLEAR MEDICINE — 1932

Scientific and Technical Background

			Ref.
1. Basic	— J. CHADWICK repeats the Boethe & Joliot experiments to	[1931]	
	DISCOVER THE NEUTRON.	[1919]	Na
	— C. Anderson discovers Dirac's positron.	[1928]	Sc
	— J. Cockroft produces first "artificial" transmutation.	[1930]	Na
	— 3 days earlier E. Lawrence's 11" got 1 MeV protons.	[1930]	Bio
	— H. Urey discovers H-2 (later called deuterium).	[1931]	PR
	— E. Fermi develops a theory of beta decay.	[1928]	Bio
	— G. Uhlenberg explains "exclusion" as particle spin.	[1925]	WoA
2. Obser	— 1932 called "Second Annus Mirabilus" of physics (1913 was first).		V98
	— A. Grosse anticipates "artificial radioactive elements";	[1934]	BACS
	complains: "periodic" is chem; "transmut" is nuclear.	[1919]	BACS
	— G. Tarrant's scatter corrects "attenuation" measurements.	[1926]	PCPS
	— J. Dumond: cloud chamb. tracks are too long for ion chamber.	[1912]	Rad
	— L. Gray notes interaction of gammas and atom nucleus.	[1924]	PRSL
	— E. Butler measures cellular reaction to irradiation.	[1925]	JEB
3. # Nuc	— F. Aston: 4n + 3 series probably goes U-235 to Pb-207;	[1929]	Bk
	finds no stable isotopes of Nb or Ta.	[1931]	Bk
	— F. Aston says 18 elements remain to be mass spectrographed.	[1920]	Bk
4. # Med	—		

Organizations and Internal Politics

5. Pols	— Pres Roosevelt introduces the term "New Deal."	[1931]	AP
	— USA has 13.7 million unemployed, world est is 30 mil.	[1929]	AP
6. Socs	— F. Soddy glorifies his work in "Interpret of the Atom."	[1902]	Bk
	— J. Peters & VanSlyke pub textbk in "Quant Clin Chem."	[1918]	Bk
	— E. Thomson write history of first decade of radiology.	[1930]	AJR
7. Event	— F. Kurie brings his GM tubes to Berkeley (they had none).	[1928]	ONR
	— H. Urey separates heavy from light water by electrolysis.	[1931]	V100
	— E. Lawrence's Rad Lab (UC Berk) begins in wooden shack.	[1931]	Bio
	— W. Carothers synthesizes polyamide to be called "nylon."	[1930]	AP

Instruments, Units of Measurement, and Drugs

8. Instr	— D. Sloan develops a million volt X-ray tube at UC Berk.	[1930]	BAPS
	— Hard X-ray e− requires "energy" calibration of instrs.	[1930]	Rad
	— C. Gianturco describes X-Ray motion picture equipment.	[1931]	MCP
9. Units	— R. Glocker says modify "r" unit to include biol dose.	[1931]	Rad
	— H. Laurens says wavelength important in biol dose.	[1924]	Rad
	— J. DuMond makes distinction: Quantity = ergs/g or "r."	[1928]	Rad
	Intensity = ergs/g per second.	[1911]	
	Quality = spectral distribution.	[1928]	Rad
	— W. Mattick: methods for finding dose around Ra needle.	[1924]	Rad
	— E. Quimby describes the grouping of Ra tubes for dose.	[1925]	AJR
	— A. Dognon measures bioeffect of energy on ascaris eggs.	[1927]	CRS
	— P. Henshaw: effect on first cleavage time of invert eggs.	[1931]	AJR
10. Concp	— US, Eng, Ger, Fr bureaus resolve "r" intercomparisons.	[1921]	Rad
	— J. Haldane first to measure human natural mutation rate.	[1927]	DSB
11. Drugs	— A. Szent-Gyorgi finds Vit C, names it ascorbic acid.	[1951]	DSB
	— F. Mietzsch discovers sulfonamide.	[1935]	DSB
	— H. Emerson publishes "Effects of Alcohol Toxicity."	[1923]	Bk
	— E. Vogt shows X-Rays of Pb poisoning in infants & children.		JAMA

Radioiodine, P-32, and Radioactive Therapy

12.	I-Res	— H. Elmer gives oral KI, notes higher blood I in hypo pts.	[1951]	DAKM
		— H. Elmer disputes Sturm's blood & urine I findings.	[1928]	E
		— W. Nyiri studies absorption of iodine painted on skin.	[1985]	JPET
13.	I-Dx	—		
14.	I-Rx	—		
15.	P-Rx	—		
16.	Tele	— 3 physicists "harness" lightning in Alps, 2 return.	[1930]	V108
		— J. Weatherwax introduces "isodose charts" for 127 kVp.	[1930]	RAD
17.	Other	— A. Heublein tells story of first total body irrad trials.	[1931]	Rad

Scans and Other Tests of Function in Various Organs

18.	Brain	— W. Clark describes the structure of the thalmus.	[1929]	B
		— H. Cushing pubs "Papers Relative to Pituitary Body."	[1929]	Bk
		— E. Vogt describes encephalography in children.	[1929]	AJR
19.	Heart	— A. Grollman studies methods of measuring cardiac output.	[1928]	Bk
		— D. Bronk sees carotid body's effect on blood pressure.	[1931]	JCC
		— T. Lewis explains "Raynaud's disease."	[1934]	BMJ
		— W. Hamilton analyzes effect on circ of injection method.	[1931]	AJPh
		— W. Fray measures the heart in LPO position.	[1930]	AJR
20.	Liver	— H. Fried does cholecystograms same time as opaque meal.	[1931]	AJS
21.	Lung	— H. Pancoast gets foreign bod by broncoscope under X-Ray.	[1974]	AJR
22.	Bone	— H. Doub reviews X-Ray signs of TBC in vertebral bodies.	[1926]	AJR
		— W. Evans describes vertebral body abnormalities.	[1931]	AJR
23.	Kidney	— S. Weiss gives hemodynamics of malignant hypertension.	[1927]	ArIM
		— F. Patch compares IV and retrograde pyelography.	[1957]	CMAJ
24.	Gut	— F. Vansant studies normal gastric acid.	[1923]	ArIM
		— T. Bennet uses liver diet in ideopathic steatorrhea.	[1928]	QJM
		— B. Crohn describes a regional ileitis.	[1903]	JAMA
		— L. Cole reviews X-Ray Dx of the intestinal tract.	[1922]	AJR
		— J. Feuz describes use of opaque oil in salivary gland.	[1929]	SMW
25.	Blood	— P. Lambin notes deficient thrombins after Thorotrast.	[1928]	Sa
26.	Other	— J. Northrup crystallizes trypsin & chymotryp as protein.	[1930]	SN
		— A. Barsky visualizes parotid gland with lipiodol.	[1931]	AnS
		— K. Ehrhardt tries placentography with Thorotrast.	[1927]	KW
		— A. Lerondier describes new method for pelvimetry.	[1931]	BMSR
		— M. Hubney does Dx and Rx of persistent thymus.	[1930]	AJR

Radiation Hysteria and Health Physics   * Obituaries *

27.	Hyst	— 0.001 threshold erythema/m for 4 1/2 y has no bioeffect.	[1931]	Rad
		— A. PIRCHAM BEGINS STORY OF JOACHIMSTHAL MINERS' LUNG CANCER. 2/3 of 1930 deaths (15 y exposure) have ca of lung.	[1926]	AJC
		— P. Lenard becomes a NAZI; denounces "Jew" (Einstein) science, despite exceptional physics he loses reputation.	[1902]	AP
		— W. Stewart describes liver & spleens with Thorotrast.	[1930]	AJR
28.	React	— A. Desjardins studies action of X-rays & Ra on tissues.	[1928]	AJR
29.	Respo	—		

* * *

30.	Obits	G. Eastman (1854–1932) Am indust; photography instruments.	Bio
		— A. Hublein (1880–1932) Am radiol, first to note beta damage.	Rad

CHRONOLOGY OF NUCLEAR MEDICINE — 1933

Scientific and Technical Background

			Ref.
1. Basic	— E. Fermi describes and names neutrino, prob undetectable.	[1932]	ZfP
	— J. Oppenheimer details pair-produc: from >1.02 MeV.	[1932]	PR
2. Obser	— O. Hahn: Manitoba Rb-87 ore $T_{1/2} = 4–6 \times 10^{10}$y (now 4.8).	[1930]	Bio
	— E. Lawrence injects first H-2 into 11″ cyclotron.	[1931]	Bio
	— E. Lawrence accelerates "deutons" to 3 MeV in new 27″.	[1931]	PR
	— P. Blackett sees + & − pair in cloud chamber.	[1932]	WoA
	— J. Hudson measures the K series spectrum of tungsten.	[1928]	PNAS
	— H. Holthusen compares Ra and X-rays at third ICR in Paris.	[1928]	BJR
3. # Nuc	— 212 stable and 38 °species in Hndbk of Chem & Phys.	[1932]	HCP
4. # Med	—		

Organizations and Internal Politics

5. Pols	— c 60,000 scientists, literati, emigrate from Nazi Ger.	by 1939	AP
6. Socs	— F. Aston updates his 1924 "Mass-Spectra and Isotopes."	[1932]	Bk
	— O. Glasser's "History of the Science of Radiology" pub.	[1896]	Rad
	— O. Glasser's "William Conrad Roentgen" biography pub.	[1895]	Bk
7. Event	— A. Gettler: first gross autoradiographs after oral $RaCl_2$.	[1924]	JAMA
	— F. Kurie: how "Diplon" became "Deuton" became "Deuteron."	(1956	ONR)
	— G. Hevesy drinks Urey's D_2O, finds he is 60% water.	[1932]	ARR
	— G. Lewis gives worlds supply of hi-conc D_2O to a mouse.	[1932]	ARR

Instruments, Units of Measurement, and Drugs

8. Instr	— E. Lawrence's 27″ cyclotron achieves 2 MeV protons.	[1932]	Bio
	— E. Fermi locates a Ra-Rn cow in Rome to obtain radon.	[1928]	Bio
	— E. Fermi makes first Rn-Be neutron sources.	[1932]	Bio
9. Units	— E. Quimby marks "Threshold Erythema" at 540 r at 200 kVp.	[1930]	AJR
	— J. Hudson's physical dose is energy absorbed /unit vol.	[1929]	GSR
	— J. Hudson: biol dose = phys dose × some biological factor.	[1929]	GSR
10. Concp	— R. SCHOENHEIMER INTRODUCES CONCEPT OF "DYNAMIC STATE."	[1926]	Bk
11. Drugs	— G. Hevesy: D_2O shows all H_2O in fish replaced in hours.	[1932]	ARR
	— G. Lewis is first to make 100% D_2O.	[1931]	DSB
	— T. Reichstein synthesizes ascorbic acid, Vit C.	[1932]	DSB
	— R. Kuhn recognizes Vit B_2, riboflavin.	[1932]	DSB

Radioiodine, P-32, and Radioactive Therapy

12. I-Res	— C. Harrington pubs "Thyroid Gland, Chem & Physiology."	[1931]	Bk
13. I-Dx	—		
14. I-Rx	— H. Blumgart introduces thyroidectomy, Rx for angina pec.	[1955]	AIM
15. P-Rx	—		
16. Tele	— L. Marinelli: depth dose curves for 200, 700 kVp and Ra.	[1930]	AJR
	— G. Failla compares 200 & 700 kVp with Ra Pack for Rx.	[1930]	AJR
	— Am Roent Ray Soc symposium, "Is Hi Energy Better?" (??)	[1932]	AJR
	— G. Failla compares 200 & 700 kVp with Ra gammas.	[1929]	AJR
17. Other	— H. Holdfelder treats erythremia (PVA) with X-rays.	[1928]	Str

Scans and Other Tests of Function in Various Organs

18. Brain	— C. Heymans studies physiology of carotid sinus.	[1927] (1944	BHM)
19. Heart	— A. Stoll isolates the digitalis glucosides.	[1803]	Bk
	— A. Bogaert studies chronaxia of myocard and His bundle.	(1944	BHM)
	— W. Dressler studies tricuspid stenosis.	[1806] (1944	BHM)
	— F. Wilson studies distrib of action current in myocard.	[1928]	JGP
	— W. Dock evaluates the cause of first heart sound.	[1937]	ArIM
	— T. Lewis studies "erythromyalgia" (Reynaud's disease).	[1932]	CS
20. Liver	— L. Ericsen visualizes ca mets with Thorotrast.	[1932]	JAMA
21. Lung	— J. Myers reviews the Dx of tuberculosis by X-Ray.	[1931]	JAMA
22. Bone	—		
23. Kidney	—		
24. Gut	— H. Rawlinson says adrenals stimulate submax gland (cat).	[1924]	AR
	— A. Alley describes mucosa on gastric lesser curve.	[1930]	TRSE
	— A. Oillman relates osmotic press, blood and body fluids.	[1930]	AJR
25. Blood	— R. Gottlieb studies Thorotrast effects on blood.	[1925]	CMAJ
	— S. Whittaker measures viscosity of blood.	[1932]	JPh
26. Other	— G. Fletcher measures "loudness" in ears.	[1931]	JAAS

Radiation Hysteria and Health Physics * Obituaries *

27. Hyst	— H. Schlundt: IV Ra to 32 prisoners/dementia, 11 improve.	[1931]	AJR
	— W. Seifriz (a believer) says mitogenetic rays in disfavor.	[1931]	GSR
	— Gurwitsch rays supported by WPA, forgotten in WWII.	[1940]	PL
	— W. Yater extols use of Thorotrast in DDx of liver dis.	[1932]	AJR
28. React	— H. Muller say bkgd rad insufficient to explain the frequency of natural human genetic mutations; disputed!	[1931]	GSR
29. Respo	—		

* * *

30. Obits —

CHRONOLOGY OF NUCLEAR MEDICINE — 1934

Scientific and Technical Background

			Ref.
1. Basic	— I.& F.JOLIOT-CURIE MAKE FIRST °ISOTOPES ON NEW YEAR'S EVE;	[1932]	CRS
	announce 14m N-13, 3.25m P-30, 2.5m S-27.	(10 Feb)	Na
	— (E. Rona tells eyewitness story of discovery. Pub by ORAU 1978)		
	— C. Lauritsen makes N-13 for first confirmation.	(27 Feb)	Sc
	— E. Lawrence: second confirm, °isotopes from 9 targets.	(28 Feb)	PR
	— E. Fermi makes 14 °isotopes by neutron bombardment.	(19 May)	Na
	— C. Lauritsen makes 2 mCi C-11 in a (p, gamma) reaction.	(June)	PR
	— E. Fermi irradiates 60 elements, gets 33 + 13 °isotopes.	(25 July)	PRS
	— H. Crane (E. Lawrence) sees what must be C-14.	(July)	PR
	— M. Livingston makes first 2.04 min O-15.	(1 Aug)	PR
	— E. Rutherford discovers H-3 in a (d,p) demonstration.	[1913]	PRS
	— W. Lozier reports H with mass 3, probably stable.	[1931]	PR
	— M. Oliphant reports H-3 is weakly radioactive.	[1938]	PM
	— I. Rabi develops magnetic resonance for atomic spectra.	[1977]	WoA
	— H. Bethe publishes bremsstrahlung cross-sections.	[1967]	PCPS
	— E. Fermi: neutron & proton same but diff quantum state.	[1932]	Bio
2. Obser	— K. Guggenheimer gives name "isotones" to constant A – Z.	[1918]	GSA
	— J. Walke says all elements can be transmuted to °isotope.	[1932]	Na
	— O. Hahn believes all Fermi's °isotopes except #93.	[1939]	Bk
	— Joliot-Curies confirm Fermi's neutron °isotope product.	[1932]	CRS
	— H. Taylor compares D_2O and H_2O from chemical standpoint.	[1932]	JACS
	— Ida Noddak doubts transuranics, says it is "fission."	[1939]	GSA
	— J. Ewing describes histology of tissue reaction to Ra.	[1926]	AJR
	— Dutch team says metal corrosion is bacterial disease.	(1985	SN)
3. # Nuc	— I. & F. Joliot-Curie make 14.0m radionitrogen (9.96m N-13), 2.5m radiosilicon (4.14s Si-27), 3.25m radiophosphorus (2.49m P-30).		Na
	— E. Lawrence makes first large amt of any °isotope (Na-24).	[1948]	PR

Organizations and Internal Politics

5. Pols	— ICRU fourth meeting decrees r/min measures dose rate.	[1931]	ICRU
	— ICRU divides air (no scatter) & effective (scatter) dose.	[1928]	ICRU
6. Socs	— Am Board of Radiology becomes fifth AMA specialty board in order to cure Radiology of commercial practices.	[1925]	JAMA
	— C. Rosenblum reviews tracer techniques.	[1926]	JCE
7. Event	— Fermi's production convinces E. Lawrence of °isotopes.	[1932]	ONR
	— L. Szilard's (Chalmers') method makes elements from compounds.		Na
	— L. Szilard patents (Eng) a Be-He chain reaction (unused).	[1945]	GSA
	— R. Watson-Watt sets up first Radio Echo Equip (RADAR).	[1940]	NPL

Instruments, Units of Measurement, and Drugs

8. Instr	— E. Lawrence's 27" cyclotron produces first 5MeV deuterons.	[1933]	Bio
9. Units	— O. Hoenigschmid remeasures Ra At Wt @ 225.97 to 226.05.	[1912]	GMP
	— O. Hoenigschmid requires new radium standards, makes 20.	[1914]	GMP
	— E. Quimby calls specific gamma constant an "Eye Gamma" (I_τ)		V103
	— E. May measures isodose charts distorted by angle.	[1928]	Rad
10. Concp	— X-ray "quality" measured in Cu (Al) Half-Value-Layers.	[1931]	ICRU
	— R. Crist can determine D_2O in H_2O with 0.2% accuracy.	[1932]	JCP
	— A. Sachsse determines mole fraction of D_2O in H_2O.	[1932]	ZPC
	— F. Breusell compares natural abundances of D_2 and H_2,	[1933]	Kw
	hence, says W. Stewart, D_2 has no biological effect.	[1955]	JACS
	— J. Gamble says urea controls water economy in normals.	[1929]	AJPh

11. Drugs	— G. Hevesy drinks 250 ml of Urey's 0.46% D_2O, urine $T_{1/2}$ = 94 days.		Na
	— G. Hevesy makes a Fermi neutron source to make his first P-32.	[1933]	ARR
	— R. Schoenheimer initiates study of fats tagged with D_2O.	[1933]	Bk
	— A. Butenant isolates androsterone, first male hormone.	[1970]	CDD

Radioiodine, P-32, and Radioactive Therapy

12. I-Res	— E. Fermi's 14 °isotopes include 30m I-128 (9.1m + 12.36h I-130).		Na
	— R. Evans notes Fermi's discovery of I-128 with neutrons.	[1936]	V90
	— A. Elmer compares blood I with BMR, suggests Dx test.	[1928]	AMS
13. I-Dx	— A. Elmer injects KI, collects blood & urine for Dx test.	[1932]	E
14. I-Rx	— H. Blumgart ablates (surg) thyroid for chron heart dis.	[1932]	JAMA
16. Tele	— J. Weatherwax introduces "isodose charts" for 200 kVp.	[1932]	Rad
17. Other	— U. Portman decides that N. Senn did first deep rad therapy.	[1902]	Rad
	— W. Pussy disputes that Senn did first deep therapy.	[1902]	Rad

Scans and Other Tests of Function in Various Organs

18. Brain	—		
19. Heart	— S. Landis measures capillary pressure in cardiac muscle.	[1933]	PhR
	— M. Kissin says pain in cardiac muscle means anoxia.	[1929]	Ci
20. Liver	—		
21. Lung	—		
22. Bone	—		
23. Kidney	— H. Goldblatt causes hypertension with surgical ischemia.	[1910]	AJPh
	— A. Richards measures excretion: inulin, creatinine, xylose.	[1934]	PSEB
	— D. Van Slyke explains mechanism of urea excretion.	[1932]	AJPh
	— E. Marshall reviews comparative physiology of kidneys.	[1929]	PhR
24. Gut	— E. McDougall injects jejunal D_2O, measures blood uptake.	[1933]	Na
	— J. Sheldon describes 311 cases of hemochromatosis.	[1933]	La
	— S. Baxter finds sympthetic nerve to gastric mucosa.	[1933]	AJDD
	— C. Wilhelms says stomach & duodenum affect acidity.	[1933]	AJPh
25. Blood	— G. Pickering explains angina & intermit claud in anemia.	[1932]	CS
26. Other	— L. Rowntree studies effect of thymus extract in rats.	[1931]	JAMA

Radiation Hysteria and Health Physics * Obituaries *

27. Hyst	— W. Boyd recommends Ra bromide as oral medication.	[1933]	BJR
	— Am Com X-ray Prot recommends "tolerance dose" 0.1 R/d.	[1931]	Rad
	— ICRP adopts "tolerance dose" of 72 r/y (good evidence).	[1931]	ICRP
	— 0.2 r/d, or 1.0 r/w, or 72 r/y is "safe" whole body exp.	[1931]	Rad
	— ICRU says rad workers need 5d week & 4wk vacation.	[1928]	BJR
	G. Roussy; first evidence of ThO_2 hazard, sarcomas in rats.	[1930]	BANM
	— Phrenology machine made $200,000 at Chicago World Fair.	[1931]	AP
28. React	—		
29. Respo	—		

* * *

30. Obits	— P. Villard (1861–1934) Fr physics; originated "R" dose concept.	DSB
	— M. Curie (1867–1934) Fr chem; polonium, radium.	DSB
	— Fritz Haber (1868–1934) Ger physic chem; nitrogen fixation.	DSB
	— W. Duane (1872–1934) Am physics; first to measure X-ray quantity.	GSR

CHRONOLOGY OF NUCLEAR MEDICINE — 1935

Scientific and Technical Background			Ref.
1. Basic	— H. Hulme derives photoelectric absorption from Z = 5 to 92.	[1932]	PRS
	— O. Hahn searches but can't find stable isotope of Ra.	[1939]	Bio
	— C. Anderson finds, names "meson," a new class of partic.	[1932]	WoA
2. Obser	— R. Schoenheimer learns how to link D_2 to carbon.	[1933]	JBC
	— A. Dempster studies exact isotope distribution of Ni.	[1918]	PR
3. # Nuc	— E. Fermi discovers 22.3m Th-233.	[1934]	Na
	— A. Dempster finds AcU (7×10^6 y U-235) 4n + 3 series parent.	[1932]	PAPS
4. # Med	—		

Organizations and Internal Politics			
5. Pols	— Germany into Saar, Italy into Abyssinia, League says bad boys.		EB
6. Socs	— Am Bd of Radiol informally recognizes a few physicists.	[1920]	Rad
	— Compton & Allison's "X-rays In Theory and Experiment."	[1922]	Bk
	— D. Lea's "Action of Radiations on Living Cells" pub.	[1924]	Bk
7. Event	— N. Bohr's 50th b'day present, 60 mg Ra-Be neut howitzer.	[1933]	Bio

Instruments, Units of Measurement, and Drugs			
8. Instr	— R. Watson-Watt invents RAdioDetectionAndRanging (RADAR).	[1934]	DSB
	— Weather Bureau sends radio transmitting balloons aloft.	[1960]	SN
9. Units	— NBS gets 2 new radium standards (<1% off 1913 std):	[1934]	GMP
	20.45 mg & 38.23 mg radium element.	[1913]	GMP
10. Concp	— R. Zirkle defines lin ener trans (LET) as RBE factor.	[1931]	AJC
	— G. HEVESY DOES FIRST DISTRIB STUDY IN BABY RAT (P-32 TO MOTHER).		Na
	— I. Tronstad measures densities in ratios of D_2O to H_2O.	[1933]	Na
	— O. Reitz measures thermal conductivity of D_2O.	[1932]	ZPC
	— E. Vogt measures density of D_2O to 1 ppm accuracy.	[1932]	AJPh
11. Drugs	— R. Schoenheimer: first biochem use of D_2O (fat metab).	[1934]	JBC
	— A. Kaplan: how to separate phospholipids from organs.	[1937]	JBC
	— O. Reitz finds that algae will exchange D_2O for H_2O.	[1933]	ZPC
	— P. Karrer synthesizes riboflavin, Vit B_2.	[1931]	DSB
	— G. Domagk finds Prontosil is anti-streptococcus agent.	[1932]	Bk
	— D. Bovet: Prontosil converts to sulfanilamide in body. THE FIRST MEDICAL "CURE"	[1929]	Bk

Radioiodine, P-32, and Radioactive Therapy

12.	I-Res	— V. Trevorrow invents plasma protein bound iodine (PBI).	[1934]	JCI
		— D. Marine discusses pathogenesis of simple goiter.	[1933]	JAMA
13.	I-Dx	—		
14.	I-Rx	—		
15.	P-Rx	—		
16.	Tele	—		
17.	Other	— O. Naegeli uses smallpox vaccine in Rx of herpes simp.	[1928]	JAMA

Scans and Other Tests of Function in Various Organs

18.	Brain	— E. Keeser says barbital localizes in brain (dog).	[1950]	AEPP
19.	Heart	— C. Beck implants pectoral muscle as Rx for angina.	[1914]	AHJ
		— D. Bronk experiments: nerves to isolated carotid sinus.	[1932]	AJPh
		— G. Anrep studies capillaries in contracting muscle.	[1934]	JPh
20.	Liver	—		
21.	Lung	—		
22.	Bone	— G. Hevesy: bone is dynamic structure (e.g., epiphyses °P)	[1933]	Na
		— H. Jaffe describes Osteoid Osteoma (not accepted until 1976).		Bk
23.	Kidney	— J. Shannon measures excretion of inulin, xylose, urea.	[1934]	JCI
		— D. VanSlyke compares inulin, creat, ferrocyan, clearances.	[1934]	AJPh
24.	Gut	— H. Rawlinson paralyzes function in submax gland (cat).	[1933]	JA
		— A. Ivy reviews enterogastric (esp stomach) hormones.	[1925]	AJPh
		— A. Alley measures effect of fats on gastric secretion.	[1933]	AJDD
25.	Blood	— M. Gregersen tells blood and plasma volume before P-32.	[1928]	AJP
		— N. Rosenthal reviews Dx & Rx of leukemia with radiation.	[1924]	JAMA
26.	Other	—		

Radiation Hysteria and Health Physics * Obituaries *

27.	Hyst	— J. Lawrence thinks mouse killed in neutron beam (wrong!).	[1933]	PL
28.	React	— H. Dean: tooth caries out with F, but causes mottling.	[1980]	AJIH
29.	Respo	—		

* * *

30. Obits —

CHRONOLOGY OF NUCLEAR MEDICINE — 1936

Scientific and Technical Background

			Ref.
1. Basic	— E. Lawrence produces 11 MeV alphas in 27″ cyclotron.	[1934]	Bio
2. Obser	— H. Hall reviews photoelectric absorption theory.	[1929]	RMP
	— Cosmic rays are alphas, + & − electrons, and protons.	[1925]	SA
3. # Nuc	— L. Meitner names the nuclear "isomers" (diff in $T_{1/2}$).	[1921]	GSAE
4. # Med	—		

Organizations and Internal Politics

5. Pols	— ICRU says "r" must include "quality" specification (HVL).	[1931]	Rad
	— USA population is 127 million.	[1931]	AP
6. Socs	— P. Brown pubs "Am Martyrs . . . to Roentgen Ray" (Thomas).	[1933]	Bk
7. Event	— J. Lawrence compares effects of neutrons and X-rays.	[1935]	PNAS
	— Cyclotrons under construction at 11 univ, 6 countries.	[1930]	Bio
	— R. EVANS SUGGESTS RADIOISOTOPES FOR K. COMPTON'S LECTURE		V90
	— G. Hevesy invents "activation analysis."	[1934]	ARR
	— G. Hevesy uses first artificial isotopes (P-32 in plants).	[1923]	ARR

Instruments, Units of Measurement, and Drugs

8. Instr	— R. Evans introduces rate meter recording into medicine.	[1932]	RSI
	— R. Evans screen wire wall GM tube ups sensitivity.	[1928]	RSI
	— R. Evans builds a Ra-Be neutron source to make I-128.	[1935]	GMP
	— E. Lawrence increases cyclotron pole diameter to 37″.	[1932]	Rad
	— A. Barnes builds GM for emersion into fluid (soft betas).	[1931]	RSI
	— E. Quimby's X-ray cone theory starts collimator design.	[1983]	Rad
	— C. Gorter says nuc mag moments can be measured.	[1934]	GSA
9. Units	— L. Gray defines "J" unit of tissue absorption (ergs/cc).	[1933]	BJR
	— F. O'Brian says erythema is the ONLY biological dose.	[1933]	Rad
10. Concp	— A. Hill says "°isotopes are as important as the microscope."		IRT
	— J. Lawrence extends RBE concept: neutron vs X-ray dose.	[1933]	PNAS
	— R. McWhirter studies "protraction" of dose to skin.	[1926]	BJR
	— K. Greib finds fungi exchange D_2 and H_2 in water.	[1935]	ZPC
	— A. Oparin begins study of origin of life on earth.	[1925]	SN
11. Drugs	— J. Hamilton gives first human Na-24 dose to himself.	[1934]	PSEB
	— E. Chargaff tags first organic compound with P-32.	[1925]	Bio
	— C. King reviews Vit C physiology.	[1928]	PhR

		Radioiodine, P-32, and Radioactive Therapy		
12.	I-Res	—		
13.	I-Dx	— H. Perkin devises blood iodine test for thyroid disease.	[1934]	NEJM
		— R. EVANS SUGGESTS °I TO J. MEANS AT A MEETING AT HARVARD MED.		V90
		ANOTHER BEGINNING OF NUCLEAR MEDICINE	[1934]	V90
14.	I-Rx	—		
15.	P-Rx	—		
16.	Tele	— J. Edward says 400 + diseases can be treated with X-ray.	[1907]	Rad
17.	Other	— R. Stone gives first dose of Na-24 to a leukemia patient.	[1934]	Bio
		FIRST HUMAN °NUCLIDE DOSE AT BERKELEY		
		Scans and Other Tests of Function in Various Organs		
18.	Brain	— L. Ellis says postural hypotension occurs in CNS dis.	[1934]	ArIM
19.	Heart	— D. Bronk measures cardiac autonomy center's activity.	[1925]	AJPh
		— C. Wiggers: drugs alter coronary flow after obstruction.	[1922]	AHJ
		— H. Green measures coronary flow in aortic valve damage.	[1930]	AJPh
20.	Liver	—		
21.	Lung	— F. Parker finds structural changes in mitral stenosis.	[1930]	AJPa
22.	Bone	— J. Kulowski sees 102 pts with Pyogen Vertebr Osteomyel.	[1987]	JNM
23.	Kidney	—		
24.	Gut	— O. Naegli reviews the biology of herpes simplex.	[1935]	JAMA
25.	Blood	— L. Halpern finds RBC permeability is temp sensitive.	[1934]	JBC
		— A. Krogh: organs tend to equilibrium in sols of D_2O.	[1933]	SAP
		— M. Ishibashi uses °K to get K content of urine, saliva.	[1929]	JJC
26.	Other	—		
		Radiation Hysteria and Health Physics * Obituaries *		
27.	Hyst	— L. Ennis documents radiation hazard from dental X-Rays.	[1928]	Rad
		— P. Brown pubs 25 deaths, all from ca mets after hi-dose.	[1933]	Bk
		— H. Dean decries mottled tooth enamel after fluorine.	[1940]	AJP
28.	React	— E. Quimby notes 69% skin recovery from 400 r exposure.	[1930]	Rad
		— S. Weiss describes barbiturate toxicity.	[1923]	IC
		— AMA council advises radiotherapy in salivary gland diseases.		JAMA
29.	Respo	— G. Bell quantifies film exposure (basic to film badges).	[1924]	BJR

* * *

30.	Obits	— I. Pavlov (1849–1936) Rus physiol; conditioned reflex.	DSB
		— F. Williams (1852–1936) Am radiol; first Am radiol, first textbk.	IJO

CHRONOLOGY OF NUCLEAR MEDICINE — 1937

Scientific and Technical Background			Ref.
1. Basic	— G. Thomson gets Nobel for proving electron has wave properties.		NC
	His father, J.J., got it for proving e^- a particle.	[1898]	Bio
2. Obser	— E. Lawrence supplies Hevesy with adequate P-32 (by mail).	[1934]	ARR
	— M. Livingstone describes prep of cyclotron °isotopes.	[1934]	RMP
	— F. Bawden says tobacco mosaic virus contains RNA.	[1898]	Sc
3. # Nuc	— E. Lawrence sends °Mo cyclotron target to Fermi (Italy):	[1934]	Bio
	5.5 MeV deuterons on iron target for °Fe, °Co, °Mn.	[1936]	Bio
	— E. Segre discovers element #43, technetium on °Mo target.	[1925]	JCP
	— D. Stewart describes 55d Sr-89 as a pure beta emitter.		PR
	— A. Grosse constructs first table of 263 stable, 141 °isotopes;		
	sets format for most future °isotope tables.	[1932]	JCE
	— I. Perlman makes $_{15}P^{31} + {}_{1}D^{2}$ –to– $_{15}P^{32} + {}_{1}H^{1}$.	[1934]	JBC
4. # Med	—		

Organizations and Internal Politics			
5. Pols	— ICRP brings up subject of "genetic" dose.	[1927]	BJR
	— Japan Premier Konoye begins aggressive war policy.	[1946]	EB
6. Socs	— Canadian Assoc Radiologists founded.	[1924]	JCAR
	— W. Mayneord publishes "Significance of the Roentgen."	[1928]	IUCC
	— J.J. Thomson's "Recollections and Reflections" published.	[1898]	Bk
7. Event	— R. Evans collects used Rn needles for neutron source.	[1927]	GMP
	— J. Lawrence pubs first article on cyclotron in medicine.	[1930]	YJBM
	— Norway hydroelectric plant collects 434 kg 99.8% D_2O.	[1932]	JCE

Instruments, Units of Measurement, and Drugs			
8. Instr	— A. Trost prepares self-quenching gases for GM tubes.	[1936]	ZfP
	— I. Baumann wraps °blotting paper around 0.1 mm Al GM wall.	[1928]	JBC
	— I. Chaikoff wraps °P blotting paper around Al GM wall,	[1928]	JBC
	counts 108 atoms or 10^{-15} g of P-32.	[1936]	JBC
	— G. Failla introduces his extrapolation chamber.	[1933]	Rad
	— GM tube not popular in physics labs, all home made.	[1936]	GMP
	— C. Lauritsen invents quartz fiber electroscope.	[1924]	RSI
9. Units	— H. Parker devises Roentgen equivalent physical (Rep).	[1933]	BJR
	— W. Mayneord defines "gram roentgen" (first rad type dose).	[1908]	BJR
	— L. Gray approaches "Rad" unit with thimble chamber inst.	[1936]	BJR
	— "Curie" = 3.40 to 3.72 × 10^{10} dps (best value = 3.67).	[1910]	V101
	— ICRU recognizes difficulty with words "quantity," "dose."	[1936]	ICRU
	— ICRU redefines "r" to include gamma rays & hi-energy.	[1931]	ICRU
	— AMA says Dx dose of Thorotrast is = 3 μg radium.	[1927]	JAMA
10. Concp	— C. Artom implies "turnover" in phospholipid exchange.	[1933]	Na
	— C. Artom finds phospholipids in liver > intestine > kidney.	[1935]	AIP
	— J. HAMILTON DEVISES DIFFERENTIAL ABSORPTION		
	RATIO (DAR).	[1935]	AJP
	— R. Schoenheimer devises concept of metabolic "pools."	[1933]	HL
11. Drugs	— G. Hevesy devises a labeled fat meal (dogs).	[1935]	Na
	— H. Borsook notes excretion in urine of S-35 sulfate.	[1973]	Sc
	— R. Stone gives first dose of °iodine to man (???).	[1935]	Rad
	— G. Hevesy gives first P-32 to man. (Too little to count.)	[1936]	ARR
	— C. Elvehjem proves nicotin acid in VitB coenzyme system.	[1935]	SN
	— du Pont Co. patents Nylon.	[1932]	EB

Radioiodine, P-32, and Radioactive Therapy

12. I-Res	— S. HERTZ INJECTS FIRST I-128 INTO EAR VEIN OF RABBIT.	[1936]	V90
	— J. Means pubs "The Thyroid and Its Diseases."	[1931]	Bk
13. I-Dx	—		
14. I-Rx	— C. Eckert says thyroid moderate resistant to radiation.	[1921]	Rad
15. P-Rx	— H. Jones: neoplastic tissue (rats) has high P-32 uptake.	[1948]	JBC
	— J. LAWRENCE GIVES LEUKEMIA PATIENT FIRST THERAPEUTIC °P DOSE.		Rad
	ANOTHER BEGINNING OF NUCLEAR MEDICINE		
16. Tele	— R. Stone "cures" Lawrence's mother of "terminal pelvic ca"; uses Sloan's 2 MeV X-ray tube.	[1931]	Bio
	BEGINNING OF SUPERVOLTAGE RADIOTHERAPY		
	— R. Dresser treats first patient with Van de Graaff machine.	[1931]	RAD
17. Other	— J. Van Roojen describes cosine surface brachytherapy.	[1931]	BJR
	— J. Hamilton (R. Stone) tries Na-24 for Rx of CL Leukemia.	[1934]	Rad

Scans and Other Tests of Function in Various Organs

18. Brain	—		
19. Heart	— A. Castellanos introduces angiography in children.	(1944	BHM)
	— R. Eckstein re-evaluates cause of first heart sound.	[1933]	AJPh
	— D. Gregg studies blood pressure in unanesthetized dog.	[1935]	AJPh
	— V. Johnson studies pulmonary circulation.	[1934]	AJPh
20. Liver	— R. Wright says hepatic artery supplies all secondary ca.	[1981]	JPB
21. Lung	—		
22. Bone	— M. Dols measures P-32 uptake in rachitic animals.	[1935]	PKAW
23. Kidney	— H. Green measures renal volume in the cat.	[1935]	AJPh
	— I. Page tells hypophysectomy effects on blood pressure.	[1934]	AJPh
	— T. Findley compares H_2O metab in norm & diab insipidus.	[1934]	JCI
	— H. Smith publishes "Physiology of the Kidney."	[1935]	Bk
24. Gut	— J. Hamilton feeds °Na, °K, °Br, °Cl, °I for human absorp.	[1935]	PNAS
25. Blood	—		
26. Other	—		

Radiation Hysteria and Health Physics * Obituaries *

27. Hyst	— R. Reeves measures thorium dioxide retention by X-Ray.	[1934]	Rad
	— JAMA editorial warns, possible danger from Dx Thorotrast.	[1934]	JAMA
	— R. Taft measures gamma rad from pt after Thorotrast.	[1934]	JAMA
	— ICRU says tolerance dose is 0.2 r/day.	[1934]	ICRU
	— M. Nakaidzumi finds neutron irrad causes sterility.	[1935]	Na
28. React	— R. Evans: GM tube detects >100 ng radium body burden.	[1929]	AJR
29. Respo	— AMA refuses to accept Thorotrast with doubts on safety.	[1929]	JAMA

* * *

30. Obits	— E. Rutherford (1871–1937) Eng physics; nuclear physics.		Eve

CHRONOLOGY OF NUCLEAR MEDICINE — 1938

Scientific and Technical Background

			Ref.
1. Basic	— O. Hahn finds, doesn't recognize transuranium isotopes.	[1934]	NaW
	— A. Nier says Bi-209 is stable end of 4n + 1 series.	[1935]	GSA
2. Obser	— T. Bonner thinks H-3 is radioactive.	[1935]	PR
	— K. Classius describes thermal diffusion isotope separ.	[1921]	JBC
3. # Nuc	— F. Kurie says 9 cyclotrons (5 in Europe) operating.	[1936]	JAP
	— 271 stable isotopes (4 are ?) plus 4 very long half-lives; 212 °isotopes listed in Handbook.	[1933]	HCP
	— J. Livingood discovers 2 isomers of Co-60, 10.7m & 5.3y.	[1937]	PR
	— J. Livingood describes production of 47d °Fe (Fe-59).	[1937]	PR
	— J. LIVINGOOD DISCOVERS 8.04d I-131.	[1936]	PR
	— G. Tape discovers 12.6d I-126.	[1934]	PR
	— E. SEGRE DISCOVERS 65h Mo-99 AND 6h ISOMER OF #43-99M.	[1937]	PR
4. # Med	—		

Organizations and Internal Politics

5. Pols	— Congress passes law, replaces 1906 Pure Food & Drug Act.	[1939]	FR
	— New law says manufacturers must prove product safety.	[1931]	FDA
6. Socs	— F. Kurie explains design and technique of cyclotron.	[1937]	JAP
7. Event	— US Army Sig Corps sets up anti-aircraft echo device (radar).	[1934]	USA
	— A. Carrel achieves tissue cultures that live "forever."	[1914]	DSB
	— L. Biro invents the ball point pen.	[1931]	EB

Instruments, Units of Measurement, and Drugs

8. Instr	— V. Zworykin builds Iconoscope: e^- mag deflect on screen.	[1902]	Sn
	— I. Rabi introduces NMR in molecular beams.	[1936]	GSA
9. Units	— NBS Comm on °Standards decides to make Ra std solutions.	[1910]	GMP
10. Concp	— G. Hevesy uses activation analysis in first °rare earths.	[1936]	KDV
	— C. ARTOM INTRODUCES "TURNOVER" CONCEPT (phosphatid rate).	[1937]	AIP
	— L. Jacobsen: autopsy 5 y post-Thorotrast shows slow elim.	[1931]	Rad
	— R. Schoenheimer begins D_2O "turnover" studies.	[1937]	DSB
11. Drugs	— P. Hahn uses °Fe in anemia. (First [?] medical use of °Fe.)	[1949]	JAMA
	— J. Hamilton studies °Na, °K, °CL, °Br, °I in normal humans.	[1937]	AJP
	— I. Chaikoff studies P-32 phospholipids in rat tissue.	[1935]	JBC
	— E. Chargaff: does first synthesis of P-32 organic compound.	[1937]	JACS
	— G. Hevesy injects heavy-oxygen sulfate into rabbit.	[1937]	Na
	— R. Kuhn isolates Vit B_6 (pyridoxine) from 14,000 gal milk.	[1935]	SN
	— P. Karrer synthesizes tokopherol, Vit E.	[1937]	DSB
	— A. Myerson studies pharmacology of autonomic system.	[1936]	AHJ
	— T. Spies demonstrates Vit B deficiency in beriberi.	[1928]	TAAP
	— W. Cebrell shows riboflavin deficiency is a disease.	[1928]	PHR

		Radioiodine, P-32, and Radioactive Therapy		
12.	I-Res	— R. Evans exposes 750 ml iodide to 110 mg Ra-Be source.	[1936]	PR
		— A. Roberts concentrates Evans' 750 cc °I to 1 cc.	[1936]	PR
		— S. Hertz reports first °iodine study (in rabbits).	[1931]	PSEB
		— A. Elmer sums stable iodine detection in body fluids.	[1934]	Bk
		— S. Seidlin discovers pituitary effect on thyroid.	[1946]	V91
		— R. Evans gets Markle grant for MIT cyclotron.	[1936]	V90
		— G. Seaborg announces discovery of I-131.	[1937]	Sc
13.	I-Dx	— J. Hamilton finds 99% of oral dose °I absorbed in 90m.	[1937]	AJP
14.	I-Rx	—		
15.	P-Rx	— J. Lawrence begins study of P-32 in mice.	[1936]	PSEB
16.	Tele	—		
17.	other	— R. Stone treats first ca patient on 37" cyclotron.	[1937]	Bio
		Scans and Other Tests of Function in Various Organs		
18.	Brain	— R. Stuck says intracranial Thorotrast causes hydroceph.	[1937]	ANP
19.	Heart	— E. Lawrence shows mouth-fingertip °Na circulation time.	[1937]	Bio
		— A. Macleod times length of EKG phases of heart cycle.	[1932]	AHJ
		— K. Jochim sees auricle filling ventricle in comp block.	[1937]	AJPh
		— E. Clark reviews AV anastemoses story.	[1934]	PhR
		— K. Grant measures blood circulation in voluntary muscle.	[1928]	CS
		— J. McMichael measures cardiac output in conges failure.	[1936]	QJM
20.	Liver	—		
21.	Lung	—		
22.	Bone	— W. Cohn finds Vit D increases P-32 uptake in bone.	[1924]	JBC
23.	Kidney	— H. Chasis measures renal blood flow & GF in normals.	[1934]	JCI
		— D. Rytand sees aortic block start renal hypertension.	[1935]	CI
		— H. Smith measures normal tubular excretory mass.	[1937]	JCI
24.	Gut	— M. Dos says deficient Vit D = phospholipids up in liver.	[1937]	Na
25.	Blood	— P. Hahn begins °Fe studies in anemia.	[1937]	JAMA
26.	Other	— W. Cohn measures P-32 in various organs; DAR type study.	[1937]	JBC
		— A. Hertzman measures blood flow to skin.	[1932]	AJPh
		Radiation Hysteria and Health Physics	* Obituaries *	
27.	Hyst	— G. Hevesy shows P-32 (oral dose) excreted in goat milk.	[1969]	Na
		— G. Pfahler warns dentists of X-ray hazard.	[1936]	JADA
		— P. Muller synthesizes DDT as an insecticide.	[1944]	DSB
28.	React	— R. Taft: 107 lost Ra tubes; 59 full, 11 partial recovery.	[1914]	Bk
29.	Respo	—		

* * *

30.	Obits	— C. Guillaume (1861–1938) Swiss physics; the liter, "Invar" alloy.	DSB

CHRONOLOGY OF NUCLEAR MEDICINE — 1939

Scientific and Technical Background

			Ref.
1. Basic	— L. MEITNER DEVELOPS THEORY TO EXPLAIN HAHN'S ISOTOPES.	[1938]	Na
	— O. Frisch applies name "fission" to Meitner's theory.	[1934]	Na
	— S. Korff says C-14 comes from cosmic neutrons on N-14.	[1940]	Sc
2. Obser	— O. Hahn finds Ba isotopes on neutron bombardment of U.	[1938]	NaW
	— N. Bohr describes Meitner's fission to Am Phys Soc (N.Y.).	[1939]	Bio
	— T. Taylor sees slight diff in chem behavior of isotopes.	[1915]	Sc
	— L. Mullins notes diff in rates of exchange of Na and °Na.	[1915]	PR
	— G. Hevesy (many others) sees small chem "isotope" effect.	[1915]	ARR
	— H. Barnett thinks rad of °isotopes might change physiol.	[1950]	PR
	H. Crane: evidence of rad change has no significance.	[1932]	PR
	M. Brooks: evidence of rad change has no significance.	[1932]	PSEB
3. # Nuc	— L. Alvarz finds and proves that H-3 is radioactive.	[1934]	PR
	— L. Dubridge finds another nuclear isomer (2.7h Sr-87m).	[1936]	PR
	— M. Perey discovers AcK (21.8m Francium-223), new element.	[1938]	CRS
	— B. Karlik discovers 1.0 × 10^{-4}s At-215.	[1938]	GSA
	— W. Cohn makes $_{19}K^{41} + {}_{1}D^{2}$ –to– $_{19}K^{42} + {}_{1}H^{1}$.	[1955]	JBC

Organizations and Internal Politics

			Ref.
5. Pols	— Germany invades Poland on September 1st.	[1929]	AP
	— Politics of Uranium in 1939:		
	Jan — N. Bohr's talk on "fission" raises military use problem.		TNW
	Mar — E. Fermi almost achieves chain reaction in water.		TNW
	Mar — L. Szilard suggests carbon moderator.		TNW
	Apr — US & UK scientists withhold their atomic publications.		TNW
	Oct — Einstein's (Szilard) letter to Pres FDR starts things.		TNW
	Oct — Uranium Committee reports, gets funds for graphite & U.		TNW
	— F. Joliot-Curie begins atomic energy effort with French Gov't.		Bk
6. Socs	— A. Eve publishes definitive biography of "Rutherford."	[1937]	Bk
	— L. Pauling publishes "Nature of the Chemical Bond."	[1916]	Bk
7. Event	— E. Lawrence completes 60" cyclotron dedicated to med.	[1938]	SC
	— US Navy coast artil gets an echo finding device (radar).	[1938]	USN

Instruments, Units of Measurement, and Drugs

			Ref.
8. Instr	— R. Evans develops a count rate meter for GM tube.	[1937]	RSI
	— H. Lifschuts develops a scaling circuit for GM counts.	[1937]	RSI
	— W. Bale develops a dip-tube counter for liquid samples.	[1937]	RSI
	— P. Hahn uses a dip-tube counter in fixed geom for °Fe.	[1936]	JEM
	— W. Libby develops Evans screen-wall GM tube for C-14.	[1937]	PR
	— E. Lawrence starts 60" cyclotron at 32 MeV.	[1936]	PR
	— V. Zworykin develops first electr microscope (& TV tube).	[1928]	SN
9. Units	— J. Richardson devises a Au-198 decay scheme.	[1954]	PR
	— L. Gray suggests an ergs/gram air neutron unit.	[1932]	Na
	— L. Gray calls ion-pair production energy "W" (c32 ev).	[1900]	BJR
	— L. Gray defines an "energy unit" eu (93 ergs/g water).	[1937]	BJR
	— -. Jordan adds "saturation effect" to target theory.	[1932]	Ra
	— W. Mayneord constructs 3-dimensional dose distribution.	[1928]	BJR
10. Concp	— W. Bale electroplates small °Fe samples onto dip tube.	[1936]	JEM
	— E. Armstrong invents frequency modulation (FM).	[1928]	EB
	— L. Mullins measures °Na, °K loss in relation to concen.	[1928]	Sc
	— L. Pauling adds quantum mechanics to explain bonds.	[1916]	SA
	— P. Aebersold measures field-of-vision of MeV beam.	[1933]	Rad
	— F. Stout shows transport of °K, °Na, °P, °Br in plants.	[1923]	AJBo

11. Drugs	— G. Hevesy tracks K-42 interchange in 1 human (0.5 μCi).	[1941]	APS
	— G. Hevesy says K-42 does not enter RBC readily.	[1936]	BJ
	— W. Cohn proves that Na-24 crosses RBC membrane in vivo.	[1936]	PSEB
	— W. Cohn says Vit D doesn't change P-32 absorption (rats).	[1936]	JBC
	— I. Perlmann measures P-32 turnover in phospholipid.	[1938]	JBC
	— R. Schoenheimer initiates N-15 tagging of amino acids.	[1936]	Bk
	— E. Doisy isolates Vit K.	[1929]	SN

Radioiodine, P-32, and Radioactive Therapy

12. I-Res	— J. Hamilton finds 53–81% °I urinary excretion (24h).	[1938]	AJP
	— J. Hamilton convinces M. Soley to try °I in patients.	[1937]	V91
	— J. Means says hyperplastic thyroid concentrates much °I.	[1936]	V91
	— G. Tape: beta spectrum indicates I-131 has max 640 keV.	[1935]	PR
13. I-Dx	— MIT group uses GM tube on animal neck, measures uptake.	[1938]	V91
	— J. Hamilton puts GM tube on human pts necks for uptake.	[1938]	AJP
14. I-Rx	— D. Marine discusses physiology of the thyroid gland.	[1937]	BNYA
15. P-Rx	— J. Lawrence says greater P-32 uptake in leukemic pts.	[1937]	PSEB
	— J. Lawrence recommends P-32 Rx for CL Leuk and PVA.	[1938]	IC
	— H. Jones finds greater P-32 uptake in many neoplasia.	[1937]	JBC
	— L. Tuttle says nucleoprot °P accounts for leuk uptake.	[1938]	PSEB
17. Other	— R. Stone finds too much damage in fast neutron ca Rx.	[1938]	Rad
	— R. Gilbert reviews radiotherapy in Hodgkin's disease.	[1914]	AJR

Scans and Other Tests of Function in Various Organs

18. Brain	— R. Crouch sees autonomic functions in cerebral cortex.	[1925]	JNMD
19. Heart	— O. Orias writes monograph on clinical phonocardiography.	[1914]	Bk
	— R. Gross does surgical ligature of ductus arteriosus.	(1944	BHM)
	— G. Robb visualizes the cardiac chambers in man.	(1944	BMH)
	— S. Robinson says normal blood pressure is <140/90.	[1925]	ArIM
	— I. Starr investigates cardiac output measurements.	[1936]	AJPh
	— J. Comroe studies role of hemoreceptors in aorta.	[1938]	AJPh
22. Bone	— C. Pecher: Sr-89 is substitute for Ca (no Ca °isotope).	[1937]	PSEB
	— M. Manly finds P-32 exchange slower in teeth than bone.	[1938]	JBC
	— W. Bale studies bone growth in rats with P-32.	[1938]	JBC
23. Kidney	— M. Joseph finds K-42 urinary excretion index of metab.	[1955]	JBC
24. Gut	— H. Turner proves Jackson right with °tagged amino acids.	[1931]	PSEB
	— H. Tarver feeds methionine °S, gets cysteine °S.	[1931]	JBC
	— H. Tarver feeds sulphate °S, gets sulphate °S.	[1931]	JBC
25. Blood	— G. Hevesy studies P-32 interchange in plasma and RBC.	[1936]	KDVS
	— L. Hahn notes P-32 exchange between RBC and plasma.	[1936]	Na
	— J. Griffiths estimates fluid compart exchange with °Na.	[1937]	Na
	— P. Levine discovers Rh factor in blood.	[1926]	JAMA
26. Other	—		

Radiation Hysteria and Health Physics * Obituaries *

27. Hyst	— S. Flugge says fission energy is "enormous."	[1934]	NaW
	— L. Erf finds Sr-89 (IV inject) secreted in cow's milk.	[1937]	PSEB
	— L. Szilard initiates support for the Atom Bomb.	[1945]	AEC
28. React	— R. Evans measures radium body burden by breath analysis.	[1937]	AJR
	— A. Krebs measures radium in crematorium ash (18 normals).	[1937]	FAR
29 Respo	—		

* * *

30. Obits	— S. Freud (1856–1939) Ger cultist MD; psychiatry non-science.		JAMA

THE RADIUM DIAL PAINTERS' TRAGEDY

J. Elster & H. Geitel's measurement of F. Giesel's (the radium chemist) breath in 1904 introduced the problem of radon body burden. [See Vig1901 .E&G] But the subject wasn't public knowledge until the radium-dial painters' tragedy in the late 1920s.

Giesel had developed a luminous paint containing radium, but had not exploited the idea. Dr. Sabin A. von Sohocky had brought the idea of radioluminescent paint to the United States around 1905. By World War I the military adaptation of luminous dials was well known. After the war, fair sized businesses were set up in the US and Europe. Many thousands of radium-dial painters, mostly young women, were employed (but usually only for a few years).

The Radium Dial Painters' Tragedy

The first hint of trouble came in 1925. F.L. Hoffman told how a patient came to see a dentist in New York City with osteomyelitis of the mandible and maxilla similar to phosphorus necrosis. He described eight patients he had seen and a few, including two deaths, he had heard of. The necrosis was caused, he said, by some radioactive substance in luminous watch dial paints. He called the disease "Radium Jaw." [JAMA 85: 961, 1925]

Two weeks later H.S. Martland, Orange County, NJ, Health Service, published a paper that had been in preparation for months. He described 18 girls employed to paint clock dials with a luminous paint containing Zn Sulfide and radium. They tipped their brushes with their lips. The result after 5 years ranged in severity from a slight necrosis of the alveolar borders to destruction of the maxilla with a profound anemia. [JAMA, 85:1769, 1925

Martland used the Elster & Geitel method of collecting expired air to measure radioactivity. On one patient he put an electroscope 18 inches over the chest to measure the *"penetrative radiation coming from the body ..."* (thus beginning whole body counting). The measurement and estimation back to the original dose became "°breath analysis" to R. Evans at MIT. [AJR 37:368, 1937]

Radium Excess Leads to Body Burden Study

In the early 1940s R. Evans concluded that a body burden of 10 to 100 μCi (370 kBq to 3.7 MBq) of radium fixed in bone would produce acute radium poisoning; a level of 1 to 10 μCi (37 to 370 kBq) so fixed would, after 5–10 years, produce symptoms of chronic poisoning. Ingestion of 100 μCi (3.7 MBq), or the injection or breathing of 20 μCi (740 kBq) would be lethal in a matter of weeks.

With a natural body burden in the range of becquerels (nCi) and with toxicity appearing in the kilo-to-megabecquerel dose range, radium has a safety factor of thousands to millions. Toxicology puts such drugs in the "very safe" class. But "radium-dial-painters" became standard Sunday-Supplement-newspaper-scandal. Radium never recovered from this bad press.

The Long Term Effects of Mild "Toxicity"

Meanwhile, what happened to the thousands of radium dial-painters doomed (by newspapers) to die of bone cancer, or at least some horrible radiation death? F. Giesel, who invented radioluminescent paint, died at age 75 with, but not of, a small skin cancer on the left index finger.

Von Sohocky, who exploited radium dial paint (and was first president of U.S. Radium Corp.), died, age 48, at the beginning of the dial-painters publicity. He protested loudly that he did not have cancer as he died of typical radiation aplastic anemia. [JAMA 182:44, 1928]

In 1954 A. Polednak published a followup study of 1155 dial-painters (Am J Epidemiol). He found that, after the few deaths described by Martland, most dial-painters went on to longer lives and had fewer cancers than the rest of the population — a true radiation hormesis. In 1959 an Argonne Nat Lab study by AEC could trace only 225 of many thousand dial-painters that "must still be alive." The girls had changed their names by marriage when they quit work. Less than 5% of the group that could be traced died of cancer — a remarkable verification, in human beings, of radiation hormesis. J.N. Stannard's Radioactivity and Health (1988) sums up: "Much of the clinical information points to a level below which bone cancer does not develop. . . ."

[See Vig1948 .Bkg; Vig1981..Hor]

THE FIRST ARTICLE IN NUCLEAR MEDICINE
(Blumgart Invents a Physiological Tag)

Hermann Blumgart (1895–1977) wrote the first article in nuclear medicine 27 years before Nuclear Medicine was conceived. It was 15 articles long (1927–1931) in the Journal of Clinical Investigation. Co-authors included every faculty member of Harvard Medical School who was either interested in the velocity of blood flow, or just interested. His papers answered, very completely, the physiological problem of the velocity of blood flow. Incidental to his interests in cardiology he introduced a new physics to medicine, a new instrumentation to physics, a new radiopharmacology to science, and reinforced some old physiological principles.

The Speed of Blood Flow

While working in Walter Cannon's physiology laboratory as a student assistant, Blumgart learned that the flow of blood to a tissue, and hence the tissue's viability, depended upon the amount of blood ejected from the heart and its velocity through the arteries. On the Harvard service at Boston City Hospital in 1924 he found much interest in cardiac output, but nobody measured blood velocity. Even the great Harvey hadn't attempted an estimate. Stephan Hales in 1717 had computed blood velocity in the aorta of a horse to be 1734.9 ft/hour, but with a method (aortic excision) frowned upon for Harvard's patients.

Blumgart spent a year on cardiology services in England where he learned of a few attempts to measure flow, but they all tampered with blood vessels — physiologically forbidden. Upon his return to Harvard in 1926 he heard of William Duane's radon cow for cancer therapy. (Duane, Marie Curie's first assistant, had invented the radium-radon extraction cow to protect her orignal source.) [See Vig1915 .Cow]

Cancer was not Blumgart's immediate interest, but he observed that Duane measured radiation "dose" from outside the body. Such a remote measurement, he thought, could be the ultimate in physiologic clarity. Inject radon into a peripheral

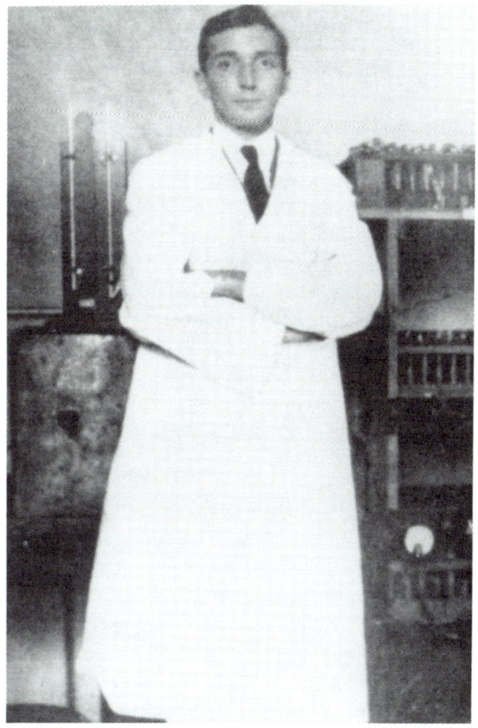

Dr. Blumgart in 1924, with the 1200 test tube battery used to prepare the radon solution for the first nuclear medicine test.

vein (the only violence to the system), and measure its arrival time at the heart; then measure its arrival time in a peripheral artery. All this could be done without disturbing blood flow.

A Few Technical Details

Radon was "known" to be non-toxic in the amount he would use. "Amount" meant amount of chemical in 1926. "Threshold Erythema" was the unit of biological effect, and a detectable amount of radon was far below this level. (Radiation hysteria was not yet a guide to safety. The newspapers had not yet discovered the radium dial painters.) [See Vig1926 .RDP] It was common knowledge that tremendous numbers of gamma rays emanated from an incredibly small "amount" of radon.

But there was a little problem — radon was very expensive for a researcher before government research grants. The answer was: use waste radon. Huntington Memorial Hospital in Boston used many 20 millicurie radium emanation tubes for cancer therapy; they were discarded at about half this value. 10 mCi was ample for Blumgart's need, and it was free.

But there was a little problem — how to get the radon gas out of a permanently sealed metal tube? Blumgart devised a tube-crusher in a gas collector flask. But another little problem arose, how to get the gas into a ml or so of sterile saline for injection? With advice from Duane, Blumgart used the Rutherford "hot" wire method. A sharpened platinum wire electrode, charged to a high voltage, collected the radon.

But still another little problem — how to charge the wire? Blumgart built 1,200 small test tube batteries to get a 2,200 volt direct current. He devised a broom stick on-off switch to prevent his own execution. After shutting off the current and adjusting the air pressure in his specially designed Hg manometer, the radon clad electrode was inserted into a fine tube of HCl. Brought to blood pH with NaOH, the solution was now 0.1 ml of radon in saline. This saline was withdrawn, with hopes for sterility, into a tuberculin syringe, ready for injection.

But there was no problem with the radon gas that escaped and the considerable contamination of equipment, the room, and his lungs. Blumgart had solved this by the Marie Curie method. He allowed no detection instruments in the area, and Health Physics hadn't been born yet.

The Real Problems are Physiological

You do not inject a substance into a vein without knowing venous pressure if you are measuring one of the parameters of pressure. Blumgart devised a three-way stopcock that permitted a verified injection of an 0.1 ml bolus at proper pressure in a fraction of a second.

You could not shield the existing electroscopes from a whole patient full of radioactivity. With advice from C.T.R. Wilson, a cloud chamber was devised for the arm-to-arm measurements. Room for the thick lead shielding was available on the arm-to-arm measurements, and timing mechanisms were attached. It worked well, but was cumbersome. But for arm-to-heart measurements the detector was too heavy. A small shielded Geiger chamber with automatic registration of time-of-arrival could be used.

Geiger tubes were a major problem — Geiger didn't invent his tube until next year! Blumgart got together with a radiation physicist, Otto Yens, and described his requirements. Yens knew the principles that Geiger was following and made a well shielded Geiger-type detection chamber.

The Study Finally Becomes Clinical

Before he could study the velocity of blood flow, Blumgart had to verify all of his assumptions. To prove he was measuring a true circulation time he measured it in 62 normal controls — a major project in itself.

Then he investigated the velocity of blood flow in patients with thyrotoxicosis, myxedema, various anemias, polycythemias, carcinomas, cardiovascular diseases, other physiological and pharmacological stresses, and in combinations of disease and stresses. Between 1926 and 1931 he published 22 articles with many collaborators, mostly in the Journal of Clinical Investigation.

In the sixth article with Soma Weiss in 1927, the famous second conclusion appeared, that has since become aphoristic in every announcement of a new nuclear medicine diagnostic technique:

> "2. *Because of the simplicity of the procedure . . . the method is well suited to its determination in man.*"
>
> [J Clin Invest 4:389, 1927]

This study of blood flow velocity in health and disease was a masterpiece of clinical science. It was also the first publication in Nuclear Medicine. For a long time it was not recognized as such for a very simple reason: it took another 27 years, the discovery of "radioisotopes," and Atomic Energy Commission moneybags, for Nuclear Medicine to get organized.

[See Vig1954 .SNM A Society. . .]

CLOUD CHAMBERS VISUALIZE NUCLEAR PHYSICS

(C.T.R. Wilson's Glass Blowing Takes Over)

C.T.R. Wilson graduated from Owens College at Manchester at age 15. He went to Cambridge for a degree and stayed on as demonstrator in chemistry and physics. Competent but not outstanding, he felt that his prospects were uncertain, and left Cambridge for a "grammar school" teaching job. During the 1894 summer holiday he spent a few weeks near the meteorological observatory at the summit of Ben Nevis (Scotland's highest peak, 4406 ft., now closed). He was tremendously impressed by the display of sunlight in the forming cloud patterns. At the age of 25 he had found his lifetime obsession: studying cloud formation in the laboratory.

With no job prospect he returned to Cambridge to his old demonstrator's job. He must have been good at it, because when two lectureships opened he was offered one at the Cavendish Laboratory. It was one of the few places in the world where a teacher was expected to do his own research. The Assistant Director was a meteorologist, and the Director, J.J. Thomson, was nearing the climax of his search for the "corpuscle" of electricity (we now say "electron").

C.T.R. Wilson Becomes a Glassblower

C.T.R. (the initials soon became the name because of another Wilson on the staff) Wilson set up an expansion chamber. Meteorologists had known since 1880 that a fog is formed in *ordinary* air if it is supersaturated, and then suddenly cooled by a volume expansion. But no fog occurs in *dust-free* air. Some "nucleus" is required around which droplets of water can be formed. ("Nucleus" was then defined as a kernel or core. The nuclear atom was still 15 years in the future.) C.T.R. made his first expansion chamber out of glass. He blew his own glass because extreme precision was required for quantitative expansion ratios.

C.T.R. was not a master glass blower, but he was the most persistent, patient and perfectionist of all glass blowers. Years later J.J. Thomson reminisced, *"Those who have tried know how exasperating glass blowing ... breaks and the work has to be done again. This never seemed to disconcert Wilson; he would take up a fresh piece of glass, perhaps say 'Oh dear', perhaps 'Dear, dear', but never anything stronger and begin again."* [J.J. Autobiog. 1937]

In 1926, after a long trip to New Zealand, Rutherford returned to the Cavendish Lab and felt he was home when he saw C.T.R. sitting at the same bench still blowing the same large glass joint.

[Eve, 1939]

The Cloud Chamber Enters Nuclear Physics

In 1896 J.J. Thomson and Rutherford were hot on the new subject of Roentgen's rays. They discovered that X-rays ionized the air and ions were charged particles. Would they, wondered C.T.R., act as nuclei in supersaturated water vapor? His cloud chamber (a new name for the expansion apparatus) was put in the path of an X-ray tube. In a dust free chamber no cloud should be formed, but a dense cloud erupted in the beam of ionized air. When J.J. Thomson saw the cloud, C.T.R. was no longer on the periphery of Cavendish research.

Wilson soon discovered that droplets were formed on both positive and negative charged particles, but more on negative and at a lower expansion ratio. As his chambers became more precise he found ionization in tap water; he verified the Elster and Geitel observation of background radiation in air. [See Vig1901 .E&G] To achieve a clean baseline he shielded the chamber with sheets of lead, but even with ultra-clean water and air he still had a "residual leak" (not answered until cosmic rays were discovered).

In his small chambers the clouds always diffused uniformly throughout the expansion volume. About 1910 C.T.R. made the discovery that changed "cloud chamber" to "Wilson tracks." He wanted to see how the cloud was formed at the instant of its formation. He built a 16 cm diameter chamber under a sheet of glass. Its volume expanded to 760 cc when the plunger activated a Leyden Jar discharge through mercury vapor. The instantaneous spark of light automatically exposed a photographic plate [PRSL 87A:277, 1912] In his 1927

Nobel lecture Wilson described the result, *"... the cloud chamber filled with little wisps and threads of cloud showing the path of electrons ejected from the atoms of air by the X-rays."* [WoA, p. 678]

Wilson Tracks Are High-Energy Physics

A pin point dipped in a weak radium solution was inserted into a chamber. After expansion the photograph showed distinctive alpha tracks. Wilson tried a beta source. Soon he could easily distinguish beta and gamma tracks. He added a stereoscopic attachment to see tracks in 3-dimensions. He added magnetic fields to deflect the tracks.

During the 1920s, cosmic rays became the most popular subject in Sunday Supplement physics. Cosmic rays were electromagnetic rays, or they were high energy particles, depending upon which Nobel Laureate you believed. Victor Hess first saw them on a balloon ride in 1913, but Sunday supplement stories during the late 1920s always featured a cloud chamber photograph. High school students (I was one of them) could distinguish alphas and betas from gamma rays. [See Vig1913 .VH]

Essential Improvements Answer Problems

The foremost problem was that hundreds of films were exposed in order to capture one cosmic event. The Japanese physicist T. Shimizu (in England at the time) added production line techniques by priming the expansion chamber with an electric motor and snapping the pictures on moving film. He gave physicists the job of looking at thousands of pictures and kept them off the streets at night.

Then P.M.S. Blackett (also at The Cavendish) corrected this problem by rigging two collimated GM tubes above and below the cloud chamber. Activation in coincidence by a cosmic ray triggered expansion of the chamber and a photograph. Now every picture was snapped by a cosmic ray, but most went through the chamber like it was Swiss cheese. Most cosmic ray pictures showed nothing.

In 1927 a Russian physicist solved this problem. D. Skobelzyn inserted a sheet of lead inside the chamber to slow down the cosmic ray and insure an interaction whose results were measured in the intense magnetic field of the new automatic-multiplate-cloud-chamber.

An Example of Discovery by Cloud Chamber

In 1930 R.A. Millikan at Cal Tech got one of his students, Carl Anderson, to build one of the new automatic-multiplate-cloud-chambers, but with an intense magnetic field. *"On August 2, 1932, ... photographing cosmic-ray tracks produced in a vertical cloud chamber (magnetic field of 15,000 Gauss) ... tracks were obtained interpretable only on the basis of the existence of a particle carrying a positive charge but having the mass of a free negative electron."* [PR43:491, 1932]

In a review of 1300 cosmic ray photos, 15 showed positive particles penetrating the 6 mm lead plate in his chamber with a curvature radius of a positive electron. He called the new particle a "positron." At first he did not associate his particle with Dirac's 1930 predicted anti-matter annihilation, but soon noticed that all of his positive electron tracks ended abruptly. Millikan was impressed and had Anderson write up the story and immediately send it to PHYSICAL REVIEW. It was good advice; the Cavendish researchers were only days behind him.

Dirac's Positive-Negative Electron Pair

Paul Dirac, Lucasian professor of math at St. John's College next door to Cavendish Laboratory, had, in 1930, predicted that a positive-negative pair of electrons would occur in very high energy collisions. An energy so high (>1.22 MeV) as to be unobtainable in the laboratory. Why not look, suggested Dirac, at cosmic ray interactions? This is exactly what was going on next door. P.M.S. Blackett and G.P.S. Occhialini had taken Dirac's prediction seriously and were looking for proof of a fundamental Dirac thesis: some concepts of quantum mechanics have no analog in classical physics but can predict the result of an experimental observation. Finding a self-annihilating positron would prove Dirac's point.

Unfortunately for them, Carl Anderson published first and got the Nobel prize. [See Vig1930 .Dir]

THE ROENTGEN IS DEFINED
(The Only Measurable Unit of Quantity)

When J.J. Thomson first read the Times' story of Roentgen's discovery (6 January 1896), the reference to a Crookes tube caught his eye. Having used the tubes for many years, his knee-jerk response was to repeat the experiment. He soon achieved some fine X-Rays of frogs. The first scientific problem, however, was to find out what emanated from the tubes.

Already conducting experiments on the passage of electricity through gases, Thomson found, to his great delight, that X-rays made air a conductor of electricity. His graduate student, Ernest Rutherford, was given the job of setting up electroscopes to measure penetration of X-rays through sheets of metal, but by fall term Rutherford was spending full time separating and measuring positive and negative ions formed in air.

Thomson Names "Ionizing Radiation"

Thomson adapted Faraday's name "ions" (carriers of charge thru liquids) to the positive and negative "ions" that were formed in air by X-rays. Rutherford showed that ions could be swept into and through a glass tube in a current of air, trapped in a wad of cotton, or be deflected to the opposite charge in a parallel plate electrometer. In the Nov 1896 Philosophical Magazine Thomson and Rutherford published the simple theory that X-rays were "ionizing radiation." To quantify, you measured electric charge.

Villard Suggests a Unit of Amount

By this time Becquerel's rays were added to ionizing radiation phenomena. Rutherford named three kinds of ionizing rays emanating from uranium: alpha, beta, and rays that were non-deviable in a magnetic field. Rutherford concentrated on radiation from uranium. Paul Villard in Paris was first to describe the gamma rays from uranium, but concentrated on machine-generated Roentgen rays.

By 1908, after years of unsatisfactory (to him) measurements of "amounts of radiation," Villard described a new instrument in the ARCHIVES OF THE ROENTGEN RAY: a "Quantitometer," parallel metal plates hooked up to a quadrant electrometer. It measured ionization in air at a quarter of the amount detected by the pastilles in current use.

Villard had calibrated his instrument in Holzknecht clinical units, but suggested that a unit could be defined in the cgs system of units: *"The quantity of rays capable of liberating 1 cgs unit of electricity in a cubic centimeter of air at a pressure of ... 750 mmHg."* He shined the rays through one of the metal plates in his electroscope to get to the cc of air and thus added a tremendous "wall effect." William Duane at Harvard had shown in 1905 that electrons from the walls of any measuring instrument were an appreciable source of ionization.

This definition of the roentgen would undergo many technical modifications, but the idea behind Villard's suggestion never changed. Duane's parallel plate device to correct the wall-effect was a laboratory, not a clinical, instrument. A unit of radiation quantity would not be accepted by clinicians until a "clinical" instrument was available.

Duane Invents an Instrument

But Villard's unit was the only good measure of quantity. In 1914 Duane overcame the "wall-effect" by turning Villard's plate Quantitometer on its side and shining the beam of X-rays through the centimeter gap between the plates. A one centimeter active area on the plates insured measuring the charge in 1 cm^3 volume of air without the beam of X-rays ever touching metal. This invention of the "parallel plate" wall-less ionization chamber is still, in the 1980s, the final word in all measurements of the roentgen.

Friedrich Demands a Clinical Instrument

Walter Friedrich, the German physicist who had proved the similar wave nature of X-rays, gammas, and light, worked closely with German radiotherapists on measurement of intensity and dose. Duane had used Villard's unit charge/cc of air as "intensity," (E) and E• second as "dose." Unaware of Duane's work (in 1918 Germany), Friedrich designated his Villard unit "e" and made a number of small chambers to measure it. He gave two of his students, Otto Glasser and H. Behnken, the job of making what we later called a "thimble chamber." Both students almost succeeded but with one defect, no material existed for making a tissue-like ion chamber. Friedrich had tried to use animal horn, but the material did not produce the same wall effect as soft tissue.

Glasser Moves To the Crile Clinic

At the end of World War I Ursus Portmann, radiotherapist at the Crile Clinic in Cleveland, wanted to update his department along the lines of expanding radiotherapy in Boston and New York. He toured European departments but was most impressed by Friedrich's two students. He persuaded the one with the best grasp of English, Otto Glasser, to move to America (which wasn't hard in depressed Germany). The other, H. Behnken, continued improving Friedrich's thimble chambers and in 1924 convinced the German Roentgen Society to adopt a careful rewording of the Villard-Duane-Friedrich coulomb/cc (air) unit which they called the R (Roentgen).

When Glasser was settled in the Crile Clinic, his assistant, V.B. Seitz, suggested that a fairly new plastic material called Bakelite might be an answer to his thimble problem. It was composed of carbon, hydrogen, oxygen, and had about the same density as tissue. Glasser got a piece and found it had close to the same radiation attenuation and scattering properties as tissue. Glasser made some 1 cm^3 thimble chambers and solved the "clinical instrumentation" problem.

Forty years later, Ursus Portmann recalled vividly the triumphant demonstration he and Glasser made to the New Orleans Meeting of the Radiological Society. They had at last achieved a clinically acceptable instrument to measure a physically acceptable unit of radiation. In 1925 the unit was proposed to the First International Congress of Radiology in London.

Glasser had sent some Bakelite to Germany, and Behnken made his own thimble chambers. His measurements of a standard differed from Glasser's by a few percent. The Congress instructed both to reconcile their difference and report back to the next Congress. Behnken shipped his instrument to Glasser for intercomparison. There was still a difference. Behnken came to Cleveland because the difference was incredible. He found the instrument had been thrown out of adjustment in shipment. When repaired, both Glasser and Behnken measured the same X-ray sources and got the same answers every time.

The Roentgen Unit is Officially Adopted

At the Second International Congress of Radiology in Stockholm, 1928, the Villard-Duane-Friedrich-Behnken-Glasser unit was adopted:

"The unit of dose is

(from 1928 to 1954 it was a "dose" unit)

that quantity of roentgen radiation

(the r unit must be modified for gammas)

which, when the secondary electrons are fully utilized

(the cm^3 measured must be surrounded by a large volume of similarly irradiated air)

and the wall effect of the chamber is avoided,

(technically this restricts the measurement to a Duane parallel plate device or we assume that a tissue equivalent wall will be an element of "dose")

produces in 1 cc of atmospheric air

(a concern that lung air, intestinal gas or fermentations might distort dose)

at 0°C and 760 mmHg pressure

(Behnken's use of 750 mm had pointed to an appreciable error; a barometer was a required instrument in radiology.)

such a degree of conductivity that one electrostatic unit is measured under saturation conditions.

(Duane had learned that the potential between the parallel plates had to exceed 1200 volts to yield a maximum, called a saturation ionization current.)

This unit shall be called the roentgen and designated by *r*."

Within a year Gioacchino Failla, physicist at New York's Memorial Hospital, was screaming softly, "The roentgen is a unit of quantity, it is not a unit of 'dose'." Failla's threshold erythema unit of dose was already being demolished by Glasser who was measuring erythema in roentgen units and finding unacceptably wide variations. A new approach was required.

[See Vig1953 .Rad]

COCKROFT-WALTON — THE FIRST ATOM SMASHER

John Cockroft, Rutherford's chief administrative assistant at the Cavendish Lab, was an electrical engineer by training. He quit Metropolitan-Vickers Electrical Company to enroll at St. John's Cambridge to study mathematics. But his engineering background tilted him towards experimental work next door at the Cavendish. After graduation he joined P. Kapitza's group studying intense magnetic fields.

Upon reading George Gamow's paper on alpha emission from uranium nuclei, he felt he had an answer to the primary Cavendish problem: penetrating the nucleus. During a visit to Cambridge by Gamow, Cockroft outlined his idea: if a "low energy" alpha can penetrate OUT of the nucleus, why can't a low energy particle penetrate INTO it? Gamow calculated that 1 MeV protons penetrated as far as 16 MeV alphas. Light elements (Li, B) should be penetrated by protons at less than 300 keV — well within acceleration capability. With Gamow he wrote a memo to Rutherford who agreed; but Gamow wasn't worth anything in the lab, so he assigned a student to assist: E.T.S. Walton.

E.T.S. Walton had graduated from Trinity College, Dublin, with highest honors in math and experimental physics. He was at the Cavendish on the same 1851 scholarship that brought Rutherford to the Cavendish in 1895. Cockroft and Walton used a "canal ray" tube and accelerated a beam of positive H ions to a target. By 1929 they had achieved protons at 380 keV.

The target was a 5 cm diameter thin lithium wafer placed in the beam at a 45′ angle. At target level an opening in the tube was sealed shut with a ZnS scintillation screen that could be visually monitored with a low power microscope.

When the beam was turned on, the accelerating voltage was slowly increased. At about 125 keV scintillations began to appear. The scintillations were typical, to those who worked with Rutherford, and were recognized immediately as alpha particles — proved quickly by absorption measurements. The only source for alphas was the lithium target.

By various tests they proved that:

$${}^{1}_{1}H + {}^{7}_{3}Li \rightarrow {}^{8}_{4}Be \rightarrow {}^{4}_{2}He + {}^{4}_{2}He$$

The protons entered some lithium nuclei and formed unstable beryllium-8 atoms. These Be-8 atoms immediately decayed to two helium nuclei (alpha particles).

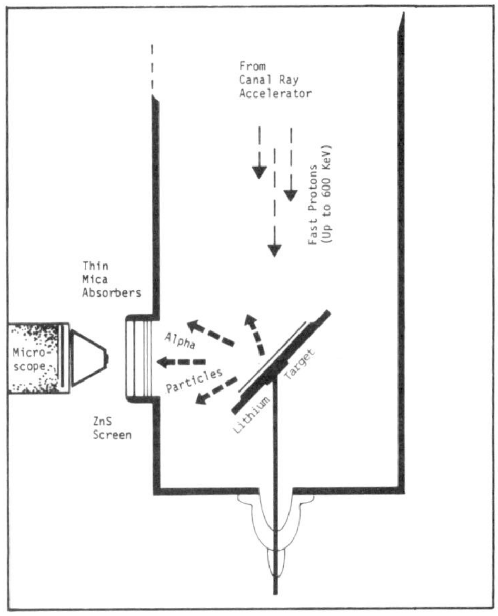

Cockroft-Walton's first "atom smasher"

Cockroft and Walton changed their targets to 16 other elements (including uranium). They used proton energies up to 600 keV (800 keV was their limit). In 1932 they published two papers. [PROC ROYAL SOC 136A:619 & 137A:229] The second paper confirmed Gamow's interpretation of breaching the Coulomb barrier of the nucleus. In a sense it also confirmed Max Born's subtle interpretation of the lifeless Schroedinger wave equations. Even the most bloodless theoretical physicist could now admit that uranium was radioactive.

The Associated Press cabled Rutherford: they would pay 2 cents/word for an interview on the meaning of Cockroft-Walton's atom-smashing (provided, of course, it was understandable). But the AP need not have spent money on an overseas cable; they could have used domestic rates. From an obscure campus on the west coast, near a city that still used cable cars, Ernest Lawrence and Stanley Livingston had submitted an article to PHYSICAL REVIEW three days before Cockroft and Walton submitted theirs to PROC ROYAL SOC. But the British set type faster and the PROC ROY SOC came out 'way ahead of the PHYS REVIEW.

[See Vig1930 .EOL. The Cyclotron]

THE STAGE IS SET FOR THE DISCOVERY OF ARTIFICIALLY PRODUCED RADIONUCLIDES

On 28 June 1914 Archduke Ferdinand's assassination ended Marie Curie's career as a seductress. [See Vig1911 .P&M] Everybody turned to war work. Marie recovered from her scandal and found good use for her skills with radiation. By sheer personality she was able to break through military (and medical) opinion against the use of X-Ray in trauma. She established a front-line semi-portable X-Ray laboratory. By the end of the war, medics found it hard to do without X-Rays.

After the war, the 1920s were a continuous triumphal tour. Marie picked up over 75 honorary scientific memberships and doctorates. Mention of her scandal was almost suppressed when she became a scientific saint among newly liberated women. The scandal disappeared but the "affair" continued. The lists of participants at the major physics conferences of the 1920s usually include both P. Langevin and M. Curie.

Paul Langevin was by now a theoretical physicist of highest international stature. He had introduced "ultrasonics" and was prominent in "relativity." Marie was primarily an historic figure. Her main contribution to science (besides Po and Ra) was becoming manifest in the 1920s: Irene Curie. By 1925 Irene was "preparature" in her mother's lab, and was being recognized as an incarnation of her father.

In 1925 Paul had two promising young students. He kept one as his own assistant and sent the other, Frederic Joliot, to be Marie's assistant. Irene did not socialize much, but she and Frederic worked together in Marie's lab. Within a year (1926) they were married, but soon adopted the name "Joliot-Curie" to keep the Curie name alive.

Both Irene and Frederic were socially and politically, as well as scientifically, influenced by Paul Langevin. Paul was deeply involved in the French Communist Party (as was Frederic which, in another 15 years, would keep him out of the American atom bomb project). Neither left-wing politics nor the abstruse algebras of the new physics affected Paul's abilities as a teacher, now at the Collége de France. Paul recommended another pupil, a young girl, as a research assistant to Marie, but this one was refused. As compensation for the girl's disappointment Paul, now pushing 60, had a son by her.

Did Irene and Frederic Make a Mistake?

In October 1933 Paul was chairing the notable Solvay Conference following the discovery of two major particles. Both the neutron and the positron confirmed P. Dirac's purely theoretical deduction. Many questions could only be answered by "atom smashing" experiments.

Cyclotrons were not yet available. Smashing was done by natural projectiles, and the Joliot-Curies had one of the best sources: clean (no betas) 5.3 MeV alpha particles from Po-210. Polonium had been Marie Curie's first discovery in July of 1898, nine months after Irene was born. Many years later Irene considered Po-210 a neglected isotope (compared to the furor over radium). In a sense polonium was her baby brother. Po-210, one of the long-lived "active deposits," was also known as radium F. Radium D (Pb-210) has a longer life, but decays to radioisotopes with further decay. Radium F (Po-210) decays to radium G (Pb-206), stable lead.

Back around 1908, when William Duane was Marie's trusted assistant, he had begun bleeding radon off of Marie's radium. The radon was stored until it decayed to 22.3 year Pb-210. After a few years radiolead could be milked for pure 138 day Po-210, the most powerful (5.3 MeV) alpha emitter known. By 1925, Irene was already the world's authority on preparation of polonium alpha sources.

When 5.3 meV alpha particles bombarded atoms of light metals, physical theory held that both positrons and neutrons should be emitted. At the 1933 Solvey conference, Frederic and Irene described some n-positron emissions they had observed after bombarding light atoms with alpha rays. Lise Meitner objected: she had done the same experiment and had noted nothing of the kind.

[See Vig1933 .F-I. Artificial °isotopes.]

THESE MEN MADE NUCLEAR MEDICINE A POSSIBILITY

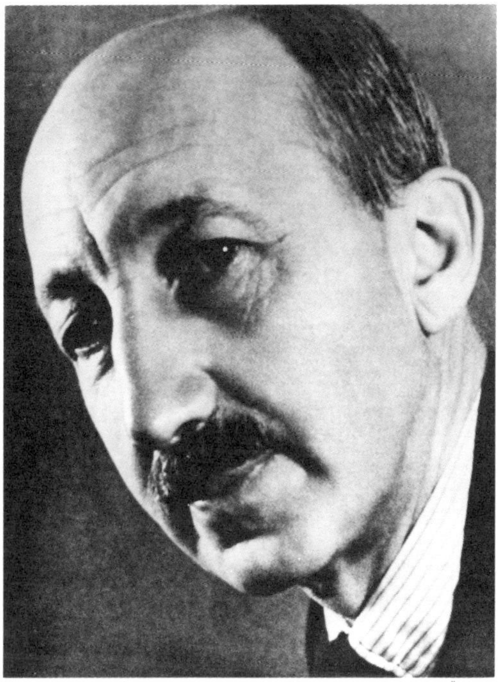

DEUTSCHES MUSEUM, MÜNCHEN

George Charles Hevesy, Ph.D., 1885–1966

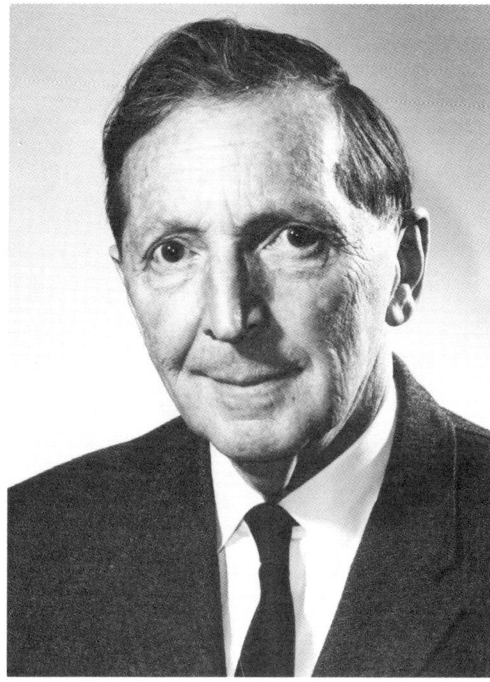

Hermann Ludwig Blumgart, M.D., 1895–1977

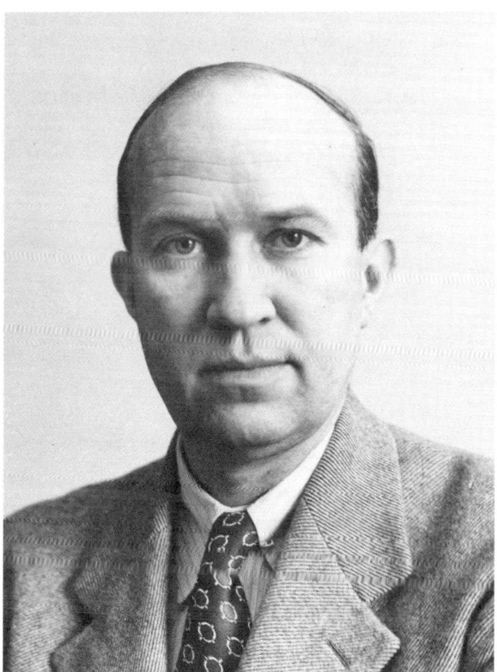

John Hundale Lawrence, M.D., 1904

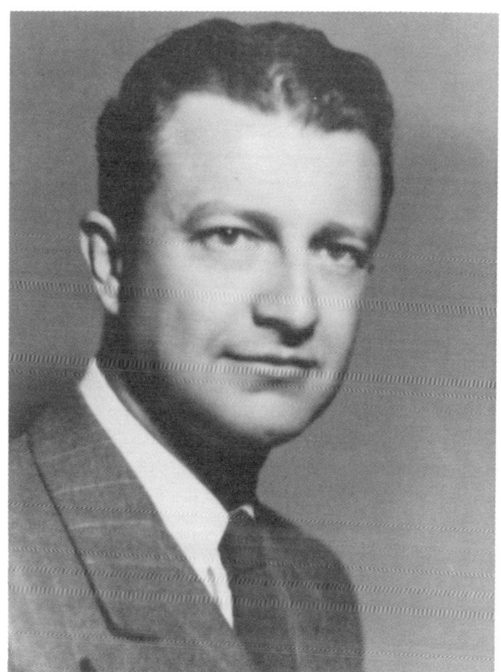

Robley Dunglison Evans, Ph.D., 1907–

DIRAC SEES A MORE SENSIBLE WORLD
The Interaction of Radiation with Matter

Frederick Soddy was an outstanding physical chemist who could see more in his own accomplishments than was actually true. In 1919 he received the Nobel prize for "Isotopes" which he knew were Kasimir Fajans' "Pleiades." After the prize he did nothing but fiddle with mathematics for which he had no feeling. He considered mathematics an "*... incredible confusion ... that followed the invention by Hindu mathematicians of negative quantities ... I am not among those who can bow down and worship the square root of minus one.*"

[Interpret. of the Atom, Putnam, 1932]

The growth of theoretical physics after 1920, particularly the Göttingen school, appalled him. Schroedinger's wave packet "particles" degenerated into Max Born's clouds of probability. They could be either inside or outside a nucleus (or both at the same time according to Einstein). These were *"the incomprehensible conceptions of the wave mechanics."* Soddy had been driven up the wall by verification of Einstein's relativity during the 1919 solar eclipse expedition.

Wilson cloud chamber tracks, Soddy said, were the only kind of direct visible evidence that could not be manipulated by theorists. He was writing this (1932) after P. Dirac had predicted that a cloud chamber would show negative energy states and anti-matter. When Soddy read the original Dirac article in 1928 he said he vomited, but much too soon. Carl Anderson was not looking for a Dirac positive-negative pair, he just described cloud chamber pictures. The only explanation for his pictures was Dirac's prediction.

The Real Reality of the Real World
(not the fake 2- & 3-dimensional worlds of Euclid, Aristotle and Newton)

Paul A.N. Dirac, Lucasian professor of math at Cambridge, agreed with Max Born that 2-valued logics, 3-valued geometries, and commutative algebras describe simplistic make-believe. The real world of quantum mechanics is an infinite sea of negative-energy electron states. These states don't exist in a false 3-dimensional pictorial language. For those of us, myself included, who cannot see physical forms in algebraic symbols, physical analogies are fundamentally inaccurate cartoons. For example:

If a gamma ray of sufficient energy (at least twice the 511 keV rest mass of the electron) collides with a negative energy state electron, it will transfer energy to the electron. When lifted to a positive state, we observe this energy as a free electron.

[WoA, chap. 69, 1966]

But this conversion leaves a hole in the negative state, a negative-negative which we observe as a positive: a positron. It has the rest mass of a free electron but has the opposite charge.

The remainder of the collision energy impels both the negative and positive particles, or pair, into visible 3-dimensional space. Hence this high energy event is called "pair production." Although the negative particle has all the characteristics of any 511 keV electron, the positron is a form of anti-matter. As soon as it meets a free electron both are annihilated. They immediately reappear as two, occasionally three, 511 keV "annihilation rays."

[Indistinguishable from gamma rays, technically they are not gammas because they do not originate in the nucleus. They are not X-rays because they do not originate in the atom's electron shells. But, once born, nobody can tell the difference.]

In the entire happening, the requirement of mass-energy conservation is maintained. The initial "photon & negative-state electron" collision can occur only at energies above 511 + 511 keV. Such photons could not be produced in the 1928 laboratory. For this reason, Dirac suggested that physicists look at cosmic ray collisions. They must be visible in a device such as a cloud chamber. (Dirac had seen the remarkable pictures that C.T.R. Wilson was taking next door to his office.)

[See Vig1927 .CTR]

Frederick Soddy's response was to publish a diatribe against theoretical physicists the same year (1932) that Carl Anderson discovered the positron in cloud chamber pictures.

[See Vig1939 .MB2]

LAWRENCE BUILDS A 4-INCH CYCLOTRON

(But Sloan's Tubes are Most Successful)

As a student (U of Minn) Merle Tuve learned that the insulation in a Tesla Coil breaks down at about 300,000 volts. In 1930, now at Carnegie Inst. in Washington, DC, he solved the problem by dunking the whole coil in an oil bath. He broke the million volt mark without breakdown.

A "million" was the magic number. European, British, and a few American groups were trying to achieve "super-voltage" radiation therapy. In 1930 C.C. Lauritsen at Cal Tech almost achieved the goal for the Los Angeles Tumor Institute. Such competition from Tinsel Town was taken seriously at UC Berkeley.

Early in April 1928 associate professor Ernest Lawrence, a physicist fresh out of Yale, was perusing the literature in the main library at Berkeley. While leafing through ARCHIV FUR ELECTROTECHNIK (1928) an article by Rolf Wideroe caught his eye. Potassium ions were passed through two metal tubes hooked up to an oscillating voltage. The ions acquired a boost in speed as they passed between the tubes to emerge at twice their entering energy. Lawrence calculated in his head: how many tubes to reach a million volts? Each tube must be longer than its predecessor because the particles accelerated. The campus wasn't long enough. Why not bend the tubes between magnetic poles to accelerate in circles. His machine was designed before he left the library.

The ions could be injected into "D" shaped hollow electrodes under vacuum. With back to back "Dee"s connected to an alternating current each passage would accelerate in an ever widening circle until ejected from the periphery at enormous energy. Such a "magnetic resonating accelerator" was limited only by the size of its magnet.

The First Cyclotrons are Built

A huge (for 1928) four inch diameter electromagnet was stored in one of the labs. Lawrence borrowed it and with his first Ph.D. graduate student, Niels Edlefsen, constructed a four inch instrument to test the principle. It worked!

But the magnet wasn't big enough to get beyond 80 keV and before they turned the machine off Lawrence was designing a million volt device. In June 1930, M.S. Livingston joined and they built an 11″ one ton magnet. They were already calling it a "cyclotron." In February 1932, with the help of "shimming" and "snouting" (mechanical adjustments to align the beam), Livingston achieved one million volts. Lawrence changed his goal to 25 million volts.

Just in Case it Didn't Work

The success of the 4-incher had been a pleasant surprise to Lawrence. Just in case his hunch was wrong he had asked another grad student, David Sloan, to make a small linear accelerator to prove Wideroe's principle. Sloan put eight 4 mm diameter nickel tubes, 1 to 5 cm long, inside a glass vacuum tube. Spaced in line about a cm apart, each tube was longer than its predecessor to allow equal time for accelerating ions in the built-in alternating electrical fields. The voltage it achieved is unknown because as soon as Lawrence saw the demonstration he called for 13 more sections which soon achieved 200 keV from 120 volt house current.

Three lines of development were ordered: one for electrons, a second for protons, and a third for heavy ions. The electron accelerator soon became known as "a helluva outfit" for producing million volt X-rays. Robert Stone, radiologist at the medical school across the bay, was intensely interested. He could now compete with Lauritsen's monstrous X-ray machine in Los Angeles.

Ernest and John Become Converts

In 1937 Ernest Lawrence's faith in the use of supervoltage X-rays to cure cancer reached unreasonable heights when Robert Stone cured Ernest's mother with the Sloan X-ray tube. She had been diagnosed at the Mayo Clinic as having terminal pelvic cancer: a "frozen pelvis" — surgically inoperable — three months prognosis. (The Mayo Clinic made mistakes, but not in diagnosis of such a well known disease.) John Lawrence, the MD younger brother of Ernest, brought his mother to California. Stone treated her with the million volt X-rays generated in Sloan's electron tube. Slowly but perceptibly the tumor got smaller. Soon it could not be detected. It was a real cure because Mrs. Lawrence outlived her son by 21 years. Some of Ernest's enthusiasm rubbed off on Bob Stone but was tempered by a "failure" (his word) with neutron therapy in 1939. John Lawrence began his lifelong search for better high voltage therapy.

[EOL biog, Dutton, 1968]

The Cyclotron is Almost Dropped

Sloan's tubes also produced 2 MeV protons and in much higher quantity than with the cyclotron. Ernest seriously considered dropping the cyclotron idea in favor of Sloan's tubes, except that the limitations of the linear device were too great: a mile long linear tube in earthquake prone California? Impossible!

In 1932 the 11 inch cyclotron was producing good physics but was too small. A friend in Engineering told Ernest of an 80-ton 37″ magnet core designed for a now obsolete radio wave generator in China. When China was invaded the core was discarded in a storage dump across the bay. Ernest got the monster and had it installed in an old two-story wooden building about to be demolished. The building, soon known as the Rad Lab, forecast things-to-come: it was closer to Chemistry than to the Physics department.

By 1933 his 27″ cyclotron had produced 2 MeV *protons*. (Lawrence hadn't used the full diameter of the magnet and after topping out at 5 MeV *deuterons* in 1934, he decided to increase the diameter to the maximum for this magnet.) In 1936 he had a 37″ cyclotron, which was the workhorse of pre-World War II nuclear science. But, in 1933, deuterons were critical.

Gilbert Lewis, Dean of Chemistry, considered the cyclotron an intellectual adjunct to his Department. He had been first to make his own supply of heavy water after its discovery, and had named H-2 the "deuton" (extension from proton). [See Vig1933 .D2] Lewis pointed out that acceleration of a one-charge-proton was the same as for a one-charge-"deuton," but the "deuton" would hit the target with a double mass. On 20 March 1933 "deutons" (now "deuterons") were accelerated in the 27″ cyclotron. Lithium was the target: "alphas" were produced of greater range than ever seen.

Chadwick thought they were his neutrons, but was this proper science? Lawrence was the only person who had both an accelerator *and* deuterium. Lawrence got Lewis to send some D_2O to Rutherford, who tried it in Cockcroft's accelerator and immediately invited Lawrence to the October 1933 Solvay Conference. (A by-invitation-only yearly meeting of the world's top physicists. Only three Americans had ever been invited.)

The Cyclotron Becomes World Class Physics

At the meeting Cockroft was still uncertain of accelerator physics. Lawrence pointed out that he wasn't talking about piddling 300 keV proton bombardments, he was describing the effects of 3,000 keV deuterons. Theoretical physicists agreed that Ernest Lawrence had started a new ball game. Overnight, very high energy accelerators had become the basic tool of nuclear physics. F. Joliot was first to request construction diagrams for a cyclotron (but he couldn't raise the money for a few years). Rutherford questioned Lawrence closely on details (the Cavendish finished theirs in 1936). E. Fermi said Rome couldn't get one with Mussolini in power. Joffe from Leningrad said they were already building a "Lawrence" (Russian for cyclotron). By 1934 Livingston had a cyclotron operating at Cornell, in 1935 Columbia's was under way. In 1936 construction was started at Birmingham, the U of Michigan, Rochester, Liverpool, Copenhagen, Stockholm, Paris, and MIT. Requests for detailed plans came from Japan and India.

One ironic twist occurred: in this seething nest of violently quantitative physicists and their algebraic overlords, the tool that ruled them did not produce particles, numbers, or formulae; it made pretty pictures. Rutherford said that a cloud chamber picture was the final arbiter of all their arguments.

[See Vig1927 .CTR, The Cloud Chamber]

HEAVY WATER IS SO HEAVY YOU CAN WEIGH THE DIFFERENCE ON A BATHROOM SCALE

(If You Have Enough Of It)

In 1914 H. Moseley proved that the ordinal number of an element in the Periodic Table (now called Z) must have physical significance. William Prout's protyle, or hydrogen, must be 1.0 atomic units exactly — but it weighed out at 1.007+. (With chemists like T. Richards at Harvard, and O. Hönigschmid in Vienna, no one questioned this accuracy.)

By 1919 a similar discrepancy in neon and chlorine had been answered as a mixture of isotopes. The gut feeling was that 1 in 4500 atoms of H was a heavy H, but nobody, not even Aston on the mass spectrograph, could demonstrate an isotope of hydrogen. It should have been detectable with a diffusion separation. The experiment was tried, and failed.

In 1931 Harold Urey at Columbia had a better idea. Vapor pressure of light and heavy hydrogen should be different. With F. Brickwedde at the National Bureau of Standards (NBS), he evaporated four liters of liquid hydrogen to 1 ml. Optical spectra of the remaining liquid showed a line precisely where H-2 should be.

To prove it was indeed H-2 required a larger sample, but not at the price of liquid hydrogen in 1931. Distilled water was cheaper. If a large volume of water is electrolyzed, the H-1 should bubble off faster than the H-2. Fortunately Urey knew of a process for making hydrogen and oxygen gas that did just that on a large scale. Urey and his NBS colleagues went to the manufacturing plant and collected samples from their electrolysis vats. As the electrolysis progressed the water got heavier and heavier. Instead of weighing 8.3 lbs/gallon, the electrolyzed water weighed over 9 lbs/gallon. Fancy spectroscopy was unnecessary; you could measure this on a bathroom scale.

Strictly speaking, because it was not a new element, Urey did not have the right to give heavy hydrogen a new name. Nevertheless, he gave the first isotope available in ponderable quantity the name diplogen (D). But D_2O was already being called "heavy water."

CHADWICK FINDS RUTHERFORD'S NEUTRON

Ernest Rutherford's second Bakerian lecture to the Royal Society in June 1920 was on artificial transmutation. (His first in 1904 had been on natural transmutation. [Vig1902 .ER2]) The nuclear atom, he pointed out, was made up of protons and electrons. But this picture is obviously incomplete. A simple look at the Periodic Table shows why. As the elements climb Moseley's staircase in single units, the positive charge goes up about half as fast. Half-charges do not exist. "*... a possible atom of mass one which has zero nuclear charge ... such an atom would have novel properties ... its external field would be practically zero ... it would be able to move freely throughout matter ... it should enter readily the structure of atoms...*"

[PRSL 97A:374, 1920]

As early as February 1920, Rutherford and James Chadwick, working with the new Cavendish scintillation detector, had noted some long range projectiles bounced out of nitrogen gas under alpha bombardment. Some went 40 cm instead of the 28 cm calculated maximum range. But more pressing things prevented a further look. When Chadwick discovered the neutron in 1932 it was not a sudden revelation. He and Rutherford had been plowing that same turf for over twelve years.

On 10 April 1925 Rutherford showed an experimental result that changed the direction of "atom smashing." A young colleague, P.M.S. Blackett, had developed a way to visualize atomic sized events in a Wilson cloud chamber. The photographic tracks of an alpha particle struck a nitrogen atom and remained inside the now oxygen nucleus, but emitted a proton:

$$^{14}_{7}N + ^{4}_{2}He \rightarrow ^{17}_{8}O + ^{1}_{1}H$$

Not only was this photo a visual proof of transmutation, it popularized a new way of balancing chemical transmutation equations. Blackett's photo was, at the time, a rare event. But throughout the world, high energy physics concentrated on "atom-smashing." Their high energy projectiles were alpha particles.

On 2 May 1932 Niels Bohr wrote to Rutherford, *"I got a very interesting letter from Madame Joliot (Irene Curie) who thought that she had evidence of [excited electron emission from nuclei] under the influence of radiation in beryllium, but I suspect that the beta ray tracks on her photographs were due to Compton effects in the [cloud chamber] rather than to nuclear excitation of gas atoms . . .”* [Eve, p. 357]

Bohr suspected wrong; this would have been a key observation if Irene (or Bohr) had been thinking of “neutrons.”

Even before Rutherford's second Bakerian lecture, Orme Mason in Australia and W.B. Harkins at the U of Chicago thought there had to be an uncharged “proton” inside the nucleus. In 1921 Harkins thought it might be an electron-proton pair; hence, it should be called a “neutral-proton” or “neutron.” But to a theorist, there was no room inside a nucleus for an elephant sized electron wave-packet (a beta particle is not a small electron until after emission from a nucleus). The key to the neutron was in Rutherford's long range “protons.” In 1930, W. Boethe and H. Becker in Germany bombarded some light elements (Be, B, Li) with polonium alphas. They noted emission of highly penetrating radiation. Rutherford's instrument saw only particles, their's favored waves; hence they reported, *“very high energy gamma rays.”* [WoA, Chap 74]

The Joliot-Curies put a sheet of paraffin in a beam of polonium alphas to check the Germans. They saw 50 MeV gammas being emitted — this was the subject of Irene's letter to Bohr. Chadwick read the report: 50 MeV gammas from 5 MeV alphas? Impossible! Chadwick had an inspired flash. He immediately repeated the experiment, but with multiple wave and particle detectors. After marshalling all the data he finished a 12 year search: *“. . . If we suppose that the radiation consists of particles of mass very nearly equal to that of the proton, all difficulties disappear. To explain great penetrating power we must assume it has no net charge . . . it consists of a proton and electron in close combination, the 'neutron' discussed by Rutherford in his Bakerian lecture of 1920.”* [PRSL 136A:692, 1932]

Enrico Fermi (Rome) read Chadwick's paper. He knew where he could get alpha particles. Add beryllium and he had neutrons. [See Vig1934 .J-C]

HOW THE DEUTERON GOT ITS NAME

(As Remembered by F.N.D. Kurie at the Dedication of the USNRDL Lab, San Francisco, Oct. 1955)

Once the heavy sister of ordinary hydrogen had been isolated by Harold Urey at Columbia, it got the name “heavy hydrogen” from its origin in “heavy water.” George Hevesy immediately recognized, in heavy water, an isotope he had wanted since 1912. He wrote to Urey for a small sample and received a few liters of 0.5 mol % heavy water by return mail. “Heavy water” was not a proper chemical name. In his first biological paper on goldfish living in heavy water, Hevesy followed Lavoisier's system: double hydrogen + oxygen = diplogen. [Zeit Physiol Chem 225:28, 1933]

G.N. Lewis, professor of chemistry at Berkeley, had also become interested in heavy hydrogen as soon as it was announced. However, he made his own, and in high concentration. He suggested substituting the heavier particle in place of the proton to Lawrence's new cyclotron group. Heavy hydrogen was a potent tool to use in artificial disintegration. They were fortunate in having Dr. Lewis supply them with what he called “deutons” (double protons) in quantities greater than available any other place in the world.

“Diplons” vs “Deutons”

Shortly thereafter, Lord Rutherford's laboratory also began working with the heavy hydrogen nucleus and — they considering themselves quite scholarly — named the particle the “diplon.” The word follows a Greek root but was probably copied from Hevesy's “diplogen.” For a few years deutons and diplons, two names for the same particle, were confusing.

The story goes that at a meeting in Canada considerable confusion occurred in papers describing one substance with two names. The English group finally conceded to change their terminology. *“I'll buy that American word,”* Ernest Rutherford said, *“if you'll put my initials in it.”* That is why heavy hydrogen is now known as the “deuteron.”

[See Vig1958 .HW Heavy Water]

MARIE CURIE'S LAST LABORATORY EXPERIENCE

(Artificial Radioactivity is Discovered, as Told By Elizabeth Rona, ORAU 1978)

At the 1933 Solvay conference Lise Meitner objected to a Joliot-Curie experiment. [See Vig1929 .Pre] Lise Meitner was major league physics, not to be taken lightly. The Joliot-Curies hurried back to their laboratory to check their notes.

Frederic and Irene Joliot-Curie's experiment had been to detect positrons and neutrons, if any, following bombardment of light elements with alpha particles. They had barely missed discovering the neutron because they misinterpreted some data. In January 1932 they had barely missed being first to see the positron. Frederic would take no chances this time. Two months later on New Year's Eve, his mistakes, if any, were totally forgotten.

Forty four years later, Elizabeth Rona, a friend of the Curie family, and one of the first to write an article on radioisotopes (G. Hevesy was co-author), told Irene's story of what happened. Although once removed it is as close to an eyewitness account as we will ever get:

"It was New Year's eve (1933–1934). The Joliot-Curies were finishing up an experiment with the cloud chamber. Alpha particles entered the chamber through a thin aluminum window to hit a target. The Joliot-Curies were ready to leave after the day's work to spend the evening with friends. They were suddenly called back to the lab by their assistant, a German scientist named W.W. Gentner, who had started to dismantle the equipment. He observed that, after he removed the radiation source, he could observe beta tracks; these disappeared after a short time.

"The first reaction of the Joliot-Curies was that the observations were a contamination. They repeated the experiment, surrounded the chamber with a magnet, and removed the alpha source. The trajectories of the electrons were still visible, slowly decreasing in number with a half-life of 3.5 minutes, and the charge on the rays was positive ... They replaced the aluminum with boron with same result except a half-life of 14 minutes ... Recognizing the importance of their observations they called Marie Curie. It was about midnight when Marie and Paul Langevin arrived to witness the new phenomenon.

"The next step was to separate the radioactive element produced. Joliot, with his usual skill, separated an active phosphorus-30 from the bombarded target aluminum. Joliot remembered with pride and affection the expression of intense joy that came over Marie's face when she held the first artificial radioactive element to the geiger counter, to hear the crackling of the rate meter."

The Initial Reaction to "Radioelements"

A report on the New Year's Eve discovery was published in NATURE on 10 Feb 1934: *"... when an aluminum foil is irradiated on a polonium preparation, the emission of positrons does not cease immediately when the active preparation is removed. The foil remains radioactive and the emission decays exponentially ... We propose for the new radio-elements ... the names radionitrogen, radiosilicon, radiophosphorus. These elements and similar ones may possibly be formed with other bombarding particles; protons, deutons, neutrons...."* Few laboratories had polonium sources of the intensity required to check the experiment. Po-210 was Irene's specialty. But the report's last sentence pointed the way. They sent telegrams to a few labs that could confirm or deny.

Elizabeth Rona continues: "Niels Bohr, when he heard of the discovery, was skeptical. Stephan Meyer (Vienna) was less skeptical. During his whole career, he had dreamed of artificial radioactivity. After receiving the telegram from the Joliot Curies announcing their discovery, he invited them to give a lecture in Vienna and so I (E. Rona) heard a first-hand report on the discovery.

"The talk was by Irene, a reception followed at the French Embassy ... I could see that both were depressed. I learned that Mme. Curie was very sick ..., the midnight trip to witness the discovery may have been Marie Curie's last visit to the laboratory. She would be dead a few months later."

[See Vig1936 .GHP & Vig1936 .°I]

A GAMOW — KAPITZA EXCHANGE
(The USSR Trades Captive Scientists)

Peter Kapitza left Russia during the Bolshevik revolution in 1921. He studied at Cambridge, received the Clark Maxwell Scholarship for 1925–26 and began studies of exceedingly high magnetic fields at very low temperatures. In one device he charged accumulators and suddenly discharged them in parallel to get a 50 kiloamp current for 0.01 sec. With an AC generator at full speed with 80 kiloamps he shorted through coils to achieve a brief 300 kilogauss field. He devised a helium liquifier on entirely new principles; also a liquid hydrogen machine yielding 25 L/hour. Inventing novel devices so enhanced his career at the Cavendish Laboratory that a special building, the Mond Laboratory, was built to house his equipment. He became a fellow of Trinity College, was elected to the Royal Society, and with his wife and children almost became a permanent feature of Cambridge society, except . . .

Kapitza is Detained in Russia

Kapitza made his peace with the communists and during the long vacations at Cambridge he often returned to Russia to visit family and fellow scientists. In 1934 he and his family visited Russia to attend a Mendeleev centenary. He was not allowed to leave Russia. (Legally he was still a Soviet citizen.)

The reason was not revealed for many years because first, it was unbelievable, and second, it involved other physicists. Thirty-eight years later, in his posthumous autobiography, Max Born told why.

[Born Autobiog, p. 279 Scribner's, 1978]

Gamow Makes a Liar Out of Einstein

It seems that the Russian theoretical physicist, George Gamow, made yearly trips to visit with western physicists. One year, probably 1932, he was refused permission to leave the USSR. He made several attempts to escape but was caught each time. Then, by mail, he somehow induced Einstein, Bohr, Langevin, and others to send letters to the Soviet government guaranteeing Gamow's return to the USSR after a short visit to Copenhagen. Gamow got the permit, he visited many European centers, then British groups on his way to finally settling down in the USA. He had had no intention of ever returning to Russia.

The Soviet government was understandably angry and considered Einstein et al, and all physicists, liars. They must pay for their treachery. The next year was the centennial of the birth of a scientist recognized as world class: the great Mendeleev. Many western scientists were invited to attend. Peter Kapitza, anxious to visit his ailing mother, took his family along to the celebration.

Kapitza Exchanged for Gamow

A few days before his return to Cambridge, Kapitza was informed that he must stay and work in Russia. Technically, the Soviets were within the law. Kapitza was still a Soviet citizen. Rutherford wrote a letter appealing that in the interests of science Kapitza be allowed to return and complete his work. With the sagacity of those who had just been cheated, the Soviets replied that of course England would like to have Kapitza, just as they would like to have Rutherford.

The new Mond laboratory apparatus without Kapitza was worthless, and Kapitza without his very special cryogenic, high voltage, and measuring instruments was handicapped. Professors Adrian and Dirac went to Russia to negotiate and interview Kapitza. Finally the Soviets purchased the apparatus for £30,000.

Kapitza was not a communist, but he loved Russia and had a loyalty to his native country. The original action of the Soviets in holding Kapitza prisoner may have been a surprise, but there is evidence that he was soon an active participant. He had privileges, conducted much research at very low temperatures. It is often said that he refused to work on the Russian A-bomb, but he never was a nuclear physicist and knew little about the subject.

[Eve, Rutherford Biog, p. 399 MacMillan 1939]

It is hard to say whether the East or the West got the best in this exchange of Kapitza for Gamow, but they didn't cheat.

[See Vig1929 .C-W]

THE BIRTHPANGS OF RADIOPHARMACEUTICALS

("°" reads "radioactive")

By Oriental tradition birth occurs when the sperm enters the ovum — but the necessary foreplay dulls the temporal precision of this moment. By Western standards birth occurs at delivery, a physiologically exciting but mathematically poor end-point. To assuage statisticians a symbolic end-point may be adopted. A noisy public relation event, the birth cry, is the "time of birth."

In dating the birth of radiopharmaceuticals we can also refer to a noisy public relations event: the birth cry was by Donalee Tabern introducing Abbott Lab's °IHSA in 1949. Delivery, however, had been long and the foreplay extensive. [See Vig1949 .Phr]

The first medical success with any radioisotope was R. Abbe's treatment of an exophthalmic goiter in 1904. (He reported it as a 6 year cure in 1911.) A sealed source of Ra had been implanted; hence technically, this might not be considered a drug. Sometime before 1913 radium salts in solution were injected in quite high doses. During the radium body burden studies of the 1950s, and with health physicists pushing public radiation hysteria, we were astonished by the size of the commercial market for intravenous radium. We were horrified by the number of elderly arthritics who sat in uranium mines for relief of pain. How could they know their pain was relieved when highly trained, government certified physicists said breathing radon will cause cancer.

°Isotopes Given to Humans Are Drugs

A "radiopharmaceutical" is given to patients to cause a biological effect. Hence, by definition IV radium is a drug, but natural background radium is not. Inhaling radon while sitting in a mine shaft, or in your home, is not ordinarily considered drug abuse, but a horde of government regulators make a fat living beating their breasts over radon.

According to pre-1980 health physics dogma, radon's longer lived daughters are among the most hazardous of °isotopes. It is never mentioned to newspapers that our population and our life span have doubled since the discovery of radon. This argument is a non sequitur until coupled with other non seqs. Those who breathed the most radon for the longest time died 10 to 20 years beyond life expectancy:

Marie Curie	67 yrs	Aplastic anemia
O. Hönigschmid	66 yrs	suicide
F. Giesel	75 yrs	lung cancer

In the late 1920s no working Joachimsthal uranium miner had lung cancer, but two thirds of the retired miners had pneumoconiosis and died of lung cancer decades above the 1920s life expectancy.

Neither radium nor X-radiation was associated with deadly danger by the public until 1946 — except in overdose. And it was difficult to achieve an overdose except by professionals.

A Primary °Isotope Problem is Production

Scattered through Rutherford's biography are tales of the need for more °sources. Crookes and Becquerel worked with miniscule smidges of °activity, as did Boltwood and Hahn. Hevesy had to separate, purify, and concentrate all of his °sources. Blumgart used radon from hospital waste. The Joliot-Curies discovered artificial °isotopes on New Year's morning in 1934, and within weeks Fermi described how to make about 16 °isotopes with neutrons.

The Union Haute Miniére made a sealed source of 600 mg of radium mixed with 2g Be in 1935. This giant neutron source was presented to Niels Bohr for his 50th birthday. Within days Hevesy was making P-32 for tracer studies in animals, but he could not make enough °activity to detect biological effects.

Sometime in 1935–36 someone gave the first dose of artificial °nuclide to a human. It may have been Hevesy (he took the first dose of D_2O in 1932), or one of the Berkeley or MIT groups. The first documented human dose was Joe Hamilton taking his own dose of °sodium to learn its biological half-time. The first use of any diagnostic agent is ethically indefensible and all such stories are apocrypha. Clinical trials couldn't begin until production of °isotopes was assured. This production grew from nothing to abundance in twenty years.

The Cyclotron Takes Over Radioisotope Production

Date	Instrument	Particle	Production	Ref
1929	Cockroft-Walton voltage multiplier	0.3 MeV protons intense beams	nuclear disintegration	GSA
1930	E.O. Lawrence 4″ cyclotron	0.8 MeV Hg ions	feasibility of high energies	Bio
1932	Berkeley 11″ cyclotron	1.2 MeV protons	proton acceleration	Bio
1934	E. Fermi Rn/Be neutron source	slow & fast neutrons	small amounts of 23 °isotopes	Na
1934	Berkeley 27″ cyclotron	4–8 MeV deuterons	millicuries of °isotopes (bio use)	PR
1935	N. Bohr giant Ra/Be neutron source	many slow & fast neutrons	microcuries P-32 Hevesy's biology	ARR
1936	R. Evans small Ra/Be neutron source	few slow & fast neutrons	few μCi °iodine thyroid studies	GMP
1937	Berkeley 37″ cyclotron	4–8 MeV many particles	few mCi °isotopes Dx & Rx studies	Bio
1939	Berkeley 60″ cyclotron	40 MeV heavy particles	many mCi °isotopes first Pu production	Bio
1940	MIT medically dedicated cyclotron	8 MeV many particles	36 hospitals get °I & °P (war time)	GMP
1942	Berkeley 184″ synchrotron	200 MeV any particle	any °isotope & transuranics	GSA
1943	Oak Ridge (secret) nuclear reactor	10^{11} flux thermal neutrons	curies of most °isotopes	GSA
1946	Oak Ridge reactor opened for °isotopes, NOT for °pharmaceuticals.			
1949	Abbott Laboratories buys "dirty" raw radioisotopes from AEC, processes them, and sells them as "clean" radiopharmaceuticals. °IHSA was the first true radioactive pharmaceutical.			

* * *

The nuclear reactor took over all °isotope production (with a miniscule exception) in 1947. In 2 years the AEC realized it had made a mistake and its Isotopes Division began sales of "non-reactor produced radioisotopes." Evergrowing rentals, then sales, of enriched stable isotopes had always come from the Oak Ridge Calutrons (gigantic cyclotrons). During the second decade of large scale °isotope use (the 1960s), the AEC began to scale down subsidy and give-away programs. With private firms taking over the °isotope business, production methods were determined on the basis of economics.

NEW RADIOISOTOPES OPEN PANDORA'S BOX

(Confirmation of Artificial °Isotopes)

Few laboratories had the tools required to confirm or deny the Joliot-Curie discovery of artificially produced °isotopes. Intense sources of 5.4 MeV polonium alpha particles were Irene's specialty, but the announcement pointed to alternate methods: "protons, deutons, neutrons." [See Vig1933 .F-I]

Unlike N. Bohr's skepticism on hearing of the discovery and S. Meyers' celebration, C.C. Lauritsen at Cal Tech immediately bombarded some Al, Li, and Mg targets for 15 minutes with 900 keV "deutons." [See Vig1933 .D$_2$] He quickly centered the targets under a GM tube. An intense activity with a half-life of 14 minutes confirmed the Joliot-Curie's boron findings, but Lauritsen considered his other findings flawed.

He bombarded a piece of carbon and immediately gave it to Carl Anderson to expose in the cloud chamber. For the first hour after bombardment every cloud chamber photograph showed positive electron tracks. On 27 February 1934 the first confirmation was submitted to *Science*. They thought they had duplicated the Joliot-Curie's N-13; or had they produced C-11, or was it a mixture of both?

In a follow-up letter to PHYSICAL REVIEW on 1 March, C.C. Lauritsen unveiled the nuclear physics problem for the next decade: identify, with certainty, what you produce. More than one transformation was usually theoretically possible. A half-life determination was insufficient evidence (in 1976 it became sufficient). The required chemical identification of a °isotope was often close to impossible.

E. Lawrence had been producing °isotopes for a few years, but didn't know it. [See Vig1934 .Kur] He and M. Livingston submitted a confirmation on 27 February 1934 to PHYSICAL REVIEW, but they didn't attempt chemical identification.

E. Fermi's Response Starts the Atom Bomb

Enrico Fermi had to respond to the Joliot-Curie telegram differently than the rich Californians. He did not have, and could never hope to get, an accelerator. But he could make neutrons — and in very large numbers (for 1934).

Fermi's early training had been in mathematics where he had been somewhat of a prodigy, but he had strong leanings towards physics. As a young physicist he had noticed with passing interest the installation of Rome's first radium cow to provide a steady supply of radon for radiotherapy. In 1926 Fermi was appointed to the first chair in theoretical physics at the Royal University of Rome, but he was equally competent in all phases of the science. He gathered a group of both theoretical and experimental young physicists which soon became known as the "Roman School of Physics."

When the discovery of the neutron was announced in 1932 his memory served him well. Chadwick had bombarded lithium with 800 keV protons. Fermi remembered the Rome radium-radon cow. He knew he could do much better with 5.5 MeV alphas from radon. He sealed up to 800 mCi of radon in 15 mm long, 6 mm diameter glass tubes filled with beryllium. Each tube produced 1000 neutrons/sec/mCi for about a week but at ever decreasing rates. Fermi made neutron sources as a lab routine.

Every Element (?) has °Isotopes

Fermi had a few neutron sources on hand when he saw the 10 February article in NATURE, but he saw a flaw (technical, not experimental). Joliot had been able to transmute ONLY light elements because he had bombarded with Po-210 alphas. The nuclear charge of anything beyond a Z of 15 would inhibit penetration by charged projectiles. But if the new uncharged neutrons were used, any nucleus should be penetrated. This experiment he would do himself and, at the same time, test Joliot's discovery.

The next morning Fermi sent his group out to find samples of every "pure" element they could find. They found 40 elements (called targets) and made them into cylinders to surround and thus maximize the geometry of the neutron tubes. After a timed exposure they could rapidly remove the neutron source and insert a small GM tube.

The Confirmation Is Far Reaching

Most targets showed exponential decay, but some were not simple. On 10 April 1934, just two months after the Joliot-Curie announcement, Fermi sent a letter to the editor of NATURE verifying their findings: P, Si, Al, Ag, I, Cr, all developed intense radioactivity. Fe was complex; Cl seemed to have a long decay period. G. Hevesy saw that "P." [See Vig1936 .GH5] R. Evans remembered the "I" two years later. [See Vig1936 .°I]

As the survey continued, Fermi's group noticed a small but persistent detail. When the target was exposed to neutrons on a wooden table, it became more radioactive than those exposed on a marble table. Fermi grasped its significance: wood had light elements, marble was heavier. Light elements, particularly hydrogen, slowed down fast neutrons by multiple non-penetrating collisions. Slow neutrons spent more time close to target atoms, hence greater likelihood of transmutation. He proved it by putting a paraffin filter between neutron source and target. Henceforth, with the neutron energy specified, each target atom had a measurable probability of capture. Fermi called it a "capture cross section."

Many elements could be made °active. (J. Walke, in the same 10 April NATURE, said on theoretical grounds all could have °isotope forms.) All of the Rome °isotopes were heavier isotopes of the neutron-bombarded element. All emitted negative; no positron emission as announced by the Joliot-Curies. Fermi was not disputing them; he was starting a new ball game. Different °isotopes are produced by neutrons than by alphas.

Alpha particles posed no threat to the cyclotron builders in Berkeley. But Fermi's neutrons were duplicating phenomena that, only weeks ago, had been in the exclusive cyclotron domain. M. Livingston immediately modified the cyclotron to bring the "deuton" beam outside its housing. Gaseous targets could now be irradiated and immediately transferred to a Lauritsen quartz fiber electroscope.

A target in nitrogen gas was bombarded with "deutons" and yielded a 12.6 sec activity — but not when the target was in oxygen, hydrogen, or argon. Fermi had said neutrons did not affect nitrogen, but a fast chemical separation showed the activity was not in the target. It was in gas. On 1 August 1934 M. Livingston dashed off a letter to PHYSICAL REVIEW. They had produced O-15 from N-14; after 12.6s $T_{1/2}$ it emitted a positron to become N-15.

Fermi had also said that sodium yielded a 40s $T_{1/2}$ moderate activity. On 1 Sep 1949 E. Lawrence dashed off another letter to PHYSICAL REVIEW. They had bombarded sodium with deutons and got many mCi of 15 hour Na-24 . . . and had verified their yield with some ultrafast homeopathic chemistry (soon to become a specialty at Berkeley).

°Isotopes Are the Road to the Bomb

In a later publication Fermi would change the face of science and, quite literally, the face of the earth. By 15 July 1934 Fermi published the completed survey which included a neutron bombardment of uranium. Following the lighter element example, U must have yielded a heavier isotope of U, or, because the chemistry did not allow such an interpretation, it must be the first transuranic element.

That is wrong, said Ida Noddack, a German chemist. The chemistry after neutron bombardment of uranium shows that the nucleus must have broken apart. She couldn't use the word "fission" because in 1934 it was a biology term. However, Otto Hahn had begun a serious search for a stable isotope of radium. In 5 more years he would be trying to identify the ashes of a Fermi type uranium irradiation and would find lighter, not heavier, elements. Lise Meitner would identify these ashes as the result of a new kind of "fission."

In 1933 the *Handbook of Chemistry and Physics* listed 212 stable and 38 °isotopes. Ten years later R. Evans listed 276 stable and 375 °isotopes. Nuclear Physics, after a decade's sojourn in theory, was suddenly back in the experimental lab. Just as before WW I, it was also back in bed with Nuclear Chemistry.

[See Appendix 1, How Many; Vig1946 .AEB]

HOW WE LEARNED ABOUT RADIOISOTOPES IN THE USA

(Radioisotopes became known to the public in 1946 after 5 years of super secrecy. I was brought up to despise "factory scientists" who were paid like prostitutes to keep secrets. My generation of scientists became used to, and now tolerates, secret science. My teachers would have blanched at the size of our lies to maintain "national security." During the 1930s scientists used international cablegrams to spread the word. The following story was told by F.N.D. Kurie at the dedication of the USNRDL lab, San Francisco, Oct. 1955.)

"E. Lawrence invited Dr. Cooksey and me to come out to Berkeley in the summer of 1932 and see if we couldn't repeat the Cockroft-Walton experiment (transmutation by accelerated particles). We came out with boxes of Geiger counters which, at that time, were not very common. The counters Cooksey and I brought out were designed for a particular job. When the job was done they were thrown away. An all-purpose Geiger counter was not known in most laboratories. The result was that even though we were simply crawling with artificial radioactivity, we were not the first to discover it.

"We learned about radioactivity one morning in 1934 when a cable came from the Joliot-Curies telling us about their experiment. We verified it. This should have been a lesson, but several months later we got a cable from Fermi telling us that he had discovered that neutrons could make things radioactive.

"These great discoveries, which really set nuclear physics on the way, were followed by a period of relative stability in which we all found an easy way to make a living: Simply bombard something new and find new radioactivity. A paper could always be written, and papers were the things that counted. So, literally, for years people would take things and bombard them; then they'd take the neighboring elements in the Periodic Table and try to figure out what the activities really were."

[See Vig1946 .Pub; First Shipment]

NEUTRONS BESMIRCHED BY A MOUSE

(The First Part is From L. Alvarez's story at the Dedication of the USNRDL lab, San Francisco, Oct 1955)

On 20 March 1933 "deutons" were accelerated in E. Lawrence's new 27″ cyclotron for the first time. In England a lithium target emitted very long range particles that Cockroft thought were his still new neutrons. In Rome, Fermi was about to produce neutrons in his Rn-Be neutron sources, but these had very low flux. Within a year Berkeley was producing enough neutrons, and they seemed to have sufficient chemical effect to worry some people.

Ernest invited his physician brother, John, to Berkeley in 1935 to look into the biological effects of neutrons. It had never been tested because nobody ever had enough neutrons. Further, as yet no unit of radiation dose or exposure had been proposed for anything but X-rays. John's obvious first experiment was to expose a mouse to a short burst of neutrons. He might then get a hint of which ballpark of toxicity he was working in.

John took a mouse to the machine shop for a fitting. They built a mouse sized brass cylinder 4 inches long with thin copper tubes at each end. From their ends rubber tubing ran to an air supply pump. The mouse had a snug but comfortable home for temporary incarceration.

The cylinder was fitted inside the cyclotron, the air tubing strung and hooked up to the pump. The mouse was then freed from its cage to be toasted by the crew as the first person to ride a neutron beam. The mouse was given a drop of the liquid to toast the crew and ever so gently put into the cylinder. After a slight warm up, the beam was turned on.

Paul Aebersold had calculated the exposure time to give a fraction of an LD_{50} roentgen exposure. (The first neutron-roentgen conversion.) The entire crew wanted to observe mouse behavior after a dose similar to what the cyclotroneers probably absorbed. The cyclotron was turned off. The crew crowded around to observe the mouse's triumphant release.

The mouse was stone dead.

You can imagine the emotional jolt to the crew of jolly physicists who had been working around the unshielded cyclotron for the past year. Neutrons would forevermore be stigmatized as "deadly." Ernest Lawrence, on the spot, ordered the entire cyclotron be shielded with a wall of water.

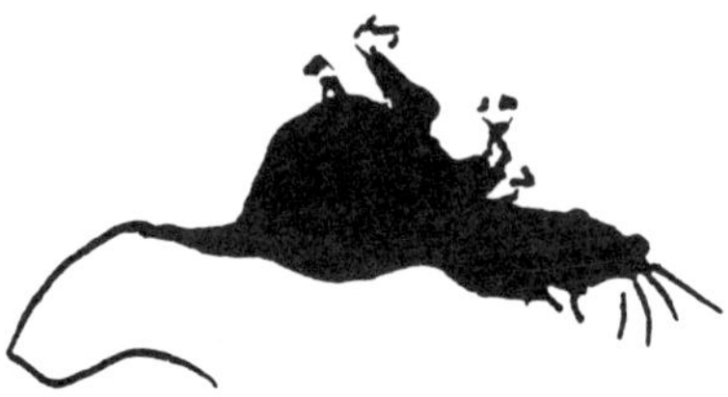

But That Wasn't the End of the Story!

Twenty-two years later Paul Aebersold told me how he had hauled a million — no, it seemed closer to a billion — five gallon cans of water to shield the cyclotron in all directions. Every physicist in sight knew that there were four directions: N, S, E, and Berkeley. Luckily the cyclotron was on the ground floor, because Aebersold more than quadrupled its weight with his foot thick floor-to-ceiling wall of water.

Even That Wasn't the End of the Story!

Joe Hamilton (an MD neurologist by training, not a physicist but highly contaminated by association) had a small mouse colony, laboratory, and his office on the second floor of the old wooden building housing Lawrence's Rad Lab. Hamilton's office was directly over the cyclotron. He died in February 1958, at age 50, with a type of leukemia compatible with excessive radiation exposure. In discussing the many exposures Hamilton had received, Aebersold remarked, *"I now think that UP is also a direction."* No ceiling of water covered the cyclotron.

This is the End of the Story!

John Lawrence retold the story to clear up a minor detail on the hazard of neutrons. [IRT:4:21, 1966] In the excitement of toasting the mouse, Aebersold had forgotten to turn on the air pump. The mouse hadn't been roasted, he had been asphyxiated.

[See Vig1954 .Rad, Unit of dose]

HOW THE "SLICE" BECAME A DOSE UNIT

Radioiodine 24 hour uptake is an accurate measure — but only in unviolated subjects. If you violate patients with a high iodine content diet they are unfit for uptake measurements for weeks. In 1969 a Birmingham group found that industrial chemists were adding so much iodine to so many foods and drugs that uptakes were unreliable. Throw a slice of bread on the table. If it doesn't become stale in a few hours it probably is laced with iodine. Irving Ariel learned this lesson in 1936.

Ariel (now a retired oncologist) became interested in the physiology of I-128 while a resident surgeon at Rochester. °Iodine was doing things to thyroid glands in the 1930s previously confined to surgery. However, to work with I-128 required purchasing cyclotron time. He needed about $400 to continue studies. Government grants were rare in 1936, but he learned of an *Iodine Educational Foundation*. He went to them for help.

During prohibition a *Chilean Nitrate Group* had shipped huge quantities of tincture of iodine into the USA as medicine. Bootleggers poured the tincture through loaves of white bread to separate the iodine from the alcohol. The waste alcohol was sold through various speakeasies, but the iodine-laden white bread, though it never got stale, had a tendency to explode when toasted. The bootleggers were thus left with a ton or so of pure iodine after prohibitions. The Iodine Educational Foundation was set up to find a market for pure iodine.

After giving his pitch for a grant, Ariel was asked to wait while the Board discussed his proposal. They were concerned that this new synthetic iodine would compete in the industrial market with their iodine. When informed that the cyclotron could produce only about one slice of bread's worth of iodine per year, Ariel got his $400. Years later, during the controversy over proper units of °I dose, Ariel proposed the "Slice." Compared to the millicurie and rad, at least it had a biological background. (Details in AJPh 1941, but not this true story.)

[See Vig1936 .°I]

THESE MEN MADE NUCLEAR MEDICINE A REALITY

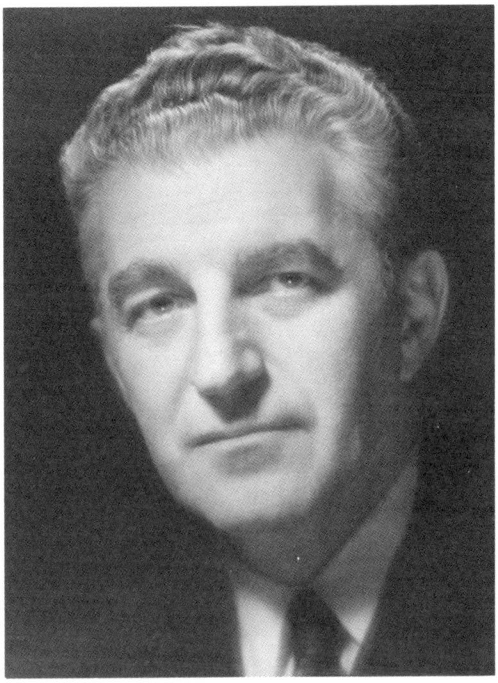

Samuel Seidlin, M.D., 1898–1955

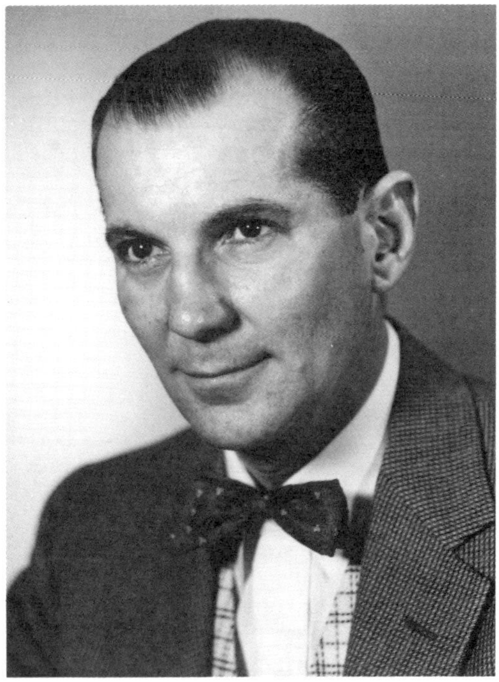

Paul Clarence Aebersold, Ph.D., 1910–1967

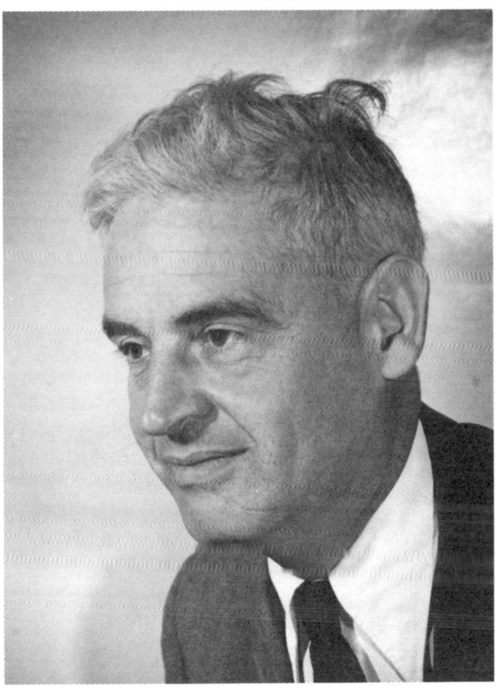

Benedict Cassen, Ph.D., 1902–1972

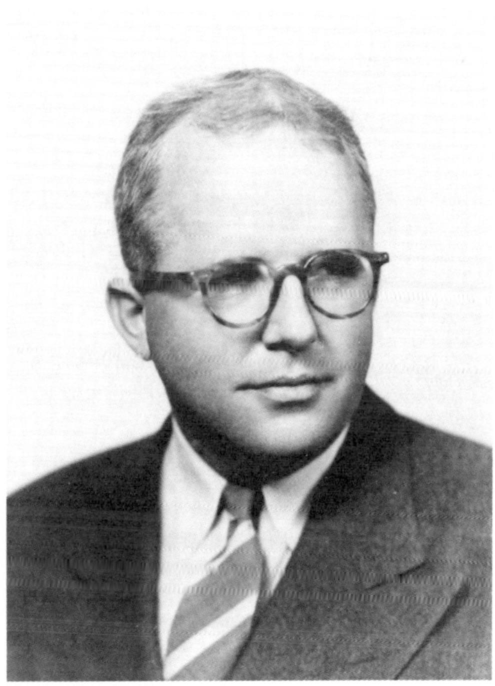

Norman Jeffries Holter, D.Sc., 1914–1983

GEORGE HEVESY INTRODUCES P-32

(Radioiron Was One Result)

Hevesy read Fermi's method of producing radioisotopes in 1934. [See Vig1934 .JC] He found a Copenhagen hospital with a Ra-Rn cow, borrowed some radon, and made a neutron source. With almost a week's exposure he made nanocuries of P-32, enough to become obsessed with the almost infinite applications of radioisotope technology in biochemistry. He had to have a much larger supply of P-32 and fortunately he found one.

Microcuries to Millicuries of P-32

Neils Bohr was due to have a 50th birthday in 1935. Somebody, probably Hevesy, dropped a hint to the Union Haute Miniére who ran the Belgian Congo uranium mine. They were appreciative and Bohr was presented with a gigantic 600 mg radium-beryllium neutron source. Hevesy had an immediate use for neutrons. He could now produce massive doses of P-32. (Microcuries were massive in 1936.) Within a year the cyclotron at Berkeley was producing millicuries. Hearing of Hevesy's needs, Ernest Lawrence asked Martin Kamen to periodically send Hevesy a few millicuries of P-32. (All done through ordinary mail.)

P-32 was an answer to a twenty year old dream. (Even more than the first experiments with heavy water.) Easy GM tube detection of P-32 beta rays was much more sensitive. P-32 allowed heretofore impossible tags of naturally occurring phosphorus compounds. With O. Chievitz, Hevesy announced the first biological use of P-32. [Nature 136:754, 1935] They fed $Na^{\circ}PO_4$ to rats and studied its distribution after a few days.

The First Use of P-32 in Humans

Because it did no harm to the rats, in the article describing their technical procedures [KDS 13:9, 1937] they included a human patient. Given 0.5 mg $Na^{\circ}PO_4$ (a few microcuries) mixed in the regular hospital diet, the patient's urine and feces were assayed for 6 days. 21.7% of the dose was eliminated via urine, and 15.5% in feces. This dose, or Joe Hamilton's first dose of Na-24 to himself, was the first use of a man-made radioisotope in humans. [See Vig1934 .Cyc]

A Label for Blood Volume Studies

In their many investigations of labeled phosphorus compounds, Hevesy found a labile pool of phosphate in plasma, and a lesser non-labile pool in red cells. The relatively permanent red cell P-32 could be, he thought, a non-destructive label for blood volume studies.

Hevesy soon learned that red cells could be labeled in vitro. Upon reinjection of the animal's own, but now radioactive, RBC all foreign body problems were avoided. It might even be a human clinical technique. He investigated the sources of error. [KDS 14:5, 1939]

Mixing time for °RBC in the blood stream was about 2½ minutes, versus about 6 minutes for the currently used dye-in-plasma methods. Loss of P-32 from RBC (about 1.5% during the testing period) was small compared to the leakage of dye from plasma. Labeling of new cells in vivo from the leaked °P was insignificant. Some °P in plasma was adsorbed on red cells without true labeling, but this was considered insignificant. Hemolysis was not a problem. [L. Hahn & G. Hevesy, APS 1940] Many years later Hevesy considered P-32 blood volumes his most significant contribution to medicine. But it doesn't match the importance of his first °isotope experiment (1913). The P-32 RBC label was a flawed "loose" label.

Fe-55 is a Much Better (Maybe?) Label

George Whipple, dean of the medical school at the U of Rochester, was not satisfied with the sloppy hematology of a "loose" label. He had heard of a °iron in Berkeley. A part of hemoglobin, °iron would be the perfect red cell tag. Labeling could be done in vivo in donor animals — no problem to hematologists. Far more difficult was the problem of measuring the soft electron capture emission of Fe-55. For this problem he hired Paul Hahn who found a major error Whipple should have seen himself. [P. Hahn & G. Whipple, JEM, 1940]

[See Vig1942 .RCV, RBC Blood Volume]

ROBLEY EVANS MAKES RADIOIODINE

(One of Two Beginnings of Nuclear Medicine)
[See Vig1937 .JL]

Before interns and medical students were paid salaries, it was traditional to treat the Harvard Medical students with a cultural event that featured the intellectual flavor of Boston. On 12 November 1936, Karl Compton, physicist president of MIT, addressed a luncheon in Vanderbilt Hall. His subject: "What Physics can do for Biology and Medicine."

Robley Evans, one of his faculty, slipped Compton some juicy physicobiological tidbits about George Hevesy's indicator-dilution studies in animals:

1913 — Isotopes are discovered;
1923 — G. Hevesy uses Bi °isotopes as tracers in animals;
1934 — Joliot-Curies produce artificial °isotopes in N, Si, P;
1936 — E. Lawrence can make millicuries of some °isotopes.

Attending Compton's lecture were James Means (whose thyroid clinic at Mass General Hospital was world famous) and two of his henchmen, Earle Chapman and Saul Hertz. They too, were students in a physics lecture, but they knew a few things outside of Compton's sphere:

1896 — E. Baumann finds iodine in the thyroid gland (lots of it);
1907 — D. Marine says iodine is essential to normal function;
1915 — E. Kendall discovers thyroxine;
1923 — J. Means studies radiation Rx for toxic goiter;
1926 — C. Harrington finds 4 iodine atoms in thyroxine molecule.

J. Means found Hevesy's P-32 work very interesting *"but,"* he asked in the post-lecture discussion, *"is there a radioisotope of iodine?"*

Robley Evans remembered one sentence from an article Fermi had written in April 1934. [See Vig1934 .J-C]

"Oh yes," Evans answered, *"Fermi found one last year."*
"How can we get some?"
"We would have to make it the same way Hevesy made his P-32."

During the next six months, Compton and Means set up a joint MIT-MGH committee to study the feasibility of making radioiodine. Chapman and Hertz represented MGH. Robley Evans represented MIT. Evans knew that neither MIT nor MGH could afford a 600 mg Ra-Be neutron generator such as Hevesy had used to make P-32. [See Vig1936 .GH5] But he knew that Fermi got the radon for his Rn-Be neutron source from a medical radium cow.

Evans also knew that the alpha particle guts of neutron sources came from radium daughters. Huntington Hospital used many radon needles from their radium cow. [See Vig1915 .Cow] After a short decay the needles were discarded. For no cost at all he could gather the discards, mix their considerable remnant activity with beryllium, and make a neutron howitzer. He put the gadget together and within a few months proudly showed Compton and Means a few nanocuries of 25 min I-128.

Compton and Means immediately raised $3,000 to start a *Joint MGH-MIT Thyroid Radioiodine Research Program.* With money to burn, Evans hired physicist Arthur Roberts to concentrate on °iodine with Saul Hertz at MGH. His first job was to make a GM tube-time clock to quantify the I-128 samples. (You didn't buy GM tubes in those days, you made them.) By late 1937 he and Hertz injected I-128 into a rabbit's ear. [PSEB 38:510, 1938]

After days of neutron irradiation they couldn't make enough I-128 for more than a teaser. Fortunately, a physician retired and donated his entire supply of radium plaques and needles. Evans got them reprocessed by a radium chemist into a 110 mg Ra-Be neutron generator. They could now produce an enormous yield of 0.05 μCi/day. Now Hertz, Roberts, and Evans could really start to study thyroid metabolism. They gave a paper on this remarkable "thyroid" tracer at a December meeting. J. Hamilton from Berkeley came to see how they did it. [PSEB 38:510, 1938]

12 Nov 1936 — K. Compton lectures and mentions °isotopes;
— J. Means asks about °I;
Apr 1937 — R. Evans makes first I-128;
May 1937 — Joint MGH-MIT Thyroid Radioiodine Program;
Sep 1937 — A. Roberts makes GM tubes;
Late 1937 — S. Hertz injects rabbit.
Late 1937 — 110 mg Ra-Be neutron source makes .05 μCi/day;

Early 1938 — J. Hamilton visits MGH;
May 1938 — First article on thyroid °I.

Joseph Hamilton had been a neurologist in a medical group near the growing Berkeley cyclotron laboratory. He found research more interesting and began his extensive studies of DAR. (Differential Absorption Ratio — the original way to compare °isotopes in bodies:

1) take a standard animal,
2) give it a standard dose,
3) sacrifice at a standard time,
4) measure cpm in each organ,
5) compare with heart = 1.00.)

He measured DARs and transfer rates of every °isotope the cyclotron produced: °Na, °K, °Cl, °Br, °Fe, and the 25 min I-128. Most of his studies were in mice, but occasionally in humans; e.g., he gave the first dose of °Na to himself. The Boston people were doing a different kind of study. Ernest Lawrence called Evans to get Hamilton a few days training.

Hamilton learned some instrumentation and much clinical thyroidology and went home clinically oriented. Evans learned that Berkeley used very large °isotope doses (compared to Boston), and threw away in a day more than MIT made. Compton and Evans went to the Markle Foundation and explained the hungry tiger they had by the tail. They needed about $30,000 to build a cyclotron; MIT would add $26,000 to house it. (Request approved the same day.) M. Livingston moved from Berkeley to Boston to build the first cyclotron dedicated to medical research.

Hamilton saw the advantages of clinical involvement. Upon his return to Berkeley he joined forces with Mayo Soley, in the thyroid clinic at UCSF across the bay. Hamilton also complained to Glenn Seaborg about the horrible short life of I-128, so Seaborg made him the first 8-day I-131. [See Vig1938 .Sea] With I-131 they had sufficient time to allow metabolism in patients. They accepted the MIT-MGH work on rabbits as adequate testing and proceeded directly to humans. Their first publication described diagnostic use of I-131 in patients with thyroid disease. I-131 was a significant achievement because it was the first to prove that °nuclides do not cause cancer. °Iodine's carcinogenicity was a mistake withdrawn by its authors but dishonestly maintained by bureaucrats. [See Vig1985 .Rum]

Spring 1938 — J. Hamilton complains about short-lived I-128;
1 June 1938 — Livingood & Seaborg find I-130 & I-131;
Fall 1938 — M. Livingston starts MIT cyclotron construction;
Early 1939 — Hamilton & Soley begin collaboration on I-131;
Oct 1939 — First article on I-131 in thyroid patients;

In 1938 tellurium had 8 stable isotopes (now 5 stable and 3 very long-lived). Bombardment of Te with deuterons produced a mixture of °iodines with yields depending upon many factors, but especially beam energy. Berkeley used 8 MeV, Michigan used 6 MeV, MIT would use 12 and later 16 MeV. Everybody made a different mixture of °iodines. Hamilton "aged" his mixture to get a "predominantly" I-131. Pure I-131 was not available until it was separated from fission products in the late 1940s.

While their cyclotron was under construction, Evans changed to I-131 and sent tellurium targets to a new cyclotron at Rochester, NY. Dean Whipple's far advanced °iron work now had its own source. [See Vig1942 .RCV] A new man entered the °iodine field. Irving Ariel, before beginning his surgical residency, was interested in the new thyroid physiology. [See Vig1936 .Ari] Early in 1940, a group in Paris brought in another medic-physicist team. The radiotherapist A. Lacassagne and Frederic Joliot (who had started °isotopes in 1934) began °iodine studies.

By July 1940 Hamilton's group published many autoradiograms to show the actual distribution of I-131 in normal, thyrotoxic, and non-toxic goiters. As an omen of an argument waiting to explode, they showed *NO* uptake in a malignant nonfunctioning thyroid tumor. Four months later the MIT cyclotron, which would remain open through World War II, produced its first sample of I-130. I-130 had a 12 hour half-life and seemed ideal for therapy.

Early 1939 — Ariel begins °I studies, and opens the °I field;
July 1940 — °I autoradiograms of human thyroids published;
1 Nov 1940 — MIT cyclotron produces I-130 and I-131 in therapeutic quantities.

[See Vig1941 .Bal]

JOHN LAWRENCE TREATS THE FIRST P-32 PATIENT

(One of Two Beginnings of Nuclear Medicine)
[See Vig1936 .°Iodine]

In 1935 G. Hevesy, then in Copenhagen, began using P-32 that he made in microcurie quantity with Bohr's giant neutron source. [See Vig1936 .GHP] His studies in P-32 metabolism naturally gravitated towards blood, the easiest precision sample he could get from living animals. His P-32 supply was inadequate for many projected studies. At a European physics conference E.O. Lawrence heard of his short supply and offered to send him a regular supply from the Berkeley cyclotron. By 1937 he began to get millicurie amounts (by ordinary mail) prepared by Martin Kamen at Berkeley. [See Vig1946 .Pub]

Millicuries of P-32 in the blood stream causes the same radiobiological effect discovered in 1903 by Gottwald Schwarz (an early Austrian radiologist). Schwarz noted that total body X-irradiation caused changes in counts of formed elements in blood. Since 1923 the Royal Society of Medicine required periodic blood counts of all X-Ray technicians, and this routine was followed (but without much enthusiasm) in California medical installations. But not at the Berkeley cyclotron, probably the most powerful radiation source in the world. All attention was on the "beam" and its target. Physicists didn't think in terms of danger. The cyclotron was not even shielded until a mouse was killed in 1935. [See Vig1935 .NBM]

But John Lawrence knew in 1936 that P-32 injected into the blood stream would kill blood cells. Therefore, diseases characterized by too many blood cells, leukemias and all of the polycythemias, might get symptomatic relief by killing a few of the cells with P-32 radiation. P-32 followed the protraction theory of H. Coutard and A. Baclere by delivering a slow steady low dose over a period of many weeks. Lawrence characterized intravenous P-32 as total body irradiation

First Treatment of Leukemia With P-32

A few trials of IV P-32 in normal and leukemic mice, and in various lymphomas in animals, convinced John Lawrence that the wide discrepancy between animal and man kept the encouraging results from proving anything. He would have to take the big step and try P-32 therapy in man. Fortunately he had a patient who could give true "informed consent." An anemic 29-year-old graduate student at Berkeley had been diagnosed in the fall of 1938 as having chronic myelogenous leukemia. He had greatly enlarged spleen and liver and understood his prognosis and the lack of any definitive therapy.

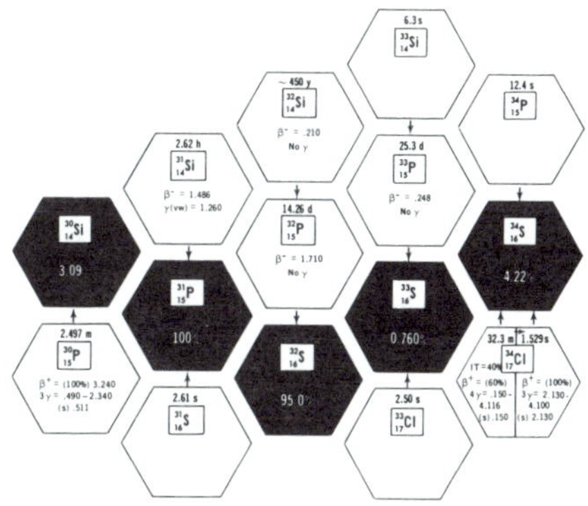

Its ease of slow neutron production, and "almost immediate" decay to non-toxic sulfur, made P-32 a perfect "tracer" in the biological sciences. (When you are accustomed to working with radium, 14 days is a very fast half-life.)

Lawrence explained the theory behind P-32 therapy to the student and how it had worked in mice. With the patient's enthusiastic support he was given 2.98 millicuries on 28 Nov 1938. The leukocyte count came down steadily each day until 12 Dec 1938 when it began to slowly rise. On 14 Jan 1939 a second dose, 2.81 millicuries of P-32, was given. The count came down even farther but began to increase on 9 May. On 15 June 1939 a third dose, this time 4.85 millicuries was followed by a decrease to normal leukocyte count levels and it stayed down. By 1940 neither liver nor spleen was palpable. The patient, symptomatically and by physical examination, was normal.

The second patient was a qualified success. By 1940 Lawrence was able to report five patients with chronic myelogenous or lymphatic leukemia treated with reasonable success, to a doubting audience of radiologists. He described the patient response as similar to that achieved by X-ray or radium. But animal studies of P-32 distribution showed that simple uniform whole body radiation was not given by P-32. The radiation was highly localized to marrow, spleen, and liver. [Rad 35:51, 1940]

A Real Hematologist Takes Over

By January 1941 P-32 therapy of chronic leukemias was taken seriously by a real hematologist. (John Lawrence never claimed expertise in hematology.) Edwin Osgood at the U of Oregon started a series in 1941 that reached 300 patients by 1961. Two thirds were chronic lymphocytic, one third granulocytic leukemias. The treatments were not an overwhelming 100% success, but were far better than anything else ever tried.

As Osgood's series extended he noticed that the dosage pattern did not make sense. He inaugurated "titrated" (meaning divided according to need) regularly spaced dosage. The amount and rate of P-32 administered was determined by the patient's response to his previous dose. This change was not a criticism of Lawrence's methods, but realization that no one in 1938 had any idea of how much should be given or how often. Lawrence started beta therapy before any unit of beta dose existed. Not even extrapolation from X-ray therapy dose was possible until Leo Marinelli invented the "e.r." (equivalent roentgen) in 1940. Osgood had the advantages of Lawrence's experience, Marinelli's dosimetry, plus his recognition as a clinical hematologist.

P-32 is a Victim of Radiation Hysteria

By the time (c1950) the new AEC had got around to making P-32 available to physicians, P-32 therapy of the chronic leukemias and of polycythemia was well accepted. Then in 1952 the Atom Bomb Casualty Commission (ABCC) described a leukemic death in 47 of 110,000 survivors. The next year L. Heilmeyer announced that he had a chemotherapy as good as P-32. In private the word was spread that chemo was better than radioactive therapy because you didn't need a special license with examinations in physics. Also AEC licensers might be snooping in your medical records, thus violating the sacred patient-physician relationship.

Radioactive fallout from A-bomb tests in Nevada was being reported in ever more hysterical terms by newspapers. Hysteria prompted Congress's Joint Committee on Atomic Energy to hold full scale hearings in 1957. In a pious display of concern for the people's health, radiation hysteria was pushed to full swing. Then headlines said 99 survivors of the atom bomb had died of leukemia (eventually it would be about 110 or 0.1%). A few of the patients who had been treated with P-32 died in acute remission; naturally, commented Lawrence, that's how most patients *not* treated with P-32 die.

The Success is "Limited" by Politics

In 1958 Lawrence pointed out that 80% of his P-32 treated lymphoblastoma patients lived a normal life span. (Ann Int Med, 1958) Osgood felt he was seeing the same thing, and hired a biostatistician to review his series. He found that chronic leukemia patients treated with P-32 had a life expectancy equal to that of the US population. (J Nuc Med 5:139, 1964)

However the NIH, already dominated by fund raising cancer societies, was pushing a new marginally successful "chemotherapy." It did not require special AEC license. During the 1950s the 0.01% of Hiroshima atom bomb survivors developed "leukemia" in the glare of world wide publicity. When added to P-32 licensure, the black stain was enough to stigmatize leukemia therapy with P-32.

A couple of offshoots of Lawrence's discovery survived. Their story concerns polcythemia, barely mentioned in Lawrence's first written report. (Rad 35:51, 1940) Polycythemia vera is still (1988) treated with P-32. Thrombocythemia P-32 treatments were added in 1958. The popularity of P-32 increases as the radiophobia of the 1970s relaxes.

[See Vig1940 .ERF, Cure of Polycythemia]

TECHNETIUM FILLS AN EMPTY SPACE

Mendeleev's periodic table was not a rigid set of boxes until late 1913, when H. Mosely gave it 92 spaces — no more, no less. (The Transuranic elements come 30 years later.) [See Vig1913 .Mos] As late as 1937 four of the spaces were glaringly empty: A# 43, 61, 85, 87. Atomic number 85 (later called astatine) and #87 (francium) were understandable because everything over bismuth (#81) was radioactive. But space #43 was surrounded by well known stable metals. Where was #43?

One morning in 1937 C. Perrier and E. Segré, in E. Fermi's laboratory in Rome, received in the mail a small package from Berkeley. It contained a molybdenum target that had been sent to the cyclotron lab to be bombarded with 8 Mev deuterons. As members of the Fermi team that produced the first rash of 23 °isotopes in 1934, they knew what to expect on theoretical grounds: an element to fill space #43.

Perrier and Segré dissolved the target in aqua regia. By theory the chemical homologues, rhenium and manganese in group VIIA, should carry out any #43 in the solution. They added rhenium and manganese salts, saturated the solution with hydrogen sulfide, and allowed the resulting metal sulfides to precipitate. The precipitate was radioactive. Hydrochloric acid dissolved out the manganese they had added. Concentrated HCl slowly dissolved the added rhenium. All of the radioactivity remained in a H_2O_2 solution; this was element #43. It had a half-life of 6 hours.

No wonder Mendeleev's space #43 was empty. The element was too short-lived to exist in nature. Because it had to be made artificially, Perrier and Segré gave it the name "technetium" from the Greek *technetos,* meaning "artificial."

[See Vig1934 .Cyc]

Tc-99 BECOMES Tc-99m

(As told by G. Seaborg, SNM, July 10, 1970)

In 1938 Italy had become unhealthy for intellectuals who didn't contribute to Fascism. E. Fermi took his family to see him get the Nobel Prize in 1938 and never returned to Italy. E. Segré, a member of the Rome team that had discovered element #43 (technetium), managed to convince the Italian Fascist authorities that technetium was bringing glory to Italian science (which was true). He had to visit the cyclotron in Berkeley to get more of it made (which was false). Segré did not return to Italy.

Soon after Segré's arrival in Berkeley he sought out Glenn Seaborg as a collaborator to study his new element, technetium. Within a few days they arranged for bombardment of a second molybdenum target with 8 MeV deuterons in the 37″ cyclotron. Using Segré's original techniques, a fraction was isolated that should have contained any isotope with atomic #43. Its °decay was complex.

Upon measuring its decay and absorption properties, Segré and Seaborg found an isotope that decayed by means of an isomeric transition — emission of an electron line spectrum from an almost completely internally converted gamma ray transition. This concept was so new that J. Oppenheimer and E. Lawrence suggested publication be delayed until additional measurements and interpretations were worked out.

In the meantime, Segré's former colleague B. Pontecorvo, now in Paris, observed and published a similar isomeric transition in an isotope of rhodium. His and Segré's transitions were similar to Otto Hahn's 1921 uranium pair that Lise Meitner had, in 1936, called *nuclear isomerism.*

The new isotope's $T_{1/2}$ was 6.6 hours and was the daughter of 67h Mo-99. Later Segré discovered that the ground state of Tc had a very long half-life (now 2.13×10^5 y) in a decay chain of mass 99. Following a new system of designating isomers with a symbol "m" (meaning metastable), the 6.6h Tc acquired the designation Tc-99m.

[See Vig1960 .°Tc, Richards introduces]

WHY I-131 HAS AN EIGHT-DAY HALF-LIFE
(From Seaborg, AEC News, 5 June 1964)

During the mid-thirties, Jack Livingood and I (Glenn Seaborg) were working with artificial radioactivities. Only a few hundred were known, but it seemed that anything bombarded would produce at least one new °isotope. We scoffed at the idea that any new °isotope would have any practical value.

George Whipple at Rochester, for example, wanted a reasonably long-lived °iron for hemoglobin studies. Jack bombarded iron with 5.5 MeV deuterons on the 27″ cyclotron. Around dinner time he gave me the target. You had to work fast in those days because you couldn't tell how long any new activity would last. I dissolved the target and separated the solution into cobalt, manganese, and iron fractions. I precipitated and re-precipitated all night and just as the sun rose gave Jack three purified fractions.

In the iron fraction, on his reconstructed Lauritsen quartz fiber electroscope, Jack found a new 45 day Fe-59. We made a production run, separated the °iron fraction, and sent it to Dr. Whipple for the first tracer studies of iron in blood — the first °isotope production on a doctor's prescription.

A more difficult "cyclotron radiopharmaceutical" involved an empty spot on the chart of the nuclides. One day in spring 1938 I ran into Joe Hamilton on the steps of Le Conte Hall (the physics building at Berkeley). He complained bitterly about the 28 min $T_{1/2}$ of I-128, *"Why can't you make me an iodine with a longer half-life?"*

"We can," said I, *"How long a half-life do you want?"*

"Oh, about a week."

Jack prepared tellurium targets; bombarded some with 8 MeV deuterons and some with neutrons. I went through chemical separation and identification techniques while wearing a gas mask and obstetrical gloves. This precaution was not protection from radiation, but warded off the dreaded "tellurium breath." We soon identified a new °isotope, I-131. As Joe Hamilton had ordered, it had a half-life of 8 days. [See Vig1946 .°I]

MAX BORN SAYS USE COMMON SENSE
(The Real World Is Non-Commutative)

On 30 January 1933 Hitler became Chancellor of Germany; on the following evening a torchlight parade of Nazis through the streets of Göttingen denounced Jewish civil servants. (Professors at the university were the most prominent "civil servants" in this birthplace of quantum mechanics.) On 25 April the *Göttinger Nachrichten,* a newspaper, published the names of dismissed civil servants. The Dean of the Faculty of Sciences and professor of theoretical physics, Max Born, learned thus that he was no longer employed. The next day an assistant at the astronomy lab knocked on his door and requested Born's lecture notes so that the student could continue the lectures.

By 10 May 1933 the Born family had left Göttingen and the next day left Germany for Switzerland. As his expulsion from Germany became known, he received offers from universities around the world — Born was a founder of Quantum Mechanics. One day a chauffeur-driven Rolls-Royce appeared bringing F.A. Lindemann with an offer from Oxford. Lindemann was visiting all the German universities, taking advantage of Nazi expulsions to improve the status of science at Oxford.

[Lindeman, as Lord Cherwell, became Winston Churchill's science advisor. He discouraged the new "radar" and botched up England's forays into atom bombs. In Born's opinion he was a lousy physicist, the power behind the British strategy of bombing civilians, and a snob.] [See Vig1919 .Ast]

Fortunately Born had already accepted an offer from Rutherford and became a lecturer at Cavendish Laboratory. He was invited to lecture at Edinburg by an old friend, Charles Darwin. [See Vig1913 .Mos] Darwin held the prestigious Tait Chair of Natural Philosophy, but was about to be elected Master of Christ's College Cambridge. Born was offered the Tait Chair, accepted and became a British citizen in 1939. He spent the next 17 years teaching extensions of his greatest achievement: he had freed science from the tyranny of commutative algebras.

[See Vig1925 .MB1]

CHARLES PECHER AND BONE METASTASES

In 1939, two months before WWII, Charles Pecher MD (1912–1941) came to UC Berkeley on a travel fellowship from the Belgium-American Foundation. The Pharmacology Department helped him get a small grant from the Child's Foundation to study °Ca metabolism with Joe Hamilton and Lowell Erf. Pecher was quickly caught up in the interdisciplinary whirl around the cyclotron.

Pecher wrote only six papers. Two, on the isolation of °yttrium and °rubidium, were cyclotron physical chemistry. One (with his wife) was on passage of °strontium to the fetus in pregnant mice. Nurturing their first radioactive baby mice makes Mrs. Pecher the mother of Pediatric Nuclear Medicine. The other paper traced °Sr in the milk of 2 cows. 20 years later, this paper was evidence in the 1950s fallout controversy. Pecher's last paper, dashed off before a forced return to Belgium, was finished by editor Chauncey Leake. and published posthumously.

[U Cal Publications in Pharmacology 2:117–150, 1942]

Ca-45 Leads to Sr-85 Leads to Sr-89

Upon arrival in Berkeley, Pecher reviewed the °isotopes of calcium. Only one, Ca-45, was useful, but could be made only in very small amounts. However, in pharmacological history, strontium was a good substitute for calcium. Sr-85 emitted a gamma ray good for detection, but its cyclotron yield was too low. Pecher found about 1 mCi/mouse a required dose.

> [In preparing samples from cyclotron irradiations Pecher incidentally discovered 106.6 day Y-88. It was worth a short note in PR. In those days at Berkeley anyone with a spare test tube could discover a new °isotope. Proving *what* he discovered separated the scientists from the janitors.]

Sr-89 had a better cyclotron *yield* than Sr-85 and deserved extensive investigation. *Yield* was important because of demands for cyclotron time. Also Sr-89 reached maximum °localization a few hours post-injection in mice and rabbit bones. °Phosphates were slow by comparison. Pecher used autoradiography and tissue counts to plot uptake and excretion over a few weeks post-injection. Chemical and radiation toxicity was measured and, under John Lawrence's supervision, the ultimate test was made. A few patients with metastatic bone prostate ca were selected.

Sr-89 Becomes the Third Therapeutic °Agent

Sr-89 was so confined to tumor metastases in bone that Pecher felt he could give 5 to 8 mCi without causing more than a transient leukopenia. With help from Paul Aebersold he calculated that each mCi of Sr-89 would produce 200 to 600 r in bone. Up to 10 mCi could be given to a human without damage to normal tissue. (Remember, morphine was the ONLY Rx for prostatic metastases in 1941.)

A 65-year-old patient with osteoblastic metastases was given 8.0 mCi Sr-89 lactate in three doses: Sep and Dec 1940, and in Jan 1941. His pain disappeared almost immediately and general condition improved remarkably. Serum phosphatase dropped from 42 to 6 Bodanski units by April. And then disaster!

Pecher was recalled for military duty in Belgium. His country had been under Nazi domination since May of 1940. On the way home Pecher committed suicide. His wife thought Pecher was despondent at coming so close to discovering a cure for a cancer and being stopped for organized mayhem. Even publication of his results was uncertain.

In 1946 B. Low-Beer renewed Pecher's ideas in breast tumors with P-32 (Sr-89 was out, the cyclotron had gone to war). In 1950 H. Friedell introduced P-32 for breast ca metastases to bone. In 1959 G. Bauer renewed Sr-85 as a bone agent. In 1961 Sklaroff and Charkes introduced the Sr-85 bone scan. In 1975 palliative P-32 therapy for metastases to bone was routine. By 1985 bone scans were being done at a rate of over a million/month. This is not a bad return for the effort of a man who had spent only 15 months in Nuclear Medicine research

Pecher's despondency was properly placed. Well over 10,000 papers should have listed Pecher in their bibliography. But very few give him credit.

[See Vig1959 .BoS, Bone Scan]

CHRONOLOGY OF NUCLEAR MEDICINE — 1940

Scientific and Technical Background

			Ref.
1. Basic —	RUBEN & KAMEN DISCOVER HOW TO MAKE C-14.	[1939]	PR
—	Abelson & McMillan discover first trans-U element, #93 Np.	[1939]	PR
—	Y. Nishina discovers 6.75d U-237.	[1939]	PR
—	O. Frisch experimentally proves nuclear fission.	[1939]	PT
—	J. Dunning proves that U-235 is the fissionable isotope.	[1939]	MED
2. Obser —	Seaborg & Segré require new "$T_{1/2}$ definition" of element.	[1899]	Na
—	E. Segré finds evidence of 6h °Tc in fission product.	[1938]	PR
—	L. Turner says 4n + 1 series has 11 steps to Bi-209.	[1931]	PR
—	G. Laurence (Canada) attempts to build nuclear reactor.	[1942]	CT
—	J. Loofbourow coins X* to mean radioactive form of X.	[1934]	RMP
	(confusion with footnote, X* changed to °X, Brucer)	1968	V29
3. #Nuc —	G. Seaborg tabulates 271 stable, 330 "artificial" nuclides.	[1944]	CR
—	E. Segré helps Seaborg find unstable element #85, astatine (At).		CR
—	M. Kamen discovers 5730y 0.156 meV beta emitter C-14.	[1939]	MED
—	Manhattan District says 370 °nuclides are known.	[1938]	MED
—	H. Walke describes the °isotopes of calcium.	[1939]	PR
—	J. Loofbourow lists 17 °isotopes used in biology.	[1936]	RMP

Organizations and Internal Politics

			Ref.
5. Pols —	Politics of uranium in 1940:		
	Mar — J. Dunning confirms possibility of chain reaction.		TNW
	Apr — G. Thomson sets up British committee to look at A Bomb.		TNW
	May — G. Pegram announces success of graphite moderator expts.		TNW
	May — G. Kistiakowski suggests gas diffusion U-235 separation.		TNW
	Jun — V. Bush's Nat Def Res Council takes over U work.		TNW
	Nov — E. Fermi builds small graphite pile, proves idea.		TNW
	(From R. Hewlett, The New World, Hist of AEC, Penn U Press, 1962)		
—	US Census says USA life-expectancy is 64 yrs.	(49 in 1900)	SAb
6. Socs —	J. Loofbourow details state-of-art biol °isotope use.	[1937]	RMP
7. Event —	G. Hevesy finds 20% of D_2O in rabbit after 39 days.	[1933]	APS
—	S. Hertz develops new "multiple labeling" technique.	[1938]	AJP
—	G. Seaborg uses "half-life," first (?) use of slang term.	[1900]	CR
—	M. Tuve calls °isotope production the "new alchemy."	[1939]	Rad
—	First discussion of commercial cyclotron for °isotopes.	[1939]	AG
—	D. Grodsensky cites first USSR med use of °nuclides (P-32).	[1935]	SPZ
—	US Navy adopts name RAdioDetection And Ranging (RADAR).	[1939]	USN

Instruments, Units of Measurement, and Drugs

			Ref.
8. Instr —	J. Hamilton develops °I microautoradiography of thyroid.	[1933]	AJP
—	D. Kerst builds an electron accelerator, "Betatron."	[1931]	PR
—	First Electron Microscope demonstrated by RCA.	[1939]	EB
—	MIT civilian cyclotron operating: supplies 36 hospitals.	[1937]	PL
9. Units —	W. Mayneord introduces gram-roentgen (c85 ergs/g air).	[1939]	BJR
—	P. Aebersold devises "n" and "beta-r" units, medical use.	[1939]	V103
—	NBS makes 10 std Ra solutions, 0.1–100 µg Ra in 5 ml BaCl.	[1910]	GMP
10. Concp —	W. Mayneord introduces absorbed dose concept.	[1938]	BJR
—	G. Hevesy uses "turnover" not "uptake" for P-32.	[1937]	APS
—	J. Loofbourow defines specific activity as cpm P-32/mg P.	[1938]	RMP
—	F. Overstreet describes °K ion transport in plants.	[1939]	PNAS
—	A. Brues measures °isotope uptakes in cell cultures.	[1938]	JAPh

11. Drugs	— H. Walke says °Ca is potentially useful in biology.	[1939]	PR
	— D. Greenberg studies first biological use of °Ca (rats).	[1939]	PNA
	— I. Chaikoff: "turnover" not "uptake" characterizes P-32.	[1938]	JBC
	— I. Perlmann measures phospholipid metab and turnover.	[1938]	JBC
	— C. Pecher uses a Y-88 to Sr-89 cow system for Rx doses.	[1939]	PR
	— C. Williams grows °*E. coli* in P-32 spiked medium.	[1939]	JB
	— H. Krebs works on lactic acid-CO_2 cycle in live bodies.	[1939]	DSB
	— H. Florey cures 9 patients with purified penicillin.	[1928]	Bk

Radioiodine, P-32, and Radioactive Therapy

12. I-Res	— Lacassagne & Joliot begin °I thyroid studies in Paris.	[1939]	CRS
	— S. Seidlin discovers the role of TSH in rabbits.	[1965]	E
	— MIT cyclotron makes I-126, 128, 130, 131 for non-MED use.	[1936]	AJP
13. I-Dx	— S. Hertz devises a "thyroid index" (not external cpm).	[1939]	AJP
	— J. Hamilton shows autoradiograms of goitrous glands.	[1933]	RAD
14. I-Rx	— R. Evans makes first 12.5h I-130, primarily for thyroid Rx.	[1939]	V90
	— Mortality from surgical thyroidectomy is 2% to 10%.	[1939]	JAMA
15. P-Rx	— J. Lawrence gives preliminary report on polycythemia Rx.	[1939]	Rad
	— A. Marshak: P-32 tumor uptake due to mitotic activity.	[1904]	Sc

Scans and Other Tests of Function in Various Organs

22. Bone	— G. Hevesy measures rate of P-32 exchange in animals.	[1939]	BJ
	— D. Greenberg uses first biological °Ca in rats.	[1939]	PNA
	— J. Volker uses first biological F-18 in bone chips.	[1939]	JBC
24. Gut	— L. Erf feeds cow °Sr-lactate, recovers 11% in milk in 4d.	[1938]	PSEB
25. Blood	— G. Hevesy uses in vitro P-32RBC label (rabbit bld vol).	[1935]	APS
	— P. Hahn says plasma °Fe doesn't exchange with hemoglobin.	[1939]	Sc
	— A. Eisenman labels blood with Na°PO_4 for blood volume.	[1935]	JBC
	— P. Hahn labels donor RBC (°Fe) for RBC mass (dogs).	[1938]	JXM
	— L. Miller notes °Fe in RBC a few hours after oral dose.	[1938]	JBC
26. Other	— L. Flexner says growth rate changes placental °Na (cats).	[1935]	PSEB

Radiation Hysteria and Health Physics * Obituaries *

27. Hyst	— W. Gaunt locates Thorotrast after IV inject (animals).	[1937]	JID
	— Mitogenetic (Gurwitch) rays peter out of existence.	[1931]	SR
	— T. Lysenko becomes head of genetics in USSR.	[1955]	AP
28. React	— RSNA Tech Bull #1: first American radiation regulation.	[1925]	CNT
	— H. Jackson writes "leukemia" & "agranulocytosis" chapters in Cecil's textbook of med without mentioning radiation.	[1914]	Bk

* * *

30. Obits	— J.J. Thomson (1856–1940) Eng physics; electron, mass spectrum.		DSB
	C. Regaud (1870–1940) Fr medic; pioneer in rad therapy.	(1977	IJO)

CHRONOLOGY OF NUCLEAR MEDICINE — 1941

Scientific and Technical Background

			Ref.
1. Basic	— G. Flerov discovers spontaneous fission.	[1939]	WoA
2. Obser	— W. Schumb estimates earth's K-40 abundance (background).	[1901]	JACS
	— P. Selwood tells story of Urey's heavy water discovery.	[1938]	JCE
3. # Nuc	— J. Livingood assigns places for Co-59, -60m, -60.	[1938]	PR
	— J. Hamilton compares Eka-iodine (At #85) with I-131.	[1940]	JAP
	— E. Lawrence uses 37″ cyclotron to make U-235 sample.	[1940]	Bio
	— C. Pecher separates 18.7 d Rb-86 from Sr-89 doses.	[1939]	Pr
	— O. Hahn's group gets fission products from a weak source.	[1940]	Bio
	— G. Seaborg discovers second trans U, 24,000y Pu-239. (report 1946		PR)
4. # Med	—		

Organizations and Internal Politics

5. Pols	— Politics of uranium in 1941:		
	May — British set up "Tube Alloys" project to build A-Bomb.		TNW
	Jun — V. Bush organizes Off Sci Res Dev (OSRD), takes U work.		TNW
	Jul — E. Lawrence reports on alternate use of plutonium.		TNW
	Jul — NRDC funds $267,000 to evaluate military use of U-235.		TNW
	Nov — A. Compton reports A-Bomb will need 2 to 100 kg U-235.		TNW
6. Socs	— P. Aebersold explains the cyclotron to medical audience.	[1927]	Rad
	— NBS Hndbk #27: Max Permis Body Burden, 0.1 μg Ra-226.	[1934]	NBS
7. Event	— PEARL HARBOR BOMBED, 7 DEC, SECRECY IMPOSED ON PUBLICATIONS.	[1939]	AP

Instruments, Units of Measurement, and Drugs

8. Instr	— A. Krebs adds photoelect counter to scintillator xtal.	[1940]	AP
	— H. Stever devises a directional GM counter.	[1936]	PR
	— C. Brown (W. Libby) makes wire mesh GM with He gas fill.	[1940]	PR
9. Units	— L. MARINELLI DERIVES A BETA "EQUIVALENT ROENTGEN" (e.r.).	[1940]	AJR
	— G. Failla measures "ergs in tissue" in parallel-plate chamber.	[1939]	AJR
10. Concp	— J. Abels says P-32 blood uptake changed by irradiation.	[1939]	CR
	— W. Fenn studies K – °K exchange in animal body.	[1940]	AJP
11. Drugs	— J. Manery sees full Cl-38 tissue penetration in minutes.	[1938]	AJP
	— W. Bale notes Na-24 tissue penetration is very fast.	[1934]	AJP
	— T. Noonan says K-42 clears plasma in hours.	[1939]	AJP
	— D. Copp does first biological study of Co-56, -57, -58.	[1938]	PNAS
	— K. Lars-Horovitz tests enteric coated pills with Na-24.	[1939]	Na
	— D. Vigneaud studies metab of C-14 labeled amino acids.	[1940]	JBC
	— J. MacKenzie notes hyperplasia in rats from sulfaguanidine.	[1935]	Sc

Radioiodine, P-32, and Radioactive Therapy

12. I-Res	— I. Perlman traces turnover of T2 & T4 with °I in normals.	[1934]	JBC
	— M. Morton says TSH increases T2 and T4 turnover.	[1938]	JBC
	— I. Ariel notes importance of time in °iodine studies.	[1939]	AJP
	— C. LeBlond says T2 (not T4) destroyed in blood in 30 min.	[1927]	AJP

13.	I-Dx	— S. Hertz finds °I uptake modified by T4.	[1930]	AJR
		— S. Hertz uses counter over neck to measure activity.	[1939]	AJR
		— E. Miller uses thigh to approximate neck background.	[1953]	Rad
14.	I-Rx	— S. HERTZ (R. EVANS) GIVES FIRST I-130 THERAPY DOSE (0.25 mCi).	[1939]	GMP
		— J. Hamilton uses I-131 in toxic, non-toxic goiter pts.	[1940]	JAP
		— V. Frantz studies thyroid ca mets with °iodine.	[1939]	AS
		— R. Ball manually scans ca mets °I on morning of 7 Dec.	[1949]	PL
15.	P-Rx	— L. Erf announces P-32 therapy of polycythemia vera (PVA).	[1940]	AIM
		— L. Tuttle says nucleoprotein causes leukemics °P uptake.	[1939]	JCI
		— A. Marshak: P-32 uptake increases in fast-grow tumors.	[1940]	JGP
		— L. Marinelli measures P-32 uptake in malignant tumors.	[1939]	Rad
		— J. Lawrence plots P-32 distrib in autopsied leukemics.	[1937]	AJM
16.	Tele	— J. Clarkson finds depth dose modified by shape of field.	[1938]	BJR
17.	Other	— C. PECHER TRIES Sr-89 THERAPY, FIRST Rx IN METS TO BONE.	[1940]	JCI
		— C. Pecher tries Ca-45 and Sr-88 in osteogenic sarcoma.	[1939]	PSEB

Scans and Other Tests of Function in Various Organs

18.	Brain	—		
19.	Heart	— J. Smith studies heart beats and vibrations with CRT.	[1937]	AHJ
		— M. Rappaport displays normal heart sounds in graph form.	[1933]	AHJ
20.	Liver	— T. Kohman finds high P-32 uptake in tumor cells.	[1939]	PSEB
21.	Lung	—		
22.	Bone	— D. Jones studies metabolism of Sr-90 in rachitic rats.	[1938]	JBC
		— W. Koss finds Na-24 in bones & teeth 24h post injection.	[1940]	JDR
		— J. Volker does first °F study; it's in teeth, not saliva.	[1940]	AJP
		— R. Soggnaes: P-32 uptake is highest in unerupted molars.	[1940]	AJPh
23.	Kidney	—		
24.	Gut	— J. Ross finds selective °Fe absorpt in iron deficiency.	[1940]	JCI
		— J. Flagg tries to label VB_{12} with Co-60 — fails.	[1950]	JACS
25.	Blood	— P. Hahn measures RBC and total blood volume with °Fe.	[1910]	Sc
26.	Other	— W. Bale measures °Na & °P in intra- & extra-cell space.	[1939]	AJP
		— C. Pecher: Ca-45 in pregnant mice, measured in babies.	[1940]	PSEB
		— N. Kaltreider measures Na-24 extracellular fluid volume.	[1939]	JEM
		— E. Lang studies metab of insulin with °I-insulin.	[1926]	Sc

Radiation Hysteria and Health Physics * Obituaries *

27.	Hyst	— L. Erf says oral °Fe is secreted in milk of cows.	[1940]	PSEB
		— E. Wigner: fission products could be used as "poison gas."	[1940]	TNW
28.	React	— NBS advis Com. sets MPC, Max Body Burden @ 0.1 μg Ra.	[1937]	NBS
29.	Respo	— F. Behounek: diff between human "Ra" & "radioactivity."	[1930]	St

* * *

30.	Obits	— W. Nernst (1864–1941) Ger phys chem; third law of thermodynamics.	DSB
		— R. Schoenheimer (1898–1941) Ger biochem; first biochem isotopes.	Sc

CHRONOLOGY OF NUCLEAR MEDICINE — 1942

Scientific and Technical Background

			Ref.
1. Basic	— E. FERMI STARTS UP FIRST NUCLEAR REACTOR (CHICAGO "PILE").	[1940]	DSB
	— Seaborg discovers Np-237, 4n + 1 parent.	[1931] (pub. 1948	PR)
	— B. Lyot notes: X-rays in sun's corona, same as in bkgnd.	[1925]	SN
2. Obser	— G. Seaborg's "ultra-microchem" makes first visible 2 μg Pu.	[1946]	Sc
3. # Nuc	— R. Evans revises table: 281 stable, 383 °isotopes = 664.	[1940]	GMP
	— E. Lawrence's 60" cyclotron can now make most °nuclides.	[1939]	Bio
	— G. Seaborg discovers 1.59 × 10^5y U-233.	[1941]	MED
4. # Med	—		

Organizations and Internal Politics

			Ref.
5. Pols	— Politics of uranium in 1942:		
	Jan — Pres FDR OKs construction of Atom Bomb.		TNW
	Jan — A. Compton sets up Metallurgical Lab at Univ Chicago.		TNW
	Jul — Oak Ridge site selected for Gas Diffusion plant.		TNW
	Sep — Col R. Marshall sets up **Manhattan Engineering District.**		TNW
	Sep — Col (soon Gen) L. Groves take over command of MED.		TNW
5a. MED	— SEP 1942 TO JAN 1947, Manhattan Engineering District (MED) will have almost complete control of SECRET NUCLEAR SCIENCE.		TNW
	Nov — Los Alamos site selected for weapons laboratory.		TNW
	3:25 PM, 7 Dec. Control rod withdrawn from first atomic "pile."		MED
6. Socs	— Laua Fermi recollects story of first "pile."	(1977	JNM)
	— C. Alardice reprints first account of first "pile."	(1962	IAEA)
	— J. Hamilton reviews °P and °I work as cover story for MED.		JCI
7. Event	— M. Burton starts "rad chemistry" group at UC Met Lab.	[1941]	MED
	— 96 sq miles set aside for Oak Ridge TN town and labs.	[1941]	MED

Instruments, Units of Measurement, and Drugs

			Ref.
8. Instr	— L. Marinelli begins external counts of P-32 in tumors.	[1939]	Rad
	— H. Stever measures "dead" & recovery time of GM tubes.	[1937]	PR
	— W. Ramsey develops "proportional counters."	[1937]	PR
9. Units	— G. Failla's extrap chamber saves "r" for all energies.	[1937]	Rad
	— D. Lea says as LET rises RBE falls in virus system.	[1936]	Par
	— F. Ellis cannot verify Mayneord's volume integral dose.	[1940]	BJR
	— L. Marinelli uses "er" for Seidlin's °I Rx dosimetry;	[1948]	AJR
	"er" will soon be "R equivalent physical" (Rep).	[1940]	AJR
	— P. Aebersold's fast neutron "n" = 1 equivalent roentgen.	[1940]	ARP
	— M. Deutsch: I-131 spectrum cascades 80 and 367 keV.	[1938]	PR
10. Concp	— L. MARINELLI DEVISES FIRST °ISOTOPE DOSIMETRY IN HUMANS.	[1975]	V26
11. Drugs	— G. Hevesy measures urine Sp Act of first human K-42 dose.	[1940]	APS
	— L. Reiner uses first °I-tagged insulin sub-Q in rabbits.	[1941]	Sc
	— J. Ely grows bacteria in P-32 agar, injects into rats.	[1940]	JFI
	— J. Kurbatov measures Y-90 properties in low concentration.	[1967]	JPC
	— I. Chaikoff reviews P-32 metabolism studies.	[1940]	PhR
	— F. Hunter tests °$AsCl_3$ in parasites.	[1940]	JPET
	— L. Reiner tags insulin with °I, measures absorption rate.	[1941]	Sc

Radioiodine, P-32, and Radioactive Therapy

			Ref.
12. I-Res	— E. Quimby tells R. Ball she knows nothing about °I dose.	[1940]	PL
	(She knew much but MED secrecy at Columbia was tight.)	[1941]	PL
	— C. Richter notes goiter in rats fed phenylthiocarbamide.	[1927]	APa

13. I-Dx	— W. Reinhart uses uptake to assess thyroidectomy.	[1941]	PSEB
	— S. Hertz: urine excretion is inverse of thyroid uptake.	[1940]	JCI
14. I-Rx	— R. Ball proves °I uptake in thyroid ca metastases.	[1946]	Sc
	— S. Hertz announces 10 hyperthyroid treatments with °I + I.	[1941]	JCI
	— J. Means requires I-127 precede all °I Rx.	[1923]	V90
	— E. Astwood: first hyperthyroid patients Rx with thiourea.	[1930]	JCEn
15. P-Rx	— E. Osgood compares P-32 chron leuk Rx with neutron Rx.	[1941]	AJMS
	— L. Craver confirms P-32 Rx in CML is equal to any other.	[1939]	CR
	— B. Low-Beer studies P-32 dose uptake & distribution.	[1941]	JLCM
16. Tele	—		
17. Other	— R. Stone: cyclotron fast neutron Rx gives mixed results.	[1939]	Rad
	— C. PECHER CURES PROSTATE METS TO BONE WITH 8 mCi Sr-89.	[1941]	V81
	— J. Lawrence reports failure of Ca-45 Rx of osteo sarc.	[1941]	PIM
	— A. Treadwell reports failure of Ca-45 Rx of osteo sarc.	[1941]	AJMS

Scans and Other Tests of Function in Various Organs

18. Brain	— D. Fishback measures circulation with fluorescein & UV.	[1931]	AJMS
	— J. Hubbard measures infant's blood velocity with Na-24.	[1938]	JCI
19. Heart	— H. Meyerson studies effect of gravity on blood pressure.	[1939]	AJPh
	— M. Rappaport repeats the "law" of auscultation.	[1941]	AHJ
	— J. Robb describes normal heart anatomy and physiology.	[1941]	AHJ
20. Liver	— K. Wakim finds only 1/4 of sinusoids open at any time;	[1941]	AR
	shows sinusoid blood flow unrelated to lobules.	[1941]	AR
21. Lung	—		
22. Bone	— P. Durbin describes metabolism of F-18 and lanthanones.	[1941]	V81
	— A. Treadwell: Sr-89 uptake in osteosarc warrants Rx.	[1941]	AJMS
23. Kidney	—		
24. Gut	—		
25. Blood	— M. Chapin: °Fe plasma & cell volumes indicate Ht error.	[1941]	AJP
	— P. Hahn: °FeRBC donor (dog) studies confirm Ht error.	[1941]	JEM
	— W. Criez shows Hb-°Fe used in new Hb on RBC destruction.	[1941]	AJP
	— W. Pommerenke studies maternal-fetal °Fe transfer, 14 pts.	[1941]	AJP
	— W. Pommerenke studies °Fe transmission to fetus.	[1941]	AJP
	— W. Balfour shows pregnant pt absorbs 2–10 × more Fe-59.	[1941]	JEM
	— G. Hevesy studies volumes with homologous P-32RBC.	[1940]	APS
	— J. Fine tags plasma protein with °I, first IHSA.	[1950]	HNM
26. Other	— I. Ariel studies As-76 distrib in rabbit epithelioma.	[1956]	AJGS
	— V. Kinsey measures °Na, °Cl, & °P movement in the eye.	[1947]	AO

Radiation Hysteria and Health Physics * Obituaries *

27. Hyst	— "Tolerance" of °gas in air set at 0.1 r/g (no cancers).	[1937]	MED
28. React	— R. Stone organizes first Health Physics unit for MED.	[1940]	MED
	"HEALTH PHYSICS" NAME FIRST USED IN MED LAB AT U CHICAGO.		
	— R. Stone says use prudent tolerance dose @ 0.1 r/8h day.	[1937]	MED
29. Respo	— R. Stone notes first health physics experiment (under HP name): mice live longer in uranium dust.	[1925]	PAPS

* * *

30. Obits	— W.H. Bragg (1862–1942) Eng physics; crystal diffrac of X-rays.	DSB
	— J. Perrin (1870–1942) Fr physics; cathode rays are particles.	DSB

CHRONOLOGY OF NUCLEAR MEDICINE — 1943

Scientific and Technical Background				Ref.
1. Basic	—	D. Lea says chromosome breaks are direct result of rad.	[1937]	BJR
	—	D. Lea: spatial distrib of ionization (LET) is important.	[1935]	BJR
2. Obser	—	Einstein's original 1905 MS auctioned at war bond rally . . . but he had destroyed it, so he wrote another (new, improved); the new "original" sells for $6,000,000.	[1905]	ONR
3. # Nuc	—			
4. # Med	—			

Organizations and Internal Politics				
5. Med	—	Politics of uranium in 1943:		
		Jan — Hanford site selected for plutonium production.		TNW
		Aug — British A-Bomb work transferred to joint Can-UK, US project.		
		U Cal gets contract to run Los Alamos, est about 30 workers.		MED
		1 FEB GROUND BROKEN, 4 NOV OAK RIDGE REACTOR GOES CRITICAL.		MED
6. Socs	—	Japan Physicist Colloquium wants to build Atom Bomb.	(1978	Sc)
7. Event	—	Penicillin becomes staple in military medicine.	[1940]	EB

Instruments, Units of Measurement, and Drugs				
8. Instr	—	C. LeBlond localizes °I in cells with micro-autoradiography.	[1933]	JA
	—	J. Mauchly builds ENIAC: first dig computer, vacuum tubes.	[1833]	FV
9. Units	—	F. Spiers searches for non-water tissue equivalents.	[1925]	BJR
	—	F. Spiers calculates a tissue "effective" atomic no.	[1929]	BJR
	—	J. Victoreen calculates accurate (?) mass absorp coefs.	[1936]	JAP
	—	W. Meredith measures depth dose from 500 kVp X-ray tube.	[1929]	BJR
10. Concp	—	J. Mitchell: bio-action related to ions in path (LET?).	[1942]	BJR
	—	W. Mayneord introduces the isodose surface concept.	[1941]	BJR
	—	D. Zilversmit introduces "turnover" theory and tech.	[1940]	JGP
11. Drugs	—	A. Winkler measures first "chloride space" (25% of body H_2O).	[1938]	AJP
	—	L. Tobin shows distrib of °dyes in tumor-bearing mice.	[1937]	JCI
	—	G. Moore plots distrib of °Br labeled trypan blue (mice).	[1937]	JCI
	—	J. Fine labels blood plasma with Br-82 for shock study.	[1942]	JCI
	—	A. Seligman labels plasma with S-35, finds a poor tag.	[1942]	JCI
	—	G. Sheline studies metabolism of Z-65 in mice and dogs.	[1949]	JBC
	—	L. Reiner measures °I-insulin absorption rates.	[1942]	JPET
	—	R. Schenck studies C-14 labeled methionine and cysteine.	[1964]	JBC
	—	Waxman & Schatz discover streptomycin.	[1040]	EB

Radioiodine, P-32, and Radioactive Therapy

12. I-Res	— C. MacKenzie introduces thioureas.	[1933]	E
	— E. Astwood says thiourea inhibits T-4 synthesis.	[1941]	E
	— E. Astwood coins term "antithyroid drug."	[1941]	E
	— H. Davenport finds °I selectively excreted by stomach.	[1957]	Ge
	— M. Morton shows I-131 will not replace I-127 in T2.	[1941]	JBC
13. I-Dx	— M. Soley differentiates hypo, hyper children by uptake.	[1942]	AJDC
14. I-Rx	— E. Astwood treats hyperthyroids with thioureas.	[1942]	JAMA
15. P-Rx	— J. Saralegui confirms P-32 Rx of leukemia in Italy.	[1942]	Ral
	— Sh. Warren notes °P retention in some tissues in leuks.	[1942]	CR
	— L. Erf says P-32 is Rx of choice in polycythemia vera.	[1942]	AIM
	— W. Tinney records rare Acute Fulm Leuk before P-32 Rx.	[1941]	MCP
16. Tele	— W. Mayneord measures and calculates isodose surfaces.	[1939]	BJR
17. Other	— W. Deutcher: skin mets from bronc ca regress by Ba-212.	[1907]	SMW

Scans and Other Tests of Function in Various Organs

18. Brain	— D. Greenberg studies which °isotopes cross bld brain barrier.	[1935]	AJP
19. Heart	— I. Starr measures venous pressure in exp heart disease.	[1941]	AHJ
	— G. Nylin tries to measure residual blood in ventricles.	[1941]	AHJ
20. Liver	— D. Copp notes °Co distrib and excretion in bile (rats).	[1930]	JBC
21. Lung	— C. Tobias: first study of C-11 in breath analy for °CO_2.	[1934]	AJP
	— W. Harnett surveys 1063 primary ca of lung patients.	[1928]	PgM
22. Bone	— J. Gunther studies P-32 bone turnover in rachitic kids.	[1941]	AJDC
23. Kidney	—		
24. Gut	— P. Hahn measures Fe-59 absorption after stable Fe meal.	[1941]	JEM
	— L. Reiner describes absorption of °I-insulin.	[1941]	JPET
25. Blood	— J. Dacie measures RBC survival in anemias with donors.	[1940]	La
26. Other	— A. Gellhorn studies Na-24 transfer across the placenta.	[1940]	AJOG
	— H. Barcroft measures vasoconstric tone in skel muscle.	[1940]	JPh

Radiation Hysteria and Health Physics * Obituaries *

27. Hyst	—		
28. React	— L. Clark: X-ray personnel wear dental film to see leaks.	[1938]	BJR
	— W. Yates can find no evidence of danger from Thorotrast.	[1938]	AnIM
29. Respo	—		

* * *

30. Obits	— N. Tesla (1856–1943) Am inventor; electricity, ac current.	Bio
	— J. Ewing (1866–1943) Am medic; pioneer in use of Ra in ca Rx.	AJR

CHRONOLOGY OF NUCLEAR MEDICINE — 1944

Scientific and Technical Background

			Ref.
1. Basic	—		
2. Obser	— A. Keston tells classic gum-ball proof of transmutation.	[1934]	GMP
	— E. Lawrence says 1 mCi I-131 takes 3–10 h cyclotron time.	[1940]	MED
	— W. Cohn makes first reactor P-32 in curie quantities.	[1942]	MED
3. # Nuc	— G. Seaborg discovers Np-241, Pu-241, Am-241, (Story in 1959 JCE); lists 267 stable, 479 °isotopes (total = 746).	[1940]	RMP
	— R. Evans lists 383 °isotopes with E and "half-period."	[1942]	GMP
4. # Med	— J. Hamilton says 21 different °isotopes tried in biol.	[1940]	GMP
	— R. Evans (MIT) supplies 36 hospitals with °isotopes.	[1942]	GMP
	— A. Keston explains poss bio use of stable H, C, N, O, S.	[1940]	GMP

Organizations and Internal Politics

5. Med	— M. Kamen (C-14) kicked off MED by Gen Groves on stupid charge.		Bio
	— Chalk River, Ontario, Canada gets a Heavy Water "Pile."	[1942]	TNW
6. Soc	— G. Hevesy gives Nobel lecture on "Isotope Indicators."	[1915]	ARR
	— P. Hahn learns to handle °Cu, °Mn, °Z, °Co, °As, °Se, and °Fe.	[1943]	GMP
	— Sh. Warren reviews histopathology of radiation lesions.	[1954]	PhR
	— O. Glasser's "Medical Physics" vol 1 published.	[1950]	GMP
7. Event	— World P-32 production: Denmark = μCi, Berk = mCi, Oak Ridge = Ci.		MED

Instruments, Units of Measurement, and Drugs

8. Instr	— C. LeBlond perfects micro-autoradiographic techniques.	[1940]	AR
	— L. Rovner reviews developed theory of GM tube physics.	[1942]	GMP
	— S. Curran adapts photomultiplier to scintil counting.	[1941]	MED
	— E. Ruska invents the electron microscope.	[1930]	SN
	— A. Martin develops paper chromatography.	[1926]	Sc
9. Units	— E. Quimby says there is no practical measurement of Rad;	[1929]	GMP
	"mg-hours," mCi-h, mCi-des, are meaningless.	[1919]	GMP
	— E. Quimby says "Threshold Erythema Dose" = 1000 r.	[1936]	GMP
	— G. Failla says W (ave energy/ion pair) is unmeasurable,	[1929]	GMP
	hence W has no physical (or biol) meaning.	[1939]	GMP
	— W. Mayneord calculates average tissue "Z" = 5.9 to 6.9.	[1943]	BJR
	— W. Meredith calculates isodoses from energy absorption.	[1943]	BJR
10. Concp	— G. Hevesy says fetal P-32 proves its maternal origin.	[1941]	ARR
	— D. Lea postulates (no evidence): a single ionizing event can destroy a sensitive molecule.	[1924]	Bk
11. Drugs	— G. Davis makes first biology use of Co-60 (in cattle feed).	[1941]	IRT
	— F. Fine introduces °I bovine serum albumin (pre-°IHSA).	[1943]	JCI
	— E. Dobson introduces °$CrPO_4$ colloid.	[1956]	CUI
	— H. JONES: COLLOID BLD CLEARANCE IS FUNCTION OF PARTICLE SIZE.		JLCI
	— H. Root tags insulin with °I, studies human absorption.	[1943]	JAMA
	— US Army uses Mullers DDT for anti-typhus in Naples.	[1938]	AP

Radioiodine, P-32, and Radioactive Therapy

12.	I-Res	— A. Keston: thyroxine iodination involves T2 & tyrosine.	[1941]	JBC
		— C. Harrington says all organic iodine either T2 or T4.	[1941]	JCS
		— E. Dempsy thinks iodate oxidation is first binding step.	[1943]	E
		— I. Chaikoff studies modifiers of PBI conversion.	[1935]	JBC
		— E. Astwood's I-depleted rats open way for PBI Dx test.	[1935]	E
		— E. Astwood uses °I to study thiouracil effect on thy I deposition.	[1943]	E
		— C. LeBlond studies °I in rats exposed to hi- & lo-temp.	[1943]	AJP
		— R. Rawson sees °I uptake changed by thio-cyanate, uracil.	[1943]	E
		— A. Franklin notes trap & binding block by sulfonamides.	[1935]	JBC
		— M. Morton notes iodide blocking of organification.	[1943]	JBC
13.	I-Dx	— B. Lowenstein correlates BMR and PBI in 32 patients.	[1935]	JCE
		— S. Seidlin collects urine from Rx pts to use in Dx pts.	[1943]	JAMA
14.	I-Rx	— S. Seidlin's first announcement of Rx of thyroid ca mets.	[1946]	JCI
		— V. Frantz: delayed paper on °I uptake in thyroid mets.	[1942]	AS
15.	P-Rx	— L. Hempelman finds one year PVA remission post-P-32 Rx.	[1943]	JLCM
		— E. Lindgren confirms P-32 leukemia Rx in Scandinavia.	[1943]	AR
16.	Tele	— L. Edling tries rotational beam therapy.	[1937]	AR
17.	Other	— H. Jones says IV CrH°PO_4 can irrad liver with betas.	[1942]	JCI
		— F. Ellis' wedge filter designs predate later collimators.	[1936]	BJR
		— J. Thygesen tries total body irradiation with Na-24.	[1932]	AR
		— J. Thygesen attempts leukemia RX with Na-24 (fails).	[1943]	AR

Scans and Other Tests of Function in Various Organs

19.	Heart	— E. Quimby measures arm-foot circulation time with °NaCl.	[1938]	SGO
24.	Gut	— C. Moore finds ferrous °Fe absorbs faster than ferric.	[1943]	JCI
		— P. Hahn measures oral °Fe absorption rates in children.	[1943]	FP
25.	Blood	— G. Nylin uses P-32 RBC, is first to estimate RBC mass.	[1942]	BHJ
		— G. Hevesy says trapping & dilution are part of Ht error.	[1942]	AMS
		— H. Jones makes Cr°PO_4 for blood volume measurement.	[1940]	JCI
		— E. Lindgren measures total body retention of Na-24.	[1932]	AR
26.	Other	— A. Gellhorn measures rate of °Na transcapillary exchange.	[1941]	JPh
		— O. Cope studies capillary permeability with °dyes.	[1915]	JCI

Radiation Hysteria and Health Physics * Obituaries *

27.	Hyst	— Contaminated fish in OR lake due to first reactor P-32.	[1943]	ORNL
		— 2,4-D introduced as herbicide; will soon cause crisis.	[1938]	SN
28.	React	— E. Lorenz notes 0.11 r (10 × MPD) irrad mice live longer.	[1942]	MED

* * *

30.	Obits	— L. Baekeland (1863–1844) Am chem; Bakelite.	DSB
		— G. Barkla (1877–1944) Eng physics; begins X-ray spectroscopy.	DSB

CHRONOLOGY OF NUCLEAR MEDICINE — 1945

	Scientific and Technical Background		Ref.
1. Basic —	W. Libby invents C-14 dating tech for biol specimens.	[1925]	Sc
2. Obser —	Both old and new (long) Periodic Tables are in new 1945 ed. Columbium is #41 Illinium is #61 Niton (or Rn) is #86 Masurium is #43 Alabamium is #85 Virginium is #87		HCP
3. # Nuc —	J. Marinsky finishes Periodic Table elements, #61 Pm.	[1869]	JACS
4. # Med —			
	Organizations and Internal Politics		
5. MED —	Col R. Nichols suggests civilian °isotope distribution.	[1942]	MED
—	MED looks for a chief of new Isotopes Branch in OR.	[1941]	MED
—	Atomic Res Center established at Harwell, Eng.	[1940]	AERE
—	Commissariate L'Energie Atomique (French AEC) organized.	[1939]	CEA
6. Socs —	H. Smyth's "Atomic Energy for Military Purposes" published.	[1941]	Bk
—	F. Dessauer writes personal hist of medical radiation.	[1905]	Ex
7. Event —	O. Hahn receives Nobel while interned as POW in England.	[1939]	Bio
—	First atomic explosion, Trinity site NM, July 16.	[1939]	MED
—	FIRST U-235 BOMB ON HIROSHIMA Aug. 6; Pu-239 ON NAGASAKI Aug. 9.		AP
—	Gen L. Groves dumps 5 Japanese cyclotrons in ocean.	[1943]	Sc
	Instruments, Units of Measurement, and Drugs		
8. Instr —	P. van Heerden reintroduces crystal counting with AgCl.	[1907]	Dis
—	H. Kallman uses wall paint and moth ball scint-crystal.	[1944]	HNM
—	M. Blau uses ZnS screen & photomultiplier, counts alphas.	[1944]	RSI
—	V. Veksler suggests the synchrocyclotron.	[1942]	WoA
—	F. Bloch develops NMR in liquids and solids.	[1938]	GSA
9. Units —	Specific Activity is defined as "Curies/gram."	[1942]	MED
—	H. PARKER DEFINES ROENTGEN EQUIVALENT PHYSICAL OR "Rep."	[1942]	BJR
	A compromise of measurements, Rep = 83 erg/g tissue.	[1942]	BJR
10. Concp —	M. Reingard approximates depth dose from exit dose.	[1943]	Rad
11. Drugs —	A. Lawton shows uptake of As-74 in rats and parasites.	[1944]	Sc
—	F. Brady finds oral °Sb goes to parasites in dogs.	[1942]	AJTM
	Radioiodine, P-32, and Radioactive Therapy		
12. I-Res —	F. Keating says TSH speeds washout of PBI from thyroid.	[1941]	E
—	E. Astwood introduces propylthiouracil.	[1943]	JCEn
—	R. Rawson: thiouracil blocks & TSH increases °I uptake.	[1944]	E
13. I-Dx —	F. Joliot-Curie: aminothiazole affects thyroid °I uptake.	[1944]	BSMH
—	F. Keating develops thyroid °I washout test.	[1941]	E
14. I-Rx —	S. Seidlin destroys thyroid mets with °I (pub unnoted).	[1938]	BNYA
—	G. Sheline finds no uptake in thyroid ca primaries.	[1942]	Rad

15.	P-Rx	— B. Hall: P-32 PVA Rx may require second dose after 8 weeks.	[1943]	AJMS
		— H. Hester fails in Rx of Hodgkins with P-32.	[1942]	JLCM
16.	Tele	— M. Deutsch deduces Co-60 decay scheme (seen by Grimmett).	[1922]	PR
		— J. Dunworth suggests med use Co-60 in secret gov report.	[1950]	NRCC
		— J. Mitchell suggests Co-60 substitute for med radium (secret).	[1955]	NRCC
		— J. Mitchell uses Ir-192 for first teletherapy (Co-60 unavailable).	[1928]	BJR
17.	Other	— J. MULLER SUSPENDS °Zn AS COLLOID FOR INTRACAVITARY THERAPY.		Ex
		— A. Forssberg confirms Low-Beer's high P-32 uptake in ca.	[1942]	AR
		— L. Hempleman: direct P-32 injection is quickly washed out.	[1948]	Cr

Scans and Other Tests of Function in Various Organs

18.	Brain	— S. Kety announces NO_2 CBF method (suggests °gas).	[1929]	AJP
		— U. Borell measures P-32 metabolism in brain segments.	[1942]	APS
19.	Heart	— G. Nylin fails to see R-L ventricle activity with P-32.	[1944]	AHJ
		— E. Quimby does 200 arm-foot circ times with Na-24.	[1944]	Rad
		— R. Shipley sees cardiac response to stimul of nerves.	[1942]	AJPh
20.	Liver	— S. Bradley announces BSP dye blood flow technique.	[1943]	JCI
21.	Lung	— C. Tobias makes first human C-11 test (CO to CO_2).	[1943]	AJP
		— J. Lawrence makes first human use of Xe-133 (narcotic ?).	[1978]	JPh
22.	Bone	— H. Singher sees IP S-35 injection localize in b-marrow.	[1937]	Sc
23.	Kidney	—		
24.	Gut	— H. Root gives first 10 human pts °I-tagged insulin.	[1943]	JAMA
25.	Blood	— G. Meneely compares ferric and ferrous °Fe in anemics.	[1938]	AJP
26.	Other	— C. Fox uses Na-24 to trace mechanism of trauma shock.	[1944]	SGO

Radiation Hysteria and Health Physics * Obituaries *

27.	Hyst	— 60 cattle exposed to 40 krep fallout from Trinity bomb.	[1984]	MED
		— Critical assembly accident at Los Alamos, death at 600 r.	[1968]	MED
		— H. Silberstein surveys internal radium poisoning lit.	[1926]	MED
		— L. Szilard (first pro-nuke) is first to bad mouth the "Bomb."	[1939]	AEC
28.	React	— S. Cantril: "tolerance dose" is a Health Physics limit.	[1942]	MED
		— First survey of "Med Effects" begins 7 weeks after Bomb.	[1969]	MM
		— MRC (Eng) publishes manual on "Radiation Hazards."	[1940]	MRC
29.	Respo	— W. Langham gives tracer dose of Pu-239 to 18 "terminally sick" patients. (Some live many years.)	[1975] (1959	HP)

* * *

30.	Obits	— T. Morgan (1866–1945) Am geneticist; chromosomes carry heredity.	DSB
		— F. Aston (1877–1945) Eng physics; mass spectrometry.	DSB
		— O. Hönigschmid (1878–1945) Ger chem; Ra primary standards.	DSB
		— H. Geiger (1882–1945) Ger physics; radioisotope detection.	DSB

CHRONOLOGY OF NUCLEAR MEDICINE — 1946

Scientific and Technical Background

			Ref.
1. Basic	— G. Seaborg announces #95 Am, #96 Cm; table is open ended.	[1913]	Sc
2. Obser	— W. Libby shows H-3 is produced from cosmic rays.	[1925]	GSA
3. # Nuc	— P. Aebersold: 150 fission products between #30 and #63.	[1941]	AJP
	— W. Sullivan puts 925 isotopes in trilinear (hexa) array.	[1944]	TC
	— G. Boyd studies basic chemistry of #43 (technetium).	[1940]	MED
	— A. Reid thinks "missing" I isotope is 1.7 × 10^7 y I-129.	[1941]	PR
	— Oak Ridge "pile" makes 200 mCi C-14 in 2 weeks @ $10,000.	[1940]	MED
	— D. Ballantine irrad Te with neutrons to produce I-131.	[1937]	MED
4. # Med	— J. Mitchell surveys 56 °isotopes of medical interest.	[1940]	BJR
	— Staf. Warren proposes civil isotope distribution (3 Jan).	[1945]	MED
	— W. Cohn writes first notice, civil isotopes available; 14 June		Sc
	— First civilian shipment of reactor isotope (C-14) on 2 Aug.		MED
	— Cyclotron cost for P-32 = $15,000/Ci. Reactor cost = $32.50.		AEC

— First 20 years of AEC, # of °isotope licenses (c65% medical):

1946 = 100	1950 = 600	1954 = 2200	1958 = 4300	1962 = 6300
1947 = 200	1951 = 1000	1955 = 3000	1959 = 5800	1963 = 7900
1948 = 300	1952 = 1300	1956 = 3700	1960 = 5900	1964 = 8600
1949 = 400	1953 = 1900	1957 = 3600	1961 = 6200	1965 = 9700

First 20 years of AEC °isotope shipments in kilocuries/year:

1946 = 1	1950 = 8	1954 = 50	1958 = 220	1962 = 550
1947 = 2	1951 = 12	1955 = 80	1959 = 300	1963 = 230
1948 = 3	1952 = 20	1956 = 110	1960 = 210	1964 = 610
1949 = 5	1953 = 30	1957 = 190	1961 = 450	1965 = 1280

Organizations and Internal Politics

5. AEC +	— PRES. TRUMAN SIGNS ATOMIC ENERGY ACT OF 1946 TO CREATE AEC.		AEC
	— NAS-AEC urge "Atom Bomb Casualty Comm" (ABCC) to study effects.		AEC
	— TRUMAN SIGNS EXECUTIVE ORDER CREATING JOINT US-JAP ABCC.		AEC
	— Pacific Atoll bomb tests begin at Bikini.	[1945]	AEC
	— R. Oppenheimer recommends to State Dept, create "IAEA."	[1957]	IRT
	— P. Aebersold becomes Chief, Isotopes Branch, MED (Jan).	[1967]	MED
	— USA population is 140 million.	[1936]	SAb
6. Socs	— G. Seaborg pubs "secret" list of "induced activities."	[1942]	Sc
	— A. Jarrett pubs statistical methods used with °activity.	[1925]	AEC
7. Event	— W. Sullivan forms "Nuclear Data Group" at ORNL & ANL.	[1949]	IRT
	— Oak Ridge & Los Alamos transfer to civilian control.	[1942]	AEC
	— M. Hawkins draws non-secret 3-bladed prop "RAD" symbol.	[1945]	AEC
	— I. Kurchatov starts up first USSR nuclear reactor.	[1942]	AEC

Instruments, Units of Measurement, and Drugs

8. Instr	— E. Lawrence starts 184" synchrocyclotron with 200 MeV D_2.	[1939]	Bio
	— R. Fredrichs: Cd sulfide crystals detect gamma rays.	[1945]	NW
	— E. Strajman makes small GM tubes for in vivo rat study.	[1942]	RSI
9. Units	— C. Wilson reviews Mayneord's integral dose concept.	[1940]	Rad
	— F. Spiers introduces new calculations for beta therapy.	[1945]	BJR
	— E. Condon (NBS) suggests Rutherford Unit (10^6 dps).	[1975]	NBS
	— D. Lea's bio dose is "lin ion dens" or "energy dissipation."	[1942]	Bk
	— W. Mayneord measures Co-60 characteristics for Rx use.	[1945]	NRCC
10. Concp	— B. Low-Beer announces P-32 surface count in breast ca.	[1942]	Sc
	— C. LeBlond's microautoradiograms become exact histology.	[1944]	E
	— F. Bush develops formulae for rad absorption by shape.	[1944]	BJR
11. Drugs	— J. Buchanan uses 20m C-11 for intermediary metabolism.	[1931]	PhR
	— H. Bloch prepares I-131 tagged organic compounds.	[1939]	JNCI

11.	Drugs	— D. Vigneaud labels penicillin with S-35 but poor yield.	[1940]	Sc
		— J. Bourhuell labels mustard gas with S-35.	[1945]	BJ
		— A. Keston makes °I-pipsyl chemical reagent.	[1944]	JACS
		— P. Hahn looks for °isotopes with specific localization.	[1939]	SMJ
		— E. Chapman: first "reverse cow," I-131 from 25 m Te-131.	[1945]	JAMA

Radioiodine, P-32, and Radioactive Therapy

13.	I-Dx	— J. Wolff says thiocyanate inhibits I-131 uptake.	[1941]	E
14.	I-Rx	— S. Hertz reviews his first 29 I-130 hyperthyroid Rx pts.	[1941]	JAMA
		— E. Chapman reviews his first 22 I-130 hyperthyroid Rx pts.	[1941]	JAMA
		— S. Seidlin's first paper delayed by doubting editors for 1 year.		JCE
		— Seidlin's second on cure of metastases starts Nuclear Medicine. THE TRUE BEGINNING OF NUCLEAR MEDICINE	[1937]	JAMA
		— High purity I-131 available from MED in large AMOUNTS.	[1940]	AEC
15.	P-Rx	— L. Erf says P-32 is Rx of choice in polycythemia vera.	[1945]	AJM
		— E. Reinhard has partial success in P-32 Rx of blood dis.	[1945]	JLCM
		— W. Graff: sufficient P-32 can wipe out all bone marrow.	[1944]	AJR
16.	Tele	— W. Mayneord makes first measurement of Co-60 @ 1.25 MeV.	[1945]	CJR
		— W. Mayneord says Co-60 is a radium substitute (secret).	[1945]	CJR
		— J. Mitchell turns to Ir-192 because Co-60 unavailable.	[1945]	BJR
17.	Other	— J. MULLER STARTS INTRACAVITARY THERAPY WITH °ZN COLLOID.	[1945]	Gyn
		— P. Hahn gets first shipment of Au-198 for ca therapy.	[1942]	AEC
		— B. Low-Beer introduces brachytherapy with P-32 blotting paper;		Rad
		dissolves Co-60 for Rx of 13 bladder ca pts.	[1945]	TAUA
		— T. Evans compares Na-24/X-ray dose in leukemic mice.	[1944]	AJR

Scans and Other Tests of Function in Various Organs

18.	Brain	— G. Moore notes IV fluorescein stains stomach ca.	[1942]	PSEB
19.	Heart	— G. Burch begins study of Na-24 in congestive failure.	[1941]	PSEB
		— E. Quimby measures °Na arm-heart circulation time.	[1945]	Rad
20.	Liver	— C. Sheppard finds exponential clearance of °Mn, °Au coll.	[1944]	SMJ
21.	Lung	— J. Lawrence autoradiographs Kr-85 dispersion, rat lung.	[1945]	JAMA
24.	Gut	— C. Moore tries IV °Fe as basis for absorption study.	[1945]	JLCM
		— P. Hahn notes depressed °Fe absorp in inflamed guts.	[1944]	PSEB
		— H. Bloch: °I-tagged dyes concentrate in pyloric region.	[1944]	Dis
		— G. Sheline measures °Co in plasma, bile and pancr juice.	[1941]	AJP
25.	Blood	— W. Peacock uses dual Fe-55–59 labeling of RBC & albumin.	[1942]	JCI
		— J. Gibson uses °Fe-RBC and °plasma to see blood distribution; measures RBC volume with °Fe.	[1942]	JCI
		— L. Jacobson studies hematic effects of long term Y-90.	[1942]	AEC
		— D. Shemin estimates 115 d RBC life span with N-15 tag Hb.	[1943]	JBC
26.	Other	— F. Moore begins total body water studies with D_2O	[1934]	Sc

Radiation Hysteria and Health Physics * Obituaries *

27.	Hyst	— Los Alamos accident causes radiation sterility; first case to be proved by sperm counts, but recovery in 2 years.	[1922]	AEC
		— A. Brues implies °isotope Rx in bone may cause osteogenic ca.		MED
		— K. Morgan introduces an unmeasurable undefinable "Rem."	[1945]	AEC
		— AEC tests atomic bomb at Bikini.	[1945]	AEC
28.	React	— S. Cantril explains MED's "Maximum Permissible Dose."	[1945]	MED
		— AEC declassifies Oak Ridge rules on radiation hazards.	[1942]	AEC
		— Am Standards Assoc publishes its X-Ray safety code.	[1945]	ASA
		— R. Stone publishes his first principles of Health Physics	[1942]	PAPS

* * *

30.	Obits	— P. Langevin (1872–1946) Fr physics; M. Curie's consort, sonar.	DSB
		— G. Lewis (1875–1946) Am chem; chem bonds and shared electrons.	DSB

CHRONOLOGY OF NUCLEAR MEDICINE — 1947

Scientific and Technical Background

			Ref.
1. Basic	— C. Anderson: cosmic neutrons on atmospheric N make C-14.	[1939]	PR
	— J. Bardeen designs a semiconductor crystal transistor.	[1928]	FV
2. Obser	— R. Overman introduces the term "activation analysis."	[1936]	AEC
	— J. Cork measures gamma rays from °Ta, °Ir, and °Au.	[1946]	PR
	— A. Grosse surveys body burden of °K, °C, and radium.	[1939]	Sc
	— T. KOHMAN INTRODUCES THE TERM "NUCLIDE" FOR ISO-TOPE-TONE-BAR.		AJP
	— J. Marinsky finds his new #61 has no stable isotopes.	[1945]	JACS
3. # Nuc	— A. English discovers Ra-225, Ac-225, At-217, Bi-213.	[1946]	PR
	— F. Hageman discovers 4.8m Fr-221.	[1946]	Sc
	— G. Boyd prepares pure metallic #43 (Tc) and #61 (Pm).	[1946]	AEC
	— L. Glendenin: Reid's lo-energy °I is probably I-125.	[1946]	PR
	— G. Seaborg say there are now 450 °isotopes.	[1944]	Sc
	— Isotopes Division now has available B-10, D_2, and D_2O.	[1934]	AEC
4. # Med	— Oak Ridge 5×10^{11} n/cm^2 is overloaded with °I, °P, °C sales.	[1946]	AEC
	— Isotopes Div's first catalog lists °isotopes >12 h $T_{1/2}$.	[1946]	AEC
	— 100 stable isotopes (29 elements) available from AEC.	[1946]	AEC
	— 945 shipments of 60 different °isotopes to 32 states.	[1946]	AEC

Organizations and Internal Politics

5. AEC +	— JAN 1, AEC FORMALLY TAKES OVER THE ENTIRE MANHATTAN ENG DIST.		AEC
	AEC CONTROLS MOST NUC MED & BIOL, MUCH NUC PHYS & CHEM.		AEC
	— Sh. Warren heads Medical Board of Review to control use.	[1946]	AEC
	— 3 Clin Res Hosp approved: Oak Ridge, Argonne, Brookhaven.	[1943]	AEC
	— ABCC organized as joint US-Japan study, Hiroshima Hq.	[1946]	AEC
6. Soc	— ABCC reports on A-Bomb effect on whole Jap population.	[1945]	ABCC
	— First Conference on °Isotopes in Agriculture at Ala Poly Inst.		AEC
	— J. Chadwick updates "Radioactivity and Radioact Substan."	[1932]	Bk
	— M. Kamen's "Radioactive Tracers in Biology" published.	[1944]	Bk
	— "Nucleonics" starts (McGraw-Hill), pubs many "firsts."	[1967]	Nuc
7. Event	— Pres Truman announces foreign distrib, some °isotopes.	[1946]	AEC
	— J. Mitchell lists 23 °isotopes of special med interest.	[1946]	BJC

Instruments, Units of Measurement, and Drugs

8. Instr	— P. Bell reviews 22 scintillators and a spectrometer.	[1946]	RSI
	— M. Eidindorf counts H-3 inside GM tube (notes 31y $T_{1/2}$).	[1946]	JACS
	— H. Kallman finds naphthalene transparent to its fluorescense.		NuT
	— L. Miller uses "magnetic lens" to find Co-60 energies.	[1946]	NBS
	— G. Pake finds H position in gypsum with NMR.	[1945]	GSA
9. Units	— G. Hine calculates ave beta energy for a few °isotopes.	[1946]	RMP
	— R. EVANS INTRODUCES THE "rhm" (r/HOUR @ 1 METER).	[1945]	Nuc
	— L. Gray uses mean linear ioniz density for biol dose.	[1946]	BJR
	— J. Mitchell finds Bi-212 (ThC) has RBE of 10.	[1942]	BJC
10. Concp	— G. Failla explains beta radiation equilib: B in = B out.	[1928]	MED
11. Drugs	— W. Cohn produces carrier-free I-131 from Te-131.	[1946]	MED
	— First I-131 labeled "drug" is chiniofon by Abbott Labs.	[1950]	AJTM
	— G. Burch finds Na-24 gross turnover rate extremely fast.	[1941]	JLCM
	— First C-14 labeled compound (methyl alcohol) available.	[1724]	AEC
	— R. Turner labels testosterone with C-14.	[1934]	Sc
	— S. Gurin labels phenylalanine at COOH with C-14.	[1941]	JBC
	— J. Bartter labels tartar emetic with Sb-122-124.	[1945]	AJTM
	— D. Axelrod labels Lewisite with As-74.	[1945]	AJPa
	— First stable labeled compound is Vitamin B_{10} with D_2O.	[1932]	IRT
	— J. Hamilton studies skin after °S-Mustard, °As-Lewisite.	[1946]	AJPa
	— 11 Authors (e.g., P. Durbin) describe metab of fission prod.	[1946]	MED

	Radioiodine, P-32, and Radioactive Therapy			
12. I-Res	— M. Stanley says thiouracil inhibits T4 for a few hours.	[1945]	E
	— J. Gross: T4 is more slowly cleared from blood than T2.	[1944]	JBC
	— L. Schiff measures °I excret in saliva and gastric juice.	[1943]	JCI
	— A. Gorbman studies radiotoxic effects in mouse thyroid.	[1937]	EBM
	— A. Taurog says iodine is "trapped" before "binding."	[1944]	JBC
13. I-Dx	— M. Stanley suggests hourly uptakes for "rate" of uptake.	[1941]	E
	— M. Stanley uses standard uptake to test antithyroid drugs.	[1942]	E
	— E. Astwood measures 36 normal early uptake "gradients."	[1941]	WJS
	— E. Quimby measures uptakes in normal & abnorm children.	[1943]	Rad
	— F. KEATING STRESSES NEED FOR "BODY BACKGROUND" CORRECTION.		JCI
	— F. Keating decides inverse of urinary excretion is best.	[1942]	AJMS
	— G. Ansell questions 50 to 200 μCi range of I-131 dose.	[1942]	BJR
	— I. Chaikoff introduces the PBI test (relates with BMR).	[1945]	E
	— G. Curtis finds PBI more reliable than BMR.	[1944]	AS
	— M. Stanley suggests inhibit °I-binding as Suppress Test.	[1944]	E
14. I-Rx	— H. BLUMGART INTRODUCES °I Rx IN NORMAL UPTAKE ANGINA.	[1934]	JAMA
	— R. Rawson says only 15% of thyroid ca will take up °I.	[1945]	JCE
	— O. Cope's autoradiograms introduce "hot" nodule concept.	[1824]	SGO
15. P-Rx	— D. Anthony: LD_{50} of P-32, rats = 4 μCi/g (man = 270 mCi).	[1937]	MED
	— H. Lisco suggests risk of bone tumors from P-32. (None!)	[1946]	Rad
	— W. Platt: some blood cells damaged after hi-dose P-32.	[1939]	APa
	— B. Low-Beer details Rx with P-32 on blotting paper.	[1937]	AJR
16. Tele	— W. Mayneord: first open publication of existence of Co-60.	[1946]	CJR
	— J. Trump devises a Van de Graaff for multi MeV therapy.	[1937]	AJR
17. Other	— P. Hahn treats 8 y old boy for Subac Lmph Leuk (Au-198).	[1946]	JLCM
	— L. Jacobsen finds As-76 of no value in tumor therapy.	[1942]	AEC
	Scans and Other Tests of Function in Various Organs		
18. Brain	— G. Moore notes fluorescein stains cancers, tries °I tag.	[1946]	Sc
19. Heart	— M. Prinzmetal uses °glass spheres to see coronary collaterals.	[1931]	AHJ
20. Liver	— J. Cain measures 0.2 ml/m lymph flow, liver to T-duct.	[1928]	SGO
21. Lung	— J. Muller shows arterial pattern by cath inj of °AuCol.	[1946]	Ex
	— T. Talbot introduces aerosol deposition with Na-24.	[1946]	AJMS
22. Bone	— H. Lisco says °Sr localizes in bone and stays put.	[1942]	Rad
24. Gut	— T. Woud crystalizes cyanocobalamin (Vit B_{12}).	[1941]	NT
25. Blood	— M. Wintrobe develops Red Cell Iron Utilization (RCIU).	[1946]	JCI
	— J. Gibson measures RBC survival in stored blood (°Fe).	[1943]	JCI
	— D. Grob uses first DF°P for RBC regeneration rate in man.	[1946]	BJHH
26. Other	— S. Seidlin uses °I in study of physiology of teeth.	[1946]	Sc
	— R. Scholz measures plasma-aque humor ratio in G-pig eye.	[1942]	AJO
	Radiation Hysteria and Health Physics * Obituaries *		
27. Hyst	— W. Bloom says C-14 is most dangerous °nuclide.	[1950]	SC
	— H. MacMahon has first doc evidence of Th-232 sarcoma.	[1940]	AJPa
	— K. Morgan develops method for calculating Max Perm Dose.	[1946]	JPCC
	— K. Morgan says "MPD" should be revised to 0.01 rd.	[1946]	JIHI
	— R. Sievert revises "Tolerance dose" to 0.01 r/d.	[1948]	BJR
28. React	— J. Lawrence says there is a safe human radiation level.	[1981]	JAMA
	— T. Leucutia says no toxic effects of °I ever been noted.	[1932]	AJR
	— J. Mitchell says no toxic effects of °I ever been noted.	[1932]	BJC
29. Respo	— V. Hess can detect 30 ng of radium in human body.	[1939]	AJR
	— F. Joliot will build French reactor without US help.	[1934]	AP
	* * *		
30. Obits	— M. Planck (1858–1947) Ger physics; quantum of energy.		DSB
	— P. Lenard (1862–1947) Ger physics; cathode rays in air.	[1932]	DSB

CHRONOLOGY OF NUCLEAR MEDICINE — 1948

	Scientific and Technical Background		Ref.
2. Obser	— M. Deutsch sets I-131 decay scheme to current pattern.	[1942]	PR
3. # Nuc	— G. Seaborg sees 4n + 1 Neptunium family (Np-237 to Bi-209).	[1942]	CEN
	— J. Jelley discovers 4.2×10^{-6} s Po-213.	[1946]	PR
	— 100 enriched stable isotopes (30 elements) available.	[1932]	AEC
	— W. Sullivan's new "Trilinear Chart" lists 1026 isotopes.	[1946]	PL
	— J. Stokley's first edit GE Chart of Isotopes lists 750.	[1946]	Bk
4. # Med	— AEC funds 185 projects on C-14 (a few in humans).	[1947]	AEC
	— AEC ships 2191 °orders to 410 depts in 236 institutions.	[1946]	AEC
	— 43 hospitals are using P-32, 38 use I-131 in Dx and Rx.	[1946]	AEC
	— P. Aebersold tells AMA 1400 (half MDs) use °isotopes.	[1946]	AEC

	Organizations and Internal Politics		
5. AEC +	— °Isotope regs pub by AEC, USPO, ICC, CAB, BE (all differ).	[1946]	FR
	— AEC (really Congress) says free ca research °isotopes.	[1952]	AEC
	— NAS-AEC sign 2 year contract for ABCC (lasted 27 years).	[1975]	AEC
	— Advisory Comm on Isotopes formed (5/12 MD members).	[1947]	AEC
	SUBCOMMITTEE ON USE IN HUMANS FORMED (CALLED SUBHUMAN COMM)		
6. Socs	— Oak Ridge 4-week °isotope training courses begin.	[1903]	AEC
	— °Isotope conferences held at Madison, Brookhaven, AMA.	[1947]	AEC
	— Manhattan District Declassified Reports (MDDC) begin.	[1946]	AEC
	— G. Seaborg "Table of Isotopes" first edition published.	[1946]	Bk
	— J. Schulman attempts first stnd glossary of nuclear terms.	[1946]	Nuc
	— L. Curtis writes first Nuclear Medicine Instrument txtbk.	[1950]	Bk
7. Event	— First French reactor "ZOE" goes critical.	[1947]	CEA
	— First "commercial" °isotope sales (I-131 and P-32).	[1947]	AEC
	— H. Willard surveys Th distribution in monazite sands.	[1980]	AC
	— Tritium (H-3) is made available outside AEC labs.	[1946]	AEC

	Instruments, Units of Measurement, and Drugs		
8. Instr	— R. HOFSTADTER INVENTS THE NaI (Tl) CRYSTAL.	[1947]	PR
	— B. Cassen puts crystal in needle to measure deep dose.	[1946]	AEC
	— N. Veall adapts GM dip tube to small liquid samples.	[1939]	BJR
	— W. Shockley transfers current across a solid-state resistor.	SN	
9. Units	— NBS standardizes the many AEC "curie" units.	[1940]	NBS
	— MRC (Eng) prepares provisional °I, °Co, °P, °Na standards.	[1910]	Na
	— NBS selects Cs-137 as best spectro-"pure" gamma source.	[1940]	AEC
	— L. Marinelli catalogs 23 "medical" °isotope dose calcs.	[1946]	AJR
	— R. Evans summarizes all med °isotope measurement units.	[1947]	AMP
	— H. Parker calculates r-equiv-mammal (rep × RBE = rem).	[1945]	BJR
	— NINTH CGPM SAYS WE NEED A NEW COHERENT SYSTEM OF UNITS;	[1889]	NBS
	adopts ampere as repulsion of 2×10^{-7} newton/m.	[1908]	NBS
10. Concp	— Argonne conference defines a "standard man" concept.	[1968]	AEC
	— E. Tompkins says "carrier-free" has daughter impurity.	[1939]	AEC
	— N. Wiener introduces cybernetics: feedback & automation.	[1943]	Bk
11. Drugs	— D. Pressman sees IV °I-antitissue antibody go to target.	[1935]	JI
	— C. Comar studies distribution of Co-60 (first biol use?).	[1944]	JBC
	— G. Vosburgh studies D_2 and °Na amniotic fluid mix.	[1943]	AJOG
	— J. Wang measures penetration of °Na, °Cl into CSF & eye.	[1947]	JGP

	Radioiodine, P-32, and Radioactive Therapy		
12. I-Res	— E. Chapman proves that fetal thyroid has I-131 uptake.	[1982]	JCE
	— C. LeBlond locates iodination site of thyroid protein.	[1945]	E
	— W. Salter discusses organic vs inorganic °I binding.	[1947]	JCE
	— D. Childs notes: 10 mg I-127 prevents uptake of I-131.	[1944]	JI CM

12. I-Res	— E. Frieden labels thyroxine with I-131.	[1915]	Sc
	— K. Fink finds monoiodotyrosine is first step in binding.	[1947]	Sc
13. I-Dx	— G. ANSELL COUNTS 32 POINTS TO MAP INTRATHORACIC GOITER.	[1949]	BJR
	— S. Werner analyzes first large series to fix 24 h uptake.	[1947]	Rad
	— D. Childes: carrier I-127 amt influences I-131 retention.	[1939]	JLCM
14. I-Rx	— F. Keating uses nonsense formula to calculate Rx dose.	[1947]	JCE
	— H. BLUMGART TREATS EUTHYROID HEART DISEASE WITH I-131.	[1933]	PSEB
	— J. Rotblat: if thyroid ca takes up °I, it can be treated.	[1947]	BJR
15. P-Rx	— D. Karnofsky finds P-32 of NO value in acute leukemia.	[1946]	NEJM
	— E. Osgood succeeds in Rx of chron leukemias with P-32.	[1946]	NM
	— J. Maxfield monitors cattle eye tumor therapy with P-32.	[1945]	TMJ
16. Tele	— G. Adams treats first patient (brain tumor) on betatron.	[1940]	AJR
17. Other	— T. Evans uses Na-24 as total body radiation on 24 pts.	[1946]	AJR
	— R. Stone attempts ca Rx with cyclotron fast neutrons,	[1942]	AJR
	thinks his neutron Rx gave bad results.	[1971]	AJR
	— W. Myers develops British Co-60 brachytherapy seeds.	[1946]	AJR
	— M. Block studies As-76 in hematopoietic malignancies.	[1947]	JLCM
	— P. Hahn announces direct tumor injection of Au-198.	[1942]	FP

Scans and Other Tests of Function in Various Organs

18. Brain	— B. Selverstone develops GM probe to localize K-42.	[1944]	TANA
	— G. Moore prepares di°iodofluorescein (D°IF) to localize tumors. INTRODUCES MULTIPOINT (GM tube) MANUAL BRAIN SCANS.	[1946]	Nuc
19. Heart	— M. Prinzmetal reports first RadioCardioGrams (400) to AMA.	[1947]	Sc
	— F. Cooper: muscles' °Na washout shows Periph Vasc Dis.	[1946]	SGO
	— R. Rohrer: °Na circ time variable in Periph Vasc Dis.	[1946]	SGO
22. Bone	— H. Dudley introduces Ga-72 for tumor localization.	[1965]	JEPT
	— W. Armstrong uses dual Ca-45 & P-32 to study bone.	[1947]	JBC
23. Kidney	— D. Cristol: P-32 uptake in bladder & prostate calculi.	[1942]	NEJM
24. Gut	— E. Smith discovers cobalt in VB_{12}, starts race to label.	[1947]	Na
	— C. Moore studies absorption-excretion of oral °Fe.	[1946]	B
25. Blood	— J. Storaasli recalls °IHSA for blood volume (dogs),	[1946]	V45
	interests Tabern (Abbott) in °IHSA bld vol.	[1946]	V45
	— L. Flexner labels plasma transferrin with °Fe (G-pigs).	[1946]	AJPh
	— C. Finch determines RBC °Fe turnover, starts RCIT study.	[1947]	JCI
	— K. Singer studies sickle cell anemia with °donor study.	[1943]	Sc
26. Other	— E. Kooyman investigates dynamic state of antibody °tags.	[1949]	JACS
	— H. Wright uses °Na to detect Deep Venous Thrombi.	[1985]	La
	— N. Pace measures "total body water" with H-3.	[1946]	JBC
	— H. Friedell sees tissue transplant viability with P-32.	[1947]	PRS

Radiation Hysteria and Health Physics * Obituaries *

27. Hyst	— J. Means restricts °I therapy to patients over age 15 y.	[1975]	BNYA
	— C. Williams lists 8 radiation hazards (hi-vac tubes).	[1938]	JIHT
	— R. Newell says "There is no antidote to radiation."	[1944]	JAMA
	— L. Dublin: 1938–42 mortality "suggests" hazard in Radiol.	[1957]	JAMA
	— P. Norris: weak relation between cosmic rays and cancer.	[1946]	Ex
	— K. Morgan says a little over 2 lbs Ra has been mined.	[1922]	AEC
28. React	— Isotope Div 3-blade propeller becomes "Radiation" symb.	[1946]	AEC
	— Shipment of >100 mg radium by mail prohibited.	[1939]	USPO
	— R. Evans writes first ICC regs on shipment of °isotopes.	[1940]	ICC
	— A. Tannenbaum's first study of uranium toxicity released.	[1944]	AEC
	— E. Chapman: Dx I-131 dose does not affect fetal thyroid.	[1982]	JCE
	— C. Tobias finds mouse LD_{50} (190 MeV D_2 beam) at 150 rep.	[1935]	AEC
	— T. Evans attempts RBE measurement, fast neutrons in mice.	[1947]	Rad

* * *

30. Obits —

CHRONOLOGY OF NUCLEAR MEDICINE — 1949

	Scientific and Technical Background		Ref.
1. Basic	— J. Cork confirms basic decay schemes of many °nuclides.	[1948]	PR
	— NBS unveils first atomic clock, accurate to 1 sec/8 mon.	[1928]	NBS
2. Obser	— B. Kern determines gamma spectra with "magnetic lens."	[1947]	PR
	— Greenwich Observatory moved to Herstmonceux, Sussex.	[1675]	Sc
4. # Med	— 3575 shipments of °nuclides to 305 institutions.	[1948]	AEC
	— 283 papers published on medical °nuclide use.	[1946]	AEC
	— P. Aebersold explains °nuclide production to med users.	[1947]	JCI

	Organizations and Internal Politics		
5. AEC +	— AEC, by law, has exclusive "artif °isotope" control.	[1946]	AEC
	— AEC begins cyclotron produc of non-reactor nuclides.	[1944]	AEC
	— Canada and England begin °isotope production.	[1947]	AEC
	— NCRP adopts Max Perm Dose (MPD) set at 0.3 R/week.	[1947]	NCRP
	— K. Way moves Nuclear Data Project to NBS in Washington.	[1948]	NBS
6. Socs	— Am Board Radiol certifies first 4 radiologic physicists.	[1935]	Rad
	— C. Behrens publishes first txtbook on "Atomic Medicine."	[1947]	Bk
	— CAB publishes its regulations on shipment of °isotopes.	[1948]	CAB
	— W. Sullivan's Trilinear Chart published (Wiley).	[1948]	Bk
7. Event	— I. Kurchatov explodes first USSR Atomic Bomb.	[1946]	AEC

	Instruments, Units of Measurement, and Drugs		
8. Instr	— P. Bell: photomult tubes sensitive to magnetic fields.	[1944]	Nuc
	— H. Slatis builds 22 tubes-in-one to up GM sensitivity.	[1947]	RSI
	— D. Copeland builds first gamma camera (too insensitive).	[1958]	Nuc
	— B. CASSEN INVENTS RECTILINEAR SCANNER (150 copies of report).		AEC
	— G. Morton perfects the photomultiplier tube.	[1945]	Nuc
	— P. Tompkins makes P-32 impregnated bakelite beta source.	[1948]	AEC
9. Units	— F. Bush derives equations for approx human organ shapes.	[1946]	BJR
	— L. Marinelli calculates specific organ doses in "er."	[1948]	JCI
	— L. Gray calculates beta/gamma emission rates (LET hint).	[1947]	BJR
	— F. Spiers begins differential bone/soft tissue dose.	[1946]	BJR
	— W. Mayneord gives geometric principles of isodoses.	[1944]	BJR
10. Concp	— Chalk River Canada conference designs a "Standard Man."	[1948]	AEC
	— G. Burch finds bio-$T_{1/2}$ (°Na) tripled in cong hrt failure.	[1947]	JLCM
	— V. Hollander develops concept of "spaces" with D_2O.	[1943]	JLCM
	— F. Burnet says antibodies formed only after exposure.	[1948]	Sc
11. Drugs	— J. Storaasli determines safety of °IHSA in 16 rats.	[1944]	FP
	— D. Hodgkin establishes structure of penicillin.	[1940]	CN
	— P. Cooper tags penicillin (C-14), sees it in staph aureus.	[1940]	Na
	— C. Moore finds first labeling error: easily degraded °Fe tag.	[1948]	JCI
	— W. Winsche develops second radioactive cow system (I-132).	[1926]	Nuc

	Radioiodine, P-32, and Radioactive Therapy		
12. I-Res	— E. Astwood solves early ??, I-131, I-127 chem identical.	[1933]	JCI
	— C. Comar proves I-131 can wipe out thyroid gland.	[1947]	Sc
	— M. Soley proves palpation est of thyroid wt 50% off.	[1948]	JCEn
	— W. Cole finds 4%–17% of nontox multinod adenomas malig.	[1928]	JCEn
13. I-Dx	— D. Clark introduces PB°I conversion ratio, avoids errors.	[1945]	S
	— H. Friedell says rate of PB°I change at 2–4 h is best Dx.	[1947]	JLCM
	— L. Hyde finds bronchial lipiodol depresses the PB°I.	[1944]	JLCM
	— E. Astwood says rate of change of uptake gives early Dx.	[1947]	JCI
	— E. Astwood gives large TSH dose for "stimulation test."	[1945]	E
	— E. Astwood gives mercaptoimidazole for "trapping test."	[1941]	E
	— F. Keating adopts 24 h thyroid uptake as routine test.	[1948]	JCI

13. I-Dx	— -. Marquez makes I-123 from Sb-121 in cyclotron.	[1985]	MP
	— E. Pochin devises a neck/thigh ratio for body bkgd fix.	[1947]	CS
	— T. Oddie uses uptake & excretion to est true body bkgd.	[1947]	BJR
	— H. Nachman reports first manual scan of lingual thyroid.	[1948]	JAMA
14. I-Rx	— R. Rawson: metastases develop uptake post-thyroidectomy.	[1945]	Ca
	— M. Stanley introduces tapazole.	[1945]	E
	— 16 articles (e.g., S. Werner) give hyperT °I Rx results.	[1946]	AJM
	— J. Trunnel introduces surgery + hi-dose I-131 Rx for thyroid ca.	[1946]	TNYA
	— G. Sheline gives post-surg °I each month until no uptake.	[1948]	Rad
	— H. Blumgart gets favorable °I Rx results in ang pect.	[1948]	TAAP
15. P-Rx	— H. Moffitt details >5 y survivals of 31 P-32 ch leuk pts.	[1948]	AIM
17. Other	— J. Muller announces first intracavitary °Zn-Colloid Rx.	[1946]	BSAM
	— D. Wallace says Co-60, Na-24 in use for brachytherapy.	[1947]	BJU
	— M. Friedman uses Co-60 "point" in balloon for bladder ca.	[1946]	Rad
	— G. Williams injects °AuColloid into tumor, it stays put.	[1945]	Nuc
	— H. Freundlich makes fission product beta applicator.	[1946]	Na

Scans and Other Tests of Function in Various Organs

18. Brain	— W. Sweet localizes P-32 in tumors with small GM tube.	[1948]	JAMA
	— G. Moore makes first brain "scans" in 12 pts (D°IF-GM tube).	[1948]	Sc
	— M. Ashkenazy locates 200 tumors (95% accuracy) with D°IF.	[1948]	JLCM
	— L. Bakay injects P-32 in CSF, measures bld-brain-barrier.	[1943]	APS
	— F. Howarth: °Na, °Br diffuse from thecal space rapidly.	[1937]	La
19. Heart	— P. Waser confirms Prinzmetal's RCG with modified tech.	[1948]	HPA
20. Liver	— H. Elias re-examines gross and micro anatomy.	[1942]	AJA
	— A. Mendeloff sees Rose Bengal in polygonal cells only.	[1930]	PSEB
	— D. Cayer studies °phospholipid metab in liver diseases.	[1937]	Sc
	— E. Dobson uses P-32 coll to measure liver blood flow.	[1945]	JLCM
22. Bone	— L. Layton attempts Dx of cartilagenous tumors with S-35.	[1945]	Ca
	— H. Dudley notes high Ga-72 uptake in skeletal tissues.	[1948]	JPET
23. Kidney	— G. Burch introduces Hg-203 in diuretic, measures plasma.	[1939]	JCI
24. Gut	— R. Braude attempts to label VB12 with Co-60, fails.	[1945]	BJN
	— P. Hahn measures gut °Fe-RBC loss in hookworm.	[1942]	Sc
	— L. Crandall detects absorption of $°BaSO_4$, not of $°IrO_2$.	[1944]	Gas
25. Blood	— C. Finch: reticulocytes take up °Fe and synthesize heme.	[1974]	Sc
	— K. Endicott: storage Fe not derived from °Fe test meal.	[1943]	JLCM
	— R. Huff measures plasma iron clearance (PIC) with °Fe.	[1948]	JLCM
	— G. Nylin begins circulation kinetics, tags RBC (P-32).	[1945]	AHJ
	— S. GRAY DETECTS TRI- AND HEXAVALENT Cr IN TISSUES.	[1932]	AEC
	— J. Storaasli measures °IHSA plasma volume in 30 pts.	[1948]	FP
26. Other	— S. Kety says °Na clearance measures regional bld flow.	[1944]	AHJ
	— T. Evans introduces fluid kinetics in eye with Na-24.	[1947]	PSEB

Radiation Hysteria and Health Physics * Obituaries *

27. Hyst	— J. Hamilton checks Pu, U, & fiss prod aerosol deposition.	[1948]	AP
	— K. Morgan reduces MPD to fake unmeasurable 0.3 rem/wk.	[1947]	AEC
	— A. Gorbman sees "tumorous" growths (mice) after hi-D I-131.	[1947]	PSEB
	— D. Uphoff finds "low intensity" genetic effect (25 r flies).	[1944]	Sc
	— MRC (Eng) revises its radiation protection standards.	[1945]	MRC
28. React	— 101 physicians deny ever seeing ca caused by I-131 Rx.	[1947]	JAMA
	— No delayed effects of radiation yet seen by ABCC.	[1945]	ABCC
	— NBS pubs Handbook #42 "Safe Handling of Radioisotopes."	[1946]	NBS
29. Respo	— L. Jacobson describes hematologic effects of radiation.	[1947]	Rad
	— R. STONE: FIRST DESCRIPTION OF "ACUTE RADIATION SYNDROME."	[1905]	JAMA

* * *

30. Obits	A. Debierne (1874–1949) Fr chem; actinium, early radioactivity.		DSB
	— M. Soley (1907–1949) Am physician; 1939 I-131 use in patients.		HNM

CHRONOLOGY OF NUCLEAR MEDICINE — 1950

Scientific and Technical Background

			Ref.
3. # Nuc	— G. Seaborg discovers #97 Berkelium and #98 Californium.	[1948]	AEC
	— F. Hagemann discovers 2.2 m Tl-209.	[1948]	PR
4. # Med	— AEC ships 5298 °isotope orders.	[1949]	AEC
	— D. Tabern (Abbott) says I-131 is most widely used.	[1946]	Nuc

Organizations and Internal Politics

			Ref.
5. AEC +	— ABCC: life span study sees 110,000 atom bomb survivors.	[1948]	ABCC
	— ICRU recommends "As Little As Possible" (ALARA). Disputed!		BJR
	— ICRP splits from ICRU; wants Health Physicists only,	[1928]	ICRU
	sets MPD at 0.3 R/week.	[1949]	ICRU
6. Socs	— Oberlin has symposium on basic effects of radiation.	[1947]	RR
	— Leeds, Eng, sympos "Biological Effects of Atomic Energy."	[1948]	Vig
	— K. Way's Nuc Data Project publishes 300 pp of data.	[1949]	NBS
	— W. Mayneord publishes "Radioisotopes in Medicine."	[1949]	BJR
	— B. Low-Beer pubs "Clinical Use of Radioactive Isotopes."	[1949]	Bk
	— S. Glasstone pubs AEC's "Sourcebook of Atomic Energy."	[1945]	Bk
7. Event	— W. Libby begins C-14 dating.	[1949]	Sc
	— ABBOTT LABS SELLS FIRST COMMERCIAL °PHARMACEUTICAL (°RISA).	[1943]	Nuc
	— AEC adopts 3-bladed propeller as °activity symbol.	[1948]	AEC

Instruments, Units of Measurement, and Drugs

			Ref.
8. Instr	— H. Kallman develops liquid scintillators.	[1947]	PR
	— E. Pochin announces first linear scanner.	[1949]	La
	— W. Mayneord is first to use NaI (Tl) crystal in medicine.	[1948]	BJR
	— H. Anger makes first crystal well scintillation counter.	[1942]	UCRL
	— B. Cassen shows his rectilinear scanner (for thyroid).	[1949]	Nuc
	— L. Marinelli invents beaker for GM counting of liquids.	[1948]	AJR
	— A. Graham makes safe pipetting apparatus for P-32 soln.	[1948]	JLCM
	— G. Burch: filter-paper count methods for biol fluids.	[1949]	JLCM
9. Units	— NBS makes a few °isotope standards available.	[1948]	NBS
	— A. Rupp makes a 10 Ci solid Cs-137 source for NBS.	[1954–48]	AEC
	— R. Hofstadter draws spectra with NaI (Tl) pulse height.	[1948]	PR
	— ICRU adopts a new "curie" unit (Ci).	[1910]	HP
	— ICRU limits "r" to X-ray energies over 400 kVp; "dose" is ergs/gram.	[1937]	HP
10. Concp	— Scintillation crystals are already replacing GM tubes.	[1949]	PL
	— E. Frank says Na-24 washout is not exponential.	[1949]	PSEB
	— G. Burch begins use of Hg-203 in diuretic studies.	[1947]	AJMS
11. Drugs	— J. Hamilton finds At-211 has iodine metabolic pattern.	[1947]	PSEB
	— B. Selverstone says P-32 goes to rapidly metabol tissue.	[1939]	JAMA
	— C. Rosenblum labels cyanocobalamine (VB_{12}) with Co-60.	[1949]	V48

Radioiodine, P-32, and Radioactive Therapy

			Ref.
12. I-Res	— E. Pochin surveys the current I-131 Dx and Rx fields.	[1949]	La
13. I-Dx	— I-131 called "atomic cocktail," therapeutic drink (Eng).	[1946]	BJR
	— H. Jaffe find I-131 uptake more accurate than BMR.	[1947]	JAMA
	— Querido & Stanbury initiate TSH stimulation test.	[1949]	JCE
14. I-Rx	— 17 authors (e.g., E. Gordon) confirm Seidlin, Chapman I-131 Rx.		JAMA
	— S. Feitelberg sees no rad sickness in 300 I-131 Rx pts.	[1947]	ArIM
	— A. Freedberg treats first pulmonary thyroid metastasis.	[1948]	JAMA
	— R. Goldberg finds parathyroids undamaged at hi-D I-131.	[1982]	E
15. P-Rx	— E. Osgood develops titrated P-32 for chronic leukemias.	[1948]	AEC
	— H. Friedell reports P-32 Rx for breast ca bone mets.	[1942]	AJR
	— H. Friedell: P-32 leg uptake predicts sympathectomy result.	[1942]	ArIM
	— H. Jaffe uses Cr°PO_4 for malignant intracav effusions.	[1946]	RiM

16. Tele	— Grimmett & Brucer report first Co-60 teletherapy design.	[1949]	AEC
	— H. Freundlich has 70d Ir-197 20 Ci 400 keV teleRx unit.	[1946]	AR
	— H. Friedell designs Sr-90 beta ray eye applicator.	[1948]	AJO
	— J. Morton uses Co-60 needles in ca of cervix.	[1948]	AJOG
17. Other	— J. Hamilton says At-211 alphas destroy thyroid.	[1947]	PSEB
	— G. LeRoy says Au-198 Colloid is fixed at injection site.	[1949]	PIM
	— A. Sherman tries direct injection Au-198 in pelvic ca.	[1949]	AJC
	— P. Hahn suggests °AuCol for malig ascites and leukemia.	[1939]	PSEB
	— D. Tabern lists 6 therapeutically useful °isotopes: Na-24, P-32, K-42, I-131, Br-82, Au-198.	[1947]	Nuc
	— D. Cara makes 290d Ru-106 surface plaque, 2.3 MeV betas.	[1949]	TRBM
	— R. Walton uses 34h Br-82 in elastic bag for bladder ca.	[1949]	BJR
	— R. Marcus treats Malig Melanoma with Cu-64 colloid.	[1985]	BJR
	— H. Goldie studies effect of °Au & °I on sarc-37 cells.	[1942]	PSEB

Scans and Other Function Tests in Various Organs

18. Brain	— Selverstone & Sweet use P-32 and K-42 to detect tumors.	[1949]	SF
	— M. Ashkenazy introduces a 32 point array of GM tubes.	[1949]	JAMA
	— R. Woolsey uses 32-point counters to see tumors (D°IF).	[1949]	JLCM
19. Heart	— J. Levi measures venous velocity in legs with Na-24.	[1945]	BJH
20. Liver	— R. Wechsler measures liver blood flow, Na-24 clearance.	[1944]	FP
	— H. Berg finds tumor makes °AuCol cold-spot-in-hot liver.	[1966]	AS
21. Lung	— F. Buckland measures lung retention of P-32 aerosols.	[1947]	Nat
22. Bone	— F. Tucker uses P-32 in Dx of avascular necros of femur.	[1943]	JBJS
23. Kidney	— Hayes & Roe label Diodrast with I-131 (for Hayes PhD).	[1965]	PSEB
24. Gut	— C. Yuile measures Fe-55 GI absorption.	[1945]	PSEB
25. Blood	— J. Storaasli describes °IHSA label for plasma volume.	[1948]	SGO
	— P. Hahn measures RBC volume with °iron tagged RBC.	[1948]	SMJ
	— K. Crispell uses combined P-32 °IHSA blood volume.	[1949]	JCI
	— J. Gray reports Cr-51 RBC tag for vol measurement (dogs).	[1949]	Sc
	— H. Nachman modifies method, in vitro P-32 label of RBC.	[1940]	JCI
26. Other	— Brown & Veal introduce °NaCl placentograms (area counts).	[1943]	JOGB
	— Roswit & Yalow measure P-32 uptake in testicle tumor.	[1945]	JU
	— J. Hardy uses D_2O to measure total body water space.	[1948]	AJMS
	— S. Hertz studies effect of testost & estrogen on P-32.	[1942]	JCI
	— L. Walker finds °colloids localize in lymph nodes.	[1945]	JLCM
	— H. Krieger notes some drain of °IHSA into lymph (dogs).	[1942]	PSEB

Radiation Hysteria and Health Physics * Obituaries *

27. Hyst	— Sweden proposes Radiation Hazard Regulations.	[1949]	AR
	— I. Doniach notes thyroid ca after I-131 in rats (false).	[1949]	BJC
	— Duffy & Fitzgerald note thyroid ca after childhood °Rx.	[1982]	JCE
	— H. March says leukemia increased in radiologists (false).	[1948]	Rad
	— L. Lewis says shoe-fitting fluoroscopes are hazardous.	[1958]	CM
	— H. Friedell says 40% of hi-dose P-32 rats get tumors.	[1949]	CR
	— D. Clark keeps age 45 restriction on I-131 thyroid Rx.	[1948]	AS
	— A. Pearl starts beta-emit syringe shield nonsense.	[1976]	JLCM
	— D. Charles estimates 1%/100 r mutations in mouse sperm.	[1959]	Rad
28. React	— ICRU adopts MPD @ 0.3r/wk.	[1949]	ICRU
	— ICRU admits r conversion to rad is physically impossible.	[1944]	ICRU
	— G. LeRoy finds no hazard in use of mCi levels of D°IF.	[1949]	JLCM
	— W. Watts cannot confirm increased lymphs in I-131 Rx	[1949]	JLCM
29. Respo	— J. Govaerts says C-14 is safest °nuclide.	(See Bloom 1947)	Sc
	— London Thyroid ca Conf: 27 experts on Seidlin's cure.	[1949]	V38
	— R. Sievert compares "Tolerance Dose" with new MPD.	[1948]	Vig
	— Emergency limits = 10 r (worker) or 25 r (public) once/life.	[1930]	AEC

* * *

30. Obits	— H. Coutard (1876–1950) Fr medic, pioneer rad therapist.	(1973	IJO)

CHRONOLOGY OF NUCLEAR MEDICINE — 1951

	Scientific and Technical Background		Ref.
1. Basic	— T. Cullen: PhD (Fordham) on "Exhalation of Rn from Earth."	[1901]	Dis
2. Obser	— First swimming pool reactor goes critical, public display.	[1948]	AEC
	— E. McMillan writes early history of trans-U elements.	[1946]	AEC
3. # Nuc	— G. Friedlander: Reid's °I is 60d 35 kev I-125.	[1946]	PR
4. # Med	— "Broad" licenses started for qualified medical users.	[1948]	AEC
	— AEC has made 6896 shipments of °nuclides, 1100 foreign.	[1947]	AEC
	— Over 1000 hyperthyroid, 1000 PVA pts treated with °I, °P.	[1950]	AEC
	— °Isotope users are 50% internists, 25% path, 12% radiol.	[1972]	RSNA
	— S. Donaldson lists 18 K X-ray units in 4242 hosps in US; 4100 radiologists take 207,500 films; give 13,200 Rx/day.	[1923]	AJR
	— AERE (Eng): 2800 °isotope shipments, US monopoly gone.	[1965]	AERE
	Organizations and Internal Politics		
5. AEC +	— First °nuclide (I-131) accepted by FDA as new drug.	[1950]	FDA
	— AEC pubs first catalog of all stable isotopes to lend.	[1948]	AEC
	— AERE (Isotopes Div) standardizes °radiography sources,	[1950]	Nuc
	displays new assay instruments at VIIth ICR.	[1950]	BJR
	— Small quantities of some °nuclides require no license.	[1948]	AEC
6. Socs	— 3250 papers have been published on °nuclides in med.	[1949]	AEC
	— T. Chalmers writes "A Short History of Radioactivity."	[1945]	TEL
	— Symposia on Nuc Engineer, Nuc Cancer Rx at AAAS (Phila).	[1950]	Sc
	— VIIth Int Cong Radiol (Copenhagen) considers Atomic E.	[1928]	Rad
7. Event	— L. Farr treats 1–6-year-old nephrotics with °isotopes.	[1944]	AEC
	— First Nuc Med division in medical school at Bonn (Ger).	[1903]	DA
	— Research reactor (OR) converted to 3×10^{13} n/cm^2.	[1947]	AEC
	— FIRST ELECTRICITY FROM EXP BREEDER REACTOR, IDAHO FALLS.	[1984]	SN
	Instruments, Units of Measurement, and Drugs		
8. Instr	— G. Moore uses 1.25" anthracene xtal for hi-sensitivity.	[1950]	Nuc
	— N. Veall shows a directional GM probe for manual scan.	[1950]	BJR
	— W. Mayneord's 1939 isodose plotter adapted to °I scans.	[1950]	Na
	— H. Anger makes the first whole body scanner (10 counters).	[1950]	AJR
9. Units	— L. Lamerton: non-uniform P-32 ARGs vitiate "Rep."	[1948]	BMJ
	— C. Wilson converts "r" to "ergs/gram."	[1950]	BJR
10. Concp	— The unmeasurable "Rem" is faked to "Roent Equiv Man."	[1948]	AEC
	— F. Spiers analyzes effect of bone spicules on dose.	[1949]	BJR
	— R. Loevinger develops counting efficiency criteria.	[1948]	Nuc
11. Drugs	— A. Rupp announces fission product I-131 in huge quant.	[1947]	AEC
	— W. Winsch announces first new °isotope cow (Te to I-132).	[1926]	Nuc
	Radioiodine, P-32, and Radioactive Therapy		
12. I-Res	— F. Keating finds injected °T2 rapidly replaces °I.	[1948]	JCE
	— F. Lahey finds only 0.68% of "hot" nodules become malig.	[1915]	JAMA
	— P. Meadows says 58% solitary cold nodules become malig.	[1949]	JAMA
13. I-Dx	— 19 articles (e.g., D. Clarke) do uptake by 19 diff methods.	[1949]	ArIM
	— 17 articles (e.g., B. Dobyns) give various Dx uses for °I.	[1950]	SGO
	— A. Freedberg: °I-uptake and PB°I in thyrotox factitia.	[1949]	AJM
	— J. Foote finds clearances differ, invalidates N/T ratio.	[1949]	La
	— D. Clarke says PB°I is an index of thyroid function.	[1949]	LCM
	— E. Man says BE°I diagnostically more effective than PB°I.	[1949]	JCI
14. I-Rx	— 14 articles (e.g., G. Crile) on hyperthyroid Rx with I-131.	[1950]	AnS
	— 12 articles (e.g., R. Coliez) on carcinoma Rx with I-131.	[1949]	JRE
	— S. Seidlin finds an uptake "rebound" after I-131 Rx.	[1950]	NYAM

15. P-Rx	— L. Erf details remission length in PVA after P-32 Rx.	[1949]	UICC
	— B. Wiseman finds no increased leukemia 10 y post-op Rx.	[1949]	AIM
16. Tele	— M. BRUCER ANNOUNCES FIRST 1000 Ci Co-60 TELETHERAPY UNIT.	[1950]	AEC
	— M. Brucer announces first fission product Cs-137 teleRx.	[1950]	AEC
17. Other	— 7 articles (e.g., I. Meschan) detail °isotope brachytherapy.	[1950]	AJR
	— R. Flocks starts Au-198 injections into prostate ca.	[1950]	JU
	— H. Elkins begins prophylactic °AuCol IP in ovarian ca.	[1950]	AJR
	— A. Sherman tries parametrial °AuCol in pelvic ca.	[1940]	AJR
	— M. Brucer declares Ga-72 Rx in osteogen sarc a failure.	[1949]	Rad
	— J. Muller develops a Sr-90 intrauterine applicator.	[1950]	PL

Scans and Other Tests of Function in Various Organs

18. Brain	— M. Ashkenazy finds "space occupying lesions" with D°If.	[1950]	JN
	— G. Moore introduces °IHSA for brain tumor localization.	[1949]	PSEB
	— F. Moore detects tumors with K-42 with external counts.	[1950]	SF
	— B. Selverstone maps P-32 in tumors with surgical probe.	[1949]	AS
	— F. Wrenn says B^+ emitters have advantage in brain scan.	[1975]	Sc
	— L. Bakay sees bld-brn-barrier with IV P-32 tissue samples.	[1949]	ANP
19. Heart	— W. MacIntyre measures cardiac output with °IHSA (dogs).	[1949]	Cir
	— G. Burch finds very short equilib time for °Na & °Cl.	[1946]	JLCM
	— N. Thyresson studies thallium-204 distrib & excretion.	[1950]	DV
20. Liver	— K. Sterling measures °IHSA turnover in cirrhosis pts.	[1950]	JCI
	— J. DeWinters notes D°If in liver after brain scan.	[1949]	BJR
21. Lung	— R. Huff tries radiobroncho-spirometry with H-3.	[1950]	JCI
22. Bone	— H. Kerman does manual scan of Ga-72, finds hot spots.	[1949]	V80
23. Kidney	— P. Handler finds P-32 excreted mainly as glomerul filt.	[1935]	AJP
	— H. Smith's "The Kidney" published (Oxf U Press).	[1935]	Bk
	— W. Goodwin: how to measure very small °I doses in urine.	[1950]	JLCM
24. Gut	— M. Brucer takes first human dose of Co-60 labeled VB_{12}.	[1950]	AEC
	— H. Friedell reports first °IHSA pancreas test meal.	[1971]	Rad
25. Blood	— W. Caton: safe to measure °FeRBC vol in pregnant women.	[1949]	AJOG
	— G. Hevesy uses in vitro K-42 RBC tag to measure bld vol.	[1941]	APS
	— 8 articles (e.g., C. Hlad) correct RBC/plasma °assay.	[1949]	AJPh
	— R. Huff does point counting to localize °Fe in patients.	[1950]	JCI
	— N. Berlin measures RBC life span in ch-leukemia and PVA.	[1947]	Sc
	— A. Dornhorst computes theoretical RBC survival curves.	[1947]	Bl
26. Other	— I. Edelman measures body water kinetics with D_2O.	[1948]	JCI
	— P. Schloerb has falling drop method for D_2O in body fluid.	[1948]	JLCM
	— P. Hahn measures °Fe absorption in 466 pregnant women.	[1904]	AJOG
	— H. Somers finds hi P-32 uptake in malig cervix tissue.	[1942]	AS
	— M. Brucer finds Hf-181 mandelate uptake in adrenal cortex.		PSEB
	— A. Perley measures Na-24 space in 53 infants and adults.	[1949]	JP
	— W. Beierwaltes says no °I, °P, or °Cu uptake in melanomas.	[1945]	JLCM

Radiation Hysteria and Health Physics * Obituaries *

27. Hyst	— J. Mitchell's canard, "no I-131 Rx except over age 45."	[1950]	BMJ
	— NBS Hbk #19 allows so much °waste/million gals sewage.	[1949]	NBS
	— I. Chaikoff says °I causes tumors in tumor-strain rats.	[1956]	PSEB
	— E. Pirkey restricts use of Thorotrast for liver X-Ray.	[1938]	AJR
28. React	— R. Evans writes definitive rules on °isotope transport.	[1949]	NRC
	— AEC reports first human H-3 distribution & excretion.	[1948]	AEC
	— C. Ruchhoft says hospitals are a remote °isotope hazard.	[1984]	NBS
	— M. Brucer outlines hospital °protection & °hazards	[1984]	JAMA
	— R. Stone describes the beginning of Health Physics.	[1945]	NNF
	— S. Thomas: 2 ca in 4325 Thorotrast inj, insignificant.	[1927]	Rad
29. Respo	— J. Clever: 5 mCi °I dose to 10 wk pregnancy, normal baby.	[1950]	AJOG
	— Hospitals may flush so many mCi/million gals sewage.	[1948]	NBS

* * *

30. Obits	— L. Grimmett (1903–1951) Eng physics; first 5 Ci Ra bomb & Co-60.		V14

CHRONOLOGY OF NUCLEAR MEDICINE — 1952

	Scientific and Technical Background		Ref.
1. Basic	— G. White calculates absorption coeff, 10 KeV to 100 MeV.	[1930]	NBS
2. Obser	— Brookhaven cosmotron accelerates protons to 2.3 GeV.	[1948]	AEC
3. # Nuc	— G. Seaborg adds Einsteinium (#99) & Fermium (#100).	[1950]	AEC
	— J. Stokley lists 1003 isotopes on new edit of GE Chart.	[1949]	Bk
4. # Med	— AEC licenses private physicians to use °isotopes.	[1951]	AEC

	Organizations and Internal Politics		
5. AEC +	— AEC, FDA, NIH fight over who controls °isotopes.	[1949]	AEC
	— AEC policy of free °isotopes changed to 20% of cost.	[1948]	AEC
	— FDA approves use of second °isotope, P-32.	[1951]	FDA
	— NSF adds a new layer of bureaucracy to "Big" science.	[1946]	AP
6. Socs	— British authors pub first bible, "Isotopes in Medicine."	[1951]	BMB
	— "Tables for Analysis of Beta Spectra" published by NBS.	[1947]	NBS
	— Radiation Research Society incorporated in Washington, DC.	[1950]	RRS
	— V. Lavrakas reviews pre-1932 history of neutron.	[1932]	JCE
	— Am Psychiatric Assn pubs first DSM (Diag & Statist Manual of Mental Disord); describes 60 mental disorders. Dx is always without any units of measurement.	[1895]	SN89
7. Event	— First thermonuclear device (H-Bomb) exploded at Eniwetok.	[1949]	AP
	— I. Kurchatov completes first USSR H-Bomb (alleged).	[1940]	AEC
	— Isoniazid is first anti-TBC agent 70 y after Koch's bacter cause.	[1876]	SN
	— ABCC reports small heads in 4–17 wk in utero exposures.	[1956]	ABCC

	Instruments, Units of Measurement, and Drugs		
8. Instr	— H. Anger introduces a pinhole gamma camera.	[1951]	Na
	— W. Mayneord's scanner has a photo-modulated display.	[1949]	BJR
	— R. Newell introduces the "honeycomb" focus collimator.	[1950]	Nuc
	— P. Bell independently invents the "honeycomb" coll.	[1950]	AEC
	— W. Lotz pubs first instruction on "Gross Autoradiography."	[1944]	Nuc
9. Units	— British °I std "mCi" up 13%, and new decay scheme used.	[1948]	Na
	— O. Glasser-Quimby mimeo notes on dosimetry widely used.	[1949]	PL
	— R. Zirkle gives name to new Linear Energy Transfer (LET).	[1949]	JCC
	— NBS calibrates Co-60, Cs-137 to 2% accuracy (ion chamber).	[1950]	NBS
10. Concp	— F. Spiers describes a hi-sensitivity whole body counter.	[1926]	BJR
	— R. Davis distinguishes total from "exchangeable" Na space.	[1949]	Na
11. Drugs	— R. Libby introduces °iodine in capsule form.	[1938]	Nuc
	— 4 articles (e.g., B. Burrows) describe °K-42 kinetics.	[1941]	JCI
	— 4 articles (e.g., S. Berson) describe °IHSA kinetics.	[1950]	JCI
	— M. Tyor notes constant °IHSA washout from blood.	[1950]	G
	— R. Wilkins introduces first tranquilizer: reserpine.	[1949]	JAMA

	Radioiodine, P-32, and Radioactive Therapy		
12. I-Res	— J. Gross discovers T3 in human plasma.	[1948]	La
	— H. Allen develops formula for gland weight from scan area, but it averages >30% error.	[1949]	Rad
	— C. Nurnberger notes °I excreted in human mother's milk.	[1941]	JAMA
13. I-Dx	— M. Morgan devises T4 Suppression Test (requires weeks).	[1949]	JCE
	— J. Stanbury introduces Perchlorate Washout Test.	[1945]	M
	— S. Berson says plasma °I clearance is test of function.	[1947]	JCI
	— G. Howard: 24% of solitary cold nodules are malignant.	[1951]	AP
	— F. Bauer describes Cassen's first thyroid gland scans.	[1950]	JLCM
	— 39 articles (e.g., S. Berson) on various thyroid °I tests.	[1949]	JCI

14.	I-Rx	— R. Nelson reports rare thyroid crisis after °I therapy.	[1942]	IMJ
		— 13 articles (e.g., A. Freedberg) on °I Rx of hyperthyroidism.	[1951]	JCEn
		— 9 articles (e.g., E. Pochin) report °I Rx of thyroid ca.	[1950]	BMJ
		— D. CLARK FINDS NO ADVERSE REACTION TO °I Rx, ANY PLACE.	[1942]	JAMA
		— H. Dietrich attempts °I Rx of lingual thyroid.	[1949]	AORL
15.	P-Rx	— E. Osgood's P-32 Rx doubles survival years of leukemics.	[1951]	JAMA
16.	Tele	— Los Angeles 400 Curie teletherapy unit in operation.	[1922]	V14
		— L. Grimmett designs 1000 Curie Co-60 teletherapy unit.	[1922]	Rad
		— M. Brucer announces design of Cs-137 teletherapy unit.	[1950]	Nuc
17.	Other	— J. Morton describes Co-60/nylon threads for brachyRx.	[1951]	V14
		— D. Smithers converts radon implantation gun to °Au seeds.	[1928]	BJR
		— E. King reports promise of Ga-72 Dx and Rx.	[1951]	ArIM
		— E. King confirms Muller's intracav Au-198 colloid Rx.	[1949]	AJR
		— R. Flocks announces °AuCol infiltration in prostate ca.	[1951]	JU
		— M. Petrohelos reports on Sr-90 beta ray Rx in eyes.	[1950]	AJO
		— W. Sweet introduces B-10 neutron-capture Rx in brain ca.	[1955]	AEC

Scans and Other Tests of Function in Various Organs

18.	Brain	— T. Fields says Ashkenazy success is "clinical, not scan."	[1951]	SMJ
19.	Heart	— W. Yates finds "holes" in heart ARGs after IV P-32.	[1962]	AFMJ
		— W. MacIntyre develops basic cardiac output RCG formula.	[1951]	Rad
		— W. Pritchard says °IHSA RadioCardioGraphy is practical.	[1949]	Cr
		— M. Cullen injects °Na into myocardium to see blood flow.	[1950]	AJPh
20.	Liver	— D. Zilversmit: °colloid clearance rests on particle size.	[1944]	JLCM
		— S. Bradley: hepatic ischemia is hallmark of cirrhosis.	[1951]	Cr
21.	Lung	— J. Muller: large particles (>50 μm) filtered out by lungs	[1945]	RIM
22.	Bone	— E. Shorr compares Sr-89 with Ca-45 in bone studies.	[1948]	BHJD
		— J. Vaughn studies °I-gamma glob in rheumatoid arthritis.	[1983]	JCI
24.	Gut	— R. Heinle studies Co-60 $VitB_{12}$ in pernicious anemia pts.	[1951]	TAAP
25.	Blood	— E. Reeve: 20% blood in small vessels makes Ht false.	[1944]	PSEB
		— M. Brucer finds Au-198 does not affect blood clotting.	[1928]	PSEB
26.	Other	— N. Berlin measures total body water with H-3.	[1948]	JCI
		— H. Wright repeats °Na Deep Venous Thrombosis detection.	[1948]	BHJ
		— H. Crammer localizes shallow lesions with P-32 & GM.	[1942]	SMW

Radiation Hysteria and Health Physics * Obituaries *

27.	Hyst	— First AEC rad accidents (Eniwetok & Chicago) not fatal.	[1946]	AEC
		— K. Corrigan spreads rumor: possible thyroid ca from °I.	[1951]	Rad
		— I. Chaikoff withdraws study of thyroid ca in °I rats.	[1951]	PSEB
		— J. Folley records 47 leukemias in ABBC continuing study.	[1950]	ABBC
		— S. Peller: leukemic deaths in radiologists is disputed.	[1950]	AJMS
		— G. Straub: medical °wastes might become health problem.	[1951]	PHB
		— ICRP hysterically warns of possible genetic effects.	[1950]	ICRP
		— ICRP dreams up accumulated lifetime dose concept.	[1950]	ICRP
28.	React	— ICRP finds no evidence to require lower MPD levels.	[1947]	ICRP
		— A. Chamberlain: occasional WBC counts are not HP screen.	[1923]	BJR
		— L. Hempleman describes the Acute Radiation Syndrome.	[1941]	AIM
		— M. Brucer explains no rad hazard in hospital path lab.	[1951]	L
		— I. Rubin reports healthy "grandson" after ovary irrad.	[1926]	JAMA
		— Arthritics sit in deep mines to ease joint pains.	[1983]	AP
		— Montana U, Au, Ag mines "cure" arthritis. (Rn = 0.8 mr/hr).	[1971]	AP
		Los Alamos discovers free beer is Rx for H-3 overexpos.	[1951]	AEC
29.	Respo	— R. Huff: chelating agent increases excretion of Fe-55.	[1949]	PSEB
		— AEC sets 3R in 10 weeks as MPD off-site in 1952 tests.	[1950]	AEC
		— F. Spiers finds human °body burden highly variable.	[1939]	Bk

* * *

30. Obits —

CHRONOLOGY OF NUCLEAR MEDICINE — 1953

	Scientific and Technical Background		Ref.
1. Basic	— F. Reines: first experimental verification of the neutrino.	[1933]	PR
2. Obser	— K. Luden measures X-ray spectrum with NaI (Tl) crystal.	[1950]	AEC

	Organizations and Internal Politics		
5. AEC +	— AEC Subhuman Comm publishes criteria for human use.	[1948]	AEC
	— L. Strauss becomes chairman of AEC (enforces secrecy).	[1947]	Bk
	— AEC announces first University (NC) reactor goes critical.	[1943]	AEC
	— FDA transferred to HEW (Dept of Health, Educ, Welfare).	[1938]	FR
6. Socs	— FIRST M.D. TNG COURSE PUB AS "RADIOISOTOPES IN MEDICINE."	[1948]	RIM
	— F. Spear's "Radiations and Living Cells" pub by Wiley.	[1935]	Bk
7. Event	— H. Jaffee successfully treats Seaborg's mother, I-131.	[1948]	HNM
	— Mallory & Co produce Heavymet: W-Cu-Ni shielding alloy.	[1903]	PL
	— Abbott Labs opens Oak Ridge radiopharmaceutical plant.	[1950]	AEC
	— Hammersmith (London) starts first med linear accelerator.	[1903]	Na
	— "Piltdown man" is found to be a scientific hoax.	[1912]	Sc

	Instruments, Units of Measurement, and Drugs		
8. Instr	— P. BELL PUTS FIRST MEDICAL SPECTROMETER IN ORINS HOSPITAL.	[1950]	AEC
	— Los Alamos liquid scint whole body counter announced.	[1952]	AEC
	— G. Brownell announces first MIT-MGH positron scanner.	[1952]	Nuc
	— G. Brownell modifies his 4-quad, 4-xtal thyroid counter.	[1952]	JCE
	— H. Anger develops "glow tube" whole body scanner.	[1952]	AEC
	— Windscale detector can measure 0.2 pCi I-131/ml water.	[1950]	AEA
	— F. Daniels invents thermoluminescent dosimetry.	[1965]	SC
	— J. Schulman introduces glass "fluorod" for internal dose.	[1965]	Sc
	— A. Martin develops gas chromatography.	[1944]	SN
	— M. Ter-Pogossian uses 2 cm × 4 cm dia NaI (Tl) crystal.	[1950]	AJR
	— NaI (Tl) scan crystals 1/2 to 1 1/2 inch dia in commercial instr; by 1956 2" dia, by 1959 3" dia, by 1964 5" dia. were common sizes; 8" dia introduced in 1966.	[1950]	JNM
9. Units	— G. Failla point source dosimetry in extrapolation chamber.	[1947]	RSI
	— ICRU accepts 100 ergs/g as "Rad," frees Curie from Ra.	[1951]	ICRU
	— ICRU says "r" is valid only up to 3 MeV.	[1937]	ICRU
10. Concp	— R. Loevinger measures point source beta dose.	[1947]	Nuc
	— H. Vetter: ext counts makes clearance studies practical.	[1950]	JCI
	— B. Cassen complains, scanning not confined to thyroid.	[1950]	AEC
	— F. Mclean confirms Krebs' body burden °activity values.	[1959]	MS
11. Drug	— B. Benacerraf finds heated IHSA forms colloid macroagg.	[1949]	BJEP
	— R. Barclay measures thallium-204 distribution in animal.	[1975]	JPET
	— W. Love finds K-42, Rb-86, Cs-134 trace K metabolism.	[1951]	JLCM

	Radioiodine, P-32, and Radioactive Therapy		
12. I-Res	— P. Starr finds hyperthyroid gland insensitive to T3 & T4.	[1950]	TAAP
	— G. Andrews: both I-131 & X-ray beams spare thyroid "rim."	[1952]	AJM
	— C. Schmidt measures I-131 bio half-time at 3–8 days.	[1940]	LI
	— H. Allen's formula for gland wt from scan area doesn't work (10 others all approach 0.33 area, all have c30% error).	[1952]	Rad
13. I-Dx	— 31 articles (e.g., M. Barry) evaluate thyroid tests.	[1952]	M
	— J. Storaasli proposes 3 hour TSH stimulated uptake test.	[1950]	NEJM
	— N. Specht finds distant metastases by scanning.	[1952]	AJM
	— K. Taber recommends whole body scanning (takes hours).	[1981]	MVMJ
	— M. Morton pushes Butanol Extractable °I (BE°I) test.	[1951]	CM
	— M. Brucer decries profusion of poor uptake techniques.	[1962]	RIA

14. I-Rx	— 12 articles (e.g., L. Seed) describe hyperthyroid Rx tech.	[1952]	JCEn
	— 10 articles (e.g., S. Wollman) describe thyroid ca Rx.	[1952]	JNCI
15. P-Rx	— L. Heilmeyer says chemotherapy as good as P-32 in leuk,	[1952]	Str
	actually better because no AEC license required.	[1947]	PL
	— M. Tubiana summarizes French use of P-32 in Rx.	[1952]	RIM
17. Other	— M. Brucer says Ga-72 of no value in Rx of bone tumors.	[1952]	Rad
	— 15 major studies confirm value of Au-198 intracav Rx.	[1951]	RIM
	— G. Andrews tries IV Au-198 for CGLeukemia (not good).	[1950]	JLCM
	— P. Harper introduces Y-90 (beads) pituitary implants.	[1976]	SF
	— H. Berg uses interstitial °Au to irradiate lymph nodes.	[1951]	ArS
	— G. Kyker irradiates lymph nodes with sub-Q °rare earths.	[1951]	RIM
	— J. Van de Erve: pigmented skin on long term thorium-X Rx.	[1947]	SMJ
	— A. Sherman uses °AuCol inject in palliative pelvic ca.	[1951]	ca

Scans and Other Tests of Function in Various Organs

18. Brain	— D. Kohl fits 18 detectors over skull for multi-points.	[1950]	Nuc
	— S. Kety measures Cerebral Blood Flow with IV Na-24.	[1949]	V51
	— E. Dobson studies °Na injection vol-vs-clearance rate.	[1949]	Cir
	— F. Bauer introduces myelogram scans with °IHSA.	[1950]	N
19. Heart	— R. Shipley gets cardiac output with MacIntyre RCG formula.	[1952]	CR
	— W. Love starts Rb-86 & Cs-134 myocardial scanning.	[1952]	JLCM
	— A. Luisada adds simultaneous ECG to RadioCardioGraphy.	[1948]	Sc
20. Liver	— E. Yuhl introduces °AuCol Kupffer's cell liver scans.	[1952]	AnS
	— E. Dobson introduces the $Cr°PO_4$ liver bld-flow measure.	[1950]	Cir
22. Bone	— R. Bernstein solves cyclotron production method of F-18.	[1940]	Nuc
	— A. Black measures P-32 turnover in bone of dairy cow.	[1943]	PSEB
23. Kidney	— C. Hlad explores inulin-vs-I-131 glomerular clearance.	[1951]	JLCM
24. Gut	— R. SCHILLING INTRODUCES °Co TEST FOR INTRINSIC FACTOR.	[1952]	JLCM
	— M. Hoffman tells method for labeling °I-fats.	[1951]	JLCM
25. Blood	— F. Ebaugh starts °CrRBC survival test (for bld storage).	[1951]	JLCM
	— G. LeRoy introduces a clinical °CrRBC survival test.	[1951]	JLCM
	— H. Chaplin finds body/venous Ht ratio constant, all Ht's.	[1952]	JCI
	— A. Feinstein devises serum iron-binding-capacity method.	[1949]	JLCM
	— N. Berlin measures P-32 blood vol in 157 pregnancies.	[1951]	SGO
26. Other	— A. Chinn uses °IHSA test meal in DX of pancreas insuff.	[1951]	JLCM
	— G. Andrews does first scans of intracavitary °AuCol.	[1950]	RIM
	— K. Stern shows lymph node uptake of interstitial $°LaCl_3$.	[1950]	JNCI
	— O. Wright finds venous flow slowed by prolonged bedrest.	[1952]	La
	— M. Brucer studies lymph node irrad with °rare earths.	[1950]	AEC

Radiation Hysteria and Health Physics * Obituaries *

27. Hyst	Pres Eisenhower proposes Int Atoms for Peace program.	[1946]	AP
	— ICRP adopts MPC for 100 °isotopes (NBS Hdbk #52).	[1950]	NBS
	— ICRP recommends 1/10 MPD for general population.	[1950]	ICRP
	— Highest fallout ever in St. George, Utah, at 1.3 $\mu Ci/m_3$.	[1957]	Nuc
	— AEC is accused of causing tornados and spring storms.	[1945]	AP
	— L. Russel suggests women's X-Rays only post-menstruation.	[1952]	JAMA
28. React	— J. Hidalgo develops syringe shield for °isotope inject.	[1950]	JAMA
	— C. Brunner notes normal baby delivered after hi-dose °I.	[1952]	SMW
	— R. Rugh reports no effect from 1 μCi/d I-131 for 6 mo.	[1952]	Bk
	— AEC finds "ultimate" waste disposal; fix °X in clay.	[1952]	AEC
29. Respo	— D. Bratt shows Windscale accident yielded only pCi.	[1962]	AEA

* * *

30. Obits	— R. Millikan (1868–1953) Am physics; charge on the electron.		DSB

LOWELL ERF AND POLYCYTHEMIA

(P-32 "Cures" Leukemias & Polycythemias)

This story was told to me over a long beer in Oklahoma City in 1952. Lowell and I were attending an "isotope" meeting, but had become fed up with sample counting trivia and had left to regain enthusiasm at the bar. Lowell was then in pediatrics because he was an expert on P-32 therapy of leukemias. Leukemia was largely geriatric and most of his patients were over 40, but there was no "senior citizen" money in those days. Most of his research funds came from childhood leukemia. In his basic science research he could get all the blood he needed from little people. Erf's primary interest was "blood," not "disease."

Lowell Erf's Formal Introduction to P-32

Fourteen years earlier, in 1938, Erf had been assigned to an internship under an unknown Dr. John Lawrence at UC–Berkeley. The new 36 inch cyclotron was producing radioisotopes faster than anybody could write papers to announce them. Hematology was also a newly recognized field. Lowell went into Hematology because patients were rarely emergencies. Hematology was quiet and clean. The only dirt would be an occasional spot of blood on his uniform.

Lowell reported to the Crocker Lab, expecting to examine patients. He was dressed in white coat and pants and had the required stethoscope hanging around his neck. In addition to the excitement of his first day as an intern — stories at medical school told of non-stop 25 hour days with hundreds of patients waiting in line — he learned that his service had one patient. But, he was told, he had the honor of being the first man in history to use a new medicine; it was called phosphorus. New interns were chosen for their strong legs and would he please climb the hill to the cyclotron lab to pick up the phosphorus.

Now Lowell had heard of phosphorus even before medical school in Boston: firecrackers, matches, sodas, that sort of stuff. But who could account for the lack of learning among Californians? He climbed the hill to what he expected to be a sparkling clean pharmacy called cyclo-something. He was directed to an old wooden building that was undoubtedly the oldest on campus. Upon entering, he was appalled by the machine shop, or was it a foundry — had anyone ever swept, let alone scrubbed, the floor?

The first to greet Erf was a small mongrel dog with an obvious, but clinically undiagnosed, diabetes insipidus. With no chairs in evidence, Lowell sat down on a small lead pot and played with the dog. "Nice doggie," said Lowell patting the dog on the head. The dog answered on the pot after the manner of his kind.

Suddenly the hum of the cyclotron died down. The sterile smell of ozone plus a touch of insolvency tainted the air, and Paul Aebersold's voice screamed out from behind a mountain of 5-gal water cans used for shielding,

"Keep that fool dog away from the pot you're sitting on!"

"Why?"

"That's the medicine for your patient."

Thus, Lowell Erf MD was introduced to the high-tech of "radioisotope medicine."

Polycythemia Vera: An Afterthought in Rx

G. Hevesy's 1935 phosphorus metabolism studies required more P-32 than the nanocuries he could make on Bohr's neutron howitzer. E.O. Lawrence furnished him with millicurie runs from the cyclotron, and got first hand reports of P-32 tracer biochemistry in return. This led Gilbert Lewis, Dean of Chemistry at Berkeley, to set up the first school of radiochemistry in conjunction with the Rad Lab at Berkeley. Martin Kamen, and then Waldo Cohn, made tremendous (for then) amounts of P-32 for the whole range of tracer chemistry. [See Vig1946 .Pub]

John Lawrence was most interested in the therapeutic possibilities of the cyclotron and the isotopes that poured out of it. [See Vig1937 .JL] In his first paper describing the therapy of chronic leukemias with P-32 he mentioned polycythemia vera therapy almost as an afterthought. It would be reported separately because this job had been assigned to Lowell Erf. (AnIM, 15:487, 1941)

Erf explained that the P-32 did not destroy red blood cells, rather it depressed hematopoiesis in bone marrow. Because of a red cell's 120 day life span, immediate relief of symptoms was not expected. Phlebotomies for immediate relief always preceded an oral dose of 3 to 4 millicuries (150 MBq). Red cell counts done frequently were expected to show a slow fall in cells in about six weeks, to a maximum effect in about three months. The RBC count may continue to fall for up to 7 months, but more often resumes a slow climb back to polycythemic levels. A second dose, usually after about 4 to 6 months, was usually required.

Reaction to P-32 Therapies

With the initial declassification of MED reports (Manhattan Engineering District Declassified Documents), D. Anthony revealed that the LD_{50} of IV P-32 for man (derived from animal data) was in the range of 270 mCi (10 GBq). Even with a tremendous error for translation from animal to man, this data made P-32 a very safe drug. By 1955 J. Harman said P-32 was the treatment of choice in England (Brit Med J, 1955). After over 15 years followup J. Lawrence said his patients were living a normal life span. In 1958 J. Fountain began treating thrombocythemia patients with equal success. (Brit Med J, 1958)

The occasional death from leukemia of an atom bomb survivor became, in 1960 newspapers, a 100% certainty of radiation leukemia after even minimal exposure to radiation. (Actually, 40 years later it turned out to be an 0.2% chance of leukemia and only in those surviving >200 R exposure.) A number of patients given P-32 were reported, in great flares of publicity, to have died of acute leukemia. In 1959 J. Lawrence pointed out that a flare-up of acute leukemia was the expected cause-of-death in polycythemia. The high incidence in patients *not* treated with P-32, and so few in patients treated, suggested that P-32 prevented the acute leukemia death. Then in 1960, E. Lesli, working from a long series of patients, gave statistical proof that P-32 prolonged the life span of polycythemia patients. (CR, 1960)

Radiophobia and the Decline of P-32

During the 1970s P-32 gradually lost its popularity for reasons easily understood. Every hematologist needed only one license to do chemotherapy; however, in order to use P-32 on even an occasional polycythemia patient he had to have an MD plus a second "license to use radioisotopes." A recent (1983) issue of Current Therapy points out that the choice therapy must be given by a physician with a special license. Along with each radioisotope license came inspection by arrogant, often insulting, inspectors and increased insurance rates.

In 1984 the Sixth International Colloquium on Radioimmunoassay at Lyons, France, reported that chemotherapy has its own morbidity; it is dreaded by many patients, and subtracts rather than adds to the life span. The major fault of radioactivity as choice therapy, they said, was government bureaucracy.

Much the same story of avoiding the stifling AEC licensure occurred after J. Fountain announced "cures" of thrombocythemia. (Brit Med J, 1958) The licensure criteria forbids use in normal patients, but the recommendation is for dosage even before the patient becomes symptomatic. Chemotherapy was slightly successful in treating the chronic leukemias, but nobody has yet repeated Osgood's feeling that his P-32 patients were actually living longer, and healthier, lives than the controls in his series.

In a 15 April 1986 NY Times story on the results of the billions of $$$ wasted in the War-on-Cancer, the GAO (General Accounting Office) found no improvement in 20 years, but much exaggeration, in the treatment of chronic leukemias. However, the patient's discomfort from chemotherapy cannot match his doctor's discomfort with the Nuclear Regulatory Commission.

A Remnant of the P-32 Success Story

Lowell Erf's first patient, as an intern on John Lawrence's service in Berkeley, was one of the first to receive therapeutic P-32. After the secrecy of all things nuclear subsided around 1950, P-32 became the world wide therapy of choice for polycythemias. After 50 years it remains so except in the USA, where an insane regulatory mania and newspaper radiophobia has minimized its use.

AN ATOMIC PILE (ALMOST) TWO YEARS BEFORE STAGG FIELD

(Or, Why Canada Uses Heavy Water Reactors)

During the first months after Hahn and Strassman's 1939 fission article, nearly 100 confirmations were printed — then publication was snuffed out. George C. Laurence at Canada's National Research Council (NRC) guessed why and felt that Canada, a prime source of uranium, should be in on it. He mobilized NRC's small physics staff and borrowed a ton of uranium from Eldorado Gold Mines Ltd.

Fermi's papers had already suggested moderators necessary to chain reaction: helium, heavy water, beryllium or carbon. The US had all the helium, D_2O was produced in droplets; beryllium was scarce; but carbon they had up to their ears in the form of petroleum coke. Laurence ordered 10 tons. The fine powder was delivered to Ottawa's NRC building in 50 lb bags — mostly broken and leaking an all-pervasive talcum of blackness. The cubical bin built to contain 10 tons received about 9. The rest coated the walls, covered desks, and clung to skin. Blonde secretaries developed a dark patina that couldn't be washed off.

A Ra-Be neutron trigger was centered between uranium oxide packages throughout the pile. Each instrument poked into the pile raised another cloud of coke. After a day of measurements the "black gang" could not wash off enough coke to be recognizable even to close friends. The pile never went critical — it wasn't meant to. But this nuclear assembly taught a lot about slow neutrons. A scientific mission from England found their measurements interesting, but did they know of the very clean work done with heavy water? And then on 2 Dec 1942 the second pile, in Chicago, went critical.

The Canadians moved everything to Chalk River. On 5 Sept 1945, a few days after Hiroshima, 5 tons of uranium metal rods and 7600 lbs of D_2O, Canada's second reactor, ZEEP, went critical. History says that the August 1943 Quebec Conference gave Canada the heavy water reactor job. But they merely ratified a conclusion. After 1942 there wasn't enough soap in all Ontario to support another carbon moderated reactor.

THE FIRST SCAN WAS OF THE WHOLE BODY

(As told by R. Ball in a 1962 letter)

"In 1939 Hamilton and Soley published studies on °iodine metabolism. [AJPH] They could detect iodine inside the body with a device called a Geiger-Müller tube. We radiology interns couldn't locate the thyroid on X-Rays.

"Shortly thereafter, rotating in radiotherapy at Presbyterian (Columbia U), I was assigned a patient with a pathological fracture of the humerus. Maude Richardson had a scar on her neck and lumps in her scalp. I aspirated some tissue from one of the scalp tumors. Microscopic section showed well differentiated thyroid with colloid.

"Walter Palmer, head of Medicine, thought Maude was perfect to find out what happened to thyroid metastases under °iodine treatment. He furnished the money and contact with MIT for °iodine. Albert Keston, a chemist, had a GM tube for some of his work. He showed us how to use the thing. Virginia Frantz, a surgical pathologist, thought the °iodine trial great fun.

"I was told to call Edith Quimby and Leo Marinelli at Memorial, for details on dosage and how to handle the stuff. Both said they knew absolutely nothing about how to calculate a °iodine dose. (A few years later I learned they were caught up in the Manhattan District Project and understood their closed mouths.)

"Maude was given her first dose of °iodine by mouth on 6 Dec 1941. The reason I remember the date so well was because I had the job of moving the GM tube slowly all over her body and marking the hot spots. It became tedious for both of us after a while and I turned on the radio. Suddenly the music stopped and a voice announced, *"Pearl Harbor has been bombed."*

"Two months later I was watching Army Training Films at Fort Meade. Having nothing else to do I published a brief report in Science (95:362, 1942). Virginia Frantz wrote Richardson's autopsy report for Annals of Surgery (119:668, 1944)."

BLOOD VOLUME AS CLINICAL PHYSIOLOGY

(Rowntree Measures a Plasma Volume)

Three items were required for the introduction of modern surgery:

1) **Bacterial sterility** (quite sophisticated procedures were available by 1915)
2) **Anesthesia** (ether was predominant in general, but many local agents were used)
3) **Fluid balance** was still esoteric in 1915 and primarily involved whole blood.

Measurement of blood volume was a laboratory rather than clinical exercise. Bischoff's 1856 decapitation method and Haldane's 1899 CO poisoning were somewhat heroic measures for clinicians. [See Vig1856 .BV] Other plasma diluents were tried: dextrin, protein, anti-toxin, acacia, but blood volume was essentially investigative until 1915. N. Keith and L. Rowntree introduced an innocuous plasma diluent dye: Vital Red, later Congo Red, that made blood volume popular. [ArIM, 1915]

Vital Red was diluted to a convenient volume and became the colorimeter standard. A measured portion was then injected into one arm vein. After 5 minutes for mixing in the body, a blood sample was withdrawn from the opposite arm. After centrifuging the blood, a sample of the plasma was decanted. The sample and standard were matched in an eyeball colorimeter. Welcker's 1854 formula gave the Plasma Volume:

$$\frac{\text{Standard}}{\text{sample}} \times \text{dilut of Std} \times \text{ml inj} = \text{PV}$$

Plasma volume multiplied by a plasmacrit was the blood volume.

In 1929 Rowntree published the definitive pre-°nuclide text, "Volume of Blood and Plasma in Health and Disease," that made the subject clinical routine. Rowntree's group recognized all of the possible errors of the technique: dye diffusion, absorption, and leakage — all except one. In 1942 Paul Hahn recognized an error visible to every medical student who looked at a tissue section through a microscope. It was an obvious plasmacrit error that was not obvious until he recognized it.

[See Vig1936 .GHP P-32 & Fe-55]

RBC BLOOD VOLUME MEASUREMENTS

By 1935, after an exhaustive search, M. Gregersen selected T-1824 (Evan's Blue) to replace Congo Red as the choice plasma dye for volume measurements. Trapping of plasma in even highly centrifuged blood was a major source of error in measuring the hematocrit. Perhaps an RBC tag should replace the plasma tag. [See Vig1936 .GHP]

So far, the only true blood volume was Welcker's 1856 body drainage — clinically unacceptable. Haldane's CO RBC label was also unacceptable. Rowntree's Congo Red plasma label was shown to be in error. Then, in 1936, Hevesy introduced P-32.

Hevesy made his own P-32 to study labile pools of phosphates in blood. He noticed a seemingly non-labile absorption of P-32 in RBC. He discovered that red cells thus labeled in vitro could be reinjected into the body. With a °isotope dilution calculation (his 1931 invention) labeled red cells allowed measurement of °P-RBC blood volume. He tried it on rabbits in 1939. [ARR 1962] Many years later Hevesy considered P-32 blood volume his great contribution to Nuclear Medicine, but it was flawed with the same hematocrit error as Rowntree's plasma label.

A graduate student in G. Whipple's pathology group (U of Rochester) had been working with °Fe in anemia studies. [AJMS 1936] Paul Hahn developed lab techniques to handle Berkeley's 47 day Fe-59 (very difficult to work with). Most problems in °Fe turnover involved a blood volume. Hahn could not match the precision of °Fe dilution with total body blood volumes. The error seemed to be in the hematocrit, so he studied its measurement.

Hahn measured both cell and plasma volumes in many animals by four independent methods:

1. Welcker's viviperfusion,
2. by phlebotomy,
3. by regeneration,
4. by donor cell dilution.

He found the 20–25% hematocrit error. Large vessel differed from small vessel hematocrits. True total body hematocrit varied widely from the usual arm vein hematocrit.

[See Vig1951 .G&S; The °Cr blood label]

THE RESEARCH INTRODUCTION OF °IHSA
(Fine & Seligman Invent a °Pharmaceutical)

World War II stimulated renewed interest in traumatic shock. Jacob Fine and Arnold Seligman were surgeons on the staff of Beth Israel Hospital and Harvard Medical School in Boston. In 1942 World War II was just beginning to empty the Boston schools and hospitals of non-war related research. MIT, for example, was already deeply involved in RADAR, then considered much more important and secret than wild ideas about "atomic energy."

Any atomic business would center around the MIT cyclotron and it was not unusually busy. It was grinding out fairly routine radioiodine for quite a few hospitals. But this work was dying down because so many physicians had gone into the armed services. Fine and Seligman, however, had a small research project started that was of direct interest to both Army and Navy.

The "Lost Plasma" Problem in Surgery

Current surgical dogma said that traumatic shock was manifested by an increased permeability of capillaries with loss of plasma from the circulating blood volume. If the loss were not an obvious hemorrhage or a weeping in burns, it might be hidden in surrounding tissues. If this "lost volume" was replaced early, shock did not occur. If >40% of plasma was lost, shock was fatal.

This nice quantification had no predictive value in trauma therapy because capillary leakage was not detectable by any known test. Hence, "lost plasma" was hypothesis only. If it were proved true, plasma replacement rather than whole blood could be used in some trauma surgery — an item of considerable importance to the military.

A Plasma Protein is Tagged with S-35

Fine and Seligman felt that any lost fluid must follow plasma protein leakage. In the intellectual excitement following Robley Evans' new MIT cyclotron, it was natural for them to consider tagging a plasma protein. Sulfur was a natural part of the protein molecule, and there was a known °isotope of sulfur. S-35 was an 87.2 day pure beta emitter.

The two surgeons synthesized some S-35 1-Cystine. After IV injection into a few normal and shocked dogs they measured °S washout in blood. It was a simple and successful experiment. But........

°Bromine Replaces °Sulfur

S-35 was available only occasionally, and in small amounts, and there was only a 2% yield of tagged protein. Fine and Seligman were not satisfied and looked for a better tag. The cyclotron people suggested °bromine. Its high cyclotron yield was matched by a high tagged protein yield. A gamma decay made °measurement much simpler. Using the falling drop method, they measured plasma volume in a series of dogs to make sure the new °bromo-protein behaved the same as the "naturally" tagged °S-protein. It did. On a series of control and shocked dogs they found washout of °plasma identical in both groups. Therefore, plasma loss into tissue was not a critical factor in shock. (JCI, 1943) But........

°Iodine Replaces °Bromine

Consistent halogenation of plasma protein required a uniform and a minimal amount of halogen. Cyclotron production of °Br required large volumes (>300 mg) of stable Br which resulted in low specific activity. Large amounts of stable bromine tended to degrade the protein it was tagging. °Iodine, on the other hand (the MIT cyclotron's best seller), was produced from tellurium targets. The volume of carrier iodine was controlled at below 5 mg. So Fine and Seligman replaced bromo-protein with a new iodo-protein to reduce the errors implicit in labeling. They repeated the entire experiment and added hemorrhagic, tourniquet, and burn shock to confirm their original conclusion with S-35.

(JCI 23:720, 1944)

Far more important, although they didn't know it, Fine and Seligman had just invented °Iodinated Serum Albumin. In six years it would become the first true radiopharmaceutical.

[See Vig1943 .°PV; Storaasli's °IHSA]

THE DISCOVERY OF °IHSA

(Storaasli Remembers Fine & Seligman)

M. Gregersen revived Evan's Blue as T-1824 (JLCM, 1938). It was the dominant blood volume agent and, up until the 1950s, was a gold standard for plasma dyes. WWII brought renewed interest in surgical shock, and the problem of "lost plasma," unmeasurable with T-1824, needed investigation. The success of P-32 RBC labeling in blood volume studies stimulated J. Fine and A. Seligman to look for a radioactive label. They tried S-35.

Synthesis of °S-plasma protein was difficult and they could get few samples of °S. (Cyclotron time was now controlled by a secret Manhattan District.) They tried a °bromo-protein and it seemed to work well, except the large amounts of carrier bromine caused the plasma protein to denature.

A carrier free °iodine could be obtained from bombarded tellurium. They devised a method for tagging bovine plasma with °iodine. (JCI 23:720, 1944) Some free °iodine was inevitable in their final product, but it was swept out of blood almost immediately by the thyroid gland. It was a very successful blood volume agent, with the exception, of course, of the availability of °I.

During the war years R. Evans supplied about 36 hospitals with small amounts of °I from the MIT cyclotron, mostly for thyroid work. But in wartime practice there was little time for innovation.

[See Vig1936 .°I]

Storaasli Remembers an Old Wartime Study

By early 1946 the Manhattan District had the capability for making megacuries of °I. A few scientists felt that °isotopes had to be made available. [See Vig1946 .Pub] In 1949 J. Storaasli remembered the Fine and Seligman work with °I labeled bovine serum albumin. He found it easy to substitute Human Serum Albumin for the objectionable bovine albumin. °Iodine was now easily available. He made a batch and called it °IHSA. (SGO 91:456, 1950)

[See Vig1949 .Phr, °Pharmaceuticles]

THE ULTIMATE IN SECRECY

(Lawrence Treats a Patient With P-32)

One morning in the fall of 1944 a DC3 and a C47 airplane left Knoxville, Tennessee airport, each with a package bound for Berkeley, California. (The DC3 and C47 were the same model airplane, but one had its passenger seats ripped out to carry Army Air Corps cargo.)

The C47 cargo was a 12 inch cube package — an unmarked cardboard box that seemed quite heavy. It contained a lead pot holding a glass vial labeled P-32. It was the regular monthly shipment of one curie from Oak Ridge (20 miles from Knoxville) to John Lawrence at the U of California cyclotron Laboratory.

Lawrence had been treating leukemia patients with P-32 for almost 7 years. His P-32 was made at the University until the Manhattan Atom Bomb Project preempted their cyclotron to make the first plutonium. In order to keep the new work secret John was instructed to continue his P-32 work with lots of papers and talks. P-32 would be supplied in lavish amounts — one curie per month — from the new reactor at Oak Ridge.

The First Package was for the Second

The second "package" that left Knoxville, on the DC3, was a child who had leukemia. In the absence of any other form of therapy his doctors had opted for a new radiation therapy being tried at the University of California. P-32 had been remarkably successful in a few adult leukemics — cures not claimed, but some were still alive.

The two packages arrived in Berkeley about the same time. The Knoxville child was treated 3000 miles from home with P-32 made in his back yard. Except that the therapy was worthless (we didn't know that in 1944), it was a successful trip. Army security was pleased with the highly publicized deception. Lawrence, though distressed at his failure, learned that P-32 was of no use in childhood leukemia. The child was said to have been thrilled by his cross-country flight.

[See Vig1940 .Erf, Polycythemia]

THE FIRST ATOM BOMB EXPOSURES

(From Final Report ORO-631 TID-4500, 6/65)

On 19 July 1945 the first atomic bomb was exploded in the desert near Alamogordo, NM. Just beyond a large test site that had been carefully cleared of all humans and large animals, a herd of Hereford cattle was grazing on the sparse desert vegetation. The radioactive cloud from the "Trinity" explosion drifted over the cattle, and the first radioactive "fallout" settled on their backs.

The unexpected exposures were not known until many hours post-explosion; hence, the dose to the cattle had to be estimated from "fallout" decay products (the first public use of the term fallout). Apparently the animals had been exposed to 150 r of total body gamma radiation and 40,000 rep of beta radiation to the skin on their backs. To an untrained observer (there were no radiation observers trained on cows) few of the animals seemed to show signs of irradiation illness. Within a few weeks the only sign of effect was patches of depigmented hair caused by beta burns.

A Study of the Cattle is Authorized

Six months after exposure — no records had been kept of the herd — the importance of observing the exposed animals was finally realized, and 60 were shipped to Oak Ridge for study of irradiation effects. Cattle are unusual laboratory animals and no knowledgeable observations were made. Two years later the U of Tennessee–AEC Agricultural Experiment Station Laboratory was formed with trained veterinary pathologists and facilities for large animal study.

An active study of fertility, reproduction, and growth of offspring was maintained from 1948 through 1951. No detrimental effects of irradiation were observed (except for the now white beta burn patches). In 1952 disaster struck: 42 of the animals developed *anaplasmosis*, a rickettsial infection of cattle transmitted by ticks (and unrelated to radiation). In compliance with state law they had to be killed. Only 11 of the original 60 cattle remained.

Breeding for Expected Genetic Damage

Out of 115 possible breeding years for the 11 cows, 98 calves were born — a rate within normal limits. Six were dead at, or shortly after birth — slightly fewer than expected. The offspring were considered an exceptionally healthy lot. The incidence of disease in the original 11 cows was normal. Squamous cell carcinoma of the eye — common in Herefords — was normal. Three cows who survived over 15 years post-irradiation — almost the life span of cows — developed small squamous cell carcinoma in the beta burn patches on their backs.

Cause of Death: Euthanasia, NOT Radiation

In 1964, 19 years post-irradiation — very old age for cattle — the remnants of the Alamogordo herd were "euthanized" because of rapidly declining old age. In November the last cow had a malignancy around the left bony orbit that did not respond to treatment. She was killed in order to save the entire skin for mounting as a museum specimen. The "beta burn" lesions were representative of the primary lesion of very high dose fallout irradiation.

The Alamogordo cattle irradiation was not a planned experiment. It was a chance event observed for any lessons that could be learned. But by the end of the 1950s many of us watching these animals saw that high dose exposure did not affect genetics or reproduction mechanisms. It did NOT shorten the life span — if anything, it fit hormesis data on increased life span. A few minor carcinomas appeared in radiation damaged skin, but only at very high dose and after almost a lifetime. Needless to say, these observations did not fit common knowledge or official cant. Cyril Comar, head of the project, and John Rust, its veterinary pathologist, already had extensive experiments on large animals in progress. They, incidentally, verified the observations on the Alamogordo cattle.

The biological effect of this first accidental exposure was verified when the Atom Bomb Casualty Commission studied the effects of the first deliberate exposure. Radiation, except at very high dose, does not cause much damage.

[See Vig1981 .Hor, Hormesis]

ISOTOPES WITHOUT RED TAPE

(The First and the Last Time it Occurred)

During the early months of 1945 a few scientists, aware of the full scope of the atom bomb effort, noticed that the project had achieved its primary goal. Hanford was making unmentioned plutonium and shipping it regularly. Los Alamos scientists had feelings of "we're-in-the-last-phase." Oak Ridge's unmentioned gas separation of enriched U-235 was in high speed, but routine, production. The race among the Oak Ridge pile drivers to make bomb materials was shifting to "how do we use this cornucopia?" [See Vig1947 .OR]

Concurrent with completion of the first atomic bombs in the spring of 1945, these scientists thought about the future of the Project's °isotope production potential. For some reason *radio*isotopes always got the glamor treatment. Stable isotopes were more important in chemistry and just as headline grabbing — witness heavy water in 1931. [See Vig1933 .D_2O] But the production cyclotrons at Y-12 in Oak Ridge did not make large volumes of stable isotopes. They slowly enriched small samples — as exciting as watching grass grow. It took almost 30 years to complete an all-element inventory.

Radioisotopes Should Be Released

Karl Compton, on the Project's advisory board, knew that Robley Evans was eking out °I to many hospitals (36 in all). Robert Stone, who watched over health physics at all locations, knew of the hidden medical demand for °isotopes. Somebody approached Col. R. Nicholls, Gen. Leslie Groves' administrator, and suggested that isotopes be released to non-project scientists.

In the spring of 1945 the decision was made to produce °isotopes for civilian use. The Oak Ridge reactor could make most of them by the megacurie. Waldo Cohn, one of the Berkeley P-32 biochemists, had made the first reactor P-32 and was among those who suggested its distribution to civilian scientists. (He wrote the first announcement of °isotope availability in Science 1946.) But he did not want the job of overseeing distribution because his interest was basic science, not in applied development.

Robert Stone, the only radiologist with hands-on experience with X-rays, neutrons, and °isotopes in human use, would not consider the job because he had never really left his Radiology Department in San Francisco. Many others were briefly considered, but by a stroke of intelligence the military brass chose the one man who already had experience in selling °isotopes.

Aebersold Becomes Chief of Isotopes

In January 1946 Paul C. Aebersold was asked to transfer from the Los Alamos Scientific Laboratory to Oak Ridge, to become Chief of the new Isotopes Branch of the Manhattan Engineering District Division of Research. Paul was a feisty PhD physicist then working in Los Alamos. He had been an early Berkeley cyclotron driver, and knew most of the chemists and biologists who had used °isotopes. He was first to try to convert neutron intensity to roentgens. [See Vig1935 .NBM] His overwhelming optimism on the ability of °isotopes to solve all measurement problems in all scientific fields (and maybe cure cancer on the side) made him top choice.

During the first months of 1946 the Isotopes Branch was a beehive of activity. There were no methods for preparation, packaging, shipment, or billing for °isotopes, or receiving funds in payment. [See Vig1953 .RPK] Neither Aebersold's superiors in Oak Ridge, nor their superiors in Washington, DC, knew anything about these small packages of "°stuff" that so many scientists and physicians wanted. So Aebersold told them how!

Aebersold Writes His Own Rules

Paul wrote memoranda on new rules for his superiors in Oak Ridge to send to their superiors in Washington. The next day he flew to Washington to be on hand when the memos were delivered. That same day he wrote the directives that his superior's superiors returned to Oak Ridge by mail. Then he flew back to Oak Ridge to receive his own directives on the new official procedure. This smooth and rapid public release of secret war-time materials has never been improved upon in the history of bureaucracy.

[See Vig1946 .Pub, First Shipment]

THE FIRST "PUBLIC" SHIPMENT OF ISOTOPES

(Part of this comes from Aebersold, the rest is O. Bizzell's story, told at the 20th anniversary of the first shipment.)

The first peacetime shipment of °isotopes from Oak Ridge occurred 2 Aug 1946. The shipment was of C-14 and went by the shortest possible route to Martin Kamen, because he had discovered C-14 in 1940 on the Berkeley cyclotron. The official history books do not tell this story because they never heard it. The truth had to be hidden from General Leslie Groves, military head of Manhattan District. Groves hated Communists but loved their system for keeping secrets. Martin had had dinner with a Communist before the war and, hence, was not allowed on the atom bomb project.

The shipment could have gone to any of 10 or 15 laboratories, but Aebersold, chief of the still new Isotopes Division, told General Groves of the public relations value of the word "CANCER." The first shipment would go to the Barnard Free Skin and Cancer Hospital in St Louis. (Incidentally, no one mentioned that Martin Kamen worked there.) Aebersold commandeered about fifty guests — all the scientists he could scrape up plus a few outsiders who had security clearance — plus, of course, a few members of the press who got their first view of still super secret Oak Ridge.

Oak Ridge is Opened — A Small Crack

In the light of the political battle then going on over the international regulation of atomic energy, the press was supposed to learn that Oak Ridge was not a bomb factory, but was now a fighter in the war against cancer. This historic First Shipment ceremony featured Eugene Wigner, scientific director of Oak Ridge, handing over a small package to Dr. E. Cowdry, representing Barnard Hospital.

The package contained 3 mg of $BaCO_3$ with 1 millicurie of C-14. Despite its small size, the contents were remarkable. This unit of C-14 was 1000 times more than had ever been produced in any single cyclotron order. It was priced at $370, about 0.1% of estimated cyclotron production cost.

The First "Shipment" was Plural

The next day Dr. Cowdry turned over his package to Martin Kamen. After converting some of it to ascorbic acid, Kamen sent the first "civilian" C-14 to P. Rothemund at Antioch College who prepared a tagged carcinogen.

But the same day another shipment of C-14 went from Oak Ridge to D. Wilson at the U of Pennsylvania who converted it to labeled sugars for a diabetes study. (Pennsylvania papers called it the first shipment.) Another shipment went to J. Franck in Physical Chemistry at the U of Chicago to study photosynthesis. (Chicago papers called it the first.) Another shipment went to W. Armstrong in Biochemistry at the U of Minnesota to trace carbon compounds in tooth enamel. (Minnesota papers hailed it as the first.) Another went to I. Chaikoff, U of Cal, to label fats (called first in California papers). About 30 orders of various °isotopes for various uses were called first shipments by local newspapers.

About fifty different °isotopes were already available at the Oak Ridge reactor. J. Christian in pharmaceutical chemistry at Purdue got the first shipment of P-32 (the many earlier lots had been to Manhattan District contractors). He used it to study absorption of phosphates in the small intestine. A Salt Lake City agricultural research group got the first shipment of S-35 to study its metabolism in plants. Both Montefiore and Memorial Hospitals in New York got the first shipments of °iodine, °antimony, °arsenic, and °cesium. With all the newspaper hoopla on cancer therapy, Paul Hahn, in biochemistry at Vanderbilt, got the first peacetime shipment of Au-198. He used it to study its uptake in colloid form — the only shipment to be directed toward the treatment of cancer.

Who got the first peacetime shipment of °isotopes from Oak Ridge? All shipments went from reactor to postoffice in the same truck — all except the symbolic millicurie of C-14. Unknown to General Groves, but perfectly obvious to his friends who prepared the C-14 in Oak Ridge, the official first shipment of a radioisotope was a loving tribute to Martin Kamen.

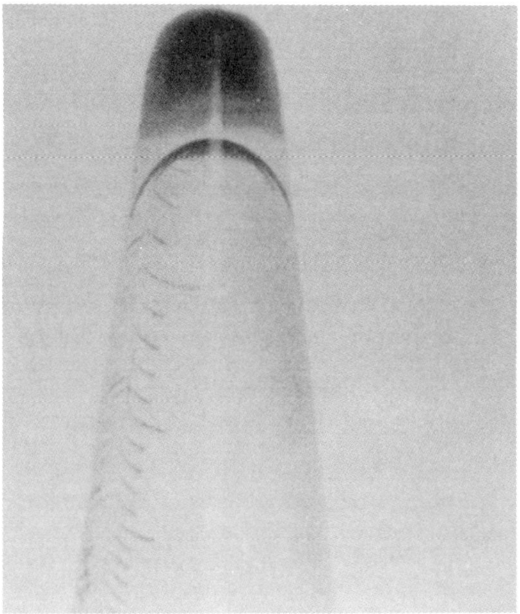

Boyd's first photomicrograph of promethium (#61) hydroxide.

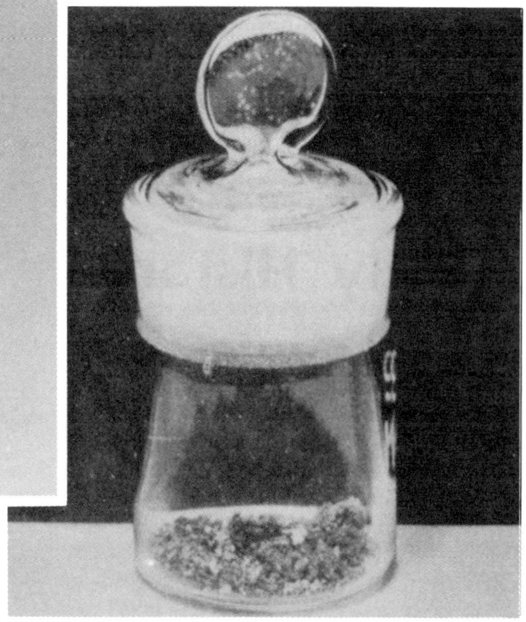

Boyd shows the first 554 mg of visible #43 (later called technetium)

MENDELEEV'S TABLE IS OFFICIALLY COMPLETED

(As told to me by G. Boyd, Japan, 1958)

An important early achievement of Manhattan Engineering District's (MED) Chemistry Division was development of Waldo Cohn's separation of high-specific-activity P-32 from reactor-irradiated sulfur. For years it was shipped from Oak Ridge to Berkeley for release as a cyclotron-produced product. This deception was considered necessary to hide its true origin. The Berkeley cyclotron was irradiating uranium for the Oak Ridge chemists who were making plutonium.

The reason for the cloak-and-dagger secrecy was that we were all convinced the Germans were ahead of us in developing the atom bomb. If, we thought, we kept them thinking that Berkeley was making medical °isotopes they wouldn't guess we were making plutonium. As it turned out at the end of the war the Germans, even Otto Hahn and Heisenberg, didn't even know plutonium existed.

°Iodine was a medically important cyclotron-produced isotope. As early as 1946 D. Ballantine was using reactor neutrons as the starting point for its production. A year or so later A. Rupp began preparing it from waste fission products.

[See Vig1953 .RPK]

An interesting sideline product was the preparation of the new element #43 (later called technetium). We all knew it had no conceivable medical use, nor did #61, promethium. But we had a directive from MED to study all of the fission products, which meant practically every element, because they were all potential reactor poisons. They might be contaminants in the very pure plutonium required in bomb production. As such they had a direct bearing on the MED war effort.

[See Vig1960 .°Tc]

Early in this strictly "practical" chemistry we prepared the first visible samples of both #43 (technetium) and #61 (promethium). Although not required by the Manhattan Project, it gave us great satisfaction to have finally completed Mendeleev's Periodic Table of the Elements.

THE TRUE $$ BEGINNING OF NUCLEAR MEDICINE
(Sam Seidlin Cures Thyroid Cancer)

At the beginning of World War II the use of °iodine was spreading beyond MIT and Berkeley. With °I being used to distinguish *hypo* from *hyper,* some measure of comparative thyroid activity was inevitable. The thyroid °iodine uptake test that would dominate Nuclear Medicine for the next generation cannot be pinpointed as a *discovery,* it just sort of grew as an obvious idea. Many of the pre-war animal studies imply the idea of uptake, but "how to do it" gradually spread by word of mouth during the 1940s.

By this time Irving Ariel was doing quantitative and *timed* organ sampling. You can't use "uptake," he concluded, unless you also mention time. Sol Hertz then threw a monkey wrench into this beautiful emerging clinical "test" by discovering that TSH modifies thyroid radioiodine uptake. By implication, his study screamed, probably other drugs affect uptake. [See Vig1953 .M°I]

Hamilton and Soley solidified the concept by measuring a thyroid uptake in 5 normal subjects. At Columbia P & S a group used °I in a metastasizing thyroid cancer. While scanning for metastases, their resident heard over the radio that Pearl Harbor had been bombed.

[See Vig1941 .Bal]

Jan 1941 — Hertz (MGH) gives first patient °I in attempt to cure Grave's disease;
Early 1941 — Ariel finds uptake is a function of time;
Mid 1941 — Hertz notes TSH modifies thyroid uptake;
Late 1941 — Hamilton & Soley measure uptake in 5 normals;
Nov 1941 — Columbia group thinks °I stored in metastases;
7 Dec 1941 — R. Ball scans whole body for °I in metastases.

World War II Insures °Isotope Production

The bombing of Pearl Harbor marks the beginning of a five year period during which scholarly priorities should not be ascribed in °iodine research. In 1940 a voluntary, and after Pearl Harbor complete, censorship affected nuclear science publication. The Berkeley cyclotron went underground to produce plutonium. The medical group was split up by the Army draft. In Boston, research acquired new priorities. The Columbia group disappeared into the Army. [See Vig1941 .Bal]

°Isotopes are Suddenly Available

During wartime secrecy the MIT cyclotron supplied millicurie to curie amounts of °iodine to 36 hospitals. By the end of the war the Oak Ridge reactor people didn't use the prefixes "micro" or "milli," they produced "megacuries." In June 1946 President Truman signed an executive order that made Oak Ridge I-131 available to qualified physicians outside the Manhattan District. Oak Ridge knew how to ship a megacurie of radioactivity; there was considerable scurrying to figure out how to ship piddling droplets, thousandths of a curie, to hospitals. [See Vig1953 .RPK]

Shortly after the bombs had been dropped (6 & 9 August 1945), Manhattan District's supersecrecy advocate, General Groves, agreed to a small distribution of virtually unlimited °isotopes. On 14 June 1946 six scientists and thirty newspapermen were invited to see the *"isotope facilities"* of Oak Ridge. Thus a science/publicity ratio was established for the next two generations.

The newspapermen were overwhelmed by elaborate and highly exaggerated safety precautions. One newspaper headlined "THE FIERY CANYONS OF DEATH" at Oak Ridge. Thus, forevermore, "radiation" was spelled "DEADLY-RADIATION" in the American press. The 1945 Smyth Report had said little about biological effects except *"It is common knowledge that the radiations . . . have deadly effects . . ."* Now, in this first publicity binge, Health Physicists could assure a remunerative place for themselves in the Atomic Age by screaming safety while waving a very large skull and crossbones flag. Groves et al wanted that reactor kept secret from the Communists (who already had one started). In Congress the "hawks," backed by generals, were demanding absolute military control of atomic energy. The "doves" wanted international sharing no matter how backward and savage the nation.

Seidlin "Cures Cancer" With Radioiodine
(And Makes Nuclear Medicine a Well Funded Science for the Next Generation)

In six weeks Congress passed the Atomic Energy Act of 1946. It was a compromise: a civilian AEC would take over, °isotopes were civilian, but "the bomb" was military with a thin wrap of civilian control. The very next day, 2 August 1946, Paul Aebersold, in charge of isotopes, staged a symbolic "First Shipment."

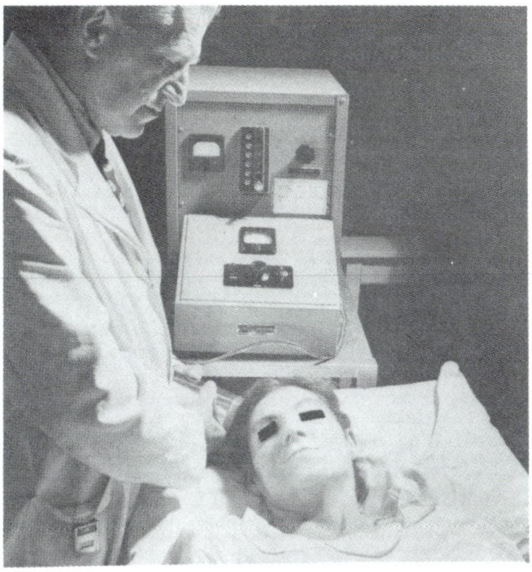

Dr. Samuel Seidlin, a New York endocrinologist, used a manual "scanning" technique during the mid-1940s, first to find metastases, then to estimate size in benign thyroid disease.

WWII — MIT cyclotron supplies 36 hospitals with °I;
[See Vig1936 .°I]

Mid 1945 — Oak Ridge reactor makes megacuries of °isotopes;
[See Vig1953 .RPK]

14 June 1946 — Executive order makes °I available from Oak Ridge
[Science 103:697, 1946];

14 June 1946 — 30 newsmen invited to a staged tour of the Oak Ridge °isotope reactor;

1 Aug 1946 — Atomic Energy Act of 1946 makes °isotopes available;

2 Aug 1946 — First civilian shipment of Oak Ridge °isotopes;
[See Vig1946 .Pub]

7 Dec 1946 — S. Seidlin announces cure of thyroid cancer.
[See Vig1950 .Lon]

On the fifth anniversary of the first crude scan of metastatic thyroid cancer, Sam Seidlin, a New York internist, published an article in the JAMA describing the complete disappearance of multiple functioning metastases in a patient who had had a thyroid cancer removed a few years earlier. This was not a description of palliation or 5-year survival. Seidlin was describing a complete cure of a cancer patient who had already been given up as terminal. Within days every Congressman heard from his constituency. Within hours the new AEC commissioners learned that they now had two priorities:

1. Build bombs under strict secrecy wraps, and to help disguise it. . .
2. Cure cancer with °isotopes with the greatest possible publicity.

Twenty four days later, 1 January 1947, the AEC officially took over all of Manhattan District.

Nuclear Medicine $tart$ With Money

Seidlin's article was the most important ever published in Nuclear Medicine. Radioiodine therapy of hyperthyroidism would undoubtedly have survived, but with cyclotron charges for the °iodine. John Lawrence's leukemia therapy and Lowell Erf's polycythemia therapy would have prospered without stupid AEC licensure requirements. But Cobalt-60 teletherapy, the most successful use of °isotopes, would never have been able to steal reactor flux from bomb making. Seidlin's cancer therapy in hopeless cancer patients captured the public's imagination and forced Congress to force AEC to act. Look at journals from the 1950s: almost every article mentioning °isotopes has a small footnote that acknowledges AEC financial support.
[See Vig1947 .Lit]

During the next twenty years a flood of AEC money supported over 95% of radiation physics, chemistry, biology, health physics, genetics, anything nuclear. Nuclear Medicine was born and nurtured on fallout from Seidlin's article.
[See Vig1949 .TRx]

EARLY NUCLEAR MEDICINE LITERATURE 1946–1951

Before World War II medical use of °isotopes was confined to areas around a few cyclotrons at Berkeley, MIT, and Rochester; and to neutron howitzers in Copenhagen and Rome. When C-14 was released its effect in all chemistry was startling. Preliminary results with P-32 and °iodine were too good to be true.

Then, suddenly, on 2 August 1946, °isotopes were on sale with a built-in promoter: Paul Aebersold of the Isotopes Division of the Manhattan District. By 1 January 1947 the super-secret District became an Atomic Energy Commission (AEC). The AEC perpetrated constant public relations to cloak secret bomb building under a thin veneer of glorious medical breakthroughs with °isotopes. Sam Seidlin's 7 December 1946 article in the JAMA on the cure of Thyroid Cancer set the stage.

The *medical* public took Seidlin at his word: an unusual cancer. But newspapers had no time for details: all cancer, including low back pain, was cured. Paul Aebersold had unlimited funds and seemingly, unlimited energy to promote an unlimited cornucopia of °isotopes. As physicians, just back from war, reestablished pre-war routines in research, the use of °isotopes grew . . . and grew . . . and kept on growing. In the first five years, 1946–51, 3200 articles extolled °isotopes.

Oak Ridge had an almost complete monopoly on °isotopes. (A few cyclotrons produced miniscule amounts.) Military control and secrecy was not relinquished easily. Civilian control was vested in a new Joint Committee on Atomic Energy in Congress. They demanded public accounting by AEC of the only thing that could be talked about: isotopes. Therefore Aebersold tried to maintain a complete list of all scientific articles on isotopes. It was published in *ISOTOPES, Three Year Summary,* then 5 and 8 year summaries.
(USGPO, 1949, '51, '55)

The monopoly was broken by England about 1954 (AERE, Atomic Energy Research Establishment). Aebersold's office staff could not keep up with the deluge of research and clinical isotope articles.

Most work done before 1947 was classified, but the AEC tried to declassify as much as possible. °Isotope decay and characteristics dominated physics journals. C-14 manipulations flooded chemistry journals. Hundreds of articles (often texts of speeches) said *"Gee whizz, look what we've got."* At least 1320 articles on physical and physiological background gave meaning to a new form of measurement in clinical medicine.

Physical & Physiological Background

	<1947	1948	1949	1950	1951	Total
A. Nuclear properties	*	8	77	136	150	371
B. Animal physiol.	88	111	196	162	301	856
C. Techniques Med use	5	7	8	19	11	50
D. Gee Whizz medical	1	2	1	18	21	43
Total	**94**	**18**	**22**	**335**	**483**	**1320**

< = some 1946; * = classified

I-131 and P-32 were dominant medical °nuclides. For a decade Nuclear Medicine was equated with the "atomic cocktail" (in England called "therapeutic drink"). The name, applied to both I-131 and P-32, originally meant a therapeutic dose but soon included diagnostic doses. After the liquid I-131 was found to partially absorb in the esophagus to botch thyroid uptake measurements, Abbott Labs introduced I-131 in capsules.

Some physicians tried to empty the capsule into a glass of water to administer partial doses. Soon Abbott was receiving complaints about empty capsules — which was true. The specific activity of I-131 was so high that a diagnostic dose barely stained a capsule's bottom. (Abbott soon added inert carrier.)

About 10 years later one hospital bought multiple dose vials of liquid and its pharmacist laboriously filled his own gelatin capsules with individual doses — incidentally, without any radiation protection. When asked why? He said *"Because hot iodine burns the esophagus."* When asked how come patients' throats had not been burned in the past? *"Oh, this is a new isotope. We just began to use it two years ago."* °Iodine therapy was then 20 years old, but I later learned that this hospital's library threw out all journals over 5 years old because they were "out of date."

Articles on Medical Use of I-131

	<1947	1948	1949	1950	1951	Total
A. General medical	1	11	9	2	3	26
B. Lab methods	7	9	10	7	12	25
C. Diagnostic uses	8	24	42	47	43	164
D. Rx-Thyroid Carcinoma	2	6	9	9	15	41
E. Rx-Hyper thyroid	1	12	25	23	24	85
Total	**19**	**62**	**95**	**88**	**97**	**361**

Articles on Medical Use of P-32

	<1947	1948	1949	1950	1951	Total
A. Lab Methods	3	5	11	13	15	47
B. Diagnostic uses	1	11	10	19	27	68
C. Rx of						
– leukemia	4	7	6	10	3	30
– polycythemia	4	3	4	5	5	21
– other ca	2	1	5	2	4	14
Total	**14**	**27**	**36**	**49**	**54**	**180**

From the number of articles written, half the medical interest was in therapy. (From my memory it was about 80%.) The Politicians gave only lip service to diagnosis and research. Seidlin's 1946 JAMA article on *curing* thyroid cancer with °iodine sparked public, and hence congressional, support of therapy with radioactive materials.

But diagnostic uses were growing. Na-24 and K-42 studies had started well before WWII. Hematology studies with °Fe got under way during the war. The use of °colloids was begun with °isotopes made on a Zurich cyclotron. In addition to the overwhelming interest in thyroid and P-32 hematology, medical interest grew rapidly in at least eight other fields.

Articles in 8 Other Medical Fields

	<1947	1948	1949	1950	1951	Total
A. Na-24 & K-42	1	10	12	10	21	54
B. Immunology studies	0	1	5	20	23	49
C. Radioiron metabolism	6	10	13	4	8	41
D. Tele- & Brachy Rx	2	2	3	5	18	27
E. Brain Tumor Dx	0	4	3	5	15	27
F. Au-198 Dx & Rx	5	5	2	3	8	23
G. °IHSA blood vol	0	0	0	4	9	13
H. °Iodinated Fats	0	0	2	2	5	9
Total	**14**	**32**	**40**	**53**	**107**	**246**

The diversity of medical interest in the use of °isotopes is best seen in the number of articles that mentioned use of specific isotopes ordered from Oak Ridge.

Articles on Specific °Isotope Use

	<1947	1948	1949	1950	1951	Total
I-131	20	64	100	97	100	389
P-32	14	29	38	51	58	190
Na-24	1	9	12	7	16	45
Fe-55, -59	6	10	13	4	8	41
Au-198	5	5	2	3	8	23
C-14 (med)	0	1	2	7	9	19
S-35	0	3	6	5	3	17
Ga-72	0	1	1	4	4	10
H-2, -3	1	1	1	3	3	9
Ca-45	0	3	2	2	2	9
K-42	0	1	0	3	5	9
Hg-203	0	0	3	5	0	8
Tc-99m	0	4	1	1	1	7
Cr-51	0	0	0	2	3	5
°As, °Br, °Cl, °N, °Zn, °Ag, °Am, °Sb, °Y, °RE & FP	0	2	3	7	10	22
Total	**47**	**133**	**184**	**201**	**238**	**803**

If "clinical medicine" is stretched to include many research attempts that never did pan out, then 25 °isotopes plus Rare Earths and Fission Products were used in the first five years.

[See Vig1950 .Co, Cobalt-60]

FOUR NATURAL RADIOACTIVE DECAY SERIES

In 1921 F. Aston's mass spectroscopy clarified the picture of an uncompleted Periodic Table. E. Rutherford saw three natural Decay Series: thorium, uranium, and actinium. A. Russell, predicted a fourth, neptunium. The traditional beginning and the stable end of each series is in bold type. Until 1907 radium was thought to be the beginning of its own series.

THE 4n + 0 THORIUM NATURAL DECAY SERIES

Date seen	Noted by	Old name	Name	Half-life	Emission
1952	Fleming		U-236	$2.4E^7$y	α
1899	**Schmidt**	**Th**	**Th-232**	**$1.4E^9$y**	α
1907	Hahn	$MeTh_1$	Ra-228	5.75y	β
1907	Hahn	$MeTh_2$	Ac-228	6.13h	β
1905	Hahn	RaTh	Th-228	1.9y	α
1902	Rutherford	ThX	Ra-224	3.66d	α
1899	Rutherford	Tn	Rn-220	55.6s	α
1910	Geiger	ThA	Po-216	0.15s	α
1902	Rutherford	AD	Pb-212	10.6h	β
1902	Rutherford	ThC	Bi-212	1.0h	36% α 64% β
1906	Hahn	ThC′	Po-212	$3.0E^{-7}$s	α
1909	Hahn	ThC″	Tl-208	3.1m	β
1913	**Boltwood**	**ThD**	**Pb-208**		**53% of stable natural lead**

THE 4n + 1 NEPTUNIUM NATURAL DECAY SERIES

Date seen	Noted by	Name	Half-life	Emission
1944	Seaborg	Np-241	16.0m	β
1944	Seaborg	Pu-241	4.4y	Wk α Stg β
1944	Seaborg	Am-241	432.2y	α
1940	Nishina	U-237	6.75d	β
1940	**Turner**	**Np-237**	**$2.1E^6$y**	α
1938	Meitner-Hahn	Pa-233	27.0d	β
1942	Seaborg	U-233	$1.6E^5$y	α
1923	Russell	Th-229	7340y	α
1947	English	Ra-225	14.8d	β
1947	English	Ac-225	10.0d	α
1947	Hagemann	Fr-221	4.8m	α
1947	English	At-217	0.03s	α
1947	English	Bi-213	45.65m	2% α 98% β
1950	Hagemann	Tl-209	2.2m	β
1948	Jelley	Po-213	$4.0E^{-6}$s	α
1949	Fajans	Pb-209	3.25h	β
1938	**Nier**	**Bi-209**		**100% of stable natural bismuth**

THE 4n + 2 URANIUM NATURAL DECAY SERIES

Date seen	Noted by	Old name	Name	Half-life	Emission
1940	Berkeley	group	Pu-242	$3.8E^5$y	α
1896	**Becquerel**	**UI**	**U-238**	**$4.5E^9$y**	α
1900	Crookes	UX_1	Th-234	24.1d	β
1913	Fajans	UX_2	Pa-234	1.17m	IT
1921	Hahn	UZ	Pa-234	6.7h	β
1911	Geiger	UII	U-234	$2.5E^5$y	α
1907	Boltwood	Ionium	Th-230	$7.7E^4$y	α
1898	**Curies**	**Radium**	**Ra-226**	**1600y**	α
1900	Dorn	Radon	Rn-222	3.82d	α
1903	Rutherford	RaA	Po-218	3.05m	99+% α Wk β
1903	Rutherford	RaB	Pb-214	6.8m	β
1903	Rutherford	RaC	Bi-214	19.8m	Wk α 99+% β
1908	Hahn	RaC′	Po-214	$1.6E^{-4}$s	α
1904	Hoffman	RaD	Pb-210	22.3y	Wk α 99+% β
1904	Meyer	RaE	Bi-210	5.0d	Wk α 99+% β
1898	Curies	RaF	Po-210	138.4d	α
1907	**Boltwood**	**RaG**	**Pb-206**		**25% of stable natural lead**

[Not shown: weak 2s At-218, 0.03s Rn-218, 1.3m Tl-210, 8.2m Hg-206, 4.2m Tl-206.]

THE 4n + 3 ACTINIUM NATURAL DECAY SERIES

Date seen	Noted by	Old name	Name	Half-life	Emission
1940	McMillan		Np-240	1.1h	β
1949	Abelson		Pu-240	$2.4E^4$y	α
1935	**Dempster**	**AcU**	**U-235**	**$7.0E^6$y**	α
1911	Antonoff	UY	Th-231	1.03d	β
1918	Hahn	Proto-Ac	Pa-231	$3.3E^4$y	α
1899	Debierne	Ac	Ac-227	21.77y	β
1906	Hahn	RaAc	Th-227	18.72d	α
1904	Godlewski	AcX	Ra-223	11.4d	α
1902	Giesel	An	Rn-219	4.0d	α
1911	Geiger	AcA	Po-215	$1.8E^{-3}$s	α
1904	Debierne	AcB	Pb-211	36.1m	β
1904	Brooks	AcC	Bi-211	2.13m	99+% α 0.3% β
1912	Soddy	AcC′	Po-211	0.56s	α
1909	Hahn	AcC″	Tl-207	4.8m	β
1913	**Boltwood**	**AcD**	**Pb-207**		**22% of stable natural lead**

[Not shown: weak 21.8m Fr-223, 54s At-219, 7.4m Bi-215, $1.0E^{-4}$s At-215.]

FOUR NATURAL RADIOACTIVE DECAY SERIES

In the beginning (1896–1912) all radioactive nuclides were distinct chemical "elements." About 1898 Bertram Boltwood at Yale began to suspect a connection between some of the radioactive species. Pierre Curie and André Debierne then found that radium would "induce activity" in cold substances. Ernest Rutherford immediately stopped this false idea; he had already shown that a gas was emitted and "deposited" further activity. In 1905 Otto Hahn demonstrated to Rutherford and Boltwood distinct genetic relationships in radioactive substances and often referred to a "muttersubstanz." [Eve, p. 166] Boltwood began seeing parent-daughter patterns of decay.

Beginning with Hahn's suggestion that radiothorium and thorium were "identical" (he was just a graduate student and this mild hint might be considered somewhat presumptuous), by 1912 most radioactivity labs saw chemical identities which soon became "isotopes." Until the 1907 discovery of ionium (Th-230), the "identities" formed into three: uranium, radium, and thorium decay patterns. The three natural decay series became two when radium became a daughter of uranium, but an actinium series was already taking its place. [Vig1907 .B&H]

In 1918 Rutherford began using high speed alpha particles from radium as projectiles to split nuclei. [See Vig1918 .ER5] In 1932 the neutron became available as a projectile against the heaviest element, uranium. Such bombardment eventually led to production of transuranic elements, which revealed the fourth natural radioactive decay series. Such a series had been predicted back in 1923 by A. Russell when he found a thorium that appeared to have an atomic weight of 229. Its half-value-period (7340 y) was too short to support "natural" decay. Radioactive decay from uranium and thorium, all the way down to lead, is primarily by alpha particles with a loss of 4 mass units in each decay. The thorium series isotopes (A = 232) all have a mass that is a multiple of 4 (or 4n). The uranium series (A = 238) all have mass 4n + 2. The actinium series (A = 235) all have a mass 4n + 3. Where, asked A. Russell, are the missing isotopes with mass 4n + 1?

12 Important Steps in Unraveling Decay

All 49 steps in the natural decay series (or 58 if you include trace decays) were important in unraveling the upper end of the Periodic Table. Twelve of the steps, however, are noteworthy:

(1) **Becquerel's** 1896 discovery must be the first step even though it did not answer questions — it raised questions. [See Vig1896 .Bq]

(2) Interest was waning in the useless discovery until **the Curies** discovered radium in 1898. It glowed in the dark (perpetual motion?) and required serious scientific study. [See Vig1898 .Ci]

(3) **G. Schmidt** of Münster discovered that thorium was also radioactive in 1899. The phenomenon was not confined to uranium ores. (Marie Curie also discovered it two months later.) [See Vig1898 .Ci]

(4) **Rutherford's** investigation of thorium activity resulted in finding a radioactive gas that led him to "half-life." [See Vig1898 .ER1]

(5) **A. Debierne** discovered actinium (1899), which implied a fourth decay series but of very low abundance. [See Vig1904 .BBB]

(6) **W. Crookes** didn't believe old friend Becquerel, and washed "all" the activity out of U into UX, and then Becquerel proved that activity grew back into U. [See Vig1900 .C&B]

(7) **E. Rutherford** sees the same regrowth phenomenon in Th and ThX. From this decay and regrowth he arrived at transmutation. [See Vig1902 .ER2]

(8) Student **O. Hahn,** while trying in 1905 to separate radium, discovered RdTh inseparable from thorium "muttersubstanz" from a radium ore. [See Vig1905 .OH1]

(9) **B. Boltwood** found the link between uranium and radium in ionium (Th-230). Hence, only three series exist: U, Th, Ac. [See Vig1907 .B&H]

(10) **K. Fajans** showed (1913) that overlapping decay chains and look-alike elements are "isotopes." [See Vig1912 .KF1]

(11) **A. Russell** saw Th-229 and asked, "Where is the 4n + 1 decay chain?" [See Vig1948 .Bkg]

(12) **E. Fermi** in 1932 used radium alphas in Be to make the new neutrons. In 1940 the Berkeley chemists used cyclotron-accelerated neutrons to transmute uranium into neptunium-237. Its 2×10^6y half-life gave its name to the 4n + 1 neptunium natural decay series. [See Vig1930 .EL1] [See Vig1956 .Bkg]

SIEVERT MEASURES RADIATION BACKGROUND

("Background" becomes "Body Burden")

Radium body burdens can be quite high in exposed persons. In 1942 Adolph Krebs (then Germany, now US) asked a pertinent question: how much radium is in the bodies of persons *never* exposed to industrial radium? Based upon "breath analysis" measurements similar to those by R. Evans, he made calculations. The figures came out quite high.

If the radium body burden is as high as Krebs said, then naturally acquired radium body burden was a large fraction of the newly forming concept of "Maximum Permissible Dose" (MPD). If you add K-40 to the dose from acquired radium, everybody had impermissible radiation. "Maximum Permissible" must be more than "naturally acquired." In 1950 a U of Rochester group tried to solve the problem. They ashed the corpses of 25 adults (and 6 stillborns). They supported Krebs' calculations.

[J. Hursch, AEC UR-119, 18 May 1950]

The Measurement of Body Burden

Breath analysis gives only an *estimated* Ra body burden, and whole-body ashing is very destructive. Two years earlier physicist Rolf Sievert, in Sweden, built an ion chamber to measure radioactivity in the living body. Ten 22 cm diameter ionization tubes 125 cm long surrounded a sliding bed. The underground instrument was shielded by concrete walls and a water tank. Many volunteers shoved into this chamber became part of the first study of "Body Background" radiation. A wide variation in natural body radioactivity (at least a factor of 5) centered around 0.5 mR/week.

[ArF 3:337, 1951]

> [Sievert, the Swedish member on the original 1928 ICRP, spent his life *measuring* radiation. After his death in 1967 he was insulted by having an unmeasurable Health Physics non-unit (the Sv) named after him.]

In October 1950 a symposium convened in Leeds, England, on "The Biological Hazards of Atomic Energy." Sievert's measurements of living bodies were impressive. His "whole-body counter" was improved upon in England with a high pressure ion chamber that could detect a body burden of 2 nanograms of radium. Normal English adults emitted 14 ng Ra-226 equivalent. One of the first discoveries was that the body's natural °K-40 accounted for the major portion of body background.

[A. Haddow, Clarendon, 1952]

By 1956 F. Spiers used his presidential address to the British Institute of Radiology to summarize the work he and others had done on measuring *The Natural Radioactivity of Man and his Environment.*

[BJR 29:409, 1956]

Fallout is a Minor Body Burden

By this time another source of radiation dominated newspapers as if no other radiation existed. Nuclear weapons testing in the atmosphere caused "deadly fallout." The AEC required measurements, primarily to answer newspaper questions. No sensible scientist considered fallout more than an exaggerated background. But the atom-bomb subcontractor at Jackass Flats, NV (the bomb test-site) was using film badges to record exposures, and every expert said, "that's too coarse."

At Los Alamos, NM, the E.C. Anderson group was trying to detect a rare neutrino interaction. They had filled a large cylinder with a liquid scintillator. A bank of photomultiplier tubes recorded and amplified any interaction within the liquid. A medical colleague noted that a slit through the axis could accommodate an adult human body. This neutrino counter was the origin of an array of liquid scintillation whole body counters. Eventually they had a sensitivity in the range of 0.1 nanocuries of any gamma emission from the body. However, the spectral resolution was not good enough to identify the radionuclide.

[PR 90:493; Na 172:4377, 1953]

Counting and Identifying Body Burden

Leo Marinelli at Argonne National Lab took a different approach. Through AEC he acquired 52 tons of pre-atom-bomb-fallout steel (from old battleships). His group constructed an 8′×8′×6′ "iron room" with 8 inch thick steel walls. (They had found that beyond 8″ the background was no longer reduced.) It was later determined that the major source of contamination in a minimum background room was the K-40 in the glass or the ceramic base of the photomultiplier tube used to measure the radiation.

In the center of this very low background room, an 8 inch diameter NaI(Tl) crystal for gamma ray spectroscopy looked at a patient in a special chair. On one of their first full spectrum recordings of a Chicago adult they saw a sharp peak at 662 keV: Cs-137 had to have originated at Jackass Flats, NV. The "hard rock" whole body counter was detecting a fraction of a nanocurie, about 10 Bq, and the spectrum was identifying it at less than half the natural K-40 level. [Sc 124:122, 1956]

Body Burden is a Background Range Risk

Back at Los Alamos the major contaminant in measuring body background in large samples of the population was the subject's clothing. From measurements of 1500 persons aged 5 to 80 years, weighing from 30 to 270 lbs, they tried to adjust to read in terms of the "reference man." The average man will emit:

at least — 50 gamma rays/second,
average — 75 gamma rays/second,
at most — 250 gamma rays/second,

all at 1.46 MeV. [Sc 125:1273, 1957]

By 1958 the Leeds group confirmed to the Second Atoms-for-Peace Conference the 12nCi K-40 emission, but added about 5 nCi of Cs-137 (135 Bq), or another hundred or so gammas/second. Within a decade well over 100 whole body counters were in operation. Every Health Physicist knew very well the levels of natural radioactivity, but with AEC grants directly proportionate to the radiation stink in the newspapers, they chose to disregard facts.

The Consequence of Health Physics

At the First Atoms-for-Peace conference (1955), an English geneticist suggested that living bodies had adapted to their radiation environment. If they had not adapted they wouldn't be alive. The genetic process had begun a few billion years ago when the earth was at least twice as radioactive as it is now. In this hot background some species have lived for millions of years with little genetic change. Some species live for over a hundred years without radiation damage. Or, he asked, is what some foolish biologists label "radiation damage" really the essence of chemical activity? We live because of, not in spite of, a radioactive earth. The recent addition of man-made radiation was an insignificant pimple in the earth's energy exchange budget.

His speech to the plenary session was unconscionable heresy. Since Muller's day X-ray mutations were "bad." The hallways at the Geneva Conference buzzed with wild speculations on fruit fly mutations and the death of all life on earth from atomic bomb fallout.

> [25 years later *Time Magazine,* Feb 1983, published pictures of West German anti-nuke protestors parading in hideous mutant costumes. The two-headed baby is still the hallmark of radiation genetics.]

At the 1958 Second Atoms-for-Peace conference, reports derived from whole-body counters proved the buildup of fallout in the human body. (And led to the 1963 atom bomb test ban treaty.) Every scientist acquainted, even remotely, with fallout data also knew that fallout body burden was far smaller than the range of variation of a person's normal background.

Eat a banana and you have ingested about a third of a nanocurie of K-40. These 12 Bq (disintegrations per second) will irradiate you for about a month. From this one banana about 28 million high energy beta particles will tunnel through your tissues. You will emit about 3 million 1.46 MeV gamma rays. Eat two eggs for breakfast each morning and you are maintaining a potassium balance equivalent in radiation to fallout body burden. Every Health Physicist and every Radiation Geneticist in 1958 knew these comparisons. Few made any attempt to stem an emerging radiation hysteria.

Hysteria exacerbated into Radiation Phobia during the 1980s. In 1981 T. Luckey revived radiation "hormesis" (small amounts are good for you), and in 1984 a US District Court dismissed the chief honcho of 1950 Health Physics as a liar. But the first step in reversing the lies of a generation of Health Physicists occurred in 1980. The proceedings of a 1978 Brazil symposium on *Natural Radiation Environment* was published. After two decades of exaggerating radiation dangers it marks the return of Health Physics to the concepts of Rolf Sievert.

[See Vig1956 .Bkg]

BRAIN TUMORS DETECTED WITHOUT SURGERY

(From G. Moore's story in Minn Med, 1948)

In 1882 P. Erlich in Germany used fluorescein to visualize fluid formation in the anterior chamber of the eye. Thirty years later, its tissue staining property was being exploited in anatomic pathology. In 1912 V. Kafka noted that fluorescein was very selective: on subcutaneous injection it would stain dura and choroid plexus, but not brain or spinal chord.

Blumgart's radon circulation time in 1927 employed a °measurement unfamiliar to physicians. A more comfortable technique, though not as accurate, was substituted. In 1931 K. Lange discovered that after IV fluorescein, under ultra violet (UV), circulation under the skin was seen. Adapted to a circulation time measurement the dye became popular.

George E. Moore, senior research fellow in Surgery at the U of Minnesota, was studying IV and IA modifications of Lange's technique. In 1946 he noted fluorescence under UV light of a stomach cancer in a patient given IV fluorescein a few hours pre-op. He repeated the observation in many tumors. Fluorescence of GI and breast tumors was variable but, with few exceptions, brain tumors all absorbed significant dye.

Microscopic exams of needle biopsies around 65 surgically exposed tumors verified his finding. Only one tumor was false-positive. In Science 106:130, 1947 he speculated that with °labeled dye, tumors might be detected before surgery.

Moore made some DiIodoFluorescein (DIF) tagged with I-131 (D°IF). Tried in 26 patients, 11 showed true-positive point-by-point manual scans, 6 showed true-negative scans (proved in subsequent surgery), 3 posterior fossa malignancies were false-negative. Benign tumors did not pick up D°IF. Moore reported a qualified success (Science 8, 1948). The odds improved with mechanical scanning, °IHSA, °Hg-203, °TcO_4 and the Camera. Within 15 years brain scans dominated Nuclear Medicine.

Then, in 1973, G. Hounsfield introduced the CAT scanner.

HOW THE ORINS MEDICAL DIVISION BEGAN

[This story is an answer to a question frequently asked me (Marshall Brucer): How did you get into Nuclear Medicine? It gives the flavor of the first five years (1948–1953) of "atomic medicine" that soon became "nuclear medicine."]

In August 1945 two bombs on Japan brought the public into the Atomic Age. (Scientists had been in the atomic age for a half century.) On 7 Dec 1946 an article in the JAMA announced the cure of a patient with metastatic cancer of the thyroid gland.

> [In a span of 2 years the patient was given almost a curie of isotopes of iodine made in the MIT cyclotron at tremendous cost. As of 2 August 1946 this same radioiodine was available from the Oak Ridge reactor for pennies plus shipping cost.]

The US Congress, at the time, was in a hassle over civilian versus military control of atomic energy, and the civilians won. On 1 January 1947 President Truman gave control of Oak Ridge, lock, stock, and slums, to a new AEC. However, the article on a "cancer cure" made a last minute adjustment necessary. The newspapers had not mentioned the unusual nature of the cancer that had been cured. They informed the public in crisp prose that cancer could be cured from the *"Fiery Canyons of Death in Oak Ridge"* (an actual newspaper headline).

Research Hospitals Are the Answer

Every congressman heard from his constituency and relayed the demands for a *cancer cure* to the new AEC. The AEC responded by authorizing three hospitals for research in the use of radioisotopes in treatment of cancer — one to be located in Oak Ridge. There was already a hospital in Oak Ridge for broken bones and babies — but nuclear research was a problem for academic medicine. However, a new, not yet complete organization, the Oak Ridge Institute of Nuclear Studies, had been set up just for this kind of problem: to close the gap between AEC (mainly ORNL's nuclear facilities) and the Southeastern universities.

The Director of ORINS, a theoretical physicist by trade, didn't know how to set up a hospital, so he called a meeting of all the Deans of all the Southeastern medical schools to get advice. The Dean at Galveston, Texas, Chauncy Leake, was in the midst of budget problems and sent me to represent him. He had been the pharmacologist at U California, Berkeley, who had edited the posthumous papers of the third man to try radioisotope therapy, and at least he knew radioisotope subject matter. I was teaching physiology and was the only faculty member who had worked with isotopes. (It was a stable isotope of oxygen and I hadn't worked with it, I just calculated the results, but I knew how to pronounce the word.)

The deans (with me as a very junior non-dean member) met in fenced-in secret Oak Ridge, deliberated, and decided that a 30-bed hospital devoted to cancer therapy with radioisotopes was feasible. If the hospital concentrated on isotopes too short-lived to be transported to their hospitals it was also desirable. (In those days 8 day I-131 was a "short-lived" marginally shippable isotope.) Then we searched for somebody to run the research: a chairman for the new ORINS Medical Division.

I Become Medical Division Chairman

By this time I had read all of the reports of the Berkeley, California, work with P-32 and the MIT, Boston, work with radioiodine. Before WWII I had published some research on blood pressure and I remembered something all the deans — and other candidates — had forgotten. Back in 1927, almost 20 years before the Atomic Age, a highly respected Harvard clinician, Hermann Blumgart, had measured the circulation time of blood with a daughter isotope of radium. In 1948 radiophosphorus and radioiodine therapy were still under contention, but nobody questioned the validity, or the value to medical science, of Blumgart's work. (It is now recognized as the first study in Nuclear Medicine.)

But radium and its daughters did not come under the supervision of the AEC in those days; only the reactor's by-products were controlled. However, every dean had radiologists on his staff who used radium in cancer therapy. The subject matter for a Medical Division for ORINS was no longer quite so outlandish. I was recommended by the deans over candidates far more experienced in the use of "officially recognized radioisotopes."

In December 1948 I moved to Oak Ridge as the first chairman of an ORINS division. The University Relations chairman hadn't moved in yet and the Training Division personnel, though in operation since June, were not yet employees of ORINS. One job I had to do quickly was to take Ralph Overman's radioisotopes course to learn about this radio-stuff that ORNL was selling.

Buildings, Fume Hoods, and Fallout

William Pollard, ORINS director, didn't know how to set up a hospital; I knew exactly as much about it as he did, but I had an MD with a license to practice medicine. A wing of the Oak Ridge community hospital had been closed down with the post-war contraction of the town's population. Because the AEC owned everything, there was no trouble getting sovereignty changed to ORINS. We began to remodel but, by state law, we had to have separate bathrooms for little Negro boys (they were not "blacks" yet) and white boys, Negro and white girls, Negro and white male and female adult patients, and of course, employees. In the closet space remaining we could house patients.

A separate laboratory building, designed specifically for large scale use of radioisotopes, was already in blueprint stage. Naturally, in remodeling the old hospital wing, I cheated quite a bit. The State had no jurisdiction over AEC, and we ended up with only two bathrooms. (If this had occurred after female liberation twenty years later, I would have cut it to one bathroom.)

Laboratory fume hoods and rooftop filters were a more difficult problem. ORNL's chemical laboratories were ten miles out of town and exhausted radioactive gases through expensive, and secret, filters that were not very good in filtering radioiodine. We were in the middle of town and radioiodine might be our primary product. A health physics consultant, a happy lot in those days before they became ambulance chasers, had a fine solution. Why not, he said, monitor twice as hard for P-32 and use ORNL prepared I-131: no problem!

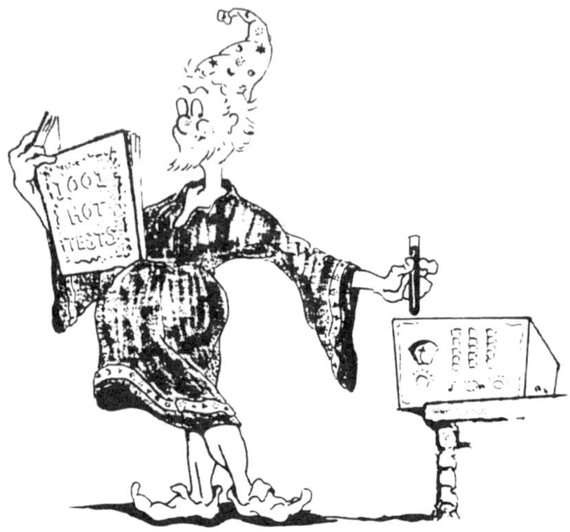

A few years later we learned how necessary our filters really were. In 1955 the Knoxville morning paper told about the Atom-bomb testing in Nevada. The AEC was shaking the gaming tables in Las Vegas, but there was no fallout because these were clean bombs. During our discussion of how you could make a "clean A-bomb," our autoradiography technician took a piece of filter paper out to our parking lot and wiped the top of my car. He put the paper on a film, exposed it for a few minutes, and showed us a picture of the fallout. Upon analysis the hot stuff turned out to contain considerable I-131. When I thought of the time, effort, and money we had put into controlling an infinitesimal fraction of the blanket of fallout radioactivity spread over Oak Ridge, I began to lose respect for the health physics numbers game. We had never had a real problem.

Cobalt-60 Is the First Research Problem

We did have a problem with Cobalt-60, the most intense medical source of radioactivity ever used — so far. When first appointed chairman of the Medical Division, I was commuting from Galveston to Oak Ridge through Houston. I stopped off in Houston to talk to an English radiation physicist, Leonard G. Grimmett, who was said to know a lot about radium. It turned out that he had helped build the first 5 curie radium "bomb" for cancer therapy back in the 1920s. Radium "bomb" cancer therapy was "supervoltage" and was very successful, relative to conventional X-rays and surgery, in many cancers. But it had a serious fault. Five curies, later 10, gave such a weak emission that patients had to be exposed for long periods of time. However, during the war he had seen reference to a new radioisotope of cobalt. This Co-60 emitted rays twice the energy of radium and, curie for curie, twice as many. Was it possible to get a 10 curie Co-60 source?

I didn't know, so I invited Grimmett to Oak Ridge for a meeting with Paul Aebersold in AEC's Isotopes Division. But Grimmett was not yet a US citizen. Security clearance was still required for plumbers to get past the gate, and this man knew more about atomic energy than most of us. After considerable hassle I was given permission to meet Grimmett at the Solway gate, bring him to the old Guest House, then to the hospital, and out the gate.

Aebersold met us at the hospital, but he was already a few months ahead of us. After Grimmett presented a summary of why we had to have this unheard-of enormous source of Co-60, Aebersold interrupted, "Why stop at ten curies, I've got a few hundred cooking in the pile." I suggested we go to a 1000 curie source to make a teletherapy machine competitive with X-ray machines. Grimmett redesigned his concept, and we started true supervoltage radiation therapy.

Unfortunately the AEC's reactors had no room for such an intense irradiation, as military priorities had precedence; we had to use a Canadian reactor. Thus the new ORINS hospital, set up to investigate short-lived radioisotopes, started working with 5 year Co-60. Set up to be near Oak Ridge's reactor, we used the Canadian reactor. Set up to try new radioactive therapies, we merely improved on a radium device from the 1920s. But in a few years we revolutionized radiotherapy. Co-60 supervoltage teletherapy was still in widespread use 35 years later, although the much higher energy linear accelerators were rapidly replacing it.

Setting Up a Research Division

The Medical Division's job was to investigate the use of short-lived (that meant <14 days) radionuclides in cancer therapy. Co-60 was an exception; it would be a machine design job with the research on patients done at any University radiology department. The best place to start short-lived isotopes in patients would be to repeat and extend John Lawrence's P-32 work and the already extensive radioiodine studies in hyperthyroidism and especially thyroid cancer.

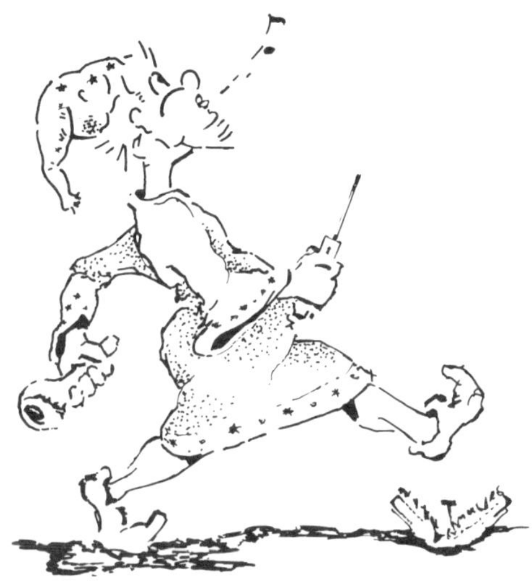

For this we needed someone to treat patients. At a polycythemia hematology meeting (U Michigan) I met Gould Andrews and convinced him he should come to Oak Ridge. He complained that he knew nothing about radioisotopes. I countered that I knew nothing about treating patients. Within a month the two of us were having the same argument with Mary Sutliff, who was about to retire from nursing. She said she knew nothing about the care of radioactive patients. We convinced her that nobody else did either, so she took a "temporary" job as head nurse that lasted over a quarter of a century. It doesn't matter what the Division's organization chart said: Gould Andrews made all final decisions on the "treatment" of patients, Mary Sutliff made all final decisions on the "care" of patients, and I kept my nose out.

Herb Kerman became the radiologist member of the clinical staff. He was the only one of us who had had formal training in radiation therapy. His first interest was Co-60 teletherapy and he wrote our first article on the subject. Lots of names were on that article, but he wrote it. Kerman brought in the U of Louisville Surgery and Pathology groups, who started lymph node localization with intradermal rare earths (W. Christofersen). Hal Berg discovered, by our new gross autoradiography procedures, that intravenous Au-198 colloid had no uptake in liver tumors — and why. These were not earth shaking ideas, but they started a diagnostic technique still, much modified, in use today. The liver studies influenced the introduction of liver scanning.

The same criteria went into the selection of the non-clinical staff. Each member had to know more about his subject than I did and he was expected to participate in the therapy of patients. Sometimes the participation was indirect, as Dave Bruner's calibration of gallium instrumentation, or it might be very direct as in Granvil Kyker's organization of our animal farm. The facility was out of town at Cyril Comar's agricultural research farm. In the early days every animal experiment was a trial of something we were about to try in a human patient.

At our regular Thursday evening conferences, human and animal data had interchangeable importance. Once we even voted on the surgical removal of a patient's leg — he had an osteogenic sarcoma — based upon the uptake of Ga-72 in animal bones. (The outcome of the vote didn't matter because Gould Andrews made his decisions on clinical grounds, but the animal data was often, with new isotopes, the only data available.)

The Thursday Evening Conferences were held on our own time because none of us had time during the work-day to compare notes. Gould Andrews pointed out that the sacrosanct Thursday Conference had been cancelled only twice: by two Jewish boys. One Thursday fell on Christmas Eve, and on the other Isaac Stern gave a concert in Oak Ridge.

Ga-72: A Most Successful Failure

Ga-72, as a therapeutic agent for osteogenic sarcoma, was the first program that really fit the Medical Division's reason for existence. A group working with Capt E.R. King of the Naval Hospital in Bethesda, MD, had discovered a remarkable uptake of Ga-72 in some bone tumors. The Navy's facilities allowed production of only a small amount of this 14-hour radioisotope — enough for a few diagnostic but no therapeutic tests. King joined our Clinical staff on a temporary Navy duty, because we could easily get therapeutic doses from the Oak Ridge reactor. We chose to study only patients with an osteogenic sarcoma in a leg and metastases to the lung. (In 1950 all such patients died in a few months.)

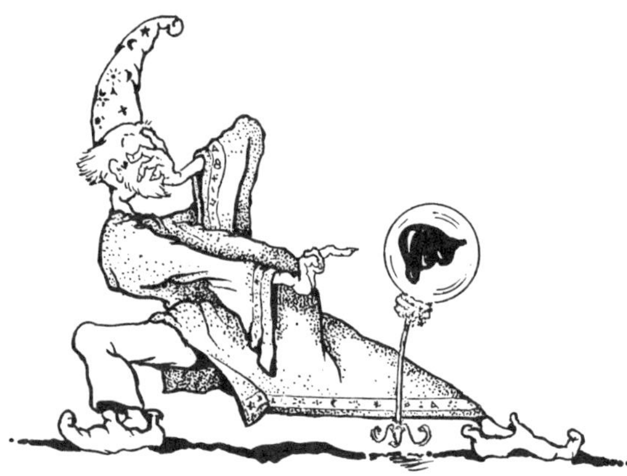

We gave the patient what we thought from animal studies was a large dose of Ga-72 and then removed the leg; amputation was standard therapy. After a few therapeutic doses a lung surgeon was called in to remove the lung metastasis — fancy but still acceptable therapy.

By 1953 the program was finished. Sixteen authors, practically our entire staff, published ten articles and a summary in the October 1951 Radiology. It detailed why Ga-72 failed as a therapeutic agent: Ga-72 dispersed, albeit unevenly, throughout a tumor mass too late for the short-lived (14 hour $T_{1/2}$) radiation to have an effect. Most of the gamma rays had been wasted on whole body irradiation. There was a serious question on the toxicity of the chemical gallium.

Ga-72 was a failure as a therapeutic agent but not necessarily as a diagnostic agent. Ray Hayes, one of the authors of the Ga-72 article, was looking at cyclotron-produced Ga-67 and Ga-68 — and Oak Ridge was getting a cyclotron. In another 15 years Hayes would introduce Ga-67 to become one of the major tumor, not bone, diagnostic scanning agents. The three year Ga-72 program was a most successful failure. It taught us how to approach a new unknown radionuclide.

> [Incidentally, one of the osteogenic sarcoma patients was still alive 20 years later. However, Shields Warren, pathologist and director of AEC's Biology & Medicine Division, who had agreed to the diagnosis of the primary, would not confirm or deny the lung metastasis origin and thus admit we had cured one of the patients.]

Intracavitary Au-198 is Successful

While the gallium program was at full speed, a U of Iowa group claimed remarkable palliation of abdominal ascites from metastatic spread to the peritoneum. The technique had been introduced during the war by a Swiss gynecologist using a colloidal radiozinc made on the Zurich cyclotron. Gould Andrews was particularly interested. We had already been using the relatively new colloidal Au-198 in some blood clearance studies. We had just received, I think it was the third, commercial scanner. I can remember seeing Gould perched high on a stool watching a scan slowly develop (it took almost an hour) of the distribution of Au-198 colloid after an intraperitoneal injection. No uniformity of distribution was evident, hence all beta dosimetry was a sham.

A few hundred questions arose on particle size of the colloid, metabolic fate, in which patients was there palliation, for how long, etc.? Intracavitary therapy was a problem for a large many-patient hospital. Low patient access limited us to a few problems, but these we did well. The particle size in the bottle was found to bear no relation to size in the patient. J. Muller, the Swiss gynecologist who introduced intracavitary radiotherapy, was also interested in the body's manipulation of different particle sizes. In connection with the first course in *"Radioisotopes in Medicine,"* Gould had Muller brought in as a guest lecturer. His Oak Ridge appearance in 1953, two years before the Atoms-for-Peace Conference, had a great influence on the popularity of intracavitary radioisotope therapy.

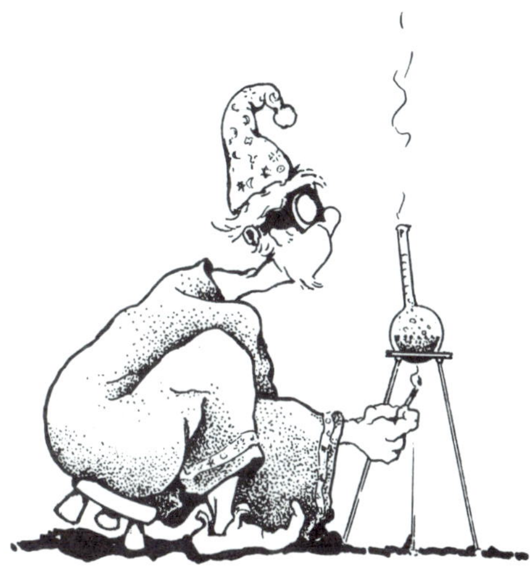

Another discovery, even older than the intracavitary use of Au-198, was its failure on intravenous injection to affect the course of childhood leukemia. Gould Andrews, who had been trained as a hematologist, was unimpressed by the stories of therapeutic doses of Au-198 colloid used in childhood leukemia; but diagnostic use was a different story.

The rate of clearance of Au-198 colloid from blood after intravenous injection seemed to have a relation to liver function. After injecting Au-198 intravenously in a last ditch attempt to save a patient with metastatic cancer, Hal Berg, a surgical consultant from the U of Louisville, discovered by autoradiography the "cold space-occupying-lesions." He would also have discovered the eventually very popular liver scan had we given him time on the scanner. (It was discovered three years later, 1954, by the UCLA group where the scanner had been invented.)

After many years of failure, in 1950 Charles Rosenblum at Merck finally succeeded in labeling Vitamin B_{12} with Co-60. Although the labeling was done primarily to aid in manufacturing, it had great significance in pernicious anemia testing. Merck had no license for human testing so they came to us. I took the first human dose.

> [Taking the first human dose is no great event when you know it is perfectly harmless. It has been done often to bypass the perverted "ethics" of bureaucrats and news media.]

After following my blood and urine clearance of Co-60 for weeks, we gave a dose to a terminal cancer patient. The autopsy survey of all tissues was the first hint of the distribution and localization of Vitamin B_{12}.

In 1951 a question remained whether radiotherapists would accept the constant adjustment of dose rate necessary with a 5 year $T_{1/2}$ Co-60 teletherapy source. We had an answer. The reactors produced, as a fission "waste" product, a large volume of Cs-137. If separated from other fission products — relatively simple but exacting chemical engineering — this cesium-137 was no longer "waste" but an intense energy source. It emitted 0.661 MeV gamma rays (about the same as the average energy of the old radium teletherapy). Its half-life was 31 years; only yearly adjustments in dose rate were required. We made the first Cs-137 teletherapy machine. It generated little attention in this country where higher energy Co-60 was easily available. About 40 units were made, and are still in use in Third World countries.

Mock Iodine and the Thyroid Uptake Test

We helped introduce P.R. Bell's (ORNL) crystal spectrometry in the mid-1950s, but it wasn't ubiquitous until the mid-1960s. Before the NaI(Tl) crystal and medical spectrometry, we measured thyroid uptake with a collimated GM tube. And, before 1953, we measured it wrong!

Thyroid Radioiodine Uptake was an exceptionally meaningful test. Physicists could intercalibrate point sources of I-131 within small fractions of a percentage point — hence "Uptake" must be accurate. Even a sloppy literature search showed that this too was wrong — many articles reported uptakes over 100%. The more scientifically oriented journals published complex mathematically derived formulae to compute uptake that were devoid of biological meaning. How could we prove this? An 8 day half-life decayed too fast for intercity comparisons (in 1952). However, by mixing 10 year $T_{1/2}$ Ba-133 (for its middle energies) with a small amount of 30 year $T_{1/2}$ Cs-137 (for its high energy), I could make a mock-I-131 that could fool every instrument except a high precision gamma ray spectrometer. (Only a couple of these existed in 1952.) "Mock Iodine" was patented in 1959 as a standard for I-131 gamma ray calibration.

We distributed Mock Iodine, firmly bound to an ion exchange resin, throughout six half-body high fashion manikins to match the I-131 body background of thyroid disease patients. In each manikin's neck a bi-lobed capsule (simulating the thyroid gland) was filled with a high intensity dose of Mock Iodine to match hypothyroid, euthyroid, and hyperthyroid patients. Each manikin was accompanied by six 100% standards matching the vials, syringes, bottles and beakers usually used as standards. Thus we could ask almost any laboratory to measure a manikin's thyroid uptake with proof that our value was correct by spectrometry and chemical analysis.

Prof. T. Oddie, radiological physicist from the U of Arkansas, took a manikin on a trip through 50 medical radioisotope laboratories in the US, getting its uptake measured. I took a manikin through 10 English labs. Eventually the manikins were shipped to over 300 labs in eleven different countries. The measurements were horrible. Only one laboratory came within 10 percentage points of the correct uptake; 50 points error was common, misreading a hypo for a hyperthyroid manikin was not unusual. The distressing point was that without using our medical spectrometer

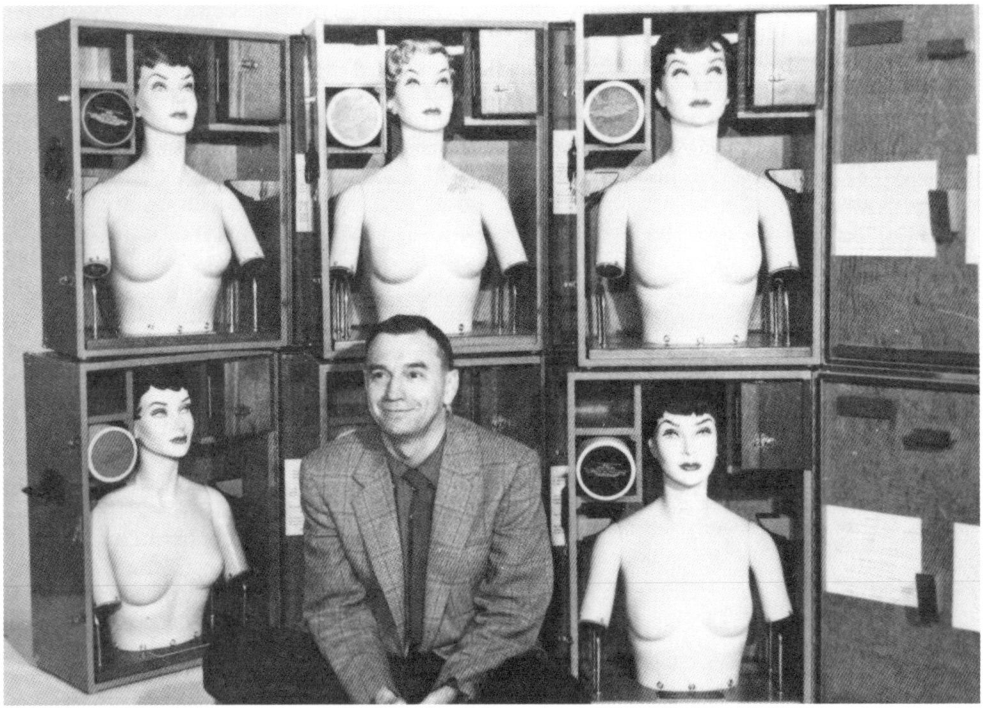

Marshall Brucer with some of the Oak Ridge manikins. Although hard to believe clinically, two thyroid uptake manikins were practically myxedematous, another two were climbing the walls. During the late 1950s most laboratories COULD detect euthyroids, but only by using fudge factor physics.

(we had the first one in existence) we could not measure the correct uptake ourselves.

To investigate the difficulty of measuring such a seemingly simple thing as an uptake, in one large room we set up every system — 18 pieces of equipment — for making the measurement we had encountered. At this time Hirotake Kakehi, an MD from U of Chiba, Japan, came for a year as visiting scientist. He took on the task of measuring the thyroid uptakes of the manikins by every method and formula until we could find a reason for the errors.

After a couple of months we detected the source of error. It was the body background and scattered gammas from the neck. If a shield, called the "B" shield, covered the gland, you could measure the body background and subtract it from the gland measurement. All of the 18 methods gave an improved thyroid uptake by this background correction.

If, in addition, the 100% standard was measured in a 10 × 10 cm right cylinder of plastic that mimicked the scatter of the neck — called a neck phantom — all 18 instrument setups gave a reasonably accurate thyroid uptake.

The manikins, phantom, and mock iodine were taken over by IAEA (International Atomic Energy Agency) as its first medical project. In 1958 an in vitro T3 blood test began an improved look at thyroid function. During the mid 1960s bakers began adding large amounts of iodine to bread, thus distorting the population's "normal" uptake. By 1980 thyroid uptake had become a test essential only in determining dosage in radioiodine therapy. It is nice to know the I-131 uptake in diagnostic scans, and it can be a physically accurate test, but it is biologically unreliable mostly because of the vagaries of dietary I-127.

Other Ideas That Blossomed or Died

Hundreds of other ideas were started, many by visiting consultants who did not have the facilities at their home university. (We paid their expenses to Oak Ridge.) For example, we measured particle sizes and its alterations in blood. With the help of Farrington Daniels we measured the exposure of the gut to I-131 with swallowed pill-shaped thermoluminescent dosimeters (published only in reports to AEC). We found a very high selective uptake of hafnium mandelate in the adrenal cortex of humans, but did not follow it up because of lack of time. Our autopsy percentage was the highest in America, over 100% — because we did autopsies on some patients who died long after leaving our hospital.

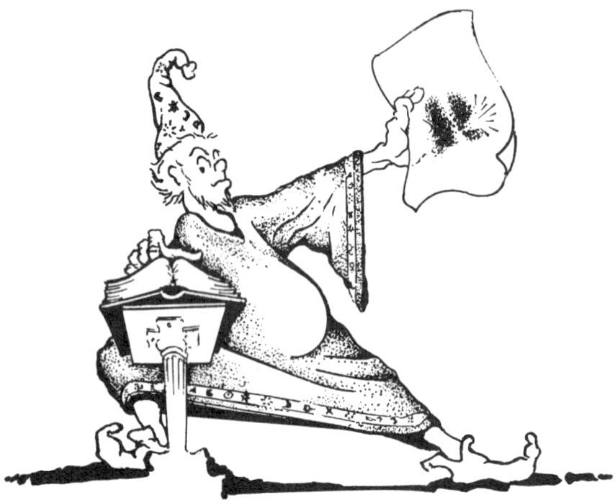

From extensive sample taking at autopsy we had the most complete set of human DARs (Differential Absorption Ratios) on more radionuclides than any other group — never published for lack of time.

One of the reasons for the chronic lack of time was "visitors." We were a non-secret installation in a still largely secret Oak Ridge lab complex, and hence, were on the AEC and State Dept "scientific tours." In one year, 1957, we counted 468 visitors; 137 were foreigners. We always had one, sometimes two visiting scientists, working on their own or on one of our projects. Our consultant staff, usually from medical school faculties, was very large but was essential. For example, we had no surgeon in residence but did complex surgery on most of our patients, usually by a surgeon from some medical school.

We gave the first course in the medical use of "radioisotopes" — they weren't "radionuclides" for another 10 years — with about half the instructors being the originators of the procedures being taught. We repeated with courses in Supervoltage Teletherapy, Radioactive Rare Earths, Thyroid Uptake, etc. Naturally, because we used consultants as instructors, we had to reciprocate by teaching at their courses back home. We also sponsored and participated in the Southeastern Society of Nuclear Medicine, and encouraged our entire staff to speak on nuclear medicine topics at the society of their specialty.

We also published, and published and published. Our list of publications in standard journals is a small portion of the output. In 1951 we hired Betty Anderson as technical editor, ostensibly to coordinate the many reports to AEC, scientific papers, and the books that grew out of our topical courses. Actually she was hired to copy read, and shame us into redoing bad writing. Our publication policy was that the person who did the work wrote the article and got his name first in multiple authors. I tried to limit the already growing trend towards listing everybody as an author of everything to spread academic Brownie points.

To summarize: How did the ORINS Medical Division get started? About 10 to 15 persons highly trained in some other branch of science tried to learn how to use "radioisotopes" and had a lot of fun learning.

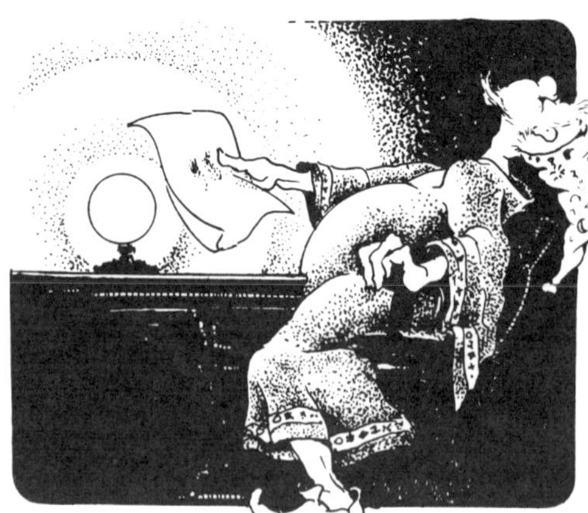

THE RUSSIANS HAD NO USE FOR MOTHBALLS

(From G. Hine's Story in JNM, 1977)

In the early 1930s Hartmut Kallman's academic activities had been suspended because of differences in political philosophy with the German Reich. He moved his research to a makeshift laboratory, formerly a horse stable for the IG Farbin Co. A new neutron photography was developed, but no German scientific journal would accept his papers. His patents are the only documentation of the early history of neutron photography. Individual scintillations produced when neutrons interacted in fluors produced light for the photos. He noticed that electron-multiplier-phototubes were more efficient than his GM tubes in detecting radiation. But then WWII erupted.

Science From Scratch, Literally

Late in 1945 Kallman returned to his old laboratory at the U of Berlin in the American sector. The USSR army had stripped the building of everything movable. Replacements were not available in the bombed-out city except, occasionally, on the black market — and then usually only for American cigarettes.

Kallman needed only three items to renew his old research: a radioactive source, a scintillator, and a radiation detector. The source was no problem: the walls of the laboratory had been painted with a lead paint. Kallman and colleague, Professor Broser, scraped the paint from the walls and concentrated the lead as compactly as possible. The crystal was no problem: the Russians in stripping the city could imagine no use for mothballs. Kallman prowled the city for all he could find, melted them, and cast large transparent blocks of naphthalene. He then scrounged a few American cigarettes and bought some photographic film.

Lucky Strike Means Photomultiplier Tube

Kallman placed the lead paint source of radium on the film for hours and achieved a mild exposure. He then put the naphthalene between source and film for the same time period. The film was black. His crystal scintillated visible light.

An official from the American Military Government found the simple efforts ludicrous and laughed heartily. Kallman chided him and said that instead of laughing he should try to be of help, by furnishing Kallman, a passionate non-smoker, with a few packs of cigarettes to buy equipment. The next morning 10,000 American cigarettes were delivered to the laboratory. Kallman was a millionaire. Years later he recalled the brand name — Lucky Strike.

He knew exactly which black market had it, and that afternoon he purchased a long desired electron-multiplier phototube. By June 1947 he demonstrated a new scintillation radiation detector at a colloquium in Berlin-Dahlem. He got good news and bad news: the good news was that his publications were no longer under Nazi censorship; the bad news was Germany no longer had scientific publications. A short note about the colloquium appeared in *Natur und Technik*.

Scintillation Counting is Introduced

A copy of Natur und Technik arrived at MIT in October 1947. Martin Deutsch translated and made the new scintillator known to American physicists. Kallman had pointed out that Rutherford counted alpha particles by their faint light flashes on interacting with zinc sulfide crystals.

His new method counted scintillations of electron or gamma ray quanta in naphthalene. They actuated a counting circuit after only moderate amplification. Not only were the number of pulses counted, but the intensity of each pulse was related to its energy. Response time was very fast: less than one microsecond.

Deutsch's abstract appeared in the 15 May 1948 issue of PHYSICAL REVIEW. It attracted world wide attention. Kallman was swamped with letters and visitors from England, France, and the US. He even received greetings from the USSR attached to a carton of cigarettes. But he wasn't tempted; rather he became professor of physics in 1949 at New York U, where cigarettes were not a form of currency. All because the Russians saw no possible use for mothballs.

[See Vig1955 .Xtl, Na(Tl) Counting]

AEBERSOLD SPOKE HERE

This story tells how Paul Aebersold left an indelible mark on Los Alamos. It was told to me by Tom Shipmann, physician in charge of industrial safety in the wartime laboratory. Los Alamos was primarily a construction camp dealing in high explosives and some unusual radiation sources. Tom took care of cuts, bruises, and pregnancies. Paul Aebersold tried to control radiation exposure.

As a graduate student, Paul had been the first man to measure neutron beams in terms of roentgens. While getting his MA in physics under Ernest Lawrence at Berkeley, when the cyclotron was being developed in 1932, he became interested in the biophysics associated with million volt X-rays. He earned a living, for awhile, teaching physics to medical students at UC medical school in San Francisco. With his earnings he returned to the Radiation Laboratory for a Ph.D.

With the 1934 discovery of artificial radioactivity, Aebersold participated in the manufacture of the first large (relatively) scale production and distribution of radioisotopes made in the only large source — the Berkeley Cyclotron. Thus, he knew most of the people who used isotopes. He earned his Ph.D. from the Radiation Lab in 1938. (To Aebersold the U of California was the Rad Lab plus a few outlying buildings of obscure use.)

Aebersold Becomes *the* Expert on Isotopes

As Research Associate in the Rad Lab in Berkeley, Aebersold investigated the properties of fast neutrons and set up some of the first biological experiments. [See Vig1935 .NBM] His was the first neutron dose unit. [See Vig1953 .Rad]. During 1939–1940 Aebersold was put in charge of operating the 60″ cyclotron in its 24-hour-a-day marathon to produce the first large (milligram) sample of plutonium. He went to Oak Ridge as a technical consultant in setting up the calutron isotope separation plants, but was called back to Los Alamos to set up neutron dosimetry and run a "health physics" program at the 16 July 1945 Trinity atom bomb explosion. He and Philip Morrison carried the plutonium core to the Trinity site.

As the Manhattan Project wound down a number of physicians and chemists, who had seen the remarkable uses for radioisotopes in biology and chemistry, suggested that radioisotopes be released to civilian scientists. [See Vig1946 .Pub] Aebersold was chosen to set up civilian radioisotope distribution. From this time on he became a salesman for radioisotopes. He spoke at every meeting of two or more scientists or physicians to extol the virtues of isotopes. No matter what field or technique was under discussion, it could be done better, or faster, or cheaper, or with greater precision, with radioisotopes. It was surprising how often he was correct, though occasionally he put a strain on the strict truth. This strain was evident in a meeting held in Los Alamos where radioisotopes were quite well known.

Three World Radioisotope Centers

When you read the post-World War II newspapers you get the impression that the atomic age headquartered in Oak Ridge, and for good reason. The Atomic Energy Commission (AEC) was highly secret. Only the Oak Ridge Isotope Division answered telephone calls from newspapers; hence, many things were attributed to Aebersold that he had nothing to do with. But he was a natural teacher and tried to explain things to the press without breaking classification. As the only AEC facility with an unclassified activity, naturally Oak Ridge became, in the press, the world source of the atom.

The Manhattan Engineering District, in its brief and profligate but highly successful lifetime (100 months and $2.2 billion), spawned three secret cities: Oak Ridge to separate U-235, Hanford to make plutonium, and Los Alamos to make the new metals into bombs. Oak Ridge was hidden in 95 square miles of backwoods hills in Tennessee (but easily plugged into TVA power). Hanford was hidden in 225 square miles of Washington desert (but with the Columbia river water supply running alongside of it). Los Alamos was isolated on top of an isolated New Mexico mesa to give the Army a feeling of secrecy.

1943 pioneers in each of these cities were among the most advanced technologists in the world. All told the same story of primitive living conditions during the project's beginnings — but each had its own flavor. Oak Ridge was put on the northwest side of Black Oak Ridge. After the bulldozers stripped the vegetation from the red Tennessee clay, normal rainfall created a morass of sticky mud that became the prime memory of "the old days." Richland, the town attached to Hanford, seldom had mud. Desert sandstorms were the primary memories of the old timers — little hills of sand blowing through every crack in a limitless landscape of nothing.

In Los Alamos, however, the early residents were sitting on top of one of the world's most beautiful landscapes — at a distance. Where they sat the Army had bulldozed a flat spot, erected some wooden tents, and forgotten to pipe in water. The early residents remember using the remains of an occasional bath to water a small garden. They remember barren dirt in the midst of plenty.

The center of the original residential Los Alamos was a shopping civic center "town square"; no sidewalks, but a dirt road went around a squared off bare patch. The road originated at a two-lane paved highway from Santa Fe, climbed over 1000 feet with numerous switchbacks, and was a thrill to ascend even after it was paved. The city was fenced with a single entrance guarded by soldiers with live ammunition. The scientists and their families were prisoners — voluntary, but still prisoners. They had their own self (almost) government.

The Army had final say, but had to keep the scientists happy, which also meant keeping their wives happy; this eventually meant getting some grass and flowers growing around town. Fertilizer would be required to get growth started in the barren tracks of the bulldozers. The acting town council requested a load of manure before the beginning of the spring rains. Everything that came into Los Alamos came by Army truck. The order went out from General Groves' Washington office on the fifth floor of the War Department: get a few loads of manure up to Los Alamos. Sante Fe procurement officers went into high gear.

Now New Mexico was not a farm and garden state, but it had ranches. The population had large manure production facilities. The Army procurement office, used to outlandish requests from scientists on the hill, sent trucks ranging the entire state of New Mexico and into Texas, buying every wisp of horse manure, with options on future production. Late one day and on into the night, it was delivered by truck convoy up the long steep road to Los Alamos.

The Meaning of Los Alamos

All of this search for horse manure occurred in the fall of 1946 shortly after the atom bomb blasts. The residents of Los Alamos now knew what their secret city was all about. Although many of the senior scientists were leaving, the job was not done. To keep the staff from leaving, the city managers held a number of public forums. Speakers were brought in to describe the golden future for Los Alamos in peacetime. It was not a "bomb factory" (which it most certainly was), but had great peacetime potential.

One of the speakers brought in was a well known former resident, Paul Aebersold. As head of the Isotopes Branch of Manhattan District he was distributing isotopes to hundreds of scientists. Radioisotopes were the *"most important scientific discovery since the invention of the microscope."* Aebersold described and showed pictures of diagnostic wonders (some true) and miraculous cures. (I-131 was miraculous to many patients.) Industry would be revolutionized by non-destructive testing. The atomic age was upon us and Los Alamos was at the center of the universe. Most of what he said had a grain of truth, but even Paul admitted that sometimes he squeezed out a little bit more blood than was originally in the turnip.

The morning after the speech the residents woke up to a clear and sunny Los Alamos day. As they walked to the Technical Area they were greeted by a monumental mound of horse manure. It filled the town square and emitted an effluvium sweet to the nose of every gardener. As they walked past they saw a small hand lettered sign posted at the base of the mound:

PAUL AEBERSOLD SPOKE HERE LAST NIGHT.

THYROID °I Rx IN SAN FRANCISCO

[Joe Hamilton visited R. Evans at MIT in 1938 to learn about °I. Upon his return to Berkeley he began thyroid studies with Mayo Soley at the Thyroid Clinic, UCSF Medical school. Earl Miller in Radiology took over when Soley went to war. Soley returned in 1945 and joined Miller in studying °I Rx of hyperthyroids. After Soley's suicide in 1949, Miller wrote up their 4 years' experience. 140 copies of the 35 page report were distributed by the Radiation Lab to AEC contractors. I abstract from this report.]

Miller reported on the first 100 patients treated for hyperthyroidism with I-131 at the Thyroid Clinic, UCSF Med School, Sep 1945 to Nov 1949. Each patient had a full clinical work-up with BMR, PBI, and serum cholesterol. (BMR is the old Basal Metabolic Rate. [See CNM1920] PBI is the Protein Bound Iodine. [See CNM1935]) No nodular thyroids were accepted for experimental °iodine therapy. (Nodularity was diagnosed by manual palpation.) The ages of the patients ranged from 5 to 65 years. Half of the patients had failed to improve after a course of anti-thyroid medication.

[Thiourea had been available since 1942, propyl since 1945, but the main therapy was still surgical. One of the reasons for trying °iodine was the lack of choice over surgery, which either failed or caused a hypothyroidism — even after hemithyroidectomy. One of the reasons for the rapid acceptance of °iodine for therapy, even in the face of a developing radiation hysteria, was the poor alternatives. A whole population of "thyroid surgeons" was wiped out in about 15 years.]

The Therapy Protocol

Each patient was given 100 μCi (Berkeley) after an overnight fast. Uptake curves were drawn from uptakes at 1, 3, 6 hours and 1, 2, 3, 4, and 5 days. Weight of the gland was estimated by palpation. From weight and uptake curve, dose was calculated by the Marinelli formula to give 6000 beta equivalent roentgens. From 3 to 9 mCi was given orally, an uptake curve remeasured, and dose recalculated. Six weeks later the patient was reexamined, another 100 μCi given, an uptake curve drawn, and the clinical response evaluated for further Rx.

The Results in 100 Patients

26 patients were considered cured after 1 dose, 46 after 2 or 3 doses, 28 after more than 3 doses. One patient was given 9, another 12 doses. It seemed that after about 4 doses another form of therapy might have been desirable. (This fear of multiple doses had no basis in fact. It was a reflection of a new Health Physics numbers game: more is bad.) On final follow-up examination in November 1949 all patients were considered cured: i.e., had no clinical signs of hyperthyroidism. There were no failures.

Measurement of "Thyroid Uptake"

Thyroid uptake was measured with a lead shielded end-window GM tube covered with a thin lead filter. The tube-gland distance was 53 cm to negate size, shape, depth of gland. In order to convert to mCi units, a radium needle standard was compared to a glass bottle containing 35 cc water + 100% of each patients' dose. BMR and PBI were used to determine patient response.

Thyroid uptake of °iodine per se was not used; it had not yet (1945) been accepted as a test of thyroid function. Rather, the 5 day curve of uptake was considered the important indicator of uptake. However, as the study progressed it became obvious that the 24 hour uptake paralleled the BMR and PBI responses to therapy.

Critiques of the Miller Report

[Miller's report was the first non-Boston area °I Rx of hyperthyroidism of a large group of patients with uniform technique. A number of meetings of AEC medical contractors were devoted to critiques of this important report. My notes of these meetings do not contain names, but most participants were non-clinical experts — for 1950 — on °isotopes in humans.]

The Problem of Dose

°Iodine dosage was calculated from the Berkeley mCi. A platinum needle containing 600 micrograms of radium was the gamma ray standard. (Every laboratory, in those days, used a different "standard" to determine curies. Remember, the "curie unit" was still *officially* confined to daughters of radium. Not until 1954 would the "curie" be *officially* accepted.) [See Vig1910 .Ci] On 1 Jan 1950 the Oak Ridge definition of "millicurie" was generally accepted by AEC subcontractors. All previous dosage studies were to be corrected to the new Oak Ridge millicurie.

Radiation dose was calculated by an adaptation of the Marinelli formula:

$$D = k\,E\,T\,C$$

E is the Energy in r/mCi • h
T is the hours since administration
C is the amount administered in mCi
k adjusts the units from r to rad

Each nuclide had an r/mCi • h value for its beta emission. For gamma dose the I_{gamma} plus geometry of absorption had to be specified. None of the details of dose calculations were well known, let alone agreed upon. But three required assumptions invalidated all dosimetry:

1. I-131 has uniform uptake throughout the gland. (They accepted no nodular thyroids, but later autoradiography showed uniformity false even in Graves disease.)
2. None of the beta particles escape from the peripheral rim of the gland. (On theoretical grounds this is a false assumption. Later experimental external beam irradiations show a rim effect. Rim sparing must have a biological cause.)
3. The weight of the gland is known. (A 1954 study of gland weight-estimation proved that this error alone vitiates all thyroid radiation dose calculations.)

Robley Evans had convinced Miller in 1947 that thyroid size must be considered in calculating administered dose. Estimation of large medium-small is obvious on neck palpation. But thyroid mass in grams cannot be "felt" within a ±50% error. Many later studies have proved this.

The Perversion of Half-Life to Half-Time

Edith Quimby (1891–1982) was known to two generations of radiologists as examiner in physics for the American Board of Radiology. She also instigated and chaired AEC's Subcommittee on the Human Use of °Isotopes (better known as the Subhuman Committee).

Exponential decay of all °isotopes was becoming well known around 1949. The handy "straight line on semilog paper," with accurate extrapolations, was being transferred to organ washouts and total body loss °isotopes. These were never simple exponentials; usually they could be approximated as three phase, short-medium-long, exponential curves. It was more precise to refer to "half-times" because they could NOT be entered in formulae that called for a half-life. (They were, of course, blindly plugged in and resulted in false answers.) Biologists began to measure the first 50% body loss as a "half-life" no matter what the next 50% decay showed.

Edith Quimby emphasized the "time" figure in the Marinelli dose formula. *"effective half-life"* = $(T_{1/2} \bullet T_{1/2Bio} / T_{1/2} + T_{1/2Bio})$. In the Miller report, a five day uptake curve, not a simple uptake, was used to calculate dose. A study of 5-day curves showed that "effective half-life" could not be averaged. The spread of biological "half-times" was so great that it had to be measured for each patient's dose.

A new branch of industrial safety devoted exclusively to radiation safety was developing at the major AEC installations. Members of this group attended the Bio-Lab AEC directors' meetings and heard us report "biological half-lives" of I-131 on euthyroid subjects from a few days to months. Imagine our surprise when K.Z. Morgan published the 1959 Tables of Maximum Permissible Concentrations of all °isotopes. The biological "half-life" for iodine was listed at 138 days, somewhat slow for the third phase body loss in a myxedematous patient. Official safety factors were adopted with an order of magnitude exaggeration of danger. This was not a mistake. It was a deliberate and dishonest act.

[See Vig1950 .Lon, London Meeting]

°PHARMACEUTICALS ARE BORN WITH °IHSA

(Tabern Introduces Storaasli's Agent)

In 1940 Hymer Friedell, a radiologist, was working with the San Francisco-Berkeley group when Bob Stone, Bertram Low-Beer, and Joe Hamilton made medical trials with the early cyclotron °isotopes: Na-24, P-32, Fe-55. He went into the army as part of Manhattan Project medical research. He moved to Cleveland in 1946 to run a radiology department at Western Reserve. When °isotopes became available after World War II he naturally continued what he had helped start in California. [See Vig1955 .Liv] One radiologist research associate in his department, John P. Storaasli, was interested in blood volume measurement.

Storaasli had resurrected the Fine-Seligman idea for labeling serum albumin as a plasma volume agent. [See Vig1942 .°PV] Because of wartime restraints on research nobody had taken up the idea — understandable in the small population in active research. Not only was academic research back to normal by 1949, but the rare ingredient in Fine-Seligman's idea, °iodine, was being given away. He substituted human for bovine serum and had a seemingly ideal plasma volume tag. His tagging method gave a reasonably stable **I**odinated **H**uman **S**erum **A**lbumin, **IHSA.** After much testing he found leakage of °IHSA out of plasma much less than T-1824 — negligible in the few minutes required for a clinical measurement.

In 1950 Storaasli published blood volume measurements of 76 humans. (SGO, 1950) °IHSA became popular overnight because, unlike Fine-Seligman's introduction of a clever technique with an esoteric practically unknown °isotope, Storaasli was talking about the well known isotope dilution principle (Hevesy 1929) using an °IHSA that was already on the market. How could it have been made available so fast?

Tabern Makes the First °Pharmaceutical

Since August 1946 the AEC had been selling raw °isotopes. They disclaimed any preparation of "medical drug." They did not even claim chemical purity. It was sold, or given away, as is.

Abbott Laboratories, on the other hand, was a pharmaceutical manufacturer. They sold nothing raw. Their reputation depended upon a guaranteed purity. One of Abbott's chemists was Donalee Tabern, the inventor of a sedative, Nembutal. With release of °iodine in 1946 he labeled "chiniofon," an intestinal amebicide, that has one iodine in its molecule. This was probably the first °labeled commercial drug, although none was sold in °active form. The ease of detecting and measuring miniscule amounts of °labeled drugs put an entirely new face on pharmacology. Even the most toxic drugs, he thought, could now be tagged with a °isotope and its metabolism studied directly in humans in homeopathic doses. Every Sunday supplement in those days had a story of some professor using "*°isotopes, the most important discovery since the microscope.*" He saw a future in making °drugs. The trouble was, there was no product to sell; the AEC was giving the stuff away.

Through Abbott sales contacts he learned that Freidell's radiology group in Cleveland was making a few °drugs. He visited Friedell and was impressed. He took note of Storaasli's clinical blood volume tests. Tabern saw its commercial possibilities. He made up a batch, tagged it with °iodine, established a standard production line, and coined the word "Radiopharmaceutical." He called it **RISA** (**R**adio-**I**odinated-**S**erum-**A**lbumin). But there were no customers.

Tabern went to every medical meeting he could get into, but not to give talks. He collared every physician individually, told him how easy it was to diagnose and even cure patients with °isotopes. Was there a problem with "nuclear" instruments? He told them which to buy, where to buy it, and which buttons to push. The roentgens, reps, milly- and micro-curies, and all that stuff? No problem! He would furnish each patient's dose in a separate bottle. What's this AEC license business? He pulled out the forms, gave the customer a souvenir ball point pen (marked Abbott), helped them fill in the silly questions, licked the stamp and mailed the letter. Somehow the local newspapers were always aware that another hospital had joined the atomic age.

[See Vig1951 .G&S, Labeling RBC]

THE 1950 LONDON THYROID CANCER MEETING

By 1949 cancer experts admitted that Sam Seidlin had cured Bernard Brunstein of widespread metastatic thyroid cancer. But the technique failed in many patients. Twenty-seven radiotherapists, endocrinologists, and physicists were invited to meet on 29 July 1950 at the University College in London. The results were never published. (I am writing this from Seidlin's notes.)

An informal discussion tried to compare combined experience on about 100 thyroid carcinomas treated with I-131. Every physician had seen at least one remarkable cure, but they all, including Seidlin, had many failures. Primary tumors did not seem to be destroyed, but consensus was quickly reached that metastases with high °I uptake were all cured. Then the meeting bogged down on a question, "How do you measure high °I uptake?"

B. Roswit of New York wanted biopsy with radioassay. H. Warrington of Manchester wanted manual point-by-point scanning. (An automatic scanner was just being introduced at UCLA.) G. Green of London wanted a thyroidectomy before measuring uptake in metastases, but J. Nicksen of New York thought he had insufficient evidence to justify such a radical procedure. W. Gilbert of Manchester gave results in 18 patients that showed no uptake post-thyroidectomy if there had been no uptake pre-surgery. He brought up the problem: "At what time post-injection do you measure uptake?"

M. Tubiana of Paris said optimum time was 36 hours. E. Miller of Sheffield said 48 hours. Seidlin said 3 days; E. Pochin of London said 4 days, "but how much I-131 do you inject?" E. Quimby of New York used no more than necessary to make the measurement: 250 microcuries. Tubiana used up to about 1 millicurie. G. Bloomfield of Sheffield said it depended upon the size of the metastasis. J. Muller of Zurich had noted a "biological reaction" with 0 millicuries.

A. Cipriani, Chalk River physicist, wondered "which millicurie: Oak Ridge, Chalk River, London, New York, Paris, California, or the Zurich millicurie?" "Millicurie" by definition specified Rn in Ra wrapped in metal. No "millicurie" of I-131 existed.

R. Tudway of Bristol pointed out the geometric difficulties in counting any dose inside the body. M. Myant of London was worried about small doses behaving like large doses. Stewart of London noted differences between tracer and therapy doses. S. Warren of Boston said a possible pathological effect of a small dose might change the biological half-value-period of a subsequent large therapy dose.

Almost every problem to plague °I uptake was brought up. Seidlin mentioned post-therapy "rebound" of blood °I. Myant countered with stimulated uptake following medical therapy, which brought up the problem of TSH stimulation, which brought up the problem of thyroidectomy prior to °I therapy, which brought up the problem of how much I-131. Seidlin used 100 mCi in divided doses. E. Quimby recommended 100 mCi repeated in 3 months if necessary. Bloomfield gave 155 mCi followed by 110 mCi in 3 months. L. Marinelli said D. Clarke at Chicago used 35 mCi every 2 weeks until uptake was abolished, but the real limit was other toxic effects.

W. Gilbert felt that patients approaching myxedema developed renal dysfunction and lymphopenia. G. Brownell had noted a drop in lymphocytes after 100 mCi. Pochin had seen 3 patients' lymphocytes fall to half their pre-treatment level after 100 mCi, but all returned to normal in 10 days. B. Roswit had a patient given 1400 mCi in $2\frac{1}{2}$ years with no drop in blood counts. Seidlin described patients given 2000 mCi with little or no blood count change.

L. Marinelli of Chicago and F. Farmer of Newcastle spoke of sensitive crystals that might replace GM tubes. G. Brownell, J. Hilton and E. Pochin mentioned a new kind of scanning to augment uptake.

Three months after the London meeting I heard Sam Seidlin ask, *"If a metastasis has high uptake we can destroy it. Now, for God's sake, when will physicists learn to measure I-131 uptake"?* Leo Marinelli murmured, *"As soon as physicians decide how much uptake is high."*

[See Vig1956 .°Rx; Hyperthyroidism]

HOW MEGACURIE Co-60 TELETHERAPY STARTED

(Grimmett Dreams of 10 Curie Teletherapy)

Leonard G. Grimmett (1903–1951) was a man of precise words. When participating in small talk he would contribute a precise "grumphh," after due consideration of course. I had worked with Grimmett for over a year before I heard the story of how he got interested in Cobalt-60. We had attended a radiobiology meeting at Oberlin College in June of 1950 and were on a train to Cincinnati to look over some teletherapy hardware. (The first kCi machine was under construction at GE in Milwaukee.) We argued Co-60 teletherapy all the way.

The argument consisted of my developing a brand new idea in brilliant detail on how to load a kilocurie source into the machine. He would say "grumphh" and then mumble 6 words: name, date, city, curies, and why it didn't work. These were all loadings of 5–10 curie Radium Bombs he was talking about. I finally asked him how you could load a big source without exposure. *"Can't. Take off film badge and work fast."* (He died before we could show him the remote control arms at ORNL.)

Supper that night was a one-sided series of abortive analyses: my expositions followed by his monosyllabic corrections. I almost went to bed at 9:00 o'clock because I was freezing cold. I told Grimmett that the coldest night I had ever spent was in an Oxford hotel room in the middle of August. He emitted an incredulous "grumphh," said he was sweltering and suggested a short walk. We walked downtown Cincinnati for about ten minutes when suddenly Grimmett stopped and pointed into a jewelry window: "Artificial star sapphires!"

Grimmett Learns About Co-60

Until about two o'clock that morning he talked continuously. Periodically I said "Grumphh." During World War II, in the London blitz, he had been immobilized night after night in an air raid shelter of his own design. As a time killing hobby he grew artificial sapphires. Ordinary gems soon became boring; he turned to an attempt at the perfect artificial star sapphire. By the end of the war his wife had a necklace of perfect stones, but he had never achieved his ambition of presenting her with a perfect star. Now somebody else had achieved it . . . well, almost. On close inspection these stars were not perfect.

After giving me a crash course in crystal chemistry, Grimmett pointed out that they could read in bomb shelters. For escapist literature he read back issues of PHYSICAL REVIEW. He came to a short note by W.V. Mayneord on the 1.25 MeV radiation of a new isotope of cobalt. It might be the answer to an old radiotherapy problem of *not enough output*. The only bombs he had known before the war was a "radium bomb" he had helped build for the Radium Beam Therapy Research, Radium Institute, London. He had increased the loading from 3 to 5 grams. Physicians complained, *"too slow, not enough output."*

Radium "bombs" were having considerable success in the treatment of cancer, but they required very long exposures. Therapists had to use very short source-skin distances and thus vitiated radium's high energy advantage. Grimmett thought back to the troubles he had had in developing the first radium bomb.

The First Radium Therapy "Bomb"

During World War I, the British Ministry of Munitions had used radium in self-luminescent gun sights, watch dials, and signs. After the war they had a surplus 5 grams of radium bromide. To get this "special handling" bother out of their warehouse, they "loaned" it to the Medical Research Committee (later Medical Research Council) until they would need it again.

The Medical Research Committee decided to determine the curative value of radium radiation in malignant disease. The work would be done in the cancer wards and research labs of Middlesex Hospital in London. In 1920 His Majesty's Treasury allowed formal transfer of radium with insured value of £72,500 to the Medical Research Council.

The 5 grams of radium bromide (about $2^1/_2$ g of radium element) was contained in

18 glass tubes, each in a second silver tube. All 18 were set in a round brass box 11.7 cm diameter by 1.7 cm deep. This brass container fitted into a 10-pound treatment box. For therapy the treatment box was fitted into a conical beam-forming applicator aimed at, and as close as possible to, the patient's tumor. When not in use the treatment box was transferred, using speed and long handles, to a 1½ ton lead block inside a safe in Middlesex Hospital's basement.

> *"The general trend of our experiments was to show that an exposure of four to five hours would probably be the limit of toleration of the skin to the radiation."* [Med Res Coun, UK, #62, 1922]

When the radiation beam was applied to skin for 7 or 8 hours, it caused blistering and epilation. But it also caused the disappearance of nodules of carcinoma.

This Radium Beam Therapy of cancer was highly successful. (The only alternative in 1925 was mutilating, usually unsuccessful, surgery.) Soon every country had its own 5–10 curie units, some of remarkable design. The design that solved the greatest number of both physical and therapeutic problems was Grimmett's transit type. The treatment head was positioned by the radiotherapist with no source in the area. When satisfied with its position, a three gram (later five gram) radium source was transferred pneumatically from a lead safe through a flexible pneumatic tube into position. The machine was highly successful to everybody except its designer. Grimmett told me of his disillusionment.

Pneumatic Transfer Has a Disadvantage

The Union Miniére Haut Katanga had loaned a five gram radium source to the Radium Beam Therapy Research unit. A group of Belgian officials were about to inspect the British use of their radium. Floors were swept, windows washed, brightwork polished, in preparation for the visit. A well meaning technician *oiled* the pneumatic transfer mechanism (a sure way to guarantee malfunction). After a talk on the inherent safety of the device, the 5 gram radium bobbin was pneumatically swished into position — but not quite. Half way through the tube it stuck and began therapeutically irradiating the inspectors.

Cobalt-60 Is a Dream Come True

Eight years later Grimmett was radiation physicist at Houston's cancer hospital, not yet a full citizen. I had just been appointed chairman of the Oak Ridge °isotope research hospital and was looking for ideas. I stopped off to see Grimmett on my way to the super-secret city of Oak Ridge and was given the complete history of all the warts on the radium bomb. Co-60 might be, Grimmett said, the answer to cancer. I invited him to Oak Ridge.

To get a foreigner — and a physicist to boot — past the gates that stopped Sen. Truman, was unheard of. After weeks of argument I got permission to let him come down one road to the guest house and the hospital. Not one peek at even the garbage dump would be allowed. Paul Aebersold, head of the peaceful Isotopes Division, would have to meet us at the still uncompleted research hospital.

We met and Grimmett explained what Co-60 was and why it could replace radium in an enormous radium bomb. If we could only get an unheard of 10 Ci source of metallic cobalt, which was theoretically possible, we could. . .

"Whadaya wanna stop at 10 for?" interrupted Aebersold, *"I've got a hundred pieces cooking in the pile that should go higher."*

Not knowing any better I pushed it up to 1000 Ci. Grimmett chose to ignore production problems and went home to design the first 1250 Ci Co-60 teletherapy machine.

Aebersold knew that he was obsoleting his unauthorized stockpile of 10 Ci slugs. I was left to deal with an international problem. AEC reactors were all busy making Pu for a different kind of bomb. We had to put the cobalt into the Chalk River reactor in Canada. The Canadians knew a money-maker when they saw it. They accepted our piece of stable cobalt and then added two pieces of their own.

[See Vig1954 .°Co, Cobalt-60 Teletherapy]

LABELING A PATIENT'S RBC WITH °CHROMIUM

(Grey & Sterling Introduce Cr-51)

While °IHSA (Iodinated Human Serum Albumin) was being introduced, a new and remarkably simple discovery changed blood volume methods. S. Gray and K. Sterling discovered that an ionic hexavalent Na_2CrO_4, incubated in vitro with whole blood, would freely cross the RBC membrane. Cationic trivalent $CrCl_3$ would not diffuse into or out of red cells. Ascorbic acid reduced Na_2CrO_4 to $CrCl_3$ and stopped RBC membrane penetration. The triad of hexavalent and trivalent chromium, and ascorbic acid, seemed to have little effect on the red cells in the doses used.

[JCI 29:1614, 1950]

The technique was simple. Incubate at room temperature a few ml of the patient's blood with hexavalent Cr-51. Within minutes equilibrium is reached inside and outside the red cells. Add ascorbic acid to convert to trivalent Cr-51, which will not pass through the red cell membrane. Wash the cells by replacing the plasma with saline to obtain an in vitro sample of the patient's own blood labeled with Cr-51 (°Cr-RBC). Reinject a measured quantity into the patient (save a sample for a standard). After a few minutes for mixing in the body, withdraw a new blood sample. The Welcker-Haldane-Rowntree-Hevesy-Hahn-Storaasli formula gives a circulating red cell volume (RCV):

$$\frac{\textbf{STANDARD}\text{ cpm}}{\textbf{SAMPLE}\text{ cpm}} \times \begin{matrix}\text{DILUTION}\\ \text{OF STANDARD}\end{matrix} \times \begin{matrix}\text{ml}\\ \text{INJ}\end{matrix} = \text{RCV}$$

Hematocrits Are an Accurate Inaccuracy

With a multiplicity of available °labels, inevitable comparison studies revealed a serious discrepancy. Blood volumes by plasma labeling did not equal blood volumes by red cell labeling. Technical errors of counting, pipetting, diluting, °labeling, etc., were well accounted for. "Leakage" from plasma and elution of red cell labels was expected, quantified, and could be predicted with reasonable accuracy.

A °Cr red cell volume plus a plasma volume should, but did not, give a total blood volume. In 1942 Paul Hahn contended that a 20% to 25% error in blood volume measurement occurred whenever a hematocrit was used. He said it had to be an error. A large vessel was different from a small vessel hematocrit. We habitually take blood from an arm vein. Its hematocrit does not represent the average total body hematocrit.

Hematocrit is Invalid for Blood Volumes

In 1952 E. Reeve summarized errors in blood volume measurement. [BMB 8:181, 1952] Technicians make most errors in dilutions, pipettings, volumes, and sample counting, which are matters of laboratory quality control. Although the hematocrit itself is an accurate measurement, it cannot be used to compute blood volumes.

Only about 80% of total blood volume is in large vessels with a high hematocrit. About 20% of blood is in vessels too small for routine blood withdrawal. These vessels have hematocrits only half as high. Peripheral venous blood yields a hematocrit not representative of the total-body. The total-body/peripheral Ht ratio has a skewed Gaussian distribution of about 0.91. The average volume error calculated with an arm vein hematocrit was 8% to 10%, no matter how accurate the cell volume measurement. In abnormal patients (when blood volume is worth knowing) the hematocrit correction also deviates wildly. There is no way to convert plasma to cell volume. Both must be measured.

Within a few years handy kits, sterile blood bags, and premeasured doses made dual °IHSA and °Cr-RBC blood volumes a truly simple clinical test.

By 1964 I. Berman reported in NATURE that the sum of separately measured plasma and cell volumes resulted in more accurate total body blood volume than any hematocrit-corrected measure. But a vexing question remained: are closed liver sinusoids included in this blood volume? Are blood sumps (e.g., spleen) included? Gregersen's definition of blood volume (JLCM 1938) comes to mind: the °Cr-RBC + °IHSA blood volume is a very accurate measure of whatever it is you are measuring.

[See Vig1846 .BV1, Blood Volume]

PLUTONIUM, BEER, & GOVERNMENT ACCOUNTING

(From a Los Alamos Story by C.C. Lushbough)

Long before there was an Office of Business and Management in Washington, DC, its duties were carried out by an even more scurrilous US Government Accounting Office (USGOA). Nothing was immune from investigation by the USGOA; it kept the small-fry crooks (anyone less powerful than a congressman) from stealing stamps and pencils from the government. That is, nothing was immune until the advent of the Manhattan Engineering District (MED) during the Japanese unpleasantness. It was rumored that General Groves had quietly informed the GAO that his guards had orders to shoot and then investigate intruders. Even Senator Truman (later President), chairman of a subcommittee investigating wartime waste, was refused entrance at the gates of Oak Ridge.

At war's end, however, when the Atomic Energy Commission (AEC) took over, the GAO moved in on Los Alamos with vengeance in their hearts.

Plutonium is as Dangerous as its Name

Plutonium was the primary product of Hanford Engineering Works, a monstrous Manhattan District facility in Washington State. It had only one customer, Los Alamos Scientific Laboratory, who neither admitted nor denied having any product at all. This plutonium was in no chemistry textbook and was mentioned in only one government report: H.D. Smyth's $2.00 *Atomic Energy for Military Purposes.*

During the first production of plutonium, stringent precautions were taken to prevent its ingestion, and for good reasons: 1. They didn't know how much they needed but no matter how much they had, it wasn't enough, 2. This was a completely unknown chemical, and 3. They were very safety conscious about anything radioactive.

When the first samples became available in sufficient quantities to handle (early chemistry had been done on microscopic amounts) hasty studies of its toxicity were run in mice. They showed that plutonium might be among the upper level toxic agents. When supplies increased and it became apparent that plutonium was going to be a permanent part of the atomic energy environment, a rash of short, medium, and long term toxicology studies got #1 priority.

The amount of plutonium ingested and inhaled by workers was so small that it was difficult to detect, let alone measure. A prime reason for development of whole body counters was to measure the plutonium body burden. (Bomb "fallout" became the first publicized measurements on whole-body counters, but health physicists were already involved in body burden studies.) Whatever the amount, or the toxicity, health physicists' first concern was: how do we get rid of it?

How to Promote Plutonium Excretion

Long before the metabolic pattern was known, or the toxicity studies completed, it had been observed that plutonium appeared in workers' urine. The more urine a worker produced, the more plutonium the worker excreted. In the absence of quantified toxicology the prudent path was to get rid of it all. Herbert Parker, chief health physicist, ordered the number of urinals at Hanford doubled. But how to assure their use?

Tom Shipmann, the chief industrial physician at Los Alamos, knew from extensive paramedical research that the best way to encourage micturition was to drink beer. He ordered free beer for all plutonium workers at Los Alamos. Hanford immediately adopted this life-saving policy. Somebody had to pay for all this beer and it became a hidden item in the budget — but the GAO sniffed it out.

The GAO was aghast! Not only was free beer non-repressive, but the workers actually followed the rules. The GAO accountants were mollified only after detailed explanation by Los Alamos medical experts. Nuclear advanced nations had a choice: either subject their plutonium workers to a lingering death from cancer, or flush out their bodies with the best diuretic known to man — free beer. It was said, on good authority, that Russian spies kept track of US plutonium production by monitoring the shipment of beer to Hanford.

°ISOTOPE PRODUCTION ON A KITCHEN TABLE

(Laundered from reminiscences of A. Rupp and E. Beauchamp at the 20th anniversary of the first °isotope shipment from Oak Ridge. [See Vig1946 .Pub])

When a June 1946 article in *Science* announced the availability of radioisotopes to the scientific public, we were not prepared for the response. No chemical engineering precedents existed for radioactive chemicals. We had to scale up research lab procedures by factors of a thousand and more. At first we supplied "units" of the popular radionuclides, but we were soon pushed into reactor neutron irradiation services. We irradiated steel piston rings, seeds, false teeth, plastics, petroleum, even diamonds.

The target material was put in a simple high purity aluminum can with a crimped lid. The can was put in a graphite "stringer" and inserted into the Clinton Pile (first name for the Oak Ridge graphite reactor). After irradiation for days or months the can was removed and sent to the customer in a shielded container. Tools to handle and open the can were sent with the shipment.

Almost immediately we were faced with devising larger scale methods for production and handling the big three: C-14, I-131, and P-32. At the same time we had to learn how to separate, purify, and process about 100 other °isotopes.

Items for irradiation had to be wrapped in aluminum as a "slug" to be placed in the stringer. One of our most difficult early problems was to remove this aluminum jacket. After many trials with remote control saws and lathes, we finally melted off the jackets in an inert-atmosphere electric-tube furnace.

The Pile Becomes a Production Reactor

Physical facilities for the °isotope program were non-existent. Any space, instruments, and tools that could be scrounged were used. Most of this work was done in an open field. Radiation safety was maintained with time-limitation and distance. Our Health Physicist was the ever-present man with the Cutie Pie and a stop watch.

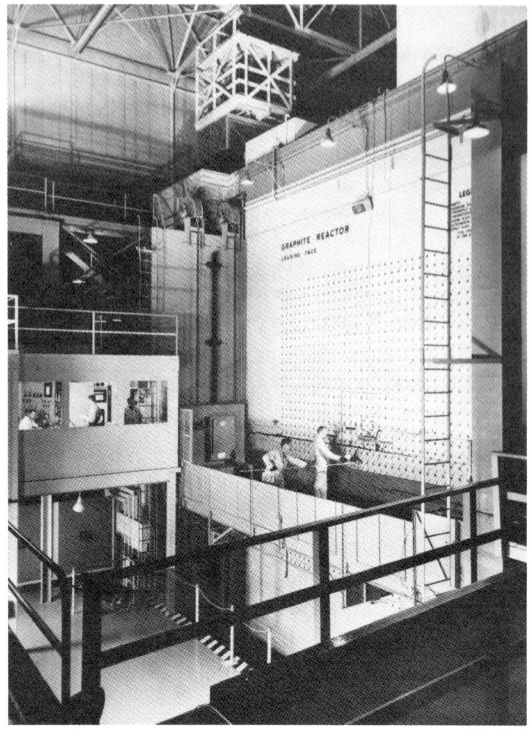

Oak Ridge National Laboratory's graphite reactor (the "Clinton Pile").

By 1949 we were already sending out 6000 shipments/year of 100 different °isotopes. Remote control had been designed and fabricated at ORNL. An "over-the-barricade-with-mirrors" served as the first packaging area. Each hot-lab man had to make his own tools. The great master-slave manipulators and hot-cells came from the remote-control group at Argonne long after we had already become a fairly large industrial facility.

The ORNL Irradiation Facility

At ORNL (Oak Ridge National Laboratory) the giant graphite reactor had a mighty 2×10^{11} n/cm^2·sec flux. (If you hadn't seen Hanford, which most people had not, it was a giant and the flux was mighty for its day.) We had hardly started production before we wanted 100 times that flux. Hundreds of $Ca(NO_3)$ slugs had to be irradiated to produce a single curie of C-14. Pounds of sulfur had to be irradiated to get a curie of P-32. Au-198 had nowhere near the desired specific activity. Our Co-60 pellets, the astounding wonder of 1950, were puny in 1951.

The really big Hanford reactors started helping us out as early as 1948, but their plutonium priority was a little higher than ours — and that damned secrecy was a pain in the neck. A new Low Intensity Test Reactor (LITR) was built at ORNL for hydraulic tests in 1951. It was soon converted into the first high flux reactor at 3×10^{13} n/cm^2 • sec. By 1955 the Materials Testing Reactor (MTR) was producing at a flux of 2×10^{14} n/cm^2 • sec. During the first decade of °isotope expansion, Oak Ridge produced over 99.99% of the °isotopes (in terms of curies) used throughout the world.

Fission Products Are NOT Waste Products

Fission products were found to be reactor poisons when the first Hanford reactor was automatically shut off by its own xenon production during the war. From the beginning it was known that ashes had to be removed from a fireplace to keep a fire going. Unlike wood and coal fires, however, the ashes of a reactor are not dirty waste (except to anti-nuke kooks). Fission products are a bountiful supply of a useful energy source.

Many radioisotopes are difficult to make in high specific activity, but are readily available carrier-free if separated as fission products. The feed for early production of I-131, Ba-140, Sr-89, Ce-141, Y-91, Xe-133 all came from the classified plutonium reactors. When the irradiation of tellurium to meet the huge demand for I-131 threatened to swamp our reactors, we went back to processing uranium fuel slugs.

Long-lived °isotopes in high specific activity are impractical to make in a reactor. Few people believed that anybody would want long-lived sources until in 1948 NBS requested a large spectrometrically pure, long-lived, gamma source for standardization purposes. The 0.661 Mev energy and 30y $T_{1/2}$ of Cs-137 fitted their requirements perfectly. We set up a Cs-alum process in the ORNL tank farm. Our equipment was so crude that the agitator in the tank was a remote-control hand-operated paddle, but a 10 Ci Cs-137 source was completed and delivered to NBS in 1950. Upon hearing of the NBS source, M. Brucer requested a Cs-137 source of at least 1000 Ci, not bigger than 2 cm diameter, for teletherapy. We improved the equipment scale and in 1954 delivered a 1500 Ci Cs-137 source properly compressed into a right cylinder about 2×2 cm.

International Competition
(From M. Brucer 1955 notes)

A sidelight on Cs-137 illustrates that the Oak Ridge monopoly on °isotope production was disappearing. At the 1953 ICR (Int Cong Radiology) Copenhagen meeting, an informal discussion of the availability of teletherapy sources was held over beer at the Tivoli Gardens. Co-60 with high specific activity was in short supply. Ir-192, tried in England, was too short-lived. Brucer mentioned Cs-137. He was measuring its gamma attenuation in tissue. "Send us your results," said William Eastwood from Harwell (the English equivalent of Oak Ridge), "we will check them with our calculations." "In our older Universities," Brucer replied, "we were taught that observations are not checked with calculations. Calculations are checked with observations." "My University (Oxford)," Eastwood replied, "wasn't established until the 1300s but we believe in the newer mathematics."

Upon my (MB) return to Oak Ridge I sent a graph of the attenuation of Cs-137 gammas by baloney sausage (tissue). It was inscribed in Latin, using Roman numerals. Eastwood returned the graph with his measurements of the I-gamma value written in Greek. We returned the graph with new measurements properly written in Japanese, using millifathom units. He returned the graph in Hebrew using millicubits as the units of length. By this time A. Rupp had a color photo of the 1500 Ci source taken in the dark using light from its own luminescence. I sent Eastwood a copy admitting I had run out of languages and anyway he mispronounced the name "aluminum." He answered by saying I misspelled it.

THE Rad UNIT OF DOSE

The roentgen is NOT a unit of radiation DOSE and its misuse as such distresses many physicists. During the 1920s a growing body of radiobiologists were beginning to study radiation bioeffects. The essential biological event, not meant to be measured with the roentgen unit, was the *energy absorbed* by a tissue during *exposure* to radiation. They assumed, as did most physicians, a high correlation between exposure and energy absorption. Two years after its 1928 adoption, Glasser proved that the r bore only a gross correlation to erythema.

The *energy* was not *absorbed* directly from an X-ray but mostly from the secondary electrons it displaced. The electrons displaced in the $cc_{(air)}$ originally visualized by the 1928 committee was a cavity of air surrounded by walls of some soft tissue. But in measuring instruments most of the ions emanated from its walls. If the walls were of iron, many electrons traversed the cavity, if of low Z material, few electrons. But for twenty years most of us read the r as a tissue dose.

The First Complaints

The French radium therapist C. Regaud had objected back in 1919 that cancers being exposed to radiation had a density orders of magnitude greater than air. Physicians thought a simple correction factor would be related to an absorption coefficient. The coefficients for X-rays then in use (except very soft radiation) were all about the same.

> (Probability of interactions in any material are about the same from 100 keV to 1000 keV rays, but with each interaction energy is lost until the rays are much less than 100 keV. Low energy interactions are highly dependant upon Z — the proton number of elements.) [Mayneord, BJR 2:373, 1929]

Mayneord's Gram-Roentgen

In the 1930s <100–250 keV energies dominated radiology. If the true meaning of "tissue dose" is to be measured with the r, a correction must include the probability of interaction in the chemical elements making up tissues. At the Royal Cancer Hospital radiotherapy center in London, W.V. Mayneord derived an average z for tissue (called bar z, or $\bar{z}$) from the Klein-Nishina formula:

$$\bar{z} = \underline{2.94}\sqrt{az_1^{2.94} + bz_2^{2.94} + cz_3^{2.94} \ldots}$$

> a, b, c, . . . are the electron contents of elements $z_1, z_2, z_3 \ldots$ [IUCC 2:271, 1937]

Mayneord's physics group calculated an effective $\bar{z}$ of air at 7.70 and of water at 7.24 (density does not enter the equation). The $\bar{z}$ of carbohydrates ($C_xH_xO_x$) was in the 6.9 range; of fats around 5.9. Proteins had $\bar{z}$ ranging from 6.3 to 6.9, but a few were unusual: thyronine (iodine inclusion) had a $\bar{z}$ of 44.6. Hence a hyperthyroid gland absorbed more radiation than a hypo gland. Hemoglobin (iron inclusion) had a $\bar{z}$ of 7.20. Such a small amount of iron is surrounded by so much globin ($\bar{z}$ = 6.6) that the $\bar{z}$ of hemoglobin (7.20) is actually less than that of air (7.70).

If the 1928 roentgen is to be used as a "dose unit" (in the medical sense of "dose = amount of drug absorbed") then, said Mayneord, we must modify the unit to say "r-dose." Although the preferred unit of absorbed energy is ergs/cc, the ionization unit "r" was an international decision. (1r = approx 0.1 erg/cc_{air}.) Mayneord proposed the dose unit be the amount of energy absorbed in a gram of tissue; hence a "gram-roentgen." [BJR 13:235, 1940]. (This unit was named the Roentgen absorbed dose (Rad) in 1954.)

Gray's "erg/cc"

Mayneord's work was centered around radiation therapy (which, after the atom bomb ended WWII, made him unpopular with anti-radiation health physicists). L.H. Gray, at Mount Vernon Hospital near London, on the other hand was studying radiation damage in animals (assuming damage at any level of radiation). Gray said, *"The most natural unit of radiation is the absolute increase in energy of the absorbing medium."* [BJR 10:721, 1937] Gray used ergs/cc as a unit, but because 1 erg = 10^{-7} joules, called it the "J." It was measured with an r meter as ions per unit volume of air.

Aebersold's "Neutron r"

At this time (1937) at UC Berkeley, R.S. Stone was using the new 61 inch cyclotron for neutron therapy of cancer. The r unit did not fit neutron irradiation so he asked physicist P.C. Aebersold to make a conversion. Aebersold measured the number of neutrons it took to produce an r (in air) and called this first conversion of particulates an "n" unit. [Rad 35:332, 1940]

Marinelli's "er"

John Lawrence was using millicuries of P-32 to treat leukemia patients in 1937. Leo Marinelli in New York said the mCi was quantity-of-substance, not a dose, so he defined the number of betas to produce an r of ionizations an "er" (equivalent roentgen). [AJR 47:210, 1942]

Gray's "eu" to Parker's "Rep"

Gray agreed with Mayneord's gram-roentgen concept and tried to adjust it to smaller animal bodies. He used water rather than air as the ionizing medium. Called "eu" (energy unit), it measured 93 ergs/gram of water. [Na 144:439, 1939] H.M. Parker, then a Manchester physicist active in radium dosimetry, measured Marinelli's beta particle "er" at 83 ergs/gram of tissue. He called this unit a Roentgen equivalent physical (Rep). [Advances in Bio Med Physics 1948]

Parker's Biological Unit

Parker's broad experience with radium therapy patient dosimetry taught him to always observe the end results of tissue irradiation. He noted the wide variation in Rep dose and relative effectiveness of alpha, beta, X and gamma rays. He proposed a modifier to the rep: the Relative Biological Effect (RBE). He called the Rep•RBE a Roentgen Equivalent Mammal (Rem). Although experimental RBE measurements were done on mice and fruit flies, many health physicists misled their press agents into calling it a Roentgen Equivalent Man (Rem).

After World War II health physics got AEC budgets directly proportional to the size of the rem dose and the fear of radiation stirred up in newspapers. The rem became known as a Roentgen Equivalent Money. With the 1960s excesses of geneticist's two-headed-babies, health physics excesses on Sr-90 watch dials, and linear extrapolations to death at De Minimus levels, the rem became known as Roentgen Equivalent Mickey Mouse. Radiobiologists can measure an RBE in 100 species and get 101 different results. (Some spoilsport always uses 2 animals.) The RBE is unmeasurable in humans, hence the rem cannot be a scientific unit.

After World War II the British Commission on Radiation Units met in 1948 to clarify the plethora of r, g-r, eu, er, Rep, Rad, Rem, ergs/g or cc of air, water, tissue. They redefined the J and Rep to be 93 ergs/g of tissue. (Gray was chairman of the commission, Parker was in America.)

The "rad" is Called the "gray"

In 1953 the ICRU made some major changes. A curie, no longer tied to radium, became exactly 3.7×10^{10} dps. The r did NOT apply to "dose." No matter what radiation was exposed to which material, the radiation absorbed dose (rad) would = 100 ergs/gram of whatever it was absorbed in. Radiotherapy was converting to supervoltage (mostly Co-60) where converting r to rad meant multiply by 1; hence, the rad became THE dose unit.

By 1975 the parent conference on weights and measures (15th CGPM), having established SI units, saw that neither the erg nor gram was coherent. The joule was the derived SI energy unit: 100 ergs = 10^{-5} joules, the kilogram = 10^3 grams; hence $10^{-5}/10^3$ = 0.01 J/kg. Such a rad is not SI acceptable. A coherent unit must have 1 J/kg and must have a new name. It could have been called the "Mayneord" because he invented the rad, but L.H. Gray had just died and had chaired the committee to define the rad. They named a 100 rad unit a gray (Gy). Now by the new rules of SI grammar all the "names" lose their caps in text but symbols named after people are capitalized: becquerel (Bq), joule (J), meter (m), second (s).

Health Physics Goes Mad

By the 1970s a radiation hysteria, fomented by geneticists and health physicists, fermented out of control. Health Physics promoted a series of unmeasurable hence non-falsifiable concepts by either legislative fiat or divine revelation. The story of the rem, the Q, Sv, Working Level Months, and dose equivalents, is a new story of a science gone mad.

[See Vig1976 rem]

THE FLOWERING OF NUCLEAR MEDICINE
1954 through 1984

FROM Jeff Holter's organization of the Montana Society of Nuclear Medicine (which never had a meeting and he was the only member), through the proliferation of at least 50 local, national, and international societies claiming at least 50,000 members . . .

FROM P-32 (a new kind of therapy), I-131 (which killed off a generation of thyroid surgeons), and Co-60 (true supervoltage therapy that saved more man-years of human life than would have been lost in many Hiroshimas), through radiopharmacies filling millions of °prescriptions by phone . . .

FROM 99.9% AEC supported research in good stuff (the Bomb was bad and very secret stuff), to a self supporting and, since about 1965, a money making business . . .

FROM Stafford Warren's observation that the ground around the Trinity explosion site was radioactive, through the fallout hysteria of the 1960s and the regulatory inspired radio-phobia of the 1970s . . .

. . . IN its third of a century lifetime, Nuclear Medicine has had Brachytherapy, Teletherapy, most wet chemistry, and RIA amputated from its body. It still survives with promise of growth of new appendages. In early days Cassen's little 1949 tap scanner visualized the thyroid gland in a physiologic mode — an astounding feat. And then a fast camera and then computers were added; and then the detection signals were changed to include positrons, sonic reflections, mathematically focused X-rays, and nuclear magnetic resonances.

Much of the human body can now be visualized in anatomic, physiologic, or biochemical mode. Nuclear Medicine minimized its original emphasis on therapy and developed a new form of physical diagnosis, a physiological "radiology" now called "imaging." All of which goes back to an off-hand remark made by Hippocrates to a student, "You really ought to look at a patient before making a diagnosis."

CNM1954 Soc of Nuc Med organized.
CNM1955 First Atoms for Peace conference.
CNM1956 1509 °isotope licenses issued.
CNM1957 Liver scan introduced.
CNM1958 First cardiac blood pool scan.
CNM1959 KY has first state AEC.
CNM1960 In vitro RIA introduced.
CNM1961 °Mo-Tc99m cow introduced.
CNM1962 "Bolus" injection introduced.
CNM1963 °IMAA lung scan introduced.
CNM1964 Med Int Rad Dose (MIRD) starts.
CNM1965 First gamma camera symposium.
CNM1966 Organ perfusion studies begin.
CNM1967 "Nuclide" replaces "isotope."
CNM1968 Gated blood pool scans begin.
CNM1969 °Xe washout measures bld flow.
CNM1970 Ventilation scans begin.
CNM1971 Ejection Fraction introduced.
CNM1972 °TcPYP takes over bone scans.
CNM1973 CAT scanning introduced.
CNM1974 Tin (in PYP) causes RBC label.
CNM1975 AEC killed by President Ford.
CNM1976 FDA says NO dose is safe
CNM1977 Tl-201 confirmed clinically.
CNM1978 °Tc-IDAs take over billiary scans.
CNM1979 TMI is news media phobia.

CHRONOLOGY OF NUCLEAR MEDICINE — 1954

	Scientific and Technical Background		Ref.
3. # Nuc —	J. Martin says Oak Ridge cyclo can make 150 °isotopes.	[1952]	AEC
—	O.R. begins multikCi fission-product separation plant.	[1946]	AEC
4. # Med —	Isotopes Div: 5000 shipments of I-131 to 400 hospitals.	[1946]	AEC
	2500 shipments of P-32 to 389 hospitals.	[1937]	AEC
	622 shipments of Au-198 to 50 hospitals.	[1946]	AEC
—	492 °labeled compounds available from 18 suppliers.	[1953]	AEC
—	3173 °isotope shipments made to 46 foreign countries.	[1947]	AEC
—	"Isotopes . . . 8-year Summary" last accurate AEC summary;	[1946]	AEC
	private and foreign suppliers are now significant.	[1950]	AEC

	Organizations and Internal Politics		
5. AEC + —	Atomic Energy Act (1948) revised: permits State & private help.		AP
—	Atomic Energy Authority Acts (Grt Brit) revised.	[1953]	AP
—	AEC plans to withdraw °isotope sales (private conflict).	[1950]	AP
—	AEC fires J. Oppenheimer as political security risk.	[1942]	AP
—	R. Zirkle edits Man Dist Declass Documents (MDDC) in Biology:		
	"Biol Effects of External X and Gamma Rad."	(1941–1946	MED)
6. Socs —	N. HOLTER ORGANIZES A SOCIETY OF NUCLEAR MEDICINE.		AP
—	Isotopes Div says 10,250 °isotope articles published	('34–54.	AEC)
—	MRC (Eng) pubs "Intro Manual, Control Health Hazards."	[1950]	MRC
—	Rad Research Soc begins pub of "Radiation Research."	[1952]	RR
7. Event —	U.N. endorses Internat atomic trade fair (Atoms-for-Peace).	[1953]	AP
—	E. Geiling (U Chi) introduces Nuclear Pharmacy concept.	[1974]	AEC
—	Ambas Lodge presents UN with AEC technical library.	[1953]	AEC
—	NBS accepts 3-bladed prop (magenta on yellow) rad symbol.	[1950]	NBS
—	USS Nautilus (first nuc sub) demonstrates power potential.	[1956]	USN
—	I. Kurchatov describes first USSR nuclear power plant:	[1949]	AEC
	5 MW_e at Oninsk on Moscow grid.	[1956] (1984	IAEA)

	Instruments, Units of Measurement, and Drugs		
8. Instr —	H. Anger makes first whole body scan (10 GM glow tubes).	[1953]	JCAE
—	E. Pochin introduces first whole body linear scanner.	[1950]	BJR
—	M. Van Dilla devises first liquid whole body (dog) counter.	[1953]	Nuc
—	R. Baskin devises well-type scintillation counter.	[1950]	Nuc
—	R. Hiebert (Packard Co) sells first liquid scint counter.	[1953]	Nuc
—	E. Gabriel introduces °IHSA zone paper electrophoresis.	[1926]	JCI
—	M. Jacobs uses "Teledeltos" paper on noisy tap scanner.	[1949]	Nuc
9. Units —	TENTH CGPM ADOPTS 6 BASIC SI UNITS		
	(seventh is held back).	[1948]	CGPM
—	CGPM accepts triple point of water as 273.16 K.	[1889]	NBS
—	NBS adopts 4-pi counter as primary standard for betas.	[1950]	NBS
—	NBS routinely calibrates 8 °isotopes (Co-60 primary).	[1948]	NBS
—	M. Brucer introduces 10y Mock-Iodine for I-131 calibration.	[1953]	AEC
10. Concp —	G. LeRoy introduces double label liquid scint counting.	[1950]	JACS
—	R. Shipley: no diff between °I & °IHSA on first pass.	[1953]	CirR
—	L. Sharney elaborates theory, multiple °Fe pools & spaces.	[1952]	PSEB
—	W. Moos finds energy-dependent effect in bacteria (LET).	[1952]	Nuc
—	R. Dudley quantifies photo-density in beta ARG.	[1953]	Nuc
—	Gamma irradiation field (to 10 Mr/h) at Idaho Test site.	[1960]	AEC
11. Drugs —	W. Tucker makes I-132 in second cow system (radon was first).	[1908]	Nuc
—	A. Bearn sees Cu-64 in blood fractions of Wilson's Dis.	[1950]	PSEB
—	N. Simon finds °AuCol particles enlarged by globulin.	[1944]	Sc
—	D. Laszlo substitutes °Y for °Au in Rx of serous effusion.	[1952]	JNCI
—	L. Farr introduces 1.8 h Kr-83 and 37.2 m Cl-38 in med.	[1952]	AEC

Radioiodine, P-32, and Radioactive Therapy

13. I-Dx	— M. Brucer starts world-wide thyroid uptake calibration.	[1953]	AEC
	— H. Thode finds I-131 very high in hypothyroid's saliva.	[1965]	NEJM
	— W. McIntyre says first deriv of uptake curve is clearance.	[1944]	AEC
	— 11 articles (e.g., T. Fields) find PB°I superior to uptake.	[1951]	JLCM
	— Abbott Labs begins sale of Dx I-131 in capsules ($1/cap).	[1950]	AP
	— D. Tabern (Ab Lab) says 24 h uptake is almost universal.	[1951]	V38
	— D. Sklaroff reports a met to thyroid from rectal ca.	[1950]	ArS
14. I-Rx	— G. Burke treats emphysema with I-131 to hypo state.	[1949]	JCI
	— 11 articles (e.g., E. Chapman) promote °I Rx of hypers.	[1953]	JCEn
	— J. Pemberton denigrates I-131 Rx of ca as "dangerous."	[1984]	ACS
16. Tele	— A. Rupp makes 1500 curie Cs-137 source for teletherapy.	[1952]	AEC
	— M. Brucer's Internat standard Co-60 source capsule accepted.	[1952]	BJR
	— 30 Co-60 teletherapy units in operation in USA.	[1952]	AEC
17. Other	— 8 articles (e.g., G. Andrews) give intracav °Au Rx results.	[1953]	AEC
	— H. Friedell summarizes 4 y Sr-90 eye tumor Rx experience.	[1952]	AJR
	— 4 articles (e.g., J. Cooper) report °AuCol prostate ca Rx.	[1953]	JU
	— L. Farr encouraged by trials of slow neutron capture Rx.	[1952]	AJR

Scans and Other Tests of Function in Various Organs

18. Brain	— N. Lassen measures cerebral blood flow with Kr-85.	[1953]	APhS
	— W. Seaman cuts scan delay time & D°IF dose: gets error.	[1950]	Rad
19. Heart	— R. Huff presents first Soc Nuc Med paper (cardiac output).	[1953]	JNM
	— N. Veall introduces precordial surface count technique.	[1952]	SRC
	— W. Love compares Rb-86 kinetics with K-42 in dog heart.	[1953]	CirR
	— G. Gigli measures Pulmonary Transit Time (PTT) on RCG.	[1948]	BSIB
	— D. Goldring introduces shunt detection by RCG.	[1948]	JPd
20. Liver	— G. Taplin introduces I-131 Rose Bengal liver testing.	[1951]	AEC
	— A. Vetter: plasma °AuCol clearance is liver blood flow.	[1953]	JCI
21. Lung	— B. Benacerraf prepares °IMMA for use in RES study.	[1953]	RH
22. Bone	— G. Bauer: P-32 dispersion is a function of bone growth.	[1939]	JBJS
	— P. Durbin studies metabolism of F-18 in bone tissues.	[1953]	JDR
24. Gut	— J. Badenoch studies oral °Fe absorption in steatorrhea.	[1951]	BJR
	— S. Callender estimates intrinsic factor by $°VB_{12}$ in feces.	[1953]	BMJ
25. Blood	— I. Weinstein introduces clinical °Cr-RBC survival test.	[1953]	BI
	— R. Read introduces the Cr-51 "closed system" RBC volume.	[1950]	NEJM
	— M. Strumia devises an improved blood preservative soln.	[1951]	AJCP
	— J. Cohen uses DF°P as RBC tag in study of RBC turnover.	[1951]	JCI

Radiation Hysteria and Health Physics * Obituaries *

27. Hyst	— R. Lange finds 65 leukemics in 76,891 A-Bomb survivors.	[1952]	ABCC
	— 82 Marshallese, 23 Jap fishman exposed Eniwetok fallout.	[1952]	JAMA
	— Public awareness of "fallout" & "°waste" begins.	[1952]	AP
	— J. Rust finds osteo sarc in muskrat exposed in °Sr dump.	[1985]	ArP
	— K. Morgan calculates MPC (70 °isotopes), explains method.	[1953]	Nuc
	— A. Upton says hi-dose irrad mice show premature aging.	[1979]	FP
28. React	— A. Polednak shows hormesis in 1155 radium dial painters.	[1931]	AJE
	— G. Burke lowers I-131 Rx age limit to 30 years.	[1951]	JCI
	— P. Aggeler relates bone marrow damage to °I dose size.	[1050]	AEC
	— A. Krebs: Ra-226 body burd in 10^{-10} range. (MPC is 10^{-7}).	[1931]	Sc
	— F. Turner: 950 Harwell workers show normal blood counts.	[1949]	AERE
29. Respo	— AEC conducts more H-bomb tests at Bikini.	[1952]	AEC

* * *

30. Obits	— E. Fermi (1901–1954) It physics; nuclear physics.		DSB

CHRONOLOGY OF NUCLEAR MEDICINE — 1955

Scientific and Technical Background

			Ref.
1. Basic	— O. Chamberlain discovers antiproton, verifies antimatter.	[1932]	PR
	— P. Bridgmann makes artif diamonds with high pressure.	[1931]	DSB
3. # Nuc	— Materials Test Reactor (MTR) to 2×10^{14} n/cm^2 flux.	[1951]	AEC
4. # Med	— MD license requires 30 h training & 10 pts experience.	[1953]	AEC
	— A. Kozlova says USSR uses °I, °P, °Au, °Co, much brachyRx.	[1952]	AfP

Organizations and Internal Politics

5. AEC +	— Am Conf Gov Indust Hygienists adopts MPD "Threshold."	[1952]	PHR
	— AEC invites Governors to form limited State AECs.	[1954]	AEC
6. Socs	— Int Labor Office (ILO) publishes its protection guide.	[1959]	ILO
	— Health Physics Soc organized at Ohio State U (200 mem).	[1954]	AP
	— Steering Com meets at RSNA to nationalize Soc Nuc Med.	[1954]	PL
	— P. Bell publishes "Medical Scintillation Spectrometry."	[1953]	Nuc
	— G. Andrew's pubs "Radioisotopes in Medicine" textbook.	[1953]	AEC
7. Event	— FIRST ATOMS-FOR-PEACE (AfP) CONFERENCE HELD IN GENEVA.	[1954]	AfP
	— First 1-month Oak Ridge foreign student training course.	[1948]	AEC
	— AEC shows first commercial reactor-produced electricity.	[1954]	AEC
	— Calder Hall reactor (Eng) produces electricity.	[1954]	AERE
	— W. Shockley manufactures integrated circuit chips.	[1948]	FV

Instruments, Units of Measurement, and Drugs

8. Instr	— G. Brownell introduces the clinical positron scanner.	[1953]	JAMA
	— Cassen, Mayneord, Brownell, Anger, Japanese scanners at Geneva.		AfP
	— L. Marinelli starts "Iron room" 8" crystal whole body counts.	[1954]	AEC
	— E. Anderson starts 4-pi "human" liquid whole body counts.	[1954]	AEC
	— Diamond crystal counter described at A-f-P conference.	[1951]	AfP
	— N. Horwitz modulates scan count rate by photoexposure.	[1952]	Nuc
	— G. Boyd pubs detail methods for gross and micro ARGs.	[1952]	Bk
9. Units	— E. Miller defines "Full Width Half Maximum" (FWHM) resolution.		Nuc
	— E. Roberts tells ICR that the "Rad" is unmeasurable.	[1944]	BJR
10. Concp	— E. Odeblad shows activation analysis of alpha emitters.	[1938]	AR
	— Leeds Body Burden Conference on Whole Body Counters.	[1954]	LBB
11. Drugs	— C. Comar finds early F-18 metabolism mimics early °Ca.	[1942]	AJP
	— G. Burch says Rb-86 good but not exact sub for K-42.	[1953]	JLCM

Radioiodine, P-32, and Radioactive Therapy

12. I-Res	— C. Tobias isolates °I-T4 on an anion exchange resin.	[1953]	ABB
	— H. Miller finds °I higher in milk/blood in lactating pt.	[1952]	La
	— F. Keating: 17% T1, 25% T2, 8% T3, 35% T4 in 9 glands.	[1951]	JCEM
	— S. BERSON SAYS PERCHLORATE STOPS °I TRAPPING, NOT WASHOUT.	[1952]	JCI
	— G. Andrews describes histology of massive dose I-131.	[1953]	AJR
13. I-Dx	— D. Tabern distributes phantom that distorts uptake.	[1953]	PL
	— S. Werner initiates a T3 suppression test for hypers.	[1952]	JCE
	— M. Perlmutter modifies (& verifies) T3 suppression test.	[1952]	JAMA
	— F. Bauer starts the TSH stim scan to find metastases.	[1953]	ca
	— M. Brucer surveys 128 US (8 Eng) labs with °I manikins;	[1953]	V39
	poor uptake calibration results in world survey.	[1953]	V39
	— L. Larsson initiates "trapping" measurements.	[1952]	AR
14. I-Rx	— D. CLARK NOTES 17% HYPOTHYROIDISM AFTER 625 °I THERAPIES.		JAMA
	— H. Blumgart gets good result in 75% of °I Rx cardiacs.	[1933]	JAMA
	— W. Hamilton gets 50% success in °I Rx of Chr Pul Insuff.	[1933]	JMAG
	— R. Rigler reports rad parotitis after hi-dose °I Rx.	[1952]	MCP

14. I-Rx — S. Seidlin reports 2 leukemia deaths after I.5 Ci °I. [1952] BNYM
— J. Buckwalter treats 78 thyroid ca children with I-131. [1951] JCEM
15. P-Rx — J. Lawrence's P-32 PV patients have normal life span. [1965] Bk
— J. Harman says P-32 is PV Rx of choice in England. [1951] BMJ
16. Tele — AEC begins large scale high sp act Co-60 production. [1954] AEC
17. Other — F. Ellis successful in Rx of bladder papillomata (°Au). [1950] BMJ
°BRACHYTHERAPY IS NO LONGER CONSIDERED "NUCLEAR MEDICINE"
— A. Sherman encouraged by °AuCol in ovarian ca ascites. [1953] AJOG
— W. Seaman: no °Au in cancerous lymph nodes on sub-Q inj. [1953] Ca
— L. Farr notes poor results in slow neutron capture Rx. [1954] Ca

Scans and Other Tests of Function in Various Organs

18. Brain — N. Lassen measures cerebral blood flow with Kr-85. [1954] APhS
— G. Nylin uses Pb-212 (Th B) for cer bld flow studies. [1953] CR
— S. Chou studies absorp of °IHSA from subarach space. [1951] N
19. Heart — G. Burch finds Cs-134 not a substitute in °K kinetics. [1953] JLCM
— R. Huff says RCG and Fick cardiac outputs match well. [1954] Cir
20. Liver — G. Taplin astounds AfP conf with °Rose Bengal test. [1954] AfP
— L. Sapirstein measures °RB clearance as plasma test. [1954] AJPh
21. Lung — H. Conn finds Xe-133 almost cleared on first lung pass. [1952] JCI
— H. Knipping measures 16 lung fields, °Xe "Thoracogram." [1951] DMW
23. Kidney — C. Hlad says 49 °I clearances more variable than inulin. [1953] JCI
— E. Cotlove's C-14 inulin: no label effect on glomerular filtration. [1951] FP
24. Gut — G. Baylin compares °I bld levels & gastric empty time. [1983] PSEB
— W. Shingleton uses °fats, °proteins in Dx of pancreas dis. [1953] NEJM
25. Blood — M. Pollycove develops ferrokinetics and ferrograms. [1951] CRP
— T. Bothwell finds diurnal variation in Fe-59 turnover. [1951] CS
— P. Mollison sees two phase curve in Cr-51 RBC survival. [1954] BJH
— D. Hodgren finds structure of cyanocobalamin (VB$_{12}$). [1954] BMJ
— C. Booth introduces Co-57 VB$_{12}$. [1954] V48
— D. Sutherland tags leuks with °Cr for in vivo survival. [1985] JLCM
— R. Schilling does ext counts of °Cr-RBC for chromigrams. [1954] CRP
— M. Morgan measures °Cr labeled platelet survival (days). [1987] JLCM
26. Other — F. Bauer measures °Na, °K kinetics in musc dystrophy pts. [1952] N
— H. Conn estimates organ's blood flow by K-42 dilution. [1952] JAPh
— K. Hultborn finds no °AuCol in cancerous lymph nodes. [1953] AR
— N. Morris measures °Na washout $T_{1/2}$ in preg uterus muscle. [1953] La

Radiation Hysteria and Health Physics * Obituaries *

27. Hyst — Now 92 of 110,000 atom bomb survivors have leukemia. [1954] ABCC
— H. Muller predicts genetic catastrophe from A-Bombs. [1920] AEC
(massive genetics funding proves him wrong in 1983 Sc)
— D. Clark notes 13 childhood thyroid ca had neck irrad. [1950] JAMA
Hempleman, Simpson, Wilson studies verify Clark's story. [1950] JAMA
— W. Libby worries about 1 µCi Ra in his wrist watch. [1959] Sc
— S. Macht finds genetic defects in radiologists' progeny. [1952] AJR
28. React — J. Crow finds no genetic diff in radiologists' progeny. [1984] AJR
— R. Stanford measures rad to gonads from Dx X-Rays. [1952] BJR
— I. Doniach finds no thyroid ca (rats) at any I-131 dose. [1952] BJC
— Symposium on hazards, dose, and genetic effects of rad. [1954] BJR
— P. Ives notes longer life span in lo-dose fruit flies. [1954] DMG
— T. Lysenko removed from USSR Inst of Genetics [1928] SN
29. Respo — No regulation of radiation by law in West Germany. [1950] RB

* * *

30. Obits — A. Einstein (1879–1955) Ger math physics; relativity. DSB
— S. Seidlin (1898–1955) Am endocrin; thyroid °iodine Rx. V36
— B. Low Beer (1900–1955) Am radiol; first surface P-32 Rx. Rad

CHRONOLOGY OF NUCLEAR MEDICINE — 1956

Scientific and Technical Background

			Ref.
1. Basic	— C. Cowan sees antineutrino to prove neutrino exists.	[1955]	Sc
	— J. Cork discovers the antineutron.	[1932]	PR
	— R. Borghgraef studies basic pharm of °Hg-chlormerodrin.	[1950]	JCI
3. # Nuc	— C. Keim says 200 stable isotopes produced in Oak Ridge.	[1951]	AEC
4. # Med	— AEC supports 210 med research projects @ $30 megabucks.	[1946]	AEC
	— °Isotope shipments mostly to commercial distributors.	[1954]	AEC
	— 1509 °isotope licenses issued to 337 med institutions.	[1955]	AEC

Organizations and Internal Politics

5. AEC +	— Texas Brd of Health passes its own rad protect rules.	[1955]	AEC
	— E. Quimby (Subhuman Comm): "Most MDs too stupid for °isotopes."		AEC
	— NBS handbk #59: same public and occupational rad limit.	[1950]	NBS
6. Socs	— SOC NUC MED BECOMES NATIONAL SOC WITH 7 REGIONAL CHAPTERS.		PN
	— AEC & NAS publish first "Biological Effects of Fallout."	[1952]	JCAE
	— c11,000 scientific papers on °isotopes since 1946 (60% Med).		AEC
	— Organized Radiol demands °isotopes to Radiologists only.	[1898]	PN
7. Event	— H-3 (Tritium) now @ $0.002/mCi (cheapest °isotope ever).	[1946]	AEC
	— Microwatt "atomic batteries" (100% reliable) on sale.	[1954]	AEC
	— Second Nuc Power plant, 5 MW$_e$, at Marcoule, France.	[1954]	(1984 IAEA)
	— Third Nuc Power plant, 55 MW$_e$, at Calder Hall, Eng.	[1957]	(1984 IAEA)

Instruments, Units of Measurement, and Drugs

8. Instr	— M. Brucer develops spectral linear whole body scanner.	[1954]	AEC
	— E. Anderson builds sensitive liquid whole body counter.	[1955]	AEC
	— C. Borkowski says 3 × 3″ NaI(Tl) scintillator most common.	[1953]	IRET
	— W. Higinbotham builds 256 chan pulse height analyser.	[1955]	IRET
	— A. Riegert develops AgPO$_4$ glass needles for dosimetry.	[1953]	Nuc
	— C. Harris makes CsI (Tl) sterilizable surg gamma probe.	[1951]	Nuc
	— DuMont Labs develops 20″ dia photomultiplier cathodes.	[1955]	IRET
9. Units	— ICRP adopts the unmeasurable Rem unit of "measurement";	[1951]	ICRP
	introduces unmeasurable "accumulated dose" concept.	[1954]	ICRP
10. Concp	— C. Miller plots precision background gamma ray spectra.	[1950]	IRET
	— E. Freiling explains difficult 2-phase curve-stripping.	[1954]	Nuc
	— R. Carter finds RBE of neutrons 1.5–2.3 >250 kVp X-ray.	[1847]	RR
	— E. Reeve finds adsorp of °IHSA on glass causes errors.	[1952]	PSEB
	— G. Palade: microsomes are rich in RNA; hence "ribosomes."	[1937]	SN
11. Drugs	— O. Daniel: IV °ZnCl localizes partly in the prostate.	[1983]	BJU
	— T. Andre labels streptomycin and tetracycline with H-3.	[1952]	AR

Radioiodine, P-32, and Radioactive Therapy

12. I-Res	— D. Doniach finds an autoantibody in Hashimoto's serum.	[1927]	La
	— M. Tubiana says °I thyroid dose cannot be calculated.	[1955]	AEC
13. I-Dx	— P. Starr detects thyroid ca pulm metastases on °I scan.	[1954]	JAMA
	— 27 articles (e.g., M. Brucer) describe tech in clin use.	[1646]	JCAE
	— E. Paulson: not every Hashimotos is low °I thyroiditis.	[1927]	MM
	— E. Martmer measures °I uptake in premature infants.	[1954]	Ped
14. I-Rx	— 7 articles (e.g., K. Fairley) discuss °I Rx of hyperthyroid.	[1954]	MJA
	— 15 articles (e.g., R. Mack) discuss thyroid ca management.	[1954]	JAMA
	— E. Pochin's ca Rx is surgical ablation + 150 mCi °I.	[1955]	BJR
	— Symposium notes post °I Rx hypothyroid in 0.2 to 30%.	[1955]	AEC
15. P-Rx	— W. Crosby: Osgood's titration in CGLeuk lower in women.	[1952]	BJH

16. Tele	— J. Nolan describes results from first Co-60 (1952) unit.	[1952]	AJOG
	— M. Brucer devises an auto-computer-control Cs-137 unit.	[1954]	AJR
	— RSNA Symposium decides 250 kVp therapy is NOT obsolete.	[1955]	Rad
17. Other	— B. Schoolman's °AuCol Rx (liver mets) causes aplas anemia.	[1953]	JAMA
	— A. Sherman's intraparametrial °AuCol is std palliat Rx.	[1955]	Bk
	— L. Orr: good palliation with Flock's °AuCol prostate Rx.	[1954]	JU
	— W. Christopherson irrad breast with subQ Lu-177 injection.	[1953]	AEC
	— R. Libby: injectate control (Cr°PO_4) is major Rx problem.	[1953]	AS
	— F. Bonte: N-Mustard as good as °AuCol in effusions Rx.	[1953]	Rad

Scans and Other Tests of Function in Various Organs

18. Brain	— L. Sapirstein: Fick principle forbids N_2O bl flow method.	[1953]	CirR
	— W. Sweet prefers As-74 positron scans to locate tumors.	[1955]	JCAE
19. Heart	— A. Hansen measures coronary (myocard ?) bld flow with Kr-85.	[1953]	SJCI
	— L. Donato measures Pulmonary Transit Time (PTT) from RCG.	[1954]	MM
20. Liver	— W. Marshall (2 others) verify Taplin's °I-RB hepatogram.	[1955]	JLCM
	— H. FRIEDELL SCANS LIVER WITH 5 AGENTS, °I-RB, °AuCol BEST.	[1953]	AJR
	— B. Halpern estimates liver bld flow from °IMAA clearance.	[1954]	CRSB
21. Lung	— J. Lammerant calculates pulm bld vol from PulTransTime.	[1954]	ACB
22. Bone	— S. Ahlstrom relates °IHSA joint-drain-time & rheum arthritis.	[1952]	ARS
23. Kidney	— J. Briggs injects IV °I-Hipp; clearance gives function.	[1951]	JCP
	— G. Taplin runs °I-Diodrast renograms on rabbits & humans.	[1950]	JLCM
	— C. Winter uses external counts for °I-Diodrast renogram.	[1950]	JU
	— 13 donor RBC & plasma studies solve Paroxy Noc Hemoglobinuria.		CS
24. Gut	— J. Halsted gets accurate °Co-VB_{12} from stool specimens.	[1954]	AJM
	— C. Booth says Co-56 VB_{12} plasma level peaks at 3-6 hour.	[1954]	BJH
	— D. Mollin finds slow Co-58 VB_{12} clearance in CMLeuk.	[1954]	Bl
	— L. Meyer measures gut hemorrhage with precise °CrRBC vol.	[1954]	JAMA
25. Blood	— F. Johnson finds 18% of dog's blood in splanchnic vasc. bed.		AJPh
	— C. Owen does ext counts of liv, spl, mar for ferrograms.	[1955]	MCNA
	— 9 donor studies (sickle into normals) use RBC life spans.		JCI
26. Other	— S. BERSON IDENTIFIES °INSULIN BINDING ANTIBODY, RIA HINT.	[1948]	JCI
	— N. DasGupta (India) confirms Low-Beer's °P uptake in ca.	[1946]	AR
	— A. Weinberg develops area count °IHSA placentography.	[1955]	OG

Radiation Hysteria and Health Physics * Obituaries *

27. Hyst	— Sh. Warren says radiologists die 5.2 y early (disputed).	[1955]	JAMA
	— P. Starr says 2 gravids given °I Rx 13th wk, babies hypo.	[1951]	SGO
	— L. vanMiddlesworth detects thyroid °I after Nev A-tests.	[1954]	Sc
	— K. Morgan says MPD is 5 Rem/y (Rem is unmeasurable).	[1954]	AEC
	— NAS starts 25 y "radiotherapy-for-maligs-only" dark age.	[1981]	NAS
	— NIH starts the cancer chemotheraphy reign of terror.	[1981]	Ca
	— A. Stewart says kids exposed in utero have more cancer.	[1970]	La
	A. Reventos considers banning radiotherapy in children.	[1950]	PMJ
	— J. Horta can list only 16 Thorotrast liver sarcomas.	[1947]	APa
28. React	— A. Freedberg finds no leukemia in 150 cardiac °I Rx pts.	[1955]	AEC
	— K. Fairley notes fertility up, in thyroid °I Rx pts.	[1955]	MJA
	— E. Uhlman: only 4 of 25 thyroid ca children had radioRx.	[1955]	JAMA
	— NAS publishes Bio Effects of Fallout; few read it.	[1954]	NAS
	— F. Farmer compares rad risks favorably with other risks.	[1955]	AfP
29. Respo	— R. Hasterlik finds 4 proofs: male rad sterility is transient.	[1946]	AEC
	— H. Schreiber; hi-dose to 14 y old's ovaries has no effect.	[1952]	BJR
	— M. Eisenbud compiles global fallout pattern.	[1954]	AEC
	G. Dunning: thyroid °I fallout dose is uncalculable.	[1954]	Nuc

* * *

30. Obits	— F. Soddy (1877–1956) Eng p chem; named the "isotopes."		Na
	— I. Joliot-Curie (1897–1956) Fr physics; first man-made °isotopes.		DoE

CHRONOLOGY OF NUCLEAR MEDICINE — 1957

Scientific and Technical Background

			Ref.
1. Basic	— Unconfirmed report of Nobelium #105 from Stockholm.	[1952]	SN
2. Obser	— W. Sullivan: gummed stamps keep Trilinear Chart current.	[1949]	TC
3. # Nuc	— 3 Sep, 100,000th AEC shipment, 75 mCi K-42 to U Iowa.	[1946]	AP
	— °Kr, °I, °Cs, °Sr, °Xe sales justify Fission Separ Plant.	[1954]	AEC
4. # Med	— New type AEC licenses to 1572 physicians & 643 hospitals.	[1956]	AEC
	— 100 private companies now distributing °isotopes.	[1954]	AEC

Organizations and Internal Politics

5. AEC +	— AMA adopts AEC policy on °isotope use in hospitals.	[1956]	JAMA
	— Fed. Register: Title 10, Part 20: Stnds for protection.	[1954]	FR
	— Fed. Register: Title 10, Part 30: Licensing procedures.	[1954]	FR
	— ICRU-ICRP joint meeting rates somatic over genetic damage.	[1952]	HP
6. Socs	— IAEA organized in Vienna with 58 member states.	[1946]	IAEA
	— UNESCO holds °isotope conf in Paris (repeats '55 AfP).	[1955]	UN
	— F. Ellinger's "Medical Radiation Biology" published.	[1954]	Bk
7. Event	— Kyoto U: 2000 Ci Co-60 irradiator to study rad effects.	[1945]	BICR
	— USSR is producing kilocuries of 75 °isotopes.	[1956]	IJAR
	— Hammersmith (Lon) installs first hospital cyclotron.	[1953]	PIEE
	— Fourth Nuc Power plant, 90 MW_e, at Shippingport, PA. Dec.	(1984	IAEA)
	— Vallecitos, 5 MW_e San Jose Nuclear license to GE, June.	[1954]	SN

Instruments, Units of Measurement, and Drugs

8. Instr	— M. Bender introduces a modulated photodot recording.	[1955]	Sc
	— E. Rapkin introduces automatic liquid sample changing.	[1954]	IJAR
	— L. Larsson demonstrates usefulness of 3/4 body scans.	[1956]	AUCC
9. Units	— G. Adams measures 70 MeV beam in H_2O @ 0.86 rads/esu•cc.	[1953]	Rad
	— R. Loevinger calculates table of beta spectra in all Z.	[1953]	PMB
	— D. Holaday introduces WL (Work Level) = 1.3×10^5 MeV alpha in air.		PHR
10. Concp	— A. Riddell warns of subjectivity of curve stripping.	[1956]	CS
11. Drugs	— H. Kroll labels DTPA with Y-90, La-140; fast & stable.	[1954]	Na
	— L. Stang makes °Mo-°Tc cow for Esso vat mixing problem.	[1938]	5CN
	— H. Fischer: stannic oxide not toxic to 350 mg/kg (rabbit).	[1977]	Rad
	— D. PRESSMAN LABELS ANTIBODIES WITH °ISOTOPE.	[1955]	NYAS

Radioiodine, P-32, and Radioactive Therapy

12. I-Res	— S. Ingbar isolates T4 binding protein on ion-exch resin.	[1955]	E
	— R. Yalow measures 30-min °I space @ 20% of body weight.	[1954]	JCE
	— M. Ferguson: same °I salivary secretion in euthyroids & hypos.	[1954]	CMAJ
	— J. Stein: constant ratio between plasma and salivary °I.	[1947]	JLCM
	— S. Newman: organic I uptake depression lasts c30 days.	[1948]	JCE
	— M. Morgan: Hashimoto's is defective organic binding.	[1956]	La
13. I-Dx	— M. Morgan sees hi-perchlorate washout, 12 Hashimoto's.	[1956]	La
	— 21 articles (e.g., T. Oddie) give details of I-131 uptake.	[1955]	MJA
	— F. Kelsey changes °I uptake with dietary iodized salt.	[1948]	ANP
	— L. Oliner measures °I uptake in 73 normal children.	[1956]	JCEM
	— M. HAMOLSKY INTRODUCES AN IN VITRO RBC °T3 BINDING TEST.	[1955]	JCE
14. I-Rx	— D. Becker tries I-133 ($T_{1/2}$ = 20 h) Rx in 8 pts — no diff.	[1953]	JCE
	— Seidlin's first °I "cancer cure" pt dies after 14 y & 2.29 Ci °I.	[1946]	AP
15. P-Rx	— H. Phillips reconfirms P-32 uptake in 10 neoplasms.	[1958]	AR
	— I. Bergstrom 7 y summary finds P-32 leukemia Rx is good.	[1956]	AR
	— H. Diamond lists 7 neoplasia in which P-32 Rx fails.	[1948]	Ca
16. Tele	— AEC reduces price of Co-60 from $50/Ci to $5/Ci.	[1955]	AEC
17. Other	— M. Carlin finds urinary complic after parametrial °Au.	[1953]	JU
	— D. Sklaroff gets good results in hemangioma Sr-90 Rx.	[1954]	Rad

Scans and Other Tests of Function in Various Organs

18.	Brain	— D. Bowsher sees °I CS fluid absorption pathways by ARG.	[1949]	AnR
		— F. Bauer's intrathecal °IHSA reduces morbidity of iodized oil.		IJAR
		— R. Rhody confirms value of °IHSA brain scan.	[1951]	JNs
		— R. Bell: °IHSA transfer diagnostic in vent-subarac block.	[1955]	JNs
19.	Heart	— A. Zacks' 3-bottle model demonstrates RCG mechanics.	[1948]	AJR
		— R. Greenspan detects shunts (dogs) by external counts.	[1954]	Rad
		— W. Love initiates myocardial scanning with IV Rb-86.	[1955]	JCI
20.	Liver	— H. FRIEDELL INTRODUCES °ROSE BENGAL BILIARY LIVER SCAN.	[1956]	AJR
		— All doing °AuCol scans note spleen & BM uptake on some.	[1953]	
		— C. Levy uses °IHSA scan to locate biopsy site.	[1951]	AJMS
		— J. Wood introduces lateral (Lp) and post (Pp) projections.	[1974]	CRP
21.	Lung	— H. Knipping monitors regional ventilation with Xe-133.	[1955]	MMW
22.	Bone	— G. Bauer finds Ba-140 bone uptake faster than Ca-45.	[1952]	AOS
		— D. Laszlo compares metabolism of Sr-85 with Ca-45.	[1952]	JCI
		— P. Rubin finds S-35 mildly toxic in growing cartilage.	[1949]	Rad
23.	Kidney	— P. Cave tries °I-acetrizoate for excretory urography.	[1956]	JFR
24.	Gut	— M. Roche measures GI bleeding in hookworm with °Cr-RBC.	[1949]	AJDG
		— G. Baylin labels fat with I-131 for oral test of absorption.	[1953]	G
		— R. Freeark gives °IHSA meal for pancreas insuff test.	[1954]	S
		— P. Beres uses °I-triolein to rate malabsorption in DDx.	[1953]	G
		— R. Bannerman measures GI bld loss by °CrRBC stool counts.	[1949]	BMJ
		— G. Jerzy-Glass develops hepatic uptake °VB_{12} for DDx.	[1956]	AnIM
		— C. Booth locates site of °VB_{12} absorp with Co-56 in rat.	[1955]	BJH
		— A. Doscherholmen makes direct plasma measure of °VB_{12}.	[1956]	BI
		— A. Miller finds best "flushing VB_{12} dose" done at 3–6 h.	[1956]	BI
		— L. Meyer measures °VB_{12} serum-bind-cap in hematic dis.	[1956]	PSEB
25.	Blood	— N. Hughs-Jones predicts splenectomy result on chromigrams.	[1955]	BJH
		— C. Finch: °Fe-PIT doesn't measure viable RBC production.	[1949]	BI
		— N. Berlin compares Fe-59, C-14, Agglut, RBC life spans.	[1953]	JLCM
26.	Other	— R. Yalow's compet binding + antigen-body reaction is RIA.	[1956]	JCI
		— P. Moore measures °Na clearance in 112 gravid uteri.	[1955]	JOGB

Radiation Hysteria and Health Physics * Obituaries *

27.	Hyst	— G. Failla begins canard "Life shorter by 1 day/r exp."	[1954]	AJR
		— ICRP stupidly suggests I-132 be required in thyroid Dx.	[1951]	CPT
		— AEC Med Advis Com hysterical about fallout hysteria.	[1955]	AEC
		— W. Court-Brown sees leuk post-RadioRx for "ankyl spondyl."	[1956]	MRC
		— Marshallese returned to Rongelap; no rad sickness.	[1954]	AEC
		— G. Baisogolov says 320 & 670 r exposures, pts well at 4 y.	[1952]	KM
		— S. Werner finds post-°I Rx leukemia a pure chance event.	[1950]	JAMA
		— FIRE IN WINDSCALE REACTOR RELEASES 20 kCi I-131. [1982]	[1947]	ICRP
28.	React	— B. Duffy finds NO evidence linking I-131 and thyroid ca.	[1956]	JCEn
		— AEC lists 46 rad accidents since 1946; safest industry.	[1952]	AEC
		— M. Duhamel reads 100,000 French film badges (1—>3 rem).	[1954]	AfP2
		— Congress holds hearings on "Fallout," pubs 2064 pages.	[1953]	JCAE
		— W. Libby: fallout is a political, not a health problem.	[1952]	AEC
		— J. Cork notes lo-dose increases flour beetle longevity.	[1956]	RR
		— R. Baxter notes lo-dose increases longevity of fleas.	[1956]	RR
		— L. Carlson notes lo-dose increases longevity in rats.	[1956]	RR
29.	Respo	— AEC begins faked health physics "Deaths from Fallout."	[1953]	AEC
		— MRC (Eng) reports no bio-effects from Windscale accident.	[1953]	MRC
		— I. Chaikoff's control rats get more ca than °I treated.	[1952]	CaR
		— F. ELLINGER'S >4500 BIBLIO SHOWS RAD BIOL MOST RESEARCHED SCI.		Bk

* * *

30.	Obits	— J. Hamilton (1907–1957) Am physician; medical use of °isotopes.		Sc

CHRONOLOGY OF NUCLEAR MEDICINE — 1958

		Scientific and Technical Background		Ref.
3.	# Nuc —	614,565 curies of °isotopes in 118,655 shipments	since 1946.	AEC
4.	# Med —	H. Allen starts first full time private Nuc Med practice.	[1951]	PL
	—	P. Buchhorn says German Nuc Med predominantly therapy.	[1951]	Str
		Organizations and Internal Politics		
5.	AEC + —	AEC kills Isotopes Div; too successful for private biz.	[1946]	AEC
	—	L. Strauss retires from chairmanship of AEC.	[1953]	AP
	—	Sen Kefauver begins attack on pharmaceutical industry.	[1954]	AP
6.	Socs —	Am Assoc of Physicists in Med (AAPM) founded, publish PMB.	[1949]	PMB
	—	Euratom founded (Belg, Fr, Ger, It, Lux, Neth) for nuc power.	[1956]	EIF
	—	Int Atom Ener Agen (IAEA) publishes its own safety regs.	[1956]	IAEA
	—	NBS publishes Handbook 59 (MPD, MPC levels).	[1956]	NBS
	—	L. Taylor writes history of ICRU, ICRP and NCRP.	[1928]	HP
	—	M. Brucer's first textbk on "Radioisotope Scanning" pub.	[1955]	AEC
	—	Soc Nuc Med begins publication of J Nuc Med, June Vol 0.	[1954]	JNM
7.	Event —	Second Int Conf on Peaceful use of Atomic Energy (A-for-P).	[1955]	AfP2
	—	First course in scanning held in Bethesda (E. King USN).	[1955]	AEC
	—	First private power reactor (Shippingport) goes critical.	[1984]	AP
		Instruments, Units of Measurement, and Drugs		
8.	Instr —	D. Kuhl introduces emiss-axial-tomography (no computer).	[1957]	JNM
	—	H. Anger introduces gamma camera, shows °Au uptake in rat.	[1949]	RSI
	—	A. Tsuya: automatic scans of collimated isoresponse curves.	[1952]	AEC
	—	J. Laughlin introduces whole body scanner (bone, Ca-47).	[1957]	Rad
9.	Units —	P. Howard-Flanders combines LET and biol target theory.	[1954]	ANM
10.	Concp —	C. Harris quantifies neutron exp on whole body linear scan.	[1956]	AEC
	—	A. Atabek says biol dose changes with divided dosage.	[1936]	PEM
	—	H. Friedell modifies scan with automatic bkgd erase.	[1955]	Rad
	—	L. Marinelli measures natural body bkgd of °K, °Cs, °Ra.	[1956]	AEC
11.	Drugs —	A. McFarlane announces method for °I-labeling proteins.	[1957]	Na
	—	H. Eiber describes synthesis and metab of S-35 heparin.	[1946]	ArIM
	—	J. Steinfeld measures degradation of brands of °IHSA.	[1953]	JLCM
	—	N. MacDonald evaluates buildup & washout of °isotopes.	[1953]	JLCM
		Radioiodine, P-32, and Radioactive Therapy		
12.	I-Res —	L. Burkinshaw's 2-plane slit collimator for thyroid wt fails.	[1953]	AR
	—	NRC sets I-127 min daily requirement at 150 micrograms.	[1928]	NAS
13.	I-Dx —	T. Oddie: manumission from I-blockers is weeks to years.	[1957]	PS
	—	A. Goolden compares I-132 to I-131 in tests (too costly).	[1951]	BJR
	—	S. Dresner introduces a 2-day T3 suppression test.	[1955]	JCEn
	—	G. Molnar reports first (?) hot solitary nodule (adenoma).	[1952]	JCEn
	—	5 thyroid °I studies from USSR (e.g., V. Lekishvili).	[1957]	PE
	—	M. Mitchell announces T3 bind resin uptake in vivo test.	[1957]	JCEn
	—	H. Farran records °I uptake for first 30 sec (early trap).	[1955]	BMJ
14.	I-Rx —	L. Seed says the "Goiter Surgeon" replaced by I-131 Rx.	[1940]	AnIM
15.	P-Rx —	J. Lawrence gets 80% lymphoblastomas to norm life span.	[1955]	AnIM
	—	J. Maxfield adds testosterone to P-32 for Rx of mets to bone.	[1950]	SMJ
	—	J. Fountain treats thrombocythemia with P-32 in 3 doses.	[1951]	BMJ
	—	R. Chodos says PVA life not prolonged by P-32 (disputed).	[1951]	AnIM
16.	Tele —	M. Brucer notes world spread of Co-60, Cs-137 at second AfP.	[1955]	AfP2
	—	M. Brucer: kCi Co-60 source leaks, requires double seal.	[1954]	JNM
17.	Other —	J. Muller lists intracav °AuCol use in 12 countries.	[1956]	IAEA
	—	I. Ariel tries palliative P-32 in inoperable lung ca.	[1956]	AJR
	—	H. Ernst tries °Au-Carbon by cath to lung site (dogs).	[1944]	Str

	Scans and Other Tests of Function in Various Organs		
18. Brain	— L. Sapirstein: °I-antipyrine crosses blood/brain barrier.	[1951]	AJPh
	— P. Crandell counts °IHSA washout over torcula for CBF.	[1954]	AfP2
	— F. Liass does myelography scans with radon in USSR.	[1953]	VN
	— S. Rothenberg measures bleeding into CSF with °CrRBC.	[1957]	JN
19. Heart	— A. REJALI: FIRST CARDIAC BLD POOL SCAN WITH °IHSA.	[1957]	AJR
	— R. Gorli: N_2O can't distinguish cor from myo bl flow.	[1956]	MMR
	— F. Dreyfuss does first mocard scan: of Na°I in infarct.	[1957]	IMJ
	— L. Donato introduces left heart only RCG with °I gas.	[1957]	AfP2
20. Liver	— A. Ganze: gelatin & plasma increase °AuCol particle size.	[1952]	JLCM
	— P. McCurdy scans °CrRBC to predict splenectomy results.	[1957]	NEJM
	— R. Nordyke counts face, liver, feces °RB for hepatogram.	[1956]	JLCM
22. Bone	— R. Heaney measures IV Ca-45: bone forms at 9 mg/kg/day.	[1952]	JCEn
	— L. Engstedt describes °AuCol dispersion in PVA marrow.	[1966]	AR
	— G. Bauer announces "Scintimetry" with Sr-85 (counts only).	[1957]	JBJS
23. Kidney	— C. Vivion: no Na-24 absorption from bladder in cystitis.	[1951]	JU
24. Gut	— N. Hughes-Jones: stool count post-IV °CrRBC for bld loss.	[1957]	BMJ
	— G. Baylin subs °triolein capsule for test meal (error).	[1957]	G
	— S. Spector uses test meal of °I-corn oil, very sensitive.	[1957]	P
	— R. Gordon introduces °IPVP exudative enteropathy test.	[1965]	JPS
	— S. Oxenhorn: $°VB_{12}$ test of choice in malabsorption synd.	[1957]	AnIM
25. Blood	— M. Strumia gives formulae for RBC volume and % survival.	[1955]	Bl
	— C. Rasch gets 13 to 22 d RBC survival in Fe-defic babies.	[1955]	JLCM
	— N. Berlin lists RBC life spans in many animal species.	[1957]	PhR
	— F. Ebaugh finds no DF°P elution from RBC, life span work.	[1957]	JLCM
26. Other	— H. Sage injects °AuCol subQ and scans lymph nodes (dogs).	[1953]	ca
	— L. Bennett verifies °IHSA placental locus by caesarian.	[1956]	SGO
	Radiation Hysteria and Health Physics * Obituaries *		
27. Hyst	— Yugoslav reactor accident; death @ 436 r, 5 live @ 425 r.	[1957]	JAMA
	— Los Alamos accident; death @ 5000 rads in 35 hours.	[1957]	AEC
	— Oak Ridge criticality accident; 5 mild expos <460 rads.	[1957]	AEC
	— 0.2 μCi Ra-dial watch adds 1% of natural bkgd to gonads.	[1955]	MRC
	— J. Haybittle's watch has 2.2 μCi; W. Libby's (1955) had 1.	[1955]	Na
	— G. Chase evaluates alleged danger from Ra-dial watches.	[1955]	Sc
	— 200 Rongelapese get 5y med followup, no abnormalities.	[1957]	AEC
	— O. Leipunskii: fallout causes 44 k genetic and 29 k leuks.	[1957]	MAE
	— A. BRILL FINDS ABCC LEUKEMIAS @ 2/MILLION >100 R EXPOSURE.	[1955]	ABCC
	— A. Stewart: increase in childhood ca after in utero rad.	[1956]	BMJ
	— A. Bell calibrates 31 shoe fit fluoros @ up to 70 r/min.	[1950]	MJA
	— United Artists shows first anti-nuke film "On The Beach."	[1957]	AP
	— FDA defines irrad a food additive, mfgr must prove safe.	[1926]	FR
	— "Delaney Clause" prohibits any "carcinogen" in anything.	[1957]	FR
	— NCRP sets MPD of 5 Rem/y occupational, 0.5 Rem/y public.	[1956]	NCRP
	Seems harmless because nobody can measure a Rem.	[1929]	
28. React	— R. Doll: no excess mortality in Brit radiol after 1920.	[1957]	BMJ
	— Rad dose to gonads from Dx X-Rays reported in	AR, Na, JAMA, & Rad	
	— S. Yass says bld transfus of no value in Acute Rad Synd.	[1952]	ASM
	— A. Burdick notes lo-dose irrad beneficial to fruit fly.	[1957]	AfP2
29. Respo	— N. KLEMPARSKAYA (USSR) SHOWS IMMUNITY IN ACUTE RAD SYND.	[1952]	Bk
	— I. Kaplan lists 541 children, 43 g-child after ovary °Rx.	[1952]	AJOG
	— P. Durbin: 8/16 pts given Pu-238 alive at 8 y.	[1945] (1985	HP)
	* * *		
30. Obits	— F. Joliot-Curie (1900–1958) Fr physics; artificial °isotopes.		DSB
	— W. Pauli (1900–1958) Aus math physics; exclusion principle.		DSB
	— E. Lawrence (1901–1958) Am physics; cyclotron.		Bio
	— C. Davisson (1881–1958) Am physics; electron wave theory.		DSB

CHRONOLOGY OF NUCLEAR MEDICINE — 1959

Scientific and Technical Background

			Ref.
1. Basic	— G. Seaborg holds symposium on new elements: 43, 61, 85, 87, 93–102.		JCE
2. Obser	— H. Parker sums current data on bkgd radiation in Rem.	[1958]	JCAE
	— R. Oliver complains, ICRP Bio-$T_{1/2}$ on °Fe is wrong.	[1963]	Na
	— J. HAMBURGER: SUPPRESS IMMUNE SYS (250 rad) FOR KIDNEY TRANSPLANTS.		LPM
4. # Med	— 5 Companies offer c1000 °label compounds (17 °nuclides).	[1957]	AEC
	— 65% of $15.6 million/y nuc instr industry is "medical."	[1948]	AIF
	— AEC has issued 2255 medical °isotope licenses.	[1957]	AEC

Organizations and Internal Politics

5. AEC +	— Radioactive Substance Act sets Nuc Med policy in Great Brit.		AEA
	— ATOMIC ENERGY ACT AMENDED TO GIVE STATES REG CONTROL.	[1954]	AEC
	— Kentucky becomes first "agreement" state with its own AEC.	[1955]	AEC
	— Fed Rad Council set up as puppet "NCRP" to Congress.	[1958]	JCAE
	— U.S. agrees to cooperate with Int Atom Energy Agency.	[1957]	IAEA
	— Protection standards not voluntary says 10 CFR part 20.	[1957]	FR
6. Socs	— ICRP pubs MaxPermConc & MPBodyBurdens for °isotopes.	[1979]	ICRP
	— Soc of Nuclear Medicine now has 14 regional chapters.	[1956]	JNM
	— IAEA holds its first scientific seminar on "Scanning."	[1958]	IAEA
	— Surg Gen US Pub Health Ser publishes its own Rad Regs.	[1958]	PHS
	— Squibb interprets obscure regulations: "Hdbk of Rules."	[1957]	
7. Event	— AEC shows a 3.5 watt Po-210 atomic battery.	[1956]	AEC
	— 3 give methods to count very low level I-131 in biol materials.	[1956]	AEA
	— S. Shimizu calibrates Kyoto's 2 kCi Co-60 rad chamber.	[1957]	BICR
	— AEC reduces price of I-131 to $0.30/500 mCi.	[1956]	AEC

Instruments, Units of Measurement, and Drugs

8. Instr	— J. Mallard introduces a rectilinear scan color printout.	[1963]	BJR
	— W. MacIntyre gets bkgd erase by variable cutoff circ's.	[1958]	.Rad
	— M. Bender introduces high-contrast video amplification.	[1957]	JNM
	— R. Libby equips scanner with events/sec readout meter.	[1966]	JNM
	— S. Albert installs magnetic tape memory for rate meter.	[1958]	JNM
	— Los Alamos builds walk-in whole body counter.	[1956]	AEC
9. Units	— ICRU declares curie = 3.7×10^{10} dps exactly, any nuclide.	[1950]	ICRU
	— H. Rossi introduces microdosimetry, to replace LET.	[1958]	RR
10. Concp	— K. Way publishes decay schemes for medical °nuclides.	[1944]	AEC
11. Drugs	— H. Bennhold finds differences in commercial °IHSAs.	[1958]	JCI

Radioiodine, P-32, and Radioactive Therapy

12. I-Res	— J. Sokal says 3% nodular glands in pop, 0.2% malignant.	[1958]	JAMA
	— M. Roche: high-uptake without goiter in Venezuela mts.	[1957]	JCE
	— R. Pitt-Rivers separates T4 on anion exchange resin.	[1957]	BJ
	— J. Gardner finds 3 kinds "trap-bind" goitrous cretinism.	[1958]	JCEM
13. I-Dx	— M. Hamolsky clinically introduces °T3 RBC binding test.	[1957]	JCE
	— R. Levy finds 10% daily variation in °I uptake.	[1957]	JCE
	— H. Ogden: Hypaque, Telepaque depress uptake, increase PB°I.	[1948]	JLCM
	— H. Groesbeck notes cold nodules in 527 scans, 9.7% malig.	[1952]	Ca
	— M. Brucer writes Std Uptake Measurement syst (ORINS-19).	[1956]	.AEC
14. I-Rx	— G. Sheline finds nodules 2 y post-°I Rx (mostly children).	[1955]	JCE
	— R. Ray treats gravid woman with °I (5th mo), baby hypo.	[1958]	AJDC
	— G. Bloomfield reports long term followup of °I hyper Rx.	[1955]	BMJ
15. P-Rx	— E. Kaplan introduces polyphosphate for Rx of bone mets.	[1958]	JNM
	— J. Lawrence: untreated leuk pts also die in acute phase.	[1958]	AJMS
16. Tele	— USSR concentrates on 400 Ci Co-60 and Cs-137 units.	[1958]	ASM

16.	Tele	— 4000 Ci Cs-137 whole body Rx room set up in Oak Ridge.	[1956]	AEC
17.	Other	— R. Richart prolongs survival, mesothelioma with IP °AuCol.	[1956]	Ca
		— L. Farr sets up medical reactor for slow neutron Rx.	[1945]	Sc

Scans and Other Tests of Function in Various Organs

18.	Brain	— R. Bell sees tumor better on 24-hour delayed °IHSA scan.	[1957]	JNM
		— D. Perese posts 162 mets deaths, multiple mets in 80%.	[1945]	ca
		— M. Blau introduces Hg-203 chlormerodrin brain scans.	[1957]	JNM
19.	Heart	— S. Weinberg measures cardiac output exercise response.	[1955]	Circ
		— P. Johnson detects third RCG wave, must be coronary flow.	[1958]	JLCM
		— B. Lourvanis finds no Na°I hot spot on myocardial scans.	[1958]	MSHJ
		— L. Rosaia confirms Pulm-Transit-Time measure from RCG.	[1952]	PmM
		— R. Greenspan uses ext counts in R-L shunts (42 children).	[1957]	JAMA
		— E. Braunwald detects L-R shunts on pulm dilution curve.	[1957]	Circ
20.	Liver	— E. Braunwald measures portal-syst circ time by RCG tech.	[1957]	SF
		— L. Bennett gets heart-to-liver trans time with °RB bolus.	[1963]	AJDD
		— Most authors disregard bile flow on °Rose Bengal scans.	[1957]	V33
21.	Lung	— C. Chidsey: first study of dispersion and fate of Kr-85.	[1957]	JAPh
22.	Bone	— G. Bauer approaches Ca-47 and Sr-85 "scintimetry."	[1958]	JBJS
		— IAEA attempts to make medical grade Ca-47 available (failed).		IAEA
		— E. Kaplan makes first high conc P-32 polyphosphate for Rx.	[1959]	IAEA
23.	Kidney	— T. Denneberg tries renogram with °I-Hypaque (not good).	[1956]	AMS
		— C. Winter introduces the vesicoureterel reflux test.	[1957]	JU
24.	Gut	— M. Schwartz confirms exudative enteropathy with °IPVP.	[1958]	La
		— G. Barlow uses Co-60 VB_{12} to assay hog intrinsic factor.	[1958]	PSEB
25.	Blood	— S. Perry labels lymphocytes with P-32: short maturation.	[1955]	Bl
		— R. Wennesland studies age, somatotype effect on bld vol.	[1954]	JCI
26.	Other	— G. Kyker irrad normal lymph nodes (not tumor) with °AuCol.	[1953]	AEC
		— E. Frolich uses clearance of subQ inj for periph flow.	[1956]	CR
		— J. Quinn unsuccessful in scanning pancreas with °Zn, °Mn.	[1953]	Rad

Radiation Hysteria and Health Physics * Obituaries *

27.	Hyst	— FDA bans sale of aminotriazole tainted cranberries.	[1906]	AP
		THE GREAT CRANBERRY CRISIS	[1960]	AP
		— G. Ochinskaya compares X & Co-60 Acute Rad Synd (mice).	[1958]	MR
		— W. Kennedy suggests I-131 Rx causes leukemia (6 pts).	[1957]	NEJM
		— E. Webster: Dx dose hazard is miniscule, but reduce dose.	[1958]	Rad
		— AEC views Sr-90 watch dial imports with jealous horror.	[1958]	AEC
		— L. Taylor says TV and fallout rad hazard at same level.	[1957]	JCAE
		— W. Hughes cites hazard from Sr-90 eye applicators.	[1954]	JAMA
		— C. Powell: Govt rad reg's have drunken driver control.	[1958]	Rad
		— Windscale reactor °I release caused no biologic damage.	[1957]	MRC
28.	React	— AEC says $70 million and 800 scientists fight fallout.	[1957]	AEC
		— Sr-90 toxicity studied in mice, rats, dogs, cows, sheep, plants.	[1954]	AEC
		— Many rad protect chemicals being studied (none work).	[1958]	AEC
		— DTPA is better than EDTA in removing Pu from rat body.	[1984]	AEC
		— D. Gustafson shows fallout is 6% over natural bkgnd.	[1957]	JCAE
		— U. Kuhn studies Acute Rad Synd in burros, breeds survivors.	[1945]	AEC
29.	Respo	— J. Loutit finds leukemia up for 30 y, hence not fallout.	[1958]	La
		— R. Greenspan shunt detection breaks AEC pediatric ban.	[1985]	JAMA
		— M. Yamagishi: bone marrow transfusion helps in ARS mice.	[1958]	BICR
		— G. Sacher finds no evidence for radiation aging effect	[1937]	CIBA
		— Search finds 225 Ra dial painters (1920s) with <5% ca.	[1939]	AEC
		— M. Brucer writes "Acute Radiation Syndrome" (ORINS-25).	[1952]	AEC

* * *

30.	Obits	— C.T.R. Wilson (1869–1959) Scot physics; the cloud chamber.		WoA
		— D. Clark (1910–1959) Am surgeon; PB°I, thyroid °I Rx.		JNM

250 kVp ORTHOVOLTAGE WILL NOT BE REPLACED
(Cobalt-60 is Just a Flash in the Pan)

In Ursus Portman's 1933 History of Roentgen Therapy (a rare history in which the historian personally knew all the participants), "skin reaction" was the first limitation. [GSR, chap XII, 1933] E. Grubbe, the first therapist, already had dermatitis when X-rays were discovered — he manufactured vacuum tubes. His "sunburn" made him think of burning away a breast cancer and its "cure" prompted him to go to medical school. (Don't laugh, this was state-of-the-art medical science in 1896.) R. Bowles first reported "sunburn" in the 12 March 1896 Lancet. Delayed epilation from a brain X-ray was reported in Science on 10 April 1896.

"Deep" Therapy Becomes Possible

W. Coolidge, an American physicist, devised a hot-cathode high-vacuum tube that produced reasonably high energy X-rays for therapy in 1913. A popular 250 kVp model had a spectrum up to 250 keV maximum. They didn't talk of "energies" until the 1950s, but used half-value-layer penetration. With added filtration and some tube-skin distance, "deep" (a few cm) therapy flourished during the 1920s. But the dose just beneath the skin was so important that "Threshold Erythema Dose" became a radiation exposure unit.

[See Vig1954 .Rad]

Solution to the problem of delivering high tumor dose without excess skin damage could be approached with radium. E. Lysholm (Sweden) collimated a narrow beam for treatment, but radium was expensive. W. Stenstrom (Minnesota) solved this with a circle of multiple thin beams of radon focused to a point under the skin. (AJR 11:176, 1924) L. Mallet (France) devised multiple X-ray beam technique. (BAM 93:146, 1925) E. Sluys-Kessler divided his radium source into multiple beam sources and focused below the skin. [Cancer, #3-4, 1925] During the 1930s a few million-volt X-ray tubes, and G. Failla's planned 50 curie radium bomb, were defining "Supervoltage."

Telecobalt Takes Over Radiotherapy

Co-60 was discovered in 1946 but in secret. Leonard Grimmett (English rad physicist) heard about it and saw an answer to the radium bomb's faults. After the war he moved to Texas and found Co-60 might be available. [See Vig1950 .Co] On 8 Nov 1949 a formal agreement was drawn up between AEC, ORINS, & U Texas to work on a "million-volt irradiator." Three weeks later L. Grimmett of UT's MD Anderson hospital and M. Brucer of ORINS submitted the first drawings of a "tele-cobalt therapy unit."

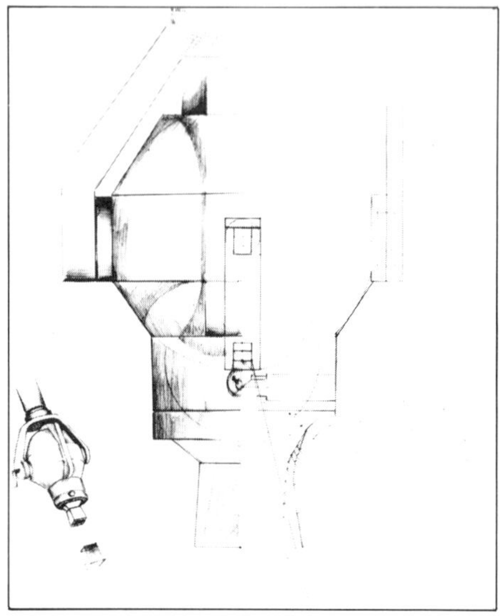

Grimmett/Brucer "telecobalt therapy unit"

On 19 Dec 1949 a contract formalized AEC's financial help. On 9 Jan 1950 sixteen 1 cm × 1 cm cylindrical c10 curie Co-60 sources were taken from Aebersold's stockpile to initiate measurements of Co-60's largely unknown characteristics.

Political Science Comes First

On 13 Feb 1950 a meeting was held in the board room of the National Academy of Sciences in Washington, DC. (We needed all the scientific backing we could get to expose humans to unheard of Co-60 "atomic" radiation.) Twenty physicists and physicians from AEC, ORINS, U-Texas, National Bureau of Standards, and the US and Canadian Nation Research Councils met by invitation. (M. Brucer had chosen this array of "unbiased" experts because he knew they all would agree to the project. A few best known radiotherapists were not invited because their response was questionable.) The history of the old radium bomb and a possible shift to cobalt-60 was explained.

No one questioned the supervoltage idea, but there was a serious Co-60 production problem because American reactors had been preempted for Pu weapons production. Canadian reactor facilities needed modification to handle such a high source intensity. The important meeting, thus, took place in Grimmett's hotel room that night. Both Canadians and Americans (Grimmett had declared for American citizenship) had details to work out. If Co-59 were to be irradiated to high intensity it had to be as large as possible and very pure. But it had to be as small as possible to be used in teletherapy.

Most of us sprawled on the floor to inspect Grimmett's calculations of gamma yield for many possible source sizes. He tossed a half dollar in the middle saying this size would repeat the mistakes of radium bombs. I caused hilarity among the reactor people when I tossed a dime on the floor. P. Aebersold said America's reactors could put 1250 curies in a dime, but not this year. H. Johns had just got a quarter in change from paying the bellboy for some booze for the group. We compromised on the size of the Canadian's quarter. We would irradiate square wafers to form a 2 cm cube at 10 Ci/g. Fifteen years later 400 C/g specific activity became commonplace. Source size could be much less than my dime.

Politics Before Science

The physical science of Co-60 was old hat, but the political science was just beginning. I made an official appeal (25 April 1950) to the Export-Import Branch of AEC explaining why we had to import an isotope. (America exported Isotopes.) Why not use American Co-60? Why couldn't less expensive I-131, also used in cancer therapy, do just as well? My appeal had to accompany CY 5812 (four copies) on Form 465 along with NRC-CR-247 (Canadian 4 copies) accompanying Form 313, under USAEC Regulations and the Agreements and Conditions subject to the Atomic Energy Regulations of Canada, to the Atomic Energy Control Board, for the import of 1250 curies of Co-60. Four copies, 1 each to four sets of lawyers: USA, Canada, Texas and ORINS. I remember swearing to the USA that I would not export any secrets of Canada's Co 60 discovery to Canada.

Grimmett Never Saw His Instrument

After nine months gestation, on 12 May 1950, a wooden mockup of Grimmett's 1000 curie Co-60 device was introduced to a cancer symposium at the Shamrock Hotel in Houston. [Tex Rep Bio Med 8:480, 1950] By 12 July the design was complete and a contract given to General Electric to build Grimmett's model for $27,000 (AEC funds). Later we learned that GE had put $40,000 of their own money into the project.

In April 1951 Grimmett and H. Kerman, our radiotherapist, went to GE's Milwaukee plant to talk finishing and cleanup. On 9 June 1951 GE announced the machine ready for delivery. The first three Co-60 sources (2 Canadian and the original American) were removed from the reactor with only about 800 curies. The Canadians chose to go ahead with inadequate output. We elected to have the source returned for another 6 months. By phone Grimmett told of a letter from John Mitchell of Cambridge: their iridium-192 teletherapy unit was working well. However, another letter from H. Freundlich, Mitchell's physicist, described their low curiage yielded *"not enough output,"* the curse of the old radium bombs. Grimmett was working on a modification to load a 2000 curie source. But on 27 May 1951 he died of a cerebral aneurysm.

The Introduction of Co-60 Teletherapy

When Co-60 teletherapy was introduced to instrument manufacturers the next year, the GE representative didn't think much of the idea and predicted only ten units would be made in the next 10 years. The most optimistic representative (the Canadian who already had five orders) predicted 300. I had inquiries from about twenty therapists, so I predicted 1000.

Co-60 supervoltage became popular in spite of organized radiology. At the 1955 annual Radiological Society meeting a symposium was held on *Supervoltage, Should we junk 250 kv?* The symposium speakers, mostly Co-60 converts, solemnly and unanimously proclaimed 250 kVp X-ray therapy not obsolete, *"it will never be replaced in radiotherapy."* [Rad 67:481, 1956]

Ten years later an international survey revealed 1750 Co-60 units in operation. Nobody manufactured 250 kVp equipment.

[See Vig1950 Co]

ORGANIZING A SOCIETY OF NUCLEAR MEDICINE

(Holter Invites Some Friends to Talk)

A few Navy doctors at Bethesda spoke of their I-131 and P-32 work as *"Atomic Medicine"* and Admiral C.F. Behrens wrote a textbook on the subject. [NY Nelson, 1949] But everything called "atomic" in 1949 meant big bombs, and we who traced our work back to R. Evans and J. Lawrence did not like the association. B. Low-Beer in San Francisco wrote a textbook on the *"Clinical Use of Radioactive Isotopes"* [Springfield, Thomas, 1950], but he called the field "Radiology." We in Oak Ridge did not agree and wrote *"Radioisotopes in Medicine."* [G. Andrews, AEC, 1953]

Bob Ball said the evidence prevailed for "radiology" as a name because when he first scanned for thyroid metastases, the Radiology Dept owned the only GM tube in the medical school. Sam Seidlin objected; he, an internist, "cured" thyroid metastases, he didn't just look at them. Sam leaned toward "isotopology." Then R.R. Newell, the doyen of organized Radiology, challenged him to name a brand of aspirin that wasn't made of isotopes.

All isotopes came from Oak Ridge in those days, and most of the users, about half medics, were trained at Oak Ridge's basic one-month course. Paul Aebersold lectured on how to order "isotopes." He used the terminology he had been taught while helping E.O. Lawrence build the first cyclotron at Berkeley. Lawrence took the word "Radioisotope" from Joliot-Curie's cable announcing their discovery. [See Vig1934 .JC]

"Jeff" Holter Dissents From Everybody

Aebersold called them "radioisotopes" because that is what they were. But one student dissented. Jeff Holter said that isotopes were plural nuclear species that occupied one place on the Periodic Table. [See Vig1912 .KF1] Is it sensible to say that iodine (one stable species) occupies itself? Holter had read Truman Kohman's 1947 proposal in the American J Physics. A new general term "nuclide," he said, would clarify the "isotone" (equal neutrons), "isotope" (equal protons), "isobar" (equal atomic weights), confusion.

Kasimir Fajans, now at U of Michigan, immediately changed his 33-year-old terminology. One of his PhD students had already submitted the first Trilinear Chart of Nuclear Species for publication and it was too late to change the title. But from then on William "H" Sullivan called it a *Chart of the Nuclides.* A rapidly growing radiopharmaceutical industry sold "radioisotopes" well into the 1960s. Only one group, an upstart Society of *Nuclear* Medicine, used "nuclear," and this was because Jeff Holter had been impressed by "fallout."

Jeff Holter Learns About Fallout

Norman "Jeff" Holter, of one of the first (historically) families of Helena, Montana, earned his Master's degree in physics at UCLA in 1937. To round out the experience while he was away from civilization (meaning Montana), he picked up a Master's in Chemistry from USC in 1938. He spent the war years with the Navy's Bureau of Ships researching ocean wave physics.

When the Navy was faced with a new kind of explosion, Holter was called back to set up the wave action and underwater instrumentation at the Bikini Atoll A-Bomb Tests. He was impressed by the similarities of fluid dynamics in water and in atmosphere. The A-bomb furnished its own tracer, and he learned how to measure radioactive fallout. Upon returning home he began charting fallout patterns from both US and USSR bombs. AEC bureaucrats stamped his measurements "secret." (All of his instruments were off-the-shelf junk.) When the first H-bomb test came up Jeff was recalled again, this time by AEC, to set up instrumentation at Eniwetok.

The Reason for a Separate Society

By the time Jeff returned to Helena in 1953, the Sunday Supplements were full of medical cures; spinoffs, they said, from the H-bomb. Jeff knew this was wrong; I-131 and P-32 dated from before the war. The new Co-60 and Cs-137 were spinoffs from fission, not fusion. He saw that his physician friends neither knew, nor cared, what "isotopes" could do in medicine. Surgeons poo-poohed any thought of treating hyperthyroidism with some kind of fake iodine. Hematologists laughed at the P-32 trials.

Radiologists hooted at 60 cobalt atoms replacing 250 kVp machines. The Medical Societies had no room on their agendas for esoterica. Isotopes were secret, hence probably quack subjects. Jeff got mad when nobody would listen. He would form his own society, and call it the Montana Society of Nuclear Medicine.

Jeff was the Northwestern States consultant and trouble-shooter for Bell Telephone and used long distance lines as though he owned them. He got on the phone to set up a central meeting place in Montana, but the Montana Society never had a chance. An internist friend from Vancouver, BC, called him to find out about a rumored meeting. Then a radiologist from Seattle, and a caller from Portland wanted in. A couple of physicists and an internist from Spokane wanted to attend the meeting. Jeff plotted the calls on a map and calculated the geographic centroid weighted by the availability of a good bar. On Tuesday, 19 January 1954, four internists, four radiologists, three physicists and a cardiac physiologist met in the Davenport Hotel in Spokane, WA. [A more complete report is in *The Heritage of Nuclear Medicine,* Soc Nuc Med 1979.]

A Society of Nuclear Medicine is Formed

"The 12 old men" decided that a new society should be formed. If they held a meeting in a bigger city they might get twenty or thirty people to attend. They elected officers, collected dues, and set up a first annual meeting for Saturday–Sunday, 29–30 May 1954. They adopted Jeff's name, Society of Nuclear Medicine, but dropped the "Montana." The place would be the big city (Seattle) where they might attract a few attendees. Asa Seeds (radiologist, Vancouver, WA) was elected secretary and wrote a letter to Paul Aebersold to invite a speech at the annual meeting, and to Abbott Labs for some commercial support. By return mail he got an application for membership from Donalee Tabern (of Abbott Labs) with a check for dues and "how could he help?"

The first meeting opened at the Benjamin Franklin Hotel on Saturday, 29 May 1954; 109 physicians, physicists, chemists, and a few technicians from 12 states were trying to get in. The first paper was presented by Rex Huff (research physician) on cardiac output measured with °IHSA. Ten papers followed through Sunday morning. A new instrument called Ben Cassen's "scanner" was described by Tyra Hutchins (internist, Portland, OR). It pecked out chicken tracks on a piece of carbon paper that were said to show the shape of the thyroid gland. Few thought it would ever amount to anything because gamma rays could not be focused. Wrong, said Bob Newell (Stanford)! He had already modified Cassen's detector with a "honey-comb" collimator. Tyra Hutchins was forecasting 80% of the next 30 years of Nuclear Medicine.

A new therapy of pleural effusions with radioactive gold was described at the Seattle meeting. Also new palliation therapy of emphysema with I-131 and an extension of P-32 therapy to serous effusions showed great promise. Therapeutic trials with Abbott's radioactive colloids were described in glowing terms by Tabern. [See Vig1949 .Phr] The physics of Co-60 and the possibility of neutron use was described. 7 of 14 papers emphasized therapy. Therapy is what "Nuclear Medicine" originally stood for. Co-60 alone (it was then a part of Nuc Med) accounted for more favorable AEC publicity than any other single subject. And that is why AEC money was the almost exclusive support during the first 10 years of Nuclear Medicine.

On Sunday noon at the closing session, Jeff Holter declared it to have been the finest meeting ever held in the history of the Society. Incidentally, there never was a second meeting of the *Montana* Society, but as its only member, Jeff told me in 1970 that he would be glad to make me a second member (he had already made about five others the "second") if I would promise never to attend a meeting.

Reverberations from the first meeting (spread by Tabern and the national sales force of Abbott) sparked a Central Society around Chicago, a Southeastern Society around Oak Ridge, a California chapter around Los Angeles, and a Southwest group spreading from New Orleans through Texas. Within two years they were clamoring for recognition. The Society had to "go national"; in 1957 it did.

[See Vig1956 .SNM]

THE MAGENTA THREE-BLADED PROPELLER

(A Universal Symbol for "Radioactive")

In 1948 ORNL (Oak Ridge Nat Lab) shipped 2191 containers of radioisotopes to 236 addresses in 32 states (about 3 kilocuries). Both Dept of Commerce and Post Office wanted these packages marked with some kind of symbol. The skull and cross bones indicating "POISON" was suggested (radiation, by definition, *is* a poison). "EXPLOSIVE" was demanded by a few (radioactivity was present in one explosive material). "DANGER," "HELLFIRE," "DEATH AND DESTRUCTION," might be used. Label everything that came out of the *"Fiery Canyons of Death in Oak Ridge."*

We were very proud of the AEC's safety record in those days. It was the second safest, second only to the corset industry, according to national statistics — and only a few accidents even remotely involved radioactivity. But radioactivity was "safe" only because we followed some simple time-distance-dilution rules. Our five physiological senses did not include a Cutie Pie, hence a visual warning symbol was appropriate, especially where large amounts of radioactivity were being handled such as at Clinton Laboratories in Oak Ridge.

An Unnamed Lab is Named, Twice

Clinton was a small East Tennessee town (pop. c3000) about 10 miles from the Gas Diffusion plant code-named K-25. It was the first railroad stop out of Knoxville and became a mailing address for supersecret Oak Ridge (pop c30,000 +), a housing and lab complex. Three major facilities were involved: K-25, an Atomic Pile at X-10 (renamed "nuclear reactor" by bureaucrats), and Calutrons, massive cyclotron "racetracks," at Y-12. These plus a ballooning Manhattan Engineering District (MED) headquarters became "Clinton Laboratories." After the diffusion process became overwhelmingly successful at separating U-235, the calutrons began separation of the stable isotopes. (They are still a prime source for enriched stable isotopes.) When AEC took over MED on 1 Jan 1947, the mailing address became "Oak Ridge." The town, however, was still behind a guarded fence for another two years.

Health Physics Needs a "Danger" Symbol

George Warlick was hired by the Health Physics Division of Clinton Laboratories in 1947. His job was to teach non-technical personnel about radioactivity and the rules for handling dangerous levels with safety. The lab was then posting areas of unacceptable radiation with a tie-on "danger" tag with red and black letters on a white background.

Before the end of 1947 ORNL was informed that their tag did not comply with the National Safety Council color codes: red was exclusively reserved for fire, blue for electrical hazards, yellow signified "caution," and green declared "safety." As a government lab ORNL must follow NSC's standards. In searching for a new symbol, a tag used at the Naval Research Laboratory in San Francisco as a warning sign came to Warlick's attention. It was a three-bladed propeller. (A whirling prop is an obvious naval hazard.) Fortunately it was meaningless in an isotope laboratory. Hence, it would not be confused with other symbols.

George Warlick had the Health Physics Division artist, Glenn Williams, prepare about 10 propeller-in-a-circle designs in different colors, but avoiding the proscribed red. A committee was appointed from lab personnel. They viewed the sample tags at 10 and 25 feet and unanimously voted for the off-red (magenta) propeller in a bright yellow circle as the most clearly visible and distinctive. The Lab adopted the symbol and attached a tag to all their shipping containers. All AEC facilities, Argonne, Los Alamos, Hanford, etc. received radioisotopes from Oak Ridge, and knowledge of the new symbol spread rapidly within the AEC.

[HP 50:678, 1968] [See Vig1953 .RPK]

But remember, ORNL was a highly secret facility. What they chose to use was known only to insiders and a few other highly secret AEC labs. One Division of AEC was highly NON-secret — the Isotopes Division. Its job was to make isotopes available to the informed public. Paul Aebersold interpreted this to mean the public had to be informed.

The Isotopes Division "Invents" a Symbol

Early in 1946 M. Hawkins (an artist who prepared the Isotopes Division's exhibits) drew up a few symbols to depict Paul Aebersold's new Isotopes Division. (It was always Aebersold's Division in those days, not yet AEC's). I have one of the original drawings. It was a 3-bladed propeller in a circle (the same symbol adopted at ORNL, but not mentioned because of secrecy). In each blade a wiggly arrow (then the common symbol for electromagnetic rays) showed radiation going out in all directions. *"Why the three blades?"* I asked Aebersold? *"Because we sell alpha, beta, and gamma radiation,"* he answered. *"Then why a gamma ray in each blade?" "Because every alpha, beta, and gamma produces another X-ray."* These wiggly arrows were soon dropped from the symbol because they were too hard to draw with symmetry. At some point the double blades were oriented upward.

[See Vig1946 .Pub; first public shipment.]

The *radioisotope* symbol must be a hazard sign but not a "DANGER" sign. The last thing Aebersold, as a salesman, wanted was a "STOP" sign. The sign should be a "hesitate-for-a-moment-and-follow-the-rules" sign. The printer who printed the first batch of signs was told to use a plum colored ink. He used an off-red ink he couldn't get rid of that he called magenta.

The 3-Bladed Propeller Becomes Official

In 1948 the AEC (I think it was Aebersold who made the decision) officially "recognized" the 3-bladed propeller in magenta on yellow as a symbol of *radiation*. The use of the word "radiation" is an error, said the AEC's ever-present lawyers. The Isotopes Division sells radioisotopes but has no jurisdiction over radiation — "Correct this at once!" By 1950 (they moved fast in those days) the AEC "officially" adopted the symbol because the lawyers thought it had already been legally adopted. Because it always had "caution" in large letters, it soon became a "public" symbol.

In 1954 the National Bureau of Standards, in a routine news release, said that they had adopted the 3 bladed magenta on yellow propeller as a standard symbol of *"radioactivity."* (Some of their own labs were already using the handy symbol for *"radiation."*)

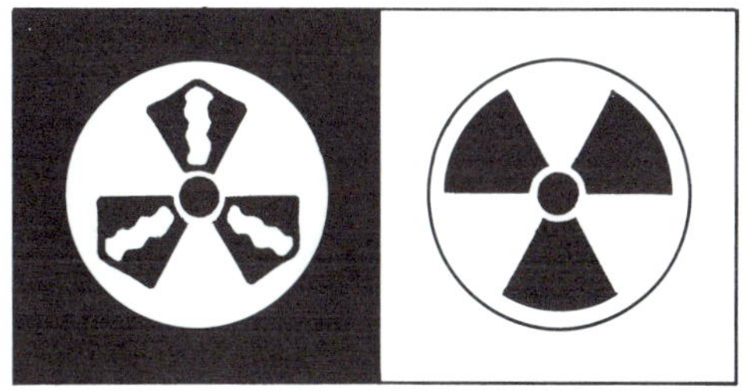

The first symbol *The final symbol*

In order to subdue the Great Radiation Hysteria fomented by the AEC, President Nixon, in 1973, split the AEC into a production and a separate regulatory division. (The same regulators used the same typewriters to spew out an ever more detailed catechism, but now they had their own executive washroom.) In January of 1975, President Ford killed the 27-year-old AEC without even a hint of its past accomplishments (which were considerable, even monumental compared to most government agencies). ERDA and NRC were born — same people but using new and improved typewriters to spew out the same regulations in new and improved gobbledygook.

The "Radioisotope," or "Radioactivity," or "Radiation" symbol by this time was imbedded in a new generation of scientists, students, teachers, advertisers, and dictionaries. It is the symbol drawn by Hawkins (lifted from Warlick's ORNL design lifted from the Office of Naval Research's lab warning sign) to accompany Aebersold's radioisotopes. It was never meant to be a "stop" or "danger" sign, but was printed in an off-red ink on a glaring yellow background to make people stop and think before opening the package.

References:

During its reign the AEC printed about 2×10^{27} news releases. I saved a few. These are now buried in my files. Anybody with a taste for archeology is welcome to dig them out. I am writing from brief notes.

In the April 1986 Health Physics Newsletter, W. Spiers gathered a number of different recollections of how the symbol got started. Some of the stories are entirely different, but not necessarily incompatible with my story. Every prime contractor to the AEC in the early years had its own highly autonomous health physics group.

[See Vig1946 .Aeb, Aebersold & red tape]

THE FIRST ATOMS-FOR-PEACE CONFERENCE GENEVA — 1955

Five major interrelated events in the field of atomic energy occurred in 1955:

1. An International Atomic Energy Agency (IAEA) proposal was drafted at the United Nations. Common knowledge said these people were not to be trusted.
2. Many bilateral agreements on atomic energy bypassing the UN were negotiated by the State Dept.
3. Training programs in the use of °isotopes, to implement the agreements, were established.
4. Whole libraries of atomic energy scientific literature were given to many countries.
5. The US dominated participation in a giant Atoms-for-Peace Conference and Trade Fair in Geneva, Switzerland.

1. Drafting IAEA

During the breakup of the Manhattan District, on 1 Feb 1946, Robert Oppenheimer suggested an international agency that would have scientific as well as political functions. The idea was prompted by a growing demand from many Manhattan Project scientists to wrest control of atomic energy from the US Military Establishment — who wouldn't let go.

Oppenheimer's proposal was presented to the United Nations by Bernard Baruch. It had been highly modified by Dean Acheson and David Lilienthal of the US State Department. State won civilian control — at least in part — and President Truman pushed the Atomic Energy Act of 1946 through Congress. United Nations action was politically stalemated into paralysis.

Six years later the US was trembling in terror over the Russian A-Bomb. Most politically active nations were terrorized by a secret thermonuclear project (secret only to the US public). The State Department wrote a speech for President Eisenhower to give to the United Nations on 8 Dec 1953. It called for the peaceful development of atomic energy. The General Assembly passed a resolution and slid back into paralysis.

2. Bilateral Agreements

Because of inaction by both the UN and the US Congress, the State Department negotiated bilateral agreements with 23 nations. The USAEC provided detailed (unclassified) information on research reactors and loaned 6 kilograms of 20% enriched U-235 (far below weapons grade). Lots of goodies on safety and the use of °isotopes, especially in medical therapy, were included. In return the 23 nations agreed to accept the gifts.

Three nations had separate treaties: Canada and the United Kingdom were already partners from World War II, and Belgium because it owned so much uranium. They got some classified documents. Switzerland was allowed to buy a swimming pool research reactor that would be the showpiece of an upcoming trade fair.

3. Training Programs

To make gifts of research reactors more than an empty gesture, the USAEC would set up a number of training programs on how to turn them on. Training programs on the use of °isotopes already operating in the US were opened to international participation. (Some of these training programs were called the most valuable part of the whole effort.)

4. Providing Libraries

On 5 Nov 1954 Henry Lodge, Ambassador to the United Nations, offered each country a technical library of unclassified USAEC documents, including many of the declassified Manhattan Project documents). Japan got the first library, then 23 other countries. The Atomic Energy Library displayed at the first Atoms-for-Peace Conference in Geneva was presented to the United Nations.

5. The Trade Fair

In December 1954 the UN General Assembly, after Eisenhower's speech, not only endorsed the idea of an International Atomic Energy Agency, but approved the holding of a giant world trade fair on the useful applications of atomic energy. Under the title Atoms-for-Peace, it was open to all countries. On 1 Feb 1955 the UN sent invitations to 84 nations to meet in Geneva on Aug 8 to 20, 1955. They were to send scientists and engineers exclusively (and this restriction was about 90% honored).

The Atoms-for-Peace Trade Fair

In the minds of the US State Department the purpose of the meeting was to change the public's word association of "atom" from "bomb" to "peaceful use." The primary exhibit for non-scientists — a stroke of public relations genius — was a swimming pool research reactor in operation. Only a handful of technicians had ever seen a reactor in operation; by the end of the fair, almost a million Europeans had seen the eerie blue light of Cherenkov radiation.

Close by was another "reactor" to explain what they had seen. A 2′ square steel box with a radium-beryllium neutron source. You gave the attendant a silver dime. He dropped it into a slot. After a few seconds the dime dropped out onto a GM tube which clicked noisily and flashed its light with every click. The coin was radioactive (for a few minutes).

The public thus learned that "atomic reactor" really meant "radioisotopes." Across the road was the main exhibit hall showing what these °isotopes could do. Electric power production was presented, but the "peaceful" nuclear submarine was played down. Agricultural and medical uses were the stars of the show.

The Science Show for Scientists

Over 1100 technical abstracts had been submitted from the participating nations (500 were from the US). Selection of papers to be read before the conference was heavily weighted favoring the non-advanced nations. The program was presented on 60 different topics. In the field of therapeutic medicine 27 papers were read. Thyroid °iodine and P-32 hematology were rehashes, but their spread throughout the world was a surprise. Co-60 supervoltage teletherapy was introduced to a world-wide audience. Although it was already old stuff in the US, Europeans learned it was in operation. Radium brachytherapy was practically made obsolete by the wide variety of papers and exhibits on new °sources.

Fifty-four papers described diagnostic techniques. The calibration of thyroid I-131 uptake was so important, and simple, that it later became the first medical project of the IAEA. The eye opener of the exhibit, however, was the introduction of nuclear scanning. Upon entering the exhibit hall visitors were overwhelmed by a gigantic portrait of Lenin marking the entrance to the Russian exhibits. An even more gigantic blowup of Hal Anger's whole body radio-iodine scan marked the US exhibit. Inside was the latest model Reed-Curtis scanner scanning the neck of a transparent plastic manikin that contained a mock-iodine "hot" thyroid gland.

The Society of Nuclear Medicine was already a year old. Many courses in Radioisotopes in Medicine had already been given in a number of countries. Many papers had already been published in a few different languages. But this first Atoms-for-Peace exhibit, showing °isotopes from reactor production through scanning to successful therapy, was the world introduction of Nuclear Medicine.

6. An Unscheduled Event

One event occurred that had not been foreseen by the planners of the conference. We didn't even know it occurred until it became obvious at the second Atoms-for-Peace conference in 1958. It was a "sleeper" — a scientific paper read by George Taplin of UCLA. Taplin had tagged a well-known liver dye, Rose Bengal, with I-131. He had measured its dynamics as it passed through the liver and was excreted. He demonstrated the variety of functional patterns in various liver diseases. Although this was just another test to Americans, the liver was the soul (and bread & butter) of European medicine.

The swimming pool reactor had proved that every country could make its own isotopes. The radioactive dimes proved them safe. The scanner proved °isotopes useful. But a liver test, if it works of course, is the real practice of medicine.

References:

The full and somewhat sordid story of the politics of Oppenheimer's proposal is in Hewlett R.G. & Anderson O.E., The New World 1939/1940. Penn State U Press 1956.

The AEC's report to Congress is in: Semi-annual Report, AEC USGPO, July 1955.

The official record by the UN is: Proceedings of the International Conference on Peaceful Uses of Atomic Energy. UN, Geneva, 1956.

URANIUM AND THORIUM KEEP THE EARTH WARM
(The Earth Exhales Radiation Background)

It is possible that in a *gedanken* experiment you might conceive a space in the universe with no ionizing radiation. However, it will be an exercise in geometry because matter implies radiation. The earth is made of 83 stable elements plus 4 chains of radioactive decay. These chains spontaneously emit the energy required to keep the earth warm and habitable. Our moon is exposed to just as much sunlight, but has a few orders of magnitude less radioactivity and hence is a cold rock uninhabitable by living things.

Four Natural Decay Series

Two of the four natural decay series start with relatively short-lived isotopes. [See Vig1947 .4n] The neptunium series starts with a 2.1×10^6 year $T_{1/2}$, hence, has already decayed to infinitesimal, almost undetectable, amounts. The actinium series stems from U-235 (7.13×10^6 year $T_{1/2}$) and is still barely detectable. In earth's 4.5 billion year history the billion year thorium and uranium series are over three quarters gone. There are people who worry that we don't have many billion years left.

Thorium as a Source of Background

The Th series starts with 1.4 billion year $T_{1/2}$ Th-232. In about 8 years half of its emissions will go through four more transitions to radon-220. This gas has only a 56 second half-life, hence is not widely dispersed. After another half-day five more transitions take the atoms to stable lead. For each Th-232 decay 6 alphas, 4 betas, at least 10 gammas (up to 1.6 MeV) and a host of X-rays accompanying each, help fill the biosphere with background radiation.

5 to 7×10^{22} Bq (200 billion curies) of thorium are widely dispersed in many minerals. Probably no very large area on earth is totally devoid of thorium, but it does tend to occur in pockets. Large concentrations occur in Kerala (India), Brazil, Scandinavia, Ceylon, Tasmania, the Urals, and at least 5 states (CO, FL, ID, NC, VA).

Uranium as a Source of Background

The U series starts with 4.5 billion year $T_{1/2}$ U-238. Within a month 3 transmutations take the atoms to a 248,000 year U-234 isotope which decays to a 77 thousand year Th-230 isotope which decays to 1600 year radium-226 which decays to radon-222. This heavy gas, highly soluble in water, has a half-life of 3.82 days, plenty of time to be exhaled by the earth and dispersed in its waters and atmosphere. After 3 more rapid transmutations the gas becomes 22.3 year Pb-210, then to 5 day Bi-210 to 108.4 day Po-210 and finally to stable lead-206. Each of the last three radionuclides lasts long enough to become trapped in the metabolism of plants and animals. Thus, each U-238 atom can eventually result in 11 long delayed alphas and 6 betas, plus at least 14 gammas in the Mev range and a horde of accompanying X-rays.

About 2×10^{22} Bq (about 60 billion curies of U, roughly a third the amount of thorium) is present in the earth's crust. It is primarily in granitic terrains, in the mountains of every continent. However, that relatively long-lived gaseous Rn daughter spreads the "fast decay" half of the series around, and makes its radiation ubiquitous.

Radiation Exposures From Natural Decay
(Recorded in Pre-1975 roentgens, 1 R = 258 μC/kg)

If distributed uniformly in the biosphere, the thorium series would deliver about twice the intensity of radiation (12 mR/y) as the uranium series (6mR/y). However, once the daughter nuclides get trapped inside a body metabolism, the uranium series becomes dominant. Unlike relatively constant cosmic irradiation [See Vig1922 .VH] the earth's exhalation is highly variable. Diurnal is superimposed on weather variations superimposed on earth disturbances (earthquakes and plowing). Exposures cannot be calculated or even averaged; they must be measured and bracketed as lows and highs. Based upon human longevity and cancer incidence, the ideal radon background in air is in the Bq/L range (nCi to μCi). The EPA has a pCi/L limit to assure their employment.

Range of Some Measured Outdoor Exposures
(Cosmic Background Subtracted)

	mR/y	
New York City	60 to	72
Berkeley, CA	48 to	98
Chiba, Japan	65 to	106
Peru, sea level	78 to	190
mountain	92 to	296
New Jersey	42 to	420
Lakeland, FL	263 to	701
Greenland	202 to	2,200
Midland, TX	44 to	4,821
Ramsar, Iran	701 to	48,200
SW France	203 to	87,660
PO_4 area, FL	58,000 to	175,000

If you live in one place on earth, your background may vary from day to day by a factor of 10, or even 100. Just by surrounding yourself with earthy materials (e.g., a house) you can double your radiation exposure:

	OUTDOORS mR/y	INDOORS mR/y
France	16 to 72	14 to 144
Sweden	30 to 77	70 to 380
Poland	53 to 105	66 to 140
Bavaria	35 to 280	14 to 134

The inside exposure rate can change by a factor of 10 within hours just by opening the windows. In Sweden, where the first extensive studies were done, the indoor exposure rate averaged 32 mR/y in wooden houses, almost doubled to 56 mR/y in brick, doubled again to 104 mR/y in concrete. Verifications filled Health Physics journals for years. In Atlanta, one study showed that indoor exposures depended upon where the builder got his materials: bricks emitted from 5 to 493 mR/y, concretes from 29 to 254 mR/y.

The Contribution from Potassium

A major source of gamma rays comes from the seventh most common element. Potassium is 2.4% of the lithosphere, and 0.0118% of its atoms have a 1.28 billion year $T_{1/2}$; 11% of decays emit a 1.46 MeV gamma ray. How much of background radiation is contributed by K-40:

	Estimates from Measured Levels
Berkeley, CA, outdoors	37%
Japan, outdoor bkg	47%
Poland, brick buildings	67–87%
Atlanta, brick buildings	85%
Western US, coal	50–67%

[See Vig1924 .°K]

Your Daily Radioactive Diet

Eat a banana. You have just added about 370 mg of potassium to your body. 0.04 mg is K-40 which means 11 Bq, or disintegrations per second (dps), will occur until you excrete and replace it with more K-40. 10 of those dps were beta rays completely absorbed in your tissues, but the eleventh was a high energy gamma that may be absorbed in the person sitting beside you. Once a K-40 atom decays to Ca-40 it is no longer radioactive, and both K-40 and Ca-40 are essential in your diet. But the U & Th and daughters ingested are a continuous source of exposure. A factor-of-10 daily variation marks the diets of most people:

		Measured Levels mBq/day
US	— Ra-226	15 to 260
Bombay, India	— K-40	44 to 444
	— Ra-226	85 to 851
Kerala, India	— Ra-226	76 to 176
	— Ra-228	4000 to 8000
20 countries	— All	15 to 407

Your Daily Radioactive Drink

When you boil water or even take a bath, dissolved radon is released into the air for you to breath. Some of it will be trapped in the lungs, decay to Pb-210, enter the circulation and be deposited permanently in your bones. An estimate of "how much" depends upon what you choose to measure. The concentration of Ra-226 varies from <4 mBq/L to over 1110 mBq/L in most of the world. A standard measure is to sample a liter of air over a body of water:

	Measured levels Bq/L(air)	
Oklahoma county	0.004 to	0.250
next county	0.433 to	0.570
Atlantic Ocean	0.004 to	2.960
Mediterranean Sea	0.370 to	7.400
Italian spas	0.370 to	1406.0
Maine wells	1.0 to	1850.0
Helsinki, Fin wells	900 kBq to	1480 kBq
schoolyard well	45,000 kBq	

In easily understood terms, you live in a sea of gamma rays, but just to make sure your environment is livable you eat and drink enough each day to assure at least a few alpha particles plowing through some tissue every second.

[See Vig1978 .Bkg]

THE EPOCHAL THIRD-AND-A-HALF YEAR SOCIETY OF NUCLEAR MEDICINE MEETING

(Palmer House, Chicago, Dec 1956)

Milo Harris (internist) presided over a small Northwest group called the Society of Nuclear Medicine (SNM), but was being pushed to open it to national membership. Three offshoots: Los Angeles, Chicago, and Southeast Societies, were already bigger than the founding group. Pittsburg, Colorado, and the Southwest chapters were organizing. They all considered themselves a part of the original Society of Nuclear Medicine.

Radiology's politicians had shoved nuclear subject matter under AMA's radiology blanket. E. Quimby pushed a regulation through AEC that all human use of radioisotopes be under local hospital control. Each hospital's "isotope committee" must be dominated by a radiologist. But most "Nuclear Medics" were not so oriented. Only a third of the NM founders were radiologists. The program that Milo had put together for the Salt Lake City third annual SNM meeting became proof that *Nuclear Medicine* was NOT *Radiology,* and could not be confined to the Northwest.

The scientific program read like a Hematology meeting: 14 papers on blood tests and therapy. Or it sounded like an Internist convention: 16 papers on heart and metabolism. Or was it Endocrinology: 7 papers on the thyroid? Health Physics accounted for 6 papers. Of 57 papers only 2 could be considered "Radiology." One was by R.R. Newell (Prof Radiology, Stanford), but he was an intellectual aberration. Newell considered both "Radiology" (X-ray tubes) and "Nuclear Medicine" (radioisotopes) far too narrow for legitimate subspecialization. Otto Glasser's 1944 text, *Medical Physics,* he thought, defined a proper medical subspecialty.

Jeff Holter (physicist who first organized "Nuclear Medicine") wanted a completely open society. "We'll drink with anybody who can pay his intellectual dues," said Jeff. [See Vig1954 .SNM] He included MDs, PhDs, technicians, osteopaths (heresy to the AMA) and commercial people (heresy to academics). Society boundaries should be neither geographic nor trade-union. At the third annual meeting Norman "Jeff" Holter was elected president with instructions to prepare for a changeover to a national society. This election also started the unwritten tradition that about every fourth president should be a physicist — at least non-MD.

The Society Goes National at the Fourth

The fourth annual meeting was scheduled for Oklahoma City. With 8 "Regional Chapters," the Society had become national geographically. An ad hoc self-appointed group met at the Radiology convention, Palmer House in Chicago in December, 1956. They were not on the program and their meeting was not advertised. We had to scrounge a room to meet in, but it was packed. A small group of radiologists, who did not realize a Nuclear Medicine Society was already formed, threatened bitter opposition to formation of upstarts who had never taken an X-Ray. They demanded that only certified radiologists be licensed to handle radioactivity. We, on the other hand, said we would not discriminate against radiologists but would not marry their sisters. A smell of sulfur filled the room.

Six months later, in Oklahoma City, the Society of Nuclear Medicine formally became a national society. M. Brucer (Chairman, Medical Division, Oak Ridge) became the first president who was not a founding member. But organized radiology struck back: before he could take office the American Board of Radiology, without his knowledge, certified him a radiology specialist in Nuclear Medicine. The Society would not get around to certification until 16 years later (1972).

It is interesting that 25 years later the Society got into the same trade-union labor dispute, but on the opposite side. Nuclear medics invented a Tl-201 myocardial ischemia test. Cardiologists saw no reason why they should not be licensed to use an innocuous dose of °nuclide. The Society screamed: too dangerous without 6 months special training. The cardiologists would settle for a month or so to learn how to turn the instruments on and off, and started their own new journal in nuclear cardiology. But the SNM was getting used to losing appendages: brachytherapy, then teletherapy, then placentography, then wet chemistry tests, then RIA. In spite of these losses, membership in the Soc Nuc Med continued to grow.

RADIOIODINE FAILS AS A CONTRACEPTIVE

(Gordon & Radioactive Family Planning)

"Radiation causes sterility" was a frequent headline quote from one Nobel geneticist. Newspaper reports of screw worm flies, sterilized by radiation to prevent a disease in cattle, was proof-positive that radiation caused impotence in man.

"Sterility" was a newspaper euphemism for "impotency" in those days. It was also, for many years, the most serious side effect of nuclear medicine. We were sitting around the lunch table at the Argonne Hospital I-131 Therapy Conference, Nov 5, 1956, discussing the evidence for radiation sterility in humans.

I told the story of a grandmother in the Oak Ridge hospital who had refused °iodine therapy for hyperthyroidism because she didn't want her grandchildren to be sterile for the rest of her life. "I can top that story," said Tom Shipmann, the medical director at Los Alamos. The Los Alamos criticality accident on the Manhattan Project was well known among experts, but medical details had been sparse.

One physicist had received an estimated 350 Rads to his gonads. Except for the usual transient lymphopenia and a sperm count of zero, he was unaffected by the accident. Los Alamos was a small town and the unfortunate childless family was a lesson to enforce Health Physics rules. About a year and a half after the accident the physicist's wife began to bulge where no bulge should appear with a sterile husband. Eyebrows went up all over town. The physicist was recalled for another sperm count and his physician leaked the confidential results widely — many sperm, and very active. At term, two years post-accident, the wife delivered a perfectly normal baby and, since then, still another.

I Rubin's successful treatment of female *infertility* with 50 r to each ovary [AJOG 1926] and large animal exposures had already proved the unreliable nature of gonad radiation sterility. But this Los Alamos case was the first documented evidence that human male radiation sterility is transient.

Dwight Clark (Surgery, U of Chicago) then told the story of a woman in her twenties being treated for thyroid carcinoma. They were finishing their standard course of 35 μCi every 2 weeks for 3 months, when she suddenly announced that she was 2 months pregnant. Tremendously upset, they warned her of thyroid ablation, leukemia, microencephaly, and recommended an immediate therapeutic abortion. She refused and in due course delivered a healthy, normal baby. The child was closely checked for all the bad predictions, but after 5 years was still perfectly normal. Since then the woman has had three more normal children.

Earl Miller (Radiology, UCSF) said he could top that story. A young married couple were admitted as patients, both with thyroid carcinoma. The wife received 50 mCi for thyroid ablation; the husband got 500 mCi. A few years later the thyroid problems had disappeared and they had become the parents of two normal healthy children.

Edgar Gordon (Internist, U of Wis) said he could top both stories. A 34-year-old woman had come to their infertility clinic after many years of disappointment. During examination a thyroid ca was discovered. Treatment was started with 80 mCi of °iodine, and instructions to return in 2 months. Two months later, while being examined for a second dose, she was found to be pregnant. Treatment was suspended until about 2 months after delivery of a carefully examined but completely normal baby. Treatment was resumed with a second 80 mCi dose of I-131. Upon her return 2 months later for followup, she again announced she was pregnant. Treatment was again suspended until about 2 months after delivery of a carefully examined but completely normal baby. Treatment was resumed with a third 80 mCi dose of I-131. Two months later she returned for her followup with the news that she was again pregnant. The treatment was naturally suspended until about two months after delivery of a carefully examined but completely normal baby. This time, however, she refused any further I-131 therapy. Her family, she said, was now complete and she thanked the doctors for the wonderful family planning.

[See Vig1985 .Rum]

HOW TO TREAT HYPERTHYROIDISM WITH °I

(Or, if confused, be glad you're not an expert)

On 5 Nov 1956 thirty-six experts on the therapeutic use of °I met at the Argonne Cancer Research Hospital (U of Chicago). Eighteen were practicing physicians and represented I-131 treatment of about 16,000 patients/year. The others were their physicists or technical advisors. They did not meet to discuss failures — °I therapy was almost too successful to believe — but because they had questions they could not answer.

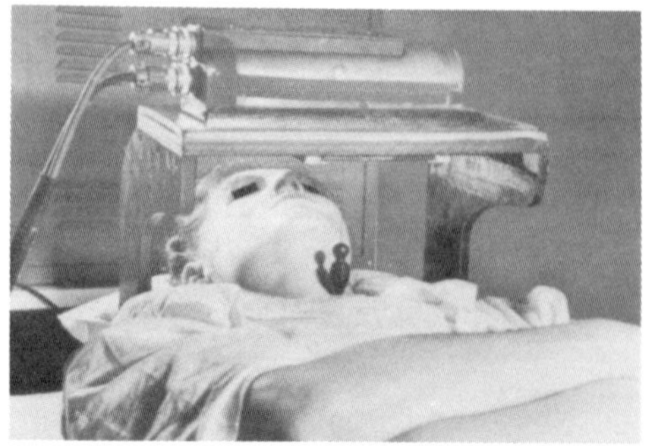

Leo Marinelli collimated this sidewall GM tube (1945) so that Seidlin could estimate the size of thyroid metastases.

The Errors in Thyroid Dosimetry

The results of the Brucer international survey of hypo, eu, and hyperthyroid manikins had just been published. It was enough to make scientists cry. One expert had measured the 65% thyroid manikin at 120%, another measured the same manikin at 45%. The range in 300 laboratories was 10% to 160%. This inaccuracy was minor when compared to results in the hypothyroid manikins. It was hard to believe the popular physical dose calculations required by editors with such variations in the basic measurement.

Further, all formulae for calculating radiation dose required an estimate of gland weight from palpation, which was known to be >100% in error. Still further, all formulae assumed a homogeneous distribution of °I in the gland which autoradiography had shown to be many orders of magnitude off the mark. Radiation dose calculations were a form of creative imagination.

Warren Sinclair (English rad physicist) led off the discussion telling how he measured thyroid uptake to calculate dose. He readily admitted a possible error of 25%–50%. F. Keating (Mayo Clinic) didn't know of any method that gave results approaching 25%–50% accuracy. M. Tubiana, an external beam therapy expert (Paris), said that although such accuracy might be achieved in homogeneous diffuse hyperthyroidism, it was certainly not true in malignant tissue. He didn't treat by "average" dose calculations, but by the minimum dose expected to reach the tissue.

The Single/Multiple Dose Controversy

J. Stanbury (Harvard) described E. Chapman's 36 patients who, in 1946, were regarded as well controlled after a single dose. They averaged weights and uptakes and chose 160 μCi/g as "a good dose." N. Larson (Stockholm) divided his patients into small, med, and large glands, recognizing that weight was even more unreliable than uptake. A.S. Freedberg (Beth Israel) and W. Van der Laan (Scripps Clinic) both used an effective half-time, measured on each patient, instead of a simple uptake.

Earl Miller (UCSF) pointed out that he and Mayo Soley, in 1945, had tried all forms of uptakes, turnovers, and half-times to determine dose — without success. Therefore, they compared the doses given patients who became hypothyroid with doses to patients who required a second dose — the correct dose must be in between.

Sidney Werner (Columbia) expanded on the patients who required retreatment: 30% of their patients required 2 doses, 14% 3 or 4 doses, a few 5 or 6. The larger glands seemed to require multiple doses. Dwight Clark (U of Chicago) described 625 patients; only 56% achieved remission on a single dose and one went up to 12 doses. Sergei Feitelberg (Mt. Sinai, NY) objected to the "number of doses" concept; it should be total dose. His patients averaged 115 μCi/g. (He did not say how he calculated 115, and he had been very high on the uptake survey.) F. Keating (Mayo) controlled hyperthyroidism on the first dose in 85% of a large series. They strove to give 200 μCi/g on the first dose (they had been low on the uptake survey) and had 31% hypothyroids.

Hypothyroidism is an Added Problem

E. McCullagh (Cleveland Clinic) tried to give 100 μCi/g on a series of 1600 patients. 75% became euthyroid on a single dose with about 10% hypothyroidism, but only temporarily. There was more hypothyroidism in the patients that received only a single dose, and the total dose bore no relationship to outcome.

Henry Jaffe (Cedars, LA) listed >3000 patients treated. They tried to give 150 μCi/g (20% off on the survey) but waited 2 or 3 months before repeating in order to reduce the incidence of hypos. (But they still had 10%.) Maurice Tubiana (Paris) aimed at 100 μCi/g on 600 patients; he reported good results on single dose with 5% becoming hypothyroid. (They were not on the survey.)

Eric Pochin (London) reported on many hospitals in England. All tried to deliver 9000 ± 1000 reps (about 100 μCi/g). This fancy calculation required many assumptions but the same uptake measurement. (5 hospitals on the survey had 20% to 30% high or low error but with physics panache.) The frequency of myxedema was about 10% no matter what the direction of their error.

Is Hypothyroidism an I-131 Problem?

Martin Sonenberg (Cornell) thought the only common denominator in all this clinical experience was that there was no common denominator. Maybe the uptake measurement was wrong, or the calculations of dose were wrong. Maybe we should look at the effective half-life. Joseph Hall (NIH) showed that the effective half-life varied from 6 hours to 7 days in a small series of patients.

Dave Becker (Cornell) pointed out the orders of magnitude variation in calculated dosages. He described the excellent results achieved in 4 patients with effective half-lives measured to prevent over or under dose from irrelevant calculations.

Sergi Feitelberg felt that hypothyroid figures were exaggerated. Cured patients in their series did not return for follow-up, but hypothyroid patients were sure to show up. Their reported 7% incidence should really be about 4%. Sidney Werner said his figures had been adjusted for that error and 7.6% became hypothyroid a year or two after I-131. Edgar Gordon (U of Wisconsin) said he had reported 2.4% hypos in his first series of 350 therapies at the 1953 Oak Ridge Symposium, but the figure had climbed to 4% since then.

Both Earle Chapman and John Stanbury (MGH) pointed out that most hypothyroidism is not severe and most patients are not diagnosed until a PBI or uptake happens to be run for some other reason. And, hypothyroidism also occurs following surgical and medical therapy. 13.9% of hyper patients surgically treated at the Brigham between 1933–1940 became hypothyroid, said Willard Vander Laan. The incidence from the literature, added Dwight Clark, runs from 0.2% to 29.7%. The natural course is those who survive hyperthroidism to become hypothyroid.

The True Cause of Hypothyroidism

Someone brought up the cases of spontaneous hypothyroidism in hypers who had received no therapy at all. If a hyperthyroid patient lives through the disease, hypothyroidism is the natural result. Rulon Rawson demurred; it might be supernatural. He remembered a patient with moderately severe hyperthyroidism. She had been a nurse at MGH back in 1912 and had seen the futility of treatment. She refused therapy of any kind.

Three years later the hyperthyroid nurse returned to the clinic. She was in a full blown myxedema and had thyroid atrophy on palpation. We asked what had happened to her. Because of her hyperthyroid distress, she replied, she had taken up Christian Science but had been overtreated with prayer.

[See Vig1950 .Lon, London]

HOW TO SAVE HUMANITY FROM GENETIC RADIATION DEFECTS

In 1952 the ICRP (Int Comm Rad Protect) became hysterical about possible genetic effects of radiation. At the 1953 International Congress of Radiology, genetic effects were not based on evidence in man — there was none. Nevertheless, genetic damage was formally recognized as the scourge of mankind. At the first Atoms-for-Peace conference the AEC made *the* big mistake that would eventually lead to its downfall in disgrace. They allowed, even encouraged, a group of Health Physicists to extrapolate data on "danger" from fruit flies to man, and from therapeutic dose levels to background radiation. (Nobody would know the range of background levels for another 30 years.) [See Vig1978 .Bkg]

Since Lea's pioneering radiobiology in the 1930s, *theoretical* dogma accepted a single ionizing event as a cause of a genetic event, e.g., a chromosome break. From this assumption, a mathematical model could be erected to bolster any biological scenario. A risk/benefit concept emerged as a political value judgement painted in "science" colors. Background radiation was "safe," or at least inescapable. Therapy doses were damaging but beneficial. Where did diagnostic doses, presumably beneficial but possibly damaging, fit? Health Physics, whose only visible means of support was radiation hysteria, trained a group of mathematical manipulators to distort biology.

In preparation for the second Atoms-for-Peace conference we were discussing new radioisotope liver tests. A health physicist of considerable stature in Oak Ridge pointed out that although a °Rose Bengal test for neonatal jaundice may be all right for patients over 40 years of age, it was immoral in babies. I admitted that all neonatal tests were done on patients under the age of 40 — and without the patient's written permission. The test would exceed the Maximum Permissible Dose, but such congenital defects, if not diagnosed and repaired, caused death. His answer was, "But at least they won't die with seared ovaries to pass on to future generations."

[See Vig1985 .Rum; Rumor]

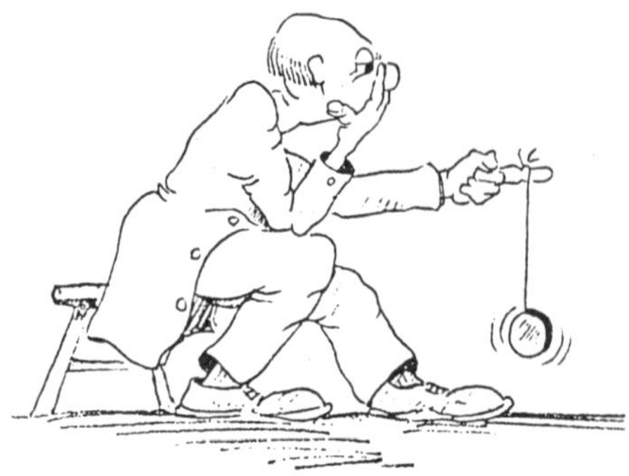

"Give me a place to sit and I can think up anything"
— Aristotle

By the end of the 1950s a group of religious zealots had parlayed a relatively minor safety problem in "possible" radiation overexposure into major public hysteria. They took over a field called "Health Physics," which had been necessary around wartime nuclear reactors. In order to perpetuate their expensive but increasingly unnecessary being, they established a rapidly metastasizing series of non-measurable "units" of radiation danger: ever-decreasing "Maximum Permissible Doses," "working levels" of every imaginable fantasy, an ALARA concept. Finally, to justify their lack of evidence they invented a "sievert."

Rolf Sievert, a Swedish radiation physicist, had been first to "measure" whole body backgrounds in 1948. The non-measurable pseudo-unit named after him is the antithesis of scientific reasoning. By 1986 even the editor of the *Health Physics Newsletter* admitted the new Federal health physics regulations, 10 CFR 20, were meaningless. [HPN 14:2, 1986] Health Physicists are no longer part of the scientific community. Like Aristotelians, they are a religious cult.

[See Vig1955 .AfP]

THESE MEN MADE NUCLEAR MEDICINE PRACTICAL

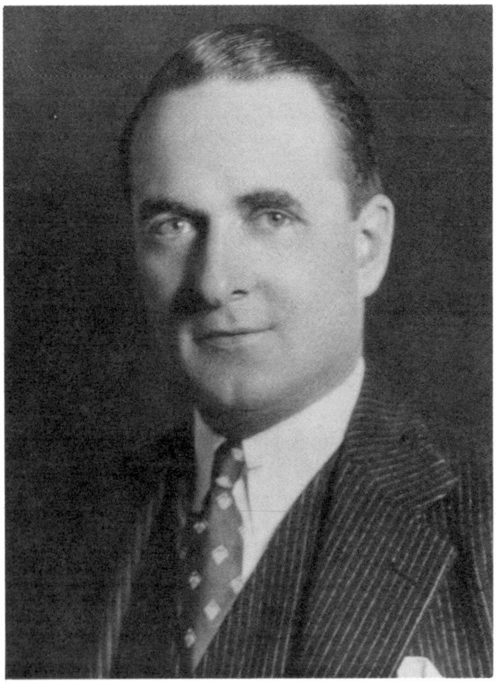

Earle MacArthur Chapman, M.D., 1903–

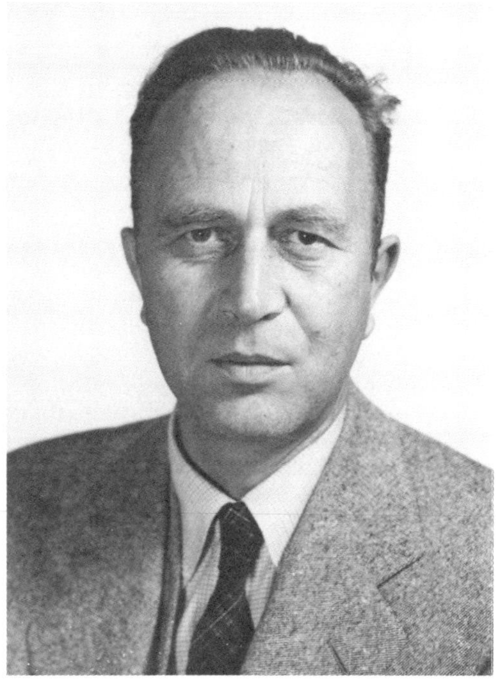

Joseph Gilbert Hamilton, M.D., 1907–1957

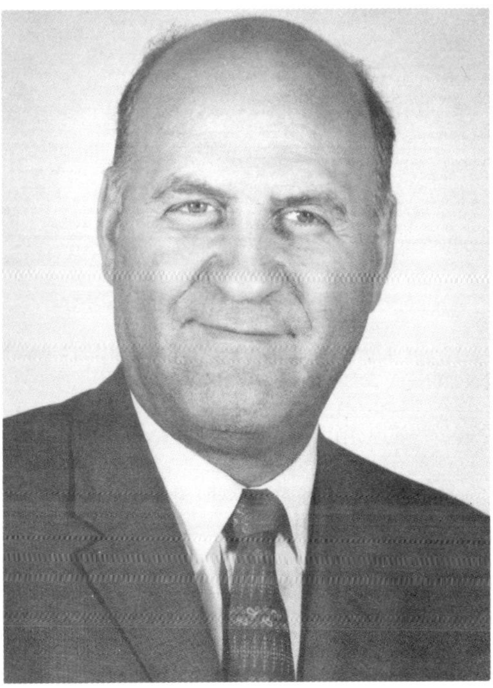

Irving Meyer Ariel, M.D., 1903–

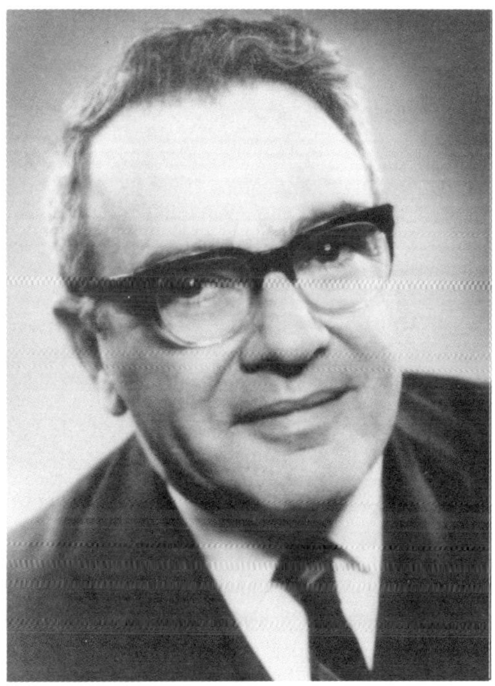

Martin David Kamen, Ph.D., 1913–

BONE SCANNING BEGINS IN THE FRUIT FLY
(Five Separate Pages in History Lead to Bone Scans)

To clear up an obscure point in P-32 history, I berated Erv Kaplan (Nuc Med, Hines, VA) for not beginning page 5 of bone scan history:

Page 1 is G. Hevesy's introduction of P-32 through Lawrence's therapy trials crowned by Charles Pecher's Sr-89.
Page 2 is the Berkeley group efforts, ending with Low-Beer's trials in P-32 brachytherapy.
Page 3 is Maxfield's booster dose with testosterone to aid Friedell's palliation of metastases to bone.
Page 4 is the Sklaroff & Charkes struggle with °Sr bone scans.

Erv Kaplan's substitution of poly- for ortho-phosphate would have started page 5 if he had noticed its applicability to scanning. But Kaplan was steeped in therapy and ends on page 3. He missed bone scans — as did all the rest of us who heard his 1960 paper. Erv became livid with nostalgia when I pointed out his near miss. *"The fruit fly,"* he insisted, *"is the beast of choice to investigate bone scanning."* The full story has many twists.

Page 2 Begins an Emphasis on Bone

Page one in the history of bone scanning must include Hevesy's discovery of how to make P-32 [See Vig1936 .GHP] through John Lawrence's first attempt to do P-32 therapy. Page 2 starts when Pecher discarded P-32 for °Ca to study metabolism in bone. He rapidly shifted to a new emphasis on treatment of then untreatable metatastases to bone.

Charles Pecher had come to U of Cal in 1939 from Belgium for postgraduate study. His field was the pharmacology of calcium using the new radioactive method. He was assigned to work across the bay with Joe Hamilton at the cyclotron lab in Berkeley. There was no good (meaning easy to make on the cyclotron) °isotope of calcium. Hamilton sold him on trying a close chemical analogue, Sr-90. It was already available, and Joe could get a new supply whenever the cyclotroneers had nothing else to do. Pecher tried it and found Sr-90 had good uptake in bone. [See Vig1939 .Pec]

After many studies he eventually tried Sr-89 in terminal cancer patients. To his surprise he found exceptional uptake in metastases to bone in patients with prostate cancer. Was it a good enough uptake for therapy? Pecher tried it in a few patients with massive (for 1939) 8 mCi doses. The results were very encouraging. This treatment was radiotherapy by any definition and caught Low-Beer's attention. But Hitler was on the loose and before Pecher finished his report he was recalled to Belgium for military duty.

Bertram Low-Beer (radiotherapist at UCSF) intended to continue Pecher's studies, but WWII had an immediate effect on cyclotron priorities. In order to keep the Germans from suspecting cyclotron hanky-panky in the atom business, scientific papers had to continue. The Manhattan District decreed that John Lawrence should receive 100 mCi of P-32 each month and produce lots of publications as a cover for secret cyclotron operations.

No more Sr-89! But Low-Beer was now up to his ears in free P-32. (John Lawrence made his bonanza freely available to any scientist.) [See Vig1944 .P32] By the end of the war Low-Beer had discovered that P-32 had high uptake in breast ca and also in its bone metastases. Hymer Friedell, one of the radiologists in the Berkeley–UCSF group, left to set up his own shop at Western Reserve. He carried with him memories of the partially finished P-32 therapy.

Page 3 Stresses Rx of Metastases to Bone

In 1950, with John Storaasli, Hymer Friedell announced the successful (quite often) palliation therapy of breast metastases to bone. J.R. Maxfield (radiologist in Dallas) extended it in 1958 to combined testosterone–P-32 palliation that improved Friedell's results.

Ervin Kaplan heard Maxfield describe the uptake of ortho-phosphate in "tumor tissue but not in other soft tissue." From his long experience with P-32 Kaplan knew this deposition could not be true. With micro-autoradiographic techniques he showed that beta cross-fire from P-32 in

Divination, once highly successful by casting bones, *Is the direct ancestor of diagnosis by bone scanning.*

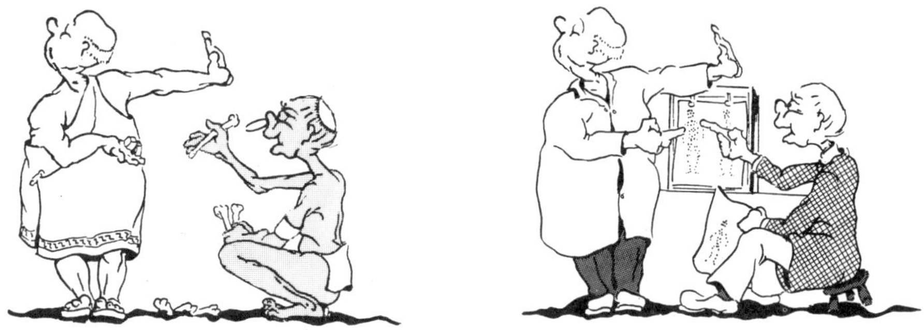

3500 years ago *3500 years later*

bone spicules surrounding the tumor must be the therapeutic agent. Hence, radiation dose would be proportional to the exchange of P-32 in bone, not in the tumor. A chemist colleague, Gordon Fells, suggested that a simple heat condensation might convert ortho- to poly-phosphate which would enhance bone uptake.

Kaplan described his findings at the 1959 Estes Park Society of Nuclear Medicine meeting. [JNM, 1959] But Kaplan saw no connection between the high uptake of polyphosphate in therapeutic use and its possible use as a scanning agent. Maxfield heard Kaplan's talk, but nothing clicked in his mind. Storaasli heard the talk but nothing clicked. Brucer's Oak Ridge group had attempted to scan bone tumors with Ga-72, but nothing clicked.

Page 4 Introduces Bone Scanning

David Sklaroff at the Einstein Medical Center in Philadelphia was impressed by the tremendous attention that radiobiologists and the newspaper-dazzled faction of health physicists were giving to strontium-90. Radioactive fallout from atom bomb testing in Nevada was spewing deadly Sr-90 all over the country. (Nobody could find dead bodies, but Sr-90 was always "deadly strontium.") Newspapers actually printed daily reports on the levels of Sr-90 in milk. Sklaroff knew this was all health physics fakery, but he was impressed by the constant reference to uptake in bone. Sr-90 was a pure beta emitter, but Sr-85 had a fine 514 keV gamma ray that could be scanned. Electron capture allowed high doses and a 65 day half-life allowed time for excretion of all not firmly bound in bone. A linear scan a week after dose could be completed in a very handy two, maybe three hours.

Sklaroff, with Norman Charkes, scanned well over 1000 patients by 1969 and had shifted to Sr-87m for some scans. They described practically every feature of bone scanning. Metastases from primaries in the prostate or breast were obvious on scan long before they could be seen on X-Ray. But a bone scan was a major undertaking, expensive in patient, laboratory, technician, and physician's time.

Page 5, A New Era in Bone Scanning

Sklaroff had heard Kaplan's 1959 talk. All of us old timers in Nuclear Medicine knew that Kaplan had described a polyphosphate with remarkable uptake in bone. But we all KNEW that P-32 could not be scanned. Not until 1972 did some new boys in the field, Raymond Marty, Gopal Subramanian, suggest the obvious — tag the polyphosphate with a °nuclide that could be scanned.

When I berated Kaplan for his lapse in perception and thus missing by a hair inaugurating page 5, the new era in bone scanning, he noted my lapse and then pointed out: *"Don't be so sure that I don't go back to page 1. I did my first bone scans in 1938 with cyclotron P-32 on the exoskeleton of the fruit fly."* But none of his fruit flies developed metastases from breast cancer.

[See Vig1960 °Tc]

THE GREAT CRANBERRY CRISIS
(Bureaucrats Learn How to Tap Fort Knox)

The greatest event in political science occurred just before the Thanksgiving holiday of 1959. The Food and Drug Administration (FDA) deliberately manufactured a major hysteria for political gain. It required a sustained confusion, and the unwitting collaboration of the news media, but FDA created the Great Cranberry Crisis of 1959 out of nothing to relieve budgetary desires. Cranberries were taken off grocery store shelves because they contained a trace of aminotriazole, a weed-killer later shown to be a natural constituent of cranberry plants. It was a lesson to all bureaucrats: your budget can be doubled by manufacturing a "crisis."

A Real Crisis Requires Preparation

In 1958 Congressman J. Delaney (D, NY) modified the Pure Food and Drug Act, and published the revision in the Federal Register (FR): *if cancer develops in any animal fed any food or drug, in any dose, for any time, the substance must be banned and its manufacturer drawn and quartered.* Scientists in the bowels of the FDA, many with academic degrees in basket weaving, were stuffing the bellies of mice to test for Delaney carcinogens. Any successful chemical was a candidate for testing. A highly successful weed-killer, aminotriazole, was known to have anti-thyroid activity in rats. The effect was easily tested. A massive dose of pure aminotriazole was rammed down a few rats' throats daily and, as expected, they all became hypothyroid.

The rats died weeks later of boredom, with little lumps in their thyroids. But in June 1959 one mouse developed a small thyroid cancer. The scientist informed his boss, who immediately notified his superior, who immediately called a committee to send a memo to the Deputy Assistant Secretary of the FDA. An ad-hoc committee was hastily organized to vitalize the Standing Committee on Research-in-Depth who went to the library. They found a book that said the offending weed-killer was used in the cranberry bogs of Massachusetts — No, that state has powerful senators, better make it the bogs of Oregon.

How to Manufacture a Crisis

Thanksgiving was only 19 days off. To prevent a carnage of mass poisoning immediate action was necessary. Thousands of FDA inspectors were alerted by emergency TWX. Then Secretary Fleming of the Dept of Health, Education, and Welfare was alerted. The Secretary briefed President Eisenhower on the third tee of Burning Tree. With Presidential approval he called a press conference and sounded the national tocsin: We are in CRISIS!

Monday, 9 November 1959: *"This is a warning not to buy either fresh or canned cranberries until further notice."*
[Chattanooga Daily Times]

Tuesday, 10 Nov 1959: *". . . it is risky for humans to eat tainted berries . . . mice developed cancer of the thyroid."* Secretary Flemming revealed that one shipment of canned cranberries had been seized, but another had been distributed.
[Knoxville News-Sentinal]

Wednesday, 11 Nov: The Secretary advises *". . . housewives be on the safe side by not buying cranberries. . . ."* Women's pages of Chattanooga and Knoxville papers recommend stuffed peaches and curried apple halves for Thanksgiving. An AP dispatch from Albany, Oregon reported a million pounds of cranberries buried.

Thursday, 12 Nov: *"The scientist from the world's foremost agricultural experimental station said that he could see no reason why people should not eat cranberries." [Knoxville News-Sentinal]*

Friday, 13 Nov: AP distributed pictures of Vice President Nixon helping himself to his fourth serving of cranberries. Presidential candidate Rockefeller had turkey a la Marco Polo with baked alaska, but no cranberries. Senator J.F. Kennedy drank a toast with Massachusetts cranberry juice. Another load of Oregon cranberries was seized by the Welfare Department of California. [AP, UPI]

Saturday, 14 Nov: AP reports another 39,000 lbs of Wisconsin berries seized, and Chicago banned the sale of all cranberries. [Chicago Daily News]

Monday, 16 Nov: President Eisenhower is asked to declare Oregon, Washington, Wisconsin, New Jersey, and Massachusetts economic disaster areas. The FDA announced that cranberries in warehouses of New Mexico, Colorado, Texas, and Utah were safe from the cancer-causing weed-killer. [Washington Post]

Tuesday, 17 Nov: HEW Secretary said most berries were not contaminated, and seized 25 cases of Wisconsin berries. [Washington Star]

Wednesday, 18 Nov: *"Those who have eaten cranberries with less than 5 ppm aminotriazole should not be apprehensive,"* said a Tennessee State Chemist, but wanted all that stuff off the market. FDA, Denver, approved 150,492 lbs of canned cranberries. [AP, Rocky Mt News]

Thursday, 19 Nov: *"The first batch of tainted cranberries from the 1958 crop turned up a few hours after the industry insisted that all berries from 1958 were safe."* [Albuquerque Journal] AP learned of the HEW plan for abundant cranberries for Thanksgiving. All the housewife has to do is look for the safety label.

Friday, 20 Nov: *"Labels for cranberries certified safe have been ordered,"* HEW Secretary tells UPI reporter.

Saturday, 21 Nov: HEW advises housewives in an AP release: Buy laboratory-approved cranberries soon because they may run out.

Sunday. 22 Nov: HEW Secretary said if he were a housewife he would be "on the safe side and wouldn't buy any." [New York Times]

Wednesday, 25 Nov: On the three days before Thanksgiving, full-page advertisements feature turkeys, bananas, applesauce, beer, but no cranberries. The A&P 100th birthday special features everything except cranberries. But on this last day the A&P openly advertised the very brand that had been found tainted 9 Nov 1959.

THANKSGIVING DAY: UPI telephotos show Secretary Flemming eating a salad made from U.S. inspected cranberries. President Eisenhower is said to have substituted applesauce.

The Aftermath

A week after Thanksgiving, SCIENCE, the weekly voice of the Am Assoc for Advance of Science, editorialized under the title "Cranberry Smash." Aminotriazole had been properly registered for years as an economic poison with the Dept of Agriculture. When used in cranberry bogs too late in the growing season, small amounts were incorporated in the berries.

Tests showed that some rats fed a lifetime diet containing 100 ppm (parts per million) of aminotriazole developed thyroid adenocarcinomas; at 50 ppm, a few developed adenomas but no carcinomas. A lifetime diet of 1 ppm caused nothing.

In 1957 the FDA had 3½ million lbs of cranberries withdrawn from the market. Industry asked for a tolerance of 1 ppm — denied. In 1958 the industry again petitioned for a 1 ppm tolerance. Again the FDA denied it, claiming misuse, but made no seizures. The SCIENCE editorial pointed out that it was hard to discuss the matter because the FDA had declared the test results *"CONFIDENTIAL official secret, vital to National Security."*

Payment for the Crisis

According to a news item spiked by most newspapers, the FDA asked Congress for an increased budget the day after Thanksgiving. [AMA News, 30 Nov 1959] It was granted and a round of promotions for the staff celebrated the deception. Before 1958 the FDA had to prove a product harmful before seizure. After the Cranberry Crisis every chemical was guilty until proved safe. Secretary Flemming pointed out that his scientists could not prove any "safe" tolerance, therefore he wanted congressional authority to specify "safe" levels. [If this does not make sense, you're out of touch with bureaucracy.]

What makes the Great Cranberry Crisis a true landmark in history is that every branch of government learned that a cancer in a mouse means money in the budget. The mouse population in Washington, DC, doubled in one year. The FDA had already started an investigation of death and illness from coal tar colors used in lipstick. [AP, 20 Nov 1959] Charcoal was listed among the deadly food additives and charcoal-broiled steak faced bureau controls; even burnt toast was suspect. [AP, 29 Nov 1959] In March 1960 the US paid $10 million in damages to cranberry growers. To mollify hurt feelings, cranberries became a big item in the free school-lunch program. The Army was instructed to buy more cranberries

The Great Cranberry Crisis was officially over when the Governor of Massachusetts declared cranberry juice the official State Drink. Then, Surgeon General Terry doubled his budget with a smoking mouse.

CHRONOLOGY OF NUCLEAR MEDICINE — 1960

Scientific and Technical Background			Ref.
1. Basic	— F. Momyer: °Xe and °Kr absorb on almost any surface.	[1957]	AEC
4. # Med	— P. Aebersold says over 135,000 shipments of °isotopes.	[1956]	AEC
	— 2500 medical licenses issued, but states taking over.	[1956]	AEC
	— France: 13 reactors, 7000 °isotope users, is 90% independent.	[1948]	CEA

Organizations and Internal Politics			
5. AEC +	— FRC publishes rehash of ICRP and NCRP data, with new titles:		FRC
	"Max Perm Dose" is out, use our "Rad Protect Guide."	[1955]	FRC
	— ICRP publishes new tables of "Max Permissible Dose."	[1955]	ICRP
	— WHO publishes its own variation of ICRP but new titles.	[1958]	WHO
	— AEC dumps unpopular inspect & enforce onto states.	[1959]	AEC
	— USA population at 179,323,000.	[1950]	SAb
6. Socs	— Journal of Nuclear Medicine begins publication.	[1959]	JNM
	— AMA recognizes "Nuclear Medicine," forms a committee.	[1934]	JAMA
	— R. Overman pubs "Radioisotope Techniques" (McG-Hill).	[1948]	Bk
7. Event	— P. Richards (Brookhaven) first describes Tc-99m for med.	[1957]	CN
	— YALOW & BERSON GIVE FIRST TRUE IN VITRO RIA PROCEDURE.	[1957]	JCI

Instruments, Units of Measurement, and Drugs			
8. Instr	— C. Amato develops photoluminesc glass needle dosimetry.	[1956]	JNM
	— M. Brucer sums 18 of the world's Whole Body Counters.	[1959]	AEC
	— Weather Bureau sends TV-Infrared-Obs Sat (TIROS) aloft.	[1935]	SN
	— LASER (Light Ampli Stim Emis Electrons) invented, USA.	[1949]	EB
9. Units	— G. Failla invents "wall-less" 200 μm ion chamber (tissues).	[1953]	RS
	— XIth CGPM ADOPTS "SYSTEME INTERNATIONAL" (SI) UNITS.	[1954]	BJC
	— CGPM adopts wavelength of krypton as length standard.	[1954]	NBS
10. Concp	— M. Argus says whole body irrad does not affect uptakes.	[1954]	BJR
	— M. Brucer: spectral, spatial, and temporal resolution.	[1935]	AEC
11. Drugs	— W. Tucker: Sr to Y-90, Te to I-132, Mo to Tc-99m cows.	[1951]	JNM
	— R. Hayes develops Cs to Ba-137 cow to teach half-life.	[1952]	JCE
	— J. Brown uses C-14 palmitate (CO_2 breath) for fat metab.	[1955]	CM
	— R. Helmkamp makes hi-specific activity °I-gamma globulin.	[1958]	CR
	— M. Tubis prepares °I-Hippurate for kid-function tests.	[1950]	PSEB

Radioiodine, P-32, and Radioactive Therapy			
12. I-Res	— R. Grayson says normal USA I-127 intake = 126–760 μg/d.	[1958]	AJM
	— R. Ekins uses competitive protein binding for T4 assay.	[1957]	CCA
13. I-Dx	— J. Crooks announces Perchlorate Suppress Test for hyper.	[1958]	La
	— T. Oddie announces T3 Suppression Test for hyperthyroid.	[1958]	JCE
	— G. Sheline proves autonomous function in thyroid nodule.	[1958]	JCE
	— W. Thomas says I-127 in drinking water cuts °I uptake.	[1958]	AEH
14. I-Rx	— E. Hammonds confirms success of I-131 Rx in cardiac dis.	[1955]	JAMA
	— C. Comas finds low dose to ovaries from thyroid therapy.	[1905]	AJR
15. P-Rx	— E. Kaplan uses poly (not ortho) phosphate in bone mets Rx.	[1959]	JNM
	— E. Leslie says P-32 prolongs life span of PVA patients.	[1959]	CR
16. Tele	— 431 Co-60 and 32 Cs-137 units known to be in operation.	[1958]	IAEA
	— M. Brucer shows a 4000 Ci Cs-137 total body irrad unit.	[1929]	AEC
17. Other	— G. Ramsay implants °Au & °Y for pituitary destruction.	[1953]	RSM
	— A. Gottschalk tries S-35 therapy in chondrosarcoma.	[1957]	JBJS

	Scans and Other Tests of Function in Various Organs		
18. Brain	— W. Oldendorf times arrival of IV bolus in hemispheres.	[1958]	Neu
	— S. Fedoruk measures cereb circ time with carotid °IHSA.	[1955]	CJS
	— S. Albert gives Kr-85 by breathing to measure CBF.	[1955]	JLCM
19. Heart	— F. Dreyfuss: Na°I uptake in infarcts not in normal myocardium.	[1959]	AJC
	— A. Courand examines R and L RadCardGrams under exercise.	[1959]	TAAP
	— J. Hakkila uses °triolein absorption in conges failure.	[1957]	AJC
	— E. Brunwald uses Kr-85 on first pass, detects R-L shunts.	[1959]	Ci
	— F. DiPietrantoni sees "index" of RadCardGraphic output.	[1955]	MN
20. Liver	— P. Johnson makes diagnostic spleen scans with Cr-51 RBC.	[1958]	Rad
21. Lung	— N. Dyson does Knipping's Kr-85 study with O-15, Xe-133.	[1957]	BMJ
	— J. West uses breath holding proc with O-15 blood flows.	[1957]	JCI
22. Bone	— S. Jacobson injects °IHSA in knee joint, measures washout.	[1956]	JNM
	— R. Guerin measures Sr-89 in femoral neck fractures.	[1952]	PM
23. Kidney	— R. Nordyke invents collimator for hippuran renogram.	[1959]	JNM
	— J. McAfee introduces Hg-203 chlormerodrin for kidney scan.	[1936]	Rad
	— W. Beierwaltes: kidney extracts °I-Hippuran from blood.	[1956]	JNM
24. Gut	— A. Cameron measures blood loss with °Cr RBC @ 1 ml/day.	[1957]	BMJ
	— E. Fedor says cholecystectomy doesn't affect °I-triolein.	[1958]	SGO
	— B. Anderson devises H-3 folic acid measurement method.	[1958]	BJH
25. Blood	— R. Huff measures rate of RBC formation with °Fe.	[1954]	MMR
	— S. Albert introduces "Unitag" bag for in vitro °CrRBC.	[1954]	JNM
	— A. Mauer labels granulocytes with DF°P.	[1959]	JCI
	— E. Brody says IV Co-58 VB_{12} cleared in 2 phase curve.	[1957]	BI
26. Other	— W. BALE TRIES °I-ANTIFIBRINOGEN Rx OF TUMORS (ANIMALS).	[1922]	CR
	— Many authors detail area count °IHSA placentography.	[1958]	JNM
	— B. Hibbard says °IHSA placental counting is routine.	[1958]	COG
	— K. Nagatani detects malig eye tumors with P-32 counting.	[1954]	AORL
	— G. Kyker starts intralymph localizing: °Au, $°YCl_2$, $°CeCl_2$.	[1959]	AEC

	Radiation Hysteria and Health Physics	* Obituaries *	
27. Hyst	— Jt Com At En hearings on Rad Protect set up FedRadCoun.	[1957]	JCAE
	— FRC rules MPD is 100 mr/y, thus outlawing Denver.	[1956]	CEN
	— W. Beierwaltes finds pCi/g levels of fallout °I in gland.	[1956]	JAMA
	— W. Looney finds 11 Thorotrast liver ca in literature.	[1934]	AJR
	— U. Minnesota holds conference on °isotopes in fallout.	[1959]	UM
	— Many authors study incorporation of °isotopes in hair.	[1959]	PSEB
	— A. Jelliffe predicts ca and leukemia from I-131 therapy.	[1978]	CR
	— Am Hrt Assoc: smoking assoc with (not cause) heart dis.	[1986]	AP
28. React	— E. CRONKITE: ALL RADIATION LEUKEMIA FROM DOSES OVER 100 R		AJM
	— Acute Radiation Syndrome LD_{50} is 450 rad.	[1959]	AFMJ
	— A. Upton: no increase in leuk (mice) after in utero rad.	[1957]	PSEB
	— I. Chaikoff: only hi-dose °I causes ca in ca-strain rats.	[1952]	AP
29. Respo	— AEC puts first Sr-90 power weather station at North Pole.	[1959]	AEC
	— Soc Nuc Med recognizes growing rad hysteria (Teller).	[1958]	JNM
	— R. Heyssel: Atom Bomb Leukemia (140 patients) has stopped.	[1955]	BI
	— H. Pabst finds no leukemia after P-32 therapy for PVA.	[1958]	SMW
	— US pays $10 million damages to cranberry growers.	[1959]	AP

30. Obits	— M. Laue (1879–1960) Ger physics; X-ray crystal diffraction.	DSB
	— L. de Broglie (1892–1960) Fr physics; wave theory of matter.	DSB
	— I. Kurchatov (1903–1960) USSR physics; nuclear physics.	DSB

CHRONOLOGY OF NUCLEAR MEDICINE — 1961

Scientific and Technical Background

			Ref.
1. Basic	— W. Mann determines half-life of C-14 at 5760y.	[1940]	Sc
2. Obser	— Word "radioisotope" improper; most use is of isobars.	[1947]	PL
3. # Nuc	— W. Sullivan's stamps give Trilinear Chart 1800 nuclides.	[1957]	
	— J. Stokley's GE chart has 1380 nuclides, 265 are stable.	[1948]	
	— >50,000 pts/y get °Dx, & 10,000 pts/y get °nuclide Rx.	[1954]	AEC
	— About 2 megacuries of °nuc have been shipped from Oak Ridge.	[1954]	AEC
4. # Med	— AEC has issued 2500 medical °nuclide licenses.	[1960]	AEC
	— AEC exempts some low-level medical uses from licensure.	[1953]	AEC

Organizations and Internal Politics

5. AEC +	— AEC, HEW, & FRC in turf battle on $$ to protect public.	[1960]	AP
	— G. Seaborg becomes Chairman of AEC; first scientist Chm.	[1958]	AP
	— AEC withdraws from routine °isotope sales – 8 private companies.	[1959]	AEC
	— AEC writes "suggested State legislation" on rad control.	[1959]	AEC
	— Arm Forc Rad Radiobiol Inst (AFRRI) formed in Bethesda.	[1960]	AP
6. Socs	— W. Sullivan writes his only article on Trilinear Chart.	[1946]	JTAS
	— G. Meneely hosts first Symposium on Whole Body Counting.	[1960]	Bk
	— A. Bartlett writes technical history of Compton scatter.	[1924]	AJP
	— G. Thomson tells the story of his father's "electron."	[1940]	PT
7. Event	— FIRST Mo-Tc 99m COW SHIPPED TO P. HARPER, U CHICAGO.	[1960]	RR
	— Largest °source (1 MCi Co-60) shpd to Army Food Process.	[1959]	AEC
	— USSR largest H-blast, 58 Megaton, Novaya Zeemlya, 10/20.	[1946]	AEC

Instruments, Units of Measurement, and Drugs

8. Instr	— S. Fedoruk builds first (?) dual head scanner (Saskatoon).	[1959]	JNM
	— c50 Whole Body Counters operating (many more building).	[1960]	IAEA
	— R. Beck: optimum °nuc energy for scanning is c100 keV.	[1958]	JNM
9. Units	— IUPAC DECREES C-12 THE NEW STANDARD FOR ATOMIC WEIGHTS.	[1894]	
10. Concp	— C. Harris says scan interpret requires 2 or more views.	[1957]	JNs
	— P. Czerniak requires 3 projections on all liver scans.	[1957]	JNM
	— M. Potsaid makes paraffin base 3-D chemical dosimeter.	[1969]	NEJM
	— P. Massini revises "absolute" beta counting methods.	[1959]	Sc
11. Drugs	— P. Harper tests I-125 for scans (then Tc-99m arrives).	[1968]	JNM
	— G. Taplin controls micro & macroaggregation of °IHSA.	[1954]	AEC
	— M. Tubis finally succeeds in labeling BSP with °I.	[1957]	JNM
	— J. Dancis studies placental transfer of °IHSA.	[1960]	AJOG
	— W. Tucker makes a 270d Ge-68 to 68m Ga-68 positron cow.	[1953]	IJAR

Radioiodine, P-32, and Radioactive Therapy

12. I-Res	— P. Meadows defines "Hot, Warm, Cool, Cold" nodules on scan.	[1960]	JAMA
	— V. Ramalingaswami notes endemic Himalayan goiter (I-131).	[1959]	La
	— E. Fowler: ca in 5.1% multiple, 8.5% single nodule glands.	[1959]	AS
	— J. Rupp hints at a T3 toxicosis from pt's plasma study.	[1970]	AJM
13. I-Dx	— Brucer manikin survey, 127 Japan hosp's show c50% error.	[1959]	IJAR
	— A. Freedberg introduces in vitro RBC T3 binding test.	[1959]	E
14. I-Rx	— R. Adrian finds remnant thyroid after "total" excisions.	[1959]	SM
	— >16 articles (e.g., R. Volpe) describe I-131 Rx for hypers.	[1958]	CMAJ
15. P-Rx	— L. Heilmeyer's thousands PVA Rx pts survive beyond life expect.	[1960]	Bkh
16. Tele	— M. Brucer: 8 (500 Ci) Cs-137 sources for total body Rx.	[1929]	Rad
	— E. King sets 60 (45 Ci) Co-60 sources for total body Rx.	[1960]	JAMA
	— M. Jacobs: 4 (300 Ci) Cs-137 sources for total body Rx.	[1960]	Rad
	— M. Brucer finds kCi Co-60 sources soon turn to powder.	[1960]	HP
17. Other	— M. Loken injects °ceramic microspheres in artery for Rx.	[1958]	S

Scans and Other Tests of Function in Various Organs

18. Brain	— G. Nylin measures brain blood flow with perfused °RBC.	[1960]	CirR
	— N. Lassen measures cereb cortex blood flow with Kr-85.	[1960]	Ex
	— W. Oldendorf use IV bolus injection to study blood flow.	[1960]	JNs
	— R. Bell measures cereb cir time, bolus (°IHSA) & ext probe.	[1960]	JNM
19. Heart	— E. Braunwald sees shunt size on RCG by precordial probe.	[1960]	SF
	— D. Rochester: cardiac outputs valid only in steady state.	[1954]	JCI
	— W. Hollander measures washout after myocard °I injection.	[1960]	JCI
	— R. Bing sees cold-spots in infarcts with °I-oleic acid.	[1960]	AJM
	— J. Applen gives method for °IHSA arterial flow in legs.	[1952]	S
20. Liver	— P. Czerniak says abscesses heal but cysts leave scar.	[1955]	JNM
	— G. Taplin sees bld flow with °AuCol, °RB sees poly cells.	[1959]	JNM
	— J. Usselidan describes post-radiotherapy scan.	[1955]	JNM
	— R. Greenlaw scans after direct °AuCol splenic injection.	[1959]	JNM
21. Lung	— R. Bing finds 10 μm °IMAA passes through lung into liver.	[1954]	AJPh
22. Bone	— W. Fleming makes first bone scans (uses °Ga).	[1961]	Rad
	— R. Goldsmith measures Ca-45 kinetics in Paget's disease.	[1959]	JNM
	— SKLAROFF & CHARKES INTRODUCE THE Sr-85 BONE SCAN.	[1957]	JNM
	— G. Wendeberg notes Sr-85 uptake at fracture site.	[1959]	AOS
23. Kidney	— A. Abt finds °I-Renografin excreted thru glomeruli.	[1955]	JU
	— A. Desgrez introduces the Hg-203 renal scan.	[1960]	JNM
	— 11 Authors (e.g., C. Winter) describe renogram in diseases.	[1960]	JU
	— J. McRae introduces °Tc-Sn- gluconate for kidney scans.	[1960]	ANZM
	— R. WITCOFSKI DISSECTS AND NAMES THE PARTS OF RENOGRAM CURVE.		Rad
24. Gut	— R. Nordyke uses °I-triolein to detect steatorrhea.	[1960]	G
	— R. Pierson finds °Cr-RBC bleeding after aspirin in 73%.	[1960]	AJM
	— K. Jeejeebhoy revives °IHSA to measure GI protein loss.	[1959]	JNM
	— D. Johns measures folic acid metabolism with H-3 label.	[1960]	JCI
25. Blood	— P. Cohen measures life span of Cr-51 labeled platelets.	[1960]	NEJM
	— P. Mollison finds Cr-51 RBC survival about 32 days.	[1958]	CS
	— B. Vaughn devises rapid H-3 assay in body fluids.	[1956]	JLCM
26. Other	— H. Antoniades thinks all hormones subj to Comp Binding.	[1957]	E
	— W. Beierwaltes introduces a Co-60 VB_{12} parathyroid scan.	[1950]	JNM
	— P. Czerniak: P-32 spermatogenesis tested by ext counts.	[1962]	JNM
	— F. Heagy localizes placenta with °IHSA blood pool scan.	[1960]	Rad
	— R. Baldwin measures 12 mg °Fe loss per menstrual period.	[1960]	AJOG
	— B. Goldberg describes Dx of eye tumors with °nuclides.	[1960]	AO

Radiation Hysteria and Health Physics * Obituaries *

27. Hyst	— Zelenko's H.R.1267 awards 90% wages for life for ANY rad exp.		FR
	— Idaho reactor construct explosion kills 3 from blast.	[1958]	AEC
	— G. Hamill gives 77 mCi to 5 mo pregnancy; baby born hypo.	[1956]	AJOG
	— R. Szepke reviews European (Polish) response to fallout rad.	[1960]	AEC
28. React	— L. Marinelli measures normal man given IV Ra-226 (1931).	[1955]	IAEA
	— First peaceful atomic detonation, 5k ton 1200 ft undergrd.	[1946]	AEC
	— W. Bost lists bibliography of 538 on Rad Protect Stds.	[1960]	AEC
	— IAEA symposium on Whole Body Counting is mostly HP.	[1960]	IAEA
	— ICRU underestimates population rad exposure in 16 countries.		ICRU
29. Respo	— S. Werner finds 10 leukemias post °I Rx, 14 expected	[1959]	JAMA
	— L. Craig: no correlation between leukemia & cosmic rays.	[1961]	BI
	— R. Newell complains: MPD is not a "health" limit	[1956]	JAMA
	— R. Sievert says people get more rad from med than bkgd.	[1960]	ICRU

* * *

30. Obits	— L. DeForest (1873–1961) Am invent; rectif & amplifier triodes.	Bio
	— E. Schroedinger (1887–1961) Aus math physics; wave theory	WoA
	— G. Failla (1891–1961) Am physics; std ion chamber, biol dose.	JNM

CHRONOLOGY OF NUCLEAR MEDICINE — 1962

Scientific and Technical Background			Ref.
1. Basic	— W. OLDENDORF INTRODUCES CONCEPT OF "BOLUS" IV INJECTION.	[1960]	JNM
2. Obser	— M. Croll finds I-125 ideal in sample (not scan) counts.	[1961]	JNM
3. # Nuc	— Oak Ridge °isotope process facility takes 15 kCi Co-60.	[1957]	AEC
4. # Med	— Radioisotope dept established in Baghdad, Iraq, hospital.	[1958]	IAEA
Organizations and Internal Politics			
5. AEC +	— IAEA tries to push Ca-47 use; fails because of Sc-47.	[1959]	IAEA
	— IAEA begins teaching survey with Mock Iodine uptakes.	[1959]	IAEA
	— New FDA Act makes prohibitive restrict on new °drugs.	[1958]	FDA
6. Socs	— AMA organizes new Com on Nuc Medicine (Radiol bias).	[1960]	JAMA
	— Society of Nuc Med of Europe organized.	[1954]	JNM
	— G. Hevesy's "Adventures in Radioisotope Research" pub (Pergamon).		Bk
	— R. Hewlett history of AEC, "The New World" pub (Penn U Press).		Bk
	— J. Chadwick edits Rutherford scientific papers (Allen & Unwin).		Bk
7. Event	— R. Carson "Silent Spring" starts hundreds of crises.	[1945]	Bk
	— Health Phys Res Reactor starts up for training & dosimetry.	[1959]	HP
	— AEC transfers 13 kg 20% enriched U to Yugoslav reactor.	[1958]	AEC
Instruments, Units of Measurement, and Drugs			
8. Instr	— C. Harris's solid gold focused collimator shows limits.	[1952]	JNM
	— D. Wolfe locates H-3 in nerve by ARG-electron-microscopy.	[1955]	Sc
	— Nuc Chicago installs first commercial scint camera.	[1958]	AP
	— M. Bender introduces the Autofluroscope scanner.	[1961]	JNM
	— H. Kakehi introduces a color display scanning system.	[1959]	AEC
	— M. Small introduces I-125 flat field transmission scans.	[1961]	JAMA
9. Units	— Specific Act. is $(0.693/T_{1/2})$ $(6.02 \times 10^{26}$/At Wt) in Bq/kg.	[1960]	V102
	— ICRU accepts the meaningless unmeasurable "Rem" unit.	[1959]	ICRU
	— J. Vennart questions ICRP model GI tract for dose calc.	[1906]	BJR
10. Concp	— J. Hidalgo finds low sp act °IHSA more stable than high.	[1959]	JNM
	— G. Hine tests accuracy, fluorescent glass rod dosimeters.	[1960]	Rad
	— T. Sargent shows possible use C-11 in W Body counter.	[1961]	IAEA
11. Drugs	— C. Neil evaluates I-132 cow, finds no clinical use.	[1958]	JNM
	— C. Kellershon (France) gets second Mo-Tc-99m cow system.	[1961]	RR
	— P. Harper clinically introduces Tc-99m for thyroid scan.	[1961]	RR
	— I. Levy introduces I-125 label for blood & fat samples.	[1961]	JNM
Radioiodine, P-32, and Radioactive Therapy			
12. I-Res	— R. Ecklund finds 75 mg T3/d stops thyroid I-131 release.	[1960]	JCE
	— AEC says fetal °I uptake at 3 mo, T4 production at 6.	[1961]	AEC
13. I-Dx	— M. Nava subs resin for RBC in in vitro T3 binding test.	[1961]	NEJM
	— C. Osorio derives "Free T4" from PBI & T3 tests.	[1959]	CS
	— O. Cohen finds saliva PB°I unreliable for thyroid func.	[1954]	JNM
	— J. Sanchez-Martin announces thiocyanate suppress test.	[1960]	JCE
	— J. Scholer announces T3 binding capacity test (TB Index).	[1961]	JNM
	— T. Oddie measures uptake in 47 infants 2 to 55 days old.	[1956]	AJDC
	— P. Skillern scans a hot nodule, finds hyperfunc adenoma.	[1960]	ArIM
14. I-Rx	— J. Müller ca Rx: ablate normal, TSH, 100 mCi °I, rescan 6 wks.	[1961]	IAEA
	— G. Sheline finds nodularity common years after °I Rx.	[1962]	JCE
	— B. Colcock notes myxedema in 11.7% after subtotal thyroidect.	[1956]	SGO
17. Other	— J. Müller lists 46 confirmations of intracav °AuCol.	[1959]	IAEA
	— M. Makin uses °AuCol in good Rx of synovial effusions.	[1960]	JAMA
	— M. Loken tries transarterial °microspheres in 21 ca pts.	[1956]	Nuc

Scans and Other Tests of Function in Various Organs

18.	Brain	— M. Blau uses Hg-203 chlormerodrin for good brain scans.	[1961]	JNM
		— G. DiChiro does intrathecal inject (°AuCol) for myelogram.	[1958]	NEJM
		— J. Mealey injects °IHSA subdurally for scan of space.	[1957]	JNs
		— I. Korolyuk uses radon or Xe-133 for myelography (USSR).	[1953]	MRM
		— L. Sapirstein: cerebr (°antipyrine) or noncerebr (°K) flow.	[1958]	JCI
		— J. Atkinson measures washout of intraventricular °IHSA.	[1961]	JNs
19.	Heart	— E. Carr looks for "cold spot" (°Rb) and "hot" (°Hg) agents.	[1961]	JNM
		— L. Donato uses °AuCol for right-heart-only RadCardGram.	[1958]	Cir
		— E. Braunwald devises "pulm dilut curves" to detect shunt.	[1961]	PCD
		— E. BRAUNWALD INTRODUCES "GATED END-SYS/DIAS" CONCEPT.	[1959]	Cir
		— J. Herd measures biphasic washout after intracor Kr-85.	[1959]	AJPh
20.	Liver	— I. Iio measures hepat-art/portal flow to liver (21% art).	[1937]	JHJ
		— R. Adams confirms hydatid cyst °AuCol scan pic in Iraq.	[1950]	JNM
		— A. Ozaeda surveys first large series (150) of met lesions.	[1950]	JNM
		— F. Feldman's 200 °RB scans illustrate CHFail artifact.	[1960]	Rad
		— H. Jammet scans spleen sequest with heat-damaged °CrRBC.	[1960]	SH
21.	Lung	— I. Ariel: first Dx of pulm embolism with °I-microspheres.	[1947]	V70
		— T. Haynie sees pulm infarct with °Hg-ceramic pellets.	[1947]	V70
		— W. Ball detects emphysema loci with Knipping °Xe study.	[1957]	JCI
		— L. Sapirstein: uniform dispersion of jugular °Sc-microspheres.	[1942]	CirR
		— F. Ghemi measures Pulm Circ Time from °IHSA RadCardGram.	[1959]	MN
		— M. Small uses I-125 source for transmission scan.	[1962]	JAMA
22.	Bone	— M. Blau introduces 1.8h F-18 as a B^+ bone scan agent.	[1955]	JNM
23.	Kidney	— T. Haynie separates tumor/vasc dis with °Hg-chlor scans.	[1961]	JAMA
		— J. Schlegel estimates effective blood flow with °I-Hipp.	[1960]	JAP
		— F. Schwartz sees slow renal blood clearance in hyperten.	[1934]	JU
		— 10 articles (e.g., R. Nordyke) detail renogram techniques.	[1961]	JAMA
		— E. Dore adds bladder probe for a renocystogram & times.	[1958]	Rad
		— I. Steinberg says iothalamate (Conray) is inulin GFR agent.	[1955]	Rad
24.	Gut	— M. Balodimos finds °I-triolein unstable in intest absorption.	[1961]	M
		— P. Welch uses stomach I-131 scans for DDx of gastric ca.	[1943]	RAC
		— A. Schwabe measures breath after C-14 labeled fat meal.	[1958]	G
25.	Blood	— J. Hidalgo computes height-weight-blood volume tables.	[1959]	S
		— N. Berlin: cohort labeling with DF°P gives RBC life span.	[1958]	Bl
		— L. Garby: 2 weeks required for DF°P RBC Survival Time.	[1961]	BH
		— W. Rosse studies a Fe-59 erythropoietin assay technique.	[1960]	PSEB
26.	Other	— P. Czerniak: surface P-32 counts give spermatogenesis test.	[1961]	AJR
		— A. Fischer traces intralymph °AuCol to region's L nodes.	[1960]	Rad
		— J. Fabricant inj °IHSA in foot vein to see venous flow.	[1961]	JNM
		— G. Rankin measures bld loss in menorrhagia with °CrRBC.	[1961]	La
		— S. Tanaka uses sub-Q °IHSA for washout measure in edema.	[1959]	NIR

Radiation Hysteria and Health Physics * Obituaries *

27.	Hyst	— J. McCanless: no deaths in 6 Puerto Rico gamma exposures.	[1961]	JAMA
		— G. Martinez: 4 deaths in Mexico chronic Co-60 exposures.	[1961]	RM
		— C. Onstead views fallout Cs-137 body burden with alarm.	[1961]	SC
		— ICRP says "any exposure to rad MAY carry some risk."	[1961]	ICRP
		— Thalidomide causes birth malformations, anti-drug hyst.	[1959]	AP
28.	React	J. Müller pubs pics of norm babies post-mother's °I Rx.	[1960]	IAEA
		— A. Brill: all 109 Atom-Bomb leukemias had > 100 rad dose	[1960]	AnIM
		— M. Brucer decries govt fallout hysteria & shelter farce.	[1960]	JAMA
29.	Respo	— J. Lindsay (Rep, NY) calls FRC Rad Prot Guides "doubletalk."	[1959]	FR

* * *

30.	Obits	— N. Bohr (1885–1962) Dan math physics; nuclear theory.	Bio
		— C. Darwin (1887–1962) Eng math; theor phys, Moseley's staircase.	DSB
		— A. Compton (1892–1962) Am physics; X-rays, Compton scatter.	DSB

CHRONOLOGY OF NUCLEAR MEDICINE — 1963

Scientific and Technical Background			Ref.
1. Basic	— M. Gell-Mann postulates quarks in makeup of protons.	[1933]	PR
3. # Nuc	— AEC withdraws from I-131 & I-125 prod (8 private companies).	[1961]	AEC
	— 1100 °nuclide shipments/month from Oak Ridge.	[1961]	AEC
4. # Med	— M. Janower: 24 teaching hosp; each do c100 °I tests/mo.	[1951]	JNM
Organizations and Internal Politics			
5. AEC +	— Hi Flux Isotopes Reactor (HFIR) begins °nuc production.	[1958]	AEC
	— FDA exempts °pharmaceuticals from Kefauver amendments.	[1958]	FDA
6. Socs	— ORINS symp on Dynamic Clinical Studies with °Isotopes.	[1960]	AEC
	— Lise Meitner recollections lecture pub by IAEA.	[1939]	IAEA
7. Event	— World's first nuc reactor (ORNL) shut down after 20 years.	[1943]	AEC
	— P. Harper describes a new scanning nuclide: Tc-99m.	[1961]	JNM
Instruments, Units of Measurement, and Drugs			
8. Instr	— E. Rapkin reviews advances in liquid scint counting.	[1957]	IRT
	— G. Hine starts 4 channel mag tape, digital recording.	[1959]	JNM
	— D. KUHL APPLIES TOMOGRAPHIC TECH TO °NUCLIDE EMISSION SCANS.		Rad
	— B. Kewin suggests digital scan display system.	[1959]	(1964 Nuc)
	— G. Uchiyama builds a color rescanning system.	[1962]	AEC
9. Units	— CGPM adopts new prefixes: tera (10^{12}), peta (10^{15}), exa (10^{18}), pico (10^{-12}), femto (10^{-15}), atto (10^{-18}).	[1960]	NBS
10. Concp	— J. Christie scans 3 levels (focused collimator) to get depth.	[1961]	AEC
	— C. Hlad devises new method to collect °sweat for counts.	[1959]	JNM
	— 6 articles (e.g., C. Lushbaugh) use whole body counters.	[1962]	JCAE
	— T. Iinuma measures bio $T_{1/2}$ of Cs-137, K-43, Na-22, Fe-59.	[1949]	Na
	— C. Miller measures K-42 body burden (whole body count).	[1955]	NYAS
11. Drugs	— N. Ackerman labels °I-atabrine and finds tumor uptake.	[1960]	SF
	— W. Tucker's new Sr-90–Y-90 cow has low Sr contamination.	[1960]	JNM
	— F. Greenwood makes high sp act °I-human growth hormone.	[1960]	BJ
	CLINICAL IN VITRO RADIOIMMUNOASSAY (RIA) BEGINS	[1960]	
	— W. Oldendorf: °Se clears blood & then is protein-bound.	[1958]	JNM
	— A. MacFarland describes bio behavior of °I-fibrinogen.	[1960]	JCI
Radioiodine, P-32, and Radioactive Therapy			
12. I-Res	— J. Phelan notes 26% Hashimoto pts had nodules, 5% ca.	[1957]	AS
	— E. Astwood notes macro nodules in 51% autopsied glands.	[1961]	JAMA
	— M. Edson finds 1% of renal ca pts get mets to thyroid.	[1954]	JAMA
	— R. Liechty finds 3.3% ca in thyroid dis pts (60% euthy).	[1961]	JAMA
13. I-Dx	— J. Stanbury: BMR still best assessment of metabol state.	[1947]	JAMA
	— T. Lemarchand finds many PB°I faults are due to low TBG.	[1951]	SMW
	— P. Guinet finds 2 hour °I uptake suppressed by T3.	[1962]	GMF
	— H. Kristensen finds 2 hour °I uptake suppressed by T3.	[1962]	AMS
14. I-Rx	— E. Astwood says dose calculations no better than guess.	[1961]	JAMA
15. P-Rx	— J. Lawrence finds normal life expect in °P Rx leuk pts.	[1961]	JNM
16. Tele	— 450 kCi Co-60 with sp act >400 Ci/g ready for sale.	[1961]	IRT
17. Other	— R. Tudway monitors P-32 during tumor response to Rx.	[1958]	PGM
	— G. Buraggi treats 39 pts with intralymph inj of °I-lipiodol.		RMT
	— A. Ratti finds no side effects from IL °I-lipiodol injection.	[1958]	MM
Scans and Other Tests of Function in Various Organs			
18. Brain	— C. Fazio measures cer bld flow with carotid inj of K-85.	[1961]	N
	— H. Glass measures "regional" not total cer bld flow.	[1962]	BMJ
	— N. Lassen measures cer blood flow by Kr-85 washout tech.	[1961]	N

18. Brain	— G. Taplin devises the cerebrogram with brain perfusion.	[1961]	JNM
	— B. Mallet measures cer bld flow with Xe-133 inhalation.	[1962]	La
	— W. Oldendorf measures °I-antipyrine Brain Transit Time.	[1962]	Nuc
	— C. Fieschi sees CO_2 effect on cerb circ from carotid °IHSA.	[1962]	CirR
	— D. Sodee introduces Hg-197 to lower rad dose of scans.	[1961]	JNM
19. Heart	— D. Gregg proves systolic coronary flow after exercise.	[1956]	AJPh
	— W. MacIntyre introduces silhouette scan in pleural effusion.	[1962]	AJR
	— E. Carr finds Cs-131 better then Rb-86 for myocard scan.	[1959]	JCI
	— E. Carr finds °Hg-chlor a hot spot myocardial scan agent.	[1962]	JNM
	— R. Bing uses Rb-84 for "index" of coronary blood flow.	[1962]	Cir
	— W. Hollander inj °I into myocard; washout gives bld flow.	[1958]	JPET
	— M. De Bakey uses artificial heart during heart repair.	[1929]	JAMA
20. Liver	— P. Czerniak: amebic lesions clear but echino cysts leave scar.	[1962]	JNM
	— M. Bender: °Au scan pos 83% accurate, scan neg 88% accurate.	[1985]	G
	— L. Sorenson sees Mo-99 in polygonal cells, first °Tc scan.	[1962]	JLCM
	— M. Crane finds portal-liver RBC transit time = 13 ± 5 sec.	[1962]	JNM
	— E. Ratzkowski introduces rectal °I + °Au dual liver scan.	[1956]	AJMS
	— L. Anghileri labels bilirubin with I-131.	[1961]	IJAR
21. Lung	— G. TAPLIN SHOWS °IMAA LUNG SCAN IN DOG AS SAFE MICROEMBOLISM.		V70
	— J. Quinn introduces the °IMAA lung scan (X-Ray required).	[1961]	Rad
	— W. Ball measures Xe-133 ventilation, 6 counter system.	[1962]	JCI
22. Bone	— W. Simpson shows first total body bone scan with Sr-85.	[1962]	CMAJ
	— S. Kofman shows Sr-85 in osteoblastic (not lytic) lesions.	[1962]	JNM
	— J. Cameron measures mineral dens, I-125 photon absorp.	[1962]	Sc
	— A. Limentani sees °IHSA in synovial fluid by ext counts.	[1960]	Rheu
23. Kidney	— >20 articles (e.g., E. Dore), renogram tech with °I-Hipp.	[1960]	JAMA
	— M. Blaufox: liver will excrete °I-Hipp in renal failure.	[1962]	AJPh
	— M. Blau details °Hg-chlor scans in some renal diseases.	[1962]	JU
24. Gut	— D. Berkowitz counts 6 abd areas after oral °I-triolein.	[1962]	JAMA
	— N. Ackerman: emulsion-surface balloons "see" P-32 in ca.	[1962]	JAMA
	— R. Nelson inserts small GM tubes into esoph & rectum.	[1948]	JNM
	— R. Hayes develops °stool assay techniques.	[1958]	AJCP
	— W. Nelp finds toadfish does NOT excrete VB_{12}.	[1960]	ChS
25. Blood	— L. Garby runs ferrograms & ferrokinetics in 27 infants.	[1956]	APe
	— Y. Najean studies thrombocytopenia with Cr-51 platelets.	[1961]	Bl
	— E. Borun: in vivo age of RBC modifies its °K, °Na, °Cr, °T3.	[1961]	JLCM
	— M. Pollycove: C-14 histadine DDx VB_{12} and folic anemia.	[1960]	Bl
	— A. Mauer: uncloned °WBC mars myeloid turnover studies.	[1960]	Bl
26. Other	— M. Croll counts °IHSA over 14 areas to locate placenta.	[1961]	JNM
	— A. Weinberg evaluates safety, 5 mCi °IHSA placental scan.	[1961]	AJOG
	— A. Weinberg replaces area counts with placental scans.	[1961]	AJOG
	— D. Seitzman cannulates lymphatics for °I-ethiodol scans.	[1962]	AJR
	— K. Winkel details abdominal °AuCol lymph node scans.	[1962]	NMG
	— W. Bale tries human fibrinogen °I-antisera in tumor pts.	[1960]	IUCC
	— M. Razzak inj IV °IHSA, counts ball of foot for circ test.	[1960]	JNM

Radiation Hysteria and Health Physics * Obituaries *

27. Hyst	— H. Mosier follows °I trap test with $KClO_4$ to prevent ca.	[1957]	P
28. React	— D. Hollingsworth: no thyroid ca in 5553 Atom Bomb pts.	[1957]	ABCC
	— J. Aleksandrowicz: less Sr 90 in leukemic autopsy tissue.	[1959]	Bl
	— D. DeLawter: normal thyroid ca incidence 10y post °I Rx.	[1961]	ca
	— H. Fisher finds no damage in fetuses irrad <70th day.	[1961]	JP
	— J. Ultman: hyperthyroid pts (no rad) have more lymphoma.	[1961]	Bl
	— AEC sees lower mortality in G-pigs after lo-dose irrad.	[1957]	AEC

* * *

30. Obits —

CHRONOLOGY OF NUCLEAR MEDICINE — 1964

Scientific and Technical Background			Ref.
1. Basic	— Dubna Inst (USSR) claims discovery of element #104.	[1962]	Sc
2. Obser	— Radioisotopes a $7.35 million export-import business.	[1963]	AEC
	— Y. Bakale says low energy I-125 unreliable for counting.	[1962]	Sc
Organizations and Internal Politics			
5. AEC +	— Third Atoms-for-Peace Conf is restricted to Nuc Power.	[1958]	AEC
	— AEC proposes all radioisotope production be private.	[1963]	AEC
6. Socs	— JAMA publishes summary of state laws on Rad Protection.	[1961]	JAMA
	— K. Way's Nuclear Data Project moves back to Oak Ridge.	[1950]	NBS
	— IAEA holds Symposium on Medical Radioisotope Scanning.	[1959]	IAEA
	— B. Goldschmidt's French history in "The Atomic Adventure" (Perg Press).		BK
	— M. Gowing's British story "Britain and Atomic Energy" (McMillan).		Bk
	— G. Thomson's "J.J. Thomson and the Cavendish Lab" pub (Nelson).		Bk
7. Event	— P. HARPER'S BAD GASTEIN PAPER MARKS START OF Tc-99m DOMINANCE.		NUC
	— Professorship in Nuc Med established at Heidelberg.	[1951]	JAMA
	— D. Brown begins use of computers in Nuclear Medicine.	[1959]	JNM
Instruments, Units of Measurement, and Drugs			
8. Instr	— New type scanning cameras are described: M. Bender — a digital autofluoroscope; W. Gross — a kinetic brain study camera; M. Ter-Pogossian — X-ray image amplifier.	[1958]	IAEA
	— G. DiChiro displays scans in sagital, coronal, axial cuts.	[1963]	JAMA
	— D. Kuhl describes cylinder and section liver scanning.	[1963]	Rad
	— D. Kuhl describes axial emission tomography of brain.	[1963]	JNM
	— P. Bell shows ideal gold scan-collimator performance.	[1962]	IAEA
	— A. Morris describes high energy (5" × 4" crystal) scanner.	[1962]	AEC
	— R. Kyle devises attachment for direct polaroid scans.	[1959]	JNM
10. Concp	— J. HIDALGO APPOINTS FIRST MED INTERNAL RAD DOSE (MIRD) COMMITTEE.		JNM
	— G. Brownell calculates Monte Carlo point source dose.	[1962]	BJR
	— 4 articles (e.g., B. Hopkins) on °isotope retention in hair.	[1958]	Sc
	— B. Roswit evaluates glass rod & thermolumin dosimeters.	[1962]	JAMA
	— M. Feldman measures low concentrate F-18 in dual well.	[1962]	JNM
11. Drugs	— J. McAfee labels HSA with Tc-99m for placental scanning.	[1960]	JNM
	— N. Mikheev designs another Mo to Tc-99m cow.	[1960]	APx
	— R. Meckelnburg introduces cow-produced Sr-87m bone scan.	[1962]	JNM
	— Y. Suzuki gets Y-90 from Sr-90 by new ion exchange cow.	[1963]	IJAR
Radioiodine, P-32, and Radioactive Therapy			
12. I-Res	— P. Heedman measures thyroid I by X-ray spectrophotometry.	[1969]	JCE
	— J. Maisterrena finds I defic goiter pop near Mexico DF.	[1961]	JCE
	— M. Van Dilla measures thyroid biol half-time @ 26-163d.	[1963]	Sc
13. I-Dx	— L. Rosenthall devises 15/5 min ratio "Trapping Index."	[1958]	JNM
	— O. Degrossi introduces thyroid °TcO_4 studies.	[1962]	RAE
	— H. Higgins measures 10m trap uptake in Hashimoto's dis.	[1957]	CMAJ
	— B. Murphy-C. Pattee introduce TBG competitive binding.	[1960]	JCE
	— >15 articles (e.g., G. McAdams) modify °I in vitro tests.	[1962]	JNM
14. I-Rx	— E. Chapman finds hypothy increases about 2%/y post Rx.	[1962]	NEMJ
15. P-Rx	— E. Osgood sums 16 of his articles on P-32 Rx in leuk.	[1958]	JNM
17. Other	— R. Flocks: 55% "cure" in 976 prostate ca, by °AuCol Rx.	[1956]	JNM
	— I. Ariel compares IL Y-90 microsp, °AuCol, °I-ethiodol.	[1963]	S

	Scans and Other Tests of Function in Various Organs		
18. Brain	— J. McAFEE ANNOUNCES BRAIN SCANNING WITH °TcO$_4$.	[1963]	JNM
	— G. DiChiro scans °IHSA injected into ventricles.	[1985]	N
	— J. Mealey scans 22 infants for subdural effusion (°IHSA).	[1962]	PSN
	— G. Brownell introduces Ga-68 positron brain scanning.	[1955]	JNM
	— R. Bell measures cer blood velocity; carotid °IHSA inj.	[1963]	JNM
19. Heart	— G. Robbins says exercise only one stress, look at drugs.	[1963]	JOM
	— D. Sklaroff detects >200 ml pericardl effus on pool scan.	[1958]	JNM
	— R. Ross: second phase intracoron °Kr washout is cor flow.	[1962]	Cir
	— R. Bing: Rb-84 coincidence count is Coronary Flow Equiv.	[1963]	Cir
	— S. Weinberg adds femoral probe to mark third wave on RCG.	[1962]	AJCr
20. Liver	— F. Netter: post WW II advances in liver micro anatomy.	[1949]	Ciba
	— P. HARPER INTRODUCES Tc-99m SULFUR COLLOID (°TcSC).	[1962]	JNM
	— L. Donato outlines anatomy on °AuCol liv structure scan.	[1962]	IAEA
	— A. Cuaron begins 6y study of amebic abscess scans.	[1963]	JNM
	— F. Gollin says °RB scan more accurate than chemistry.	[1963]	JAMA
	— H. Oeser uses rectal Na°I to see portal splanchnic flow.	[1962]	MMW
	— C. Lushbaugh proves liver blood clearance is 3 phase.	[1957]	DCS
21. Lung	— J. Quinn compares °CrRBC, °Hg-Chlor, °IHSA as scan agents.	[1963]	JNM
	— G. Taplin controls particle size from °IμAA to °IMAA.	[1961]	DCS
	— H. Wagner shows °IMAA scans of massive pulm embolism.	[1963]	JAMA
	— H. Dworkin measures °IMAA distribution and half-time.	[1963]	JNM
22. Bone	— N. Charkes studies 90 patient Sr-87m bone scan series.	[1962]	AJR
	— W. Maxfield introduces °IHSA joint scan in rheumatic dis.	[1963]	JNM
	— G. Letizia finds synovial °IHSA before X-Ray shows dis.	[1963]	RP
	— D. Van Dyke achieves camera snaps of Fe-52 in b-marrow.	[1958]	Sc
	— G. Andrews compares Au-198 & -199 in bone marrow scans.	[1960]	Bl
23. Kidney	— S. Wax studies angiotensin effect on renogram.	[1934]	SF
	— G. Taplin relates renogram second phase slope to bld flow.	[1961]	Nuc
	— G. Johnston relates renogram third phase to washout.	[1961]	JU
	— J. Trinkle shows 10 pt's renograms in renal failure.	[1961]	JU
	— J. Wenzl shows renograms in 30 renal normal children.	[1959]	JPd
	— M. Loken shows renograms following transplantation.	[1963]	JNM
	— W. Tauxe: °I-Hipp similar to PAH, °diatrizoate to inulin.	[1962]	MCP
	— M. Farmelant measure tubular passage time with °I-Hipp.	[1962]	AJSr
	— J. Concannon measures GFR with I-125 allyl inulin.	[1955]	AJR
24. Gut	— W. Clode studies localization of Na°I in stomach wall.	[1962]	IAEA
	— E. Kemp protests °IHSA, uses amberlite for protein loss.	[1961]	Gut
	— A. Iartaroglu finds ave 24h focal RBC loss is 0,78 ml.	[1961]	KW
25. Blood	— R. Walker labels DNA with P-32 to study WBC kinetics.	[1960]	Bl
	— I. Berman; dual plasma-cell vol better than Ht use.	[1962]	Na
26. Other	— H. Sage: °AuCol subQ in foot + leg counts is lymph flow.	[1963]	JNM
	— T. Haynie sees parathyroid adenoma on °Se-meth scan.	[1943]	JNM
	— W. Munck inj °Xe in uterine muscle, washout is blood flow.	[1962]	La
	Radiation Hysteria and Health Physics * Obituaries *		
27. Hyst	— Rhode Island cricality accident, 1 dead at 8800 rads.	[1962]	APa
	— Surg Gen L. Terry issues "Smoking is Evil" revelation.	[1971]	AP
28. React	— R. Sitterson shows male rad sterility is temporary.	[1956]	JAMA
	— Age limit for I 131 therapy down from 40 to 25 years.	[1954]	IMAG
	— G. Sacher: life span in mice increased after lo-dose.	[1963]	AEC
29. Respo	— Of 157 leukemics in Hiroshima, 94 not exposed to Bomb.	[1963]	ABCC
	— Euthanasia for old age, Trinity exposed cows (150 rads).	[1946]	AEC

* * *

30. Obits	— V. Hess (1883–1964) Aus physics; cosmic rays, radon cow.		DSB
	— O. Glasser (1895–1964) Am physics; the "r," edits Med Physics.		Rad

CHRONOLOGY OF NUCLEAR MEDICINE — 1965

	Scientific and Technical Background		Ref.
3. # Nuc	— Y. Yano prepares 8h 169 keV Fe-52 for medical use.	[1963]	IJAR
	— H. Seligman says nuclear power supplied "free" °sources.	[1960]	IAEA
4. # Med	— Amersham and Euratom now sell many labeled compounds.	[1959]	AEC
	— 3600 hospitals & physicians have °nuclide licenses.	[1961]	AEC
	— 3200 industrial firms have °nuclide licenses.	[1959]	AEC
	— 550 colleges & universities have °nuclide licenses.	[1964]	AWC
	— 3700 scientists (50% MDs) have taken OR basic course.	[1963]	AEC
	Organizations and Internal Politics		
5. AEC +	— AEC, in panic, stops °IHSA cisternography, alleged death.	[1957]	N
6. Soc's	— Brit Nuclear Medicine Society is proposed.	[1954]	BMJ
	— Stanford Radiol: symposium on luminescent dose devices.	[1964]	PL
	— Oak Ridge: symposium on Radioactive Pharmaceuticals.	[1963]	Bk
	— H. ANGER PRESIDES AT FIRST GAMMA SCINTILLATION CAMERA SYMPOSIUM.		JNM
	— K. Siegbahn's "Alpha, Beta, Gamma Spectroscopy" pub (N-Holland).		Bk
	— J. Quinn begins pub of "Yearbooks of Nuclear Medicine."	[1980]	YB
	— K. Way's Nuc Data Group prepares Nuc Data Sheets.	[1964]	IRT
7. Event	— Greetings to G. Hevesy on his 70th birthday published.	[1962]	IJAR
	— M. Ter-Pogossian installs cyclotron in Wash U Hospital.	[1957]	AP
	— NCC (now Mallinckrodt) sells first commercial °Tc-generator.	[1963]	JNM
	Instruments, Units of Measurement, and Drugs		
8. Instr	— E. Kaplan devises contin-monitor °Na dialysis-perfusion syst.	[1976]	JNM
	— S. Friedland explores solid state instrument for biomed.	[1955]	NUC
	— R. Spencer gets 2 channel spectrometer for dual °nuc scans.	[1961]	BJR
9. Units	— R. Huntoon reviews c.g.s. (now m.k.s.) standards.	[1960]	Sc
10. Concp	— W. Oldendorf displays a "bolus" injection technique.	[1962]	JNM
	— R. Witcofski warns of highly contaminating °TcO_4 saliva.	[1964]	JNM
	— E. Osgood ests 1 mCi P-32 IV = about 15 R total body expos.	[1963]	JNM
	— R. Hayes proves °Ga bio distribution is carrier dependent.	[1953]	JNM
11. Drugs	— M. Brucer shows 118 possible °cow systems ($T_{1/2} > 12h$).	[1964]	IRT
	— J. McAfee introduces a simple cow-kit (for °TcSC prep).	[1964]	ArIM
	— J. McAfee introduces °TcHSA (as brain scanning agent).	[1964]	IJAR
	— NEN Corp: commercial Ge-Ga-68 B^+ cow is economic flop.	[1965]	
	— K. Samsahl: 30 trace elements (nuc activ anal) in ca.	[1948]	IJAR
	— S-Y Yeh measures Kr-85, Xe-133 solubility in proteins.	[1963]	JAPh
	— L. Tothil finds 50% excretion of °IPVP in 24h (biliary).	[1959]	JNM
	Radioiodine, P-32, and Radioactive Therapy		
12. I-Res	— W. London says bread is major source of I-127 in diet.	[1960]	NEJM
	— G. Broadhead finds seasonal change in urine I-127 (Eng).	[1928]	BMJ
	— P. Czerniak finds 23% °I excreted in milk in lactation.	[1955]	Haf
	— R. Greene notes suppressible & non-supp hot nodules.	[1961]	JEA
	— A. Nicastri sees thyroid cells in normal neck lymph nodes.	[1966]	JAMA
	— L. Shane finds chronic thyroiditis in 7.3% of surg spec.	[1963]	AJMS
	— R. Liechty: 6% of solitary cold nodules are malignant.	[1963]	SGO
	— J. Müller: on 4000 scans, 6% benign, 2% malig nodules.	[1963]	Rad
13. I-Dx	— T. Lemarchand-Beraud measures serum TSH by RIA.	[1955]	SMW
	— F. CLARK CALCULATES "FREE" T4 FROM PBI & RESIN T3 TESTS.	[1962]	JCEn
	— O. DeGrossi suggests °Tc as substitute for I-131.	[1964]	NMG
	— J. Hamburger says malig rare in autonomous hot nodules.	[1960]	Rad
14. I-Rx	— D. Smithers says if °I uptake in mets, °I Rx is dramatic.	[1962]	BMJ
	— G. Crile recommends °I Rx in children; leukogen rep false.	[1962]	JAMA

15. P-Rx	— J. Smart relieves prostate mets bone pain with P-32.	[1962]	BJU
	— D. Joshi: palliation better in prostate than breast ca.	[1962]	JAMA
16. Tele	— AEC will not supply Co-60 in <100,000 Curie amounts.	[1964]	AEC
	— AEC charges $0.125/Curie for Cs-137, Sr-90 = $0.20/Ci.	[1963]	AEC
17. Other	— H. Fischer tries intralymph °AuCol in cervix ca mets.	[1956]	ca
	— F. Greenwood: no change in growth horm after pit implant.	[1960]	La
	— I. Ariel treats inop liver ca with Y-90 microspheres.	[1964]	AnS

Scans and Other Tests of Function in Various Organs

18. Brain	— H. Jaffe says true advance is 800 mCi °Tc vs 700 μCi °Hg.	[1964]	JNM
	— H. Waxman points out, time after CV accident is critical.	[1982]	JAMA
	— T. Haynie introduces a new vertex projection.	[1961]	JNM
	— W. Tauxe: °IPVP and °Tc contaminate a fresh scalp lesion.	[1961]	JNM
	— A. Johnson: CBF is first of 3 phase °Xe washout over head.	[1957]	JNM
	— R. Adams mentions occult hydrocephalus (cisternograms?).	[1962]	NEJM
19. Heart	— F. Bonte introduces °TcHSA for silhouette cardiac scans.	[1963]	Rad
	— W. Love suggests exercise may enhance abnormal scans.	[1964]	Cir
	— R. Gorton discovers import of scan time in °Hg hot spot scans.		CirR
20. Liver	— M. Pollycove: left diff than right lobe enlargement.	[1964]	JNM
	— D. BROWN INTRODUCES COMBINED LUNG-LIVER SCANS FOR ABSCESS.		AJSr
	— W. Eyler proves kidneys excrete °I-RB if poor liver function.	[1964]	AJR
	— R. Grunnert succeeds in °I-Hipp portography (°I = bad tag).	[1964]	AS
	— R. Grunnert separates portal from hepatic artery flow.	[1962]	AS
	— J. Siemsen: °AuCol uptake in spleen = portal hypertension.	[1962]	JNM
21. Lung	— A. Dawson studies regional ventilation with Xe-133.	[1963]	JCI
	— H. Ueda: absent perfusion in unilat X-Ray translucency.	[1964]	JNM
22. Bone	— D. Copp says Sr-85 blood clearance is bone blood flow.	[1981]	CirR
	— F. Harris does osteograms, pts on VitD Rx have rickets.	[1950]	CS
	— R. Hayes does first whole body bone scan (rat) with Ga-68.	[1948]	V80
23. Kidney	— >15 articles (e.g., J. Collins) evaluate renogram in dis.	[1964]	AnS
	— >10 articles (e.g., B. Warren) evaluate kidney scan in dis.	[1979]	APa
	— E. Sigman proves °I-Conray is inulin type agent.	[1964]	JIU
	— J. Green proves Hg loading dose cuts °Hg-chlor uptake.	[1963]	JNM
24. Gut	— V. Mabry says °CrHSA can measure GI protein loss.	[1964]	JNM
	— J. Sisson finds °I-triolein purity test meal no concern.	[1963]	JNM
	— J. Wetterfors measures normal albumin metab & gut leaks.	[1964]	AMS
25. Blood	— Z. Farid measures RBC survival after hookworm Rx.	[1962]	AJTM
	— L. Sharney explains ferrokinetics with pools analysis.	[1955]	JSH
	— A. Norman: life span of rad damaged WBC is 530 days.	[1964]	Sc
	— S. Robinson: life span of °H labeled WBC is >9 months.	[1964]	Bl
	— E. Adelson measures platelet survival (°H tag) $T_{1/2}$ = 2.4d.	[1963]	Bl
	— J. Inall measures °IHSA plasma vol in premature infants.	[1963]	AJDC
26. Other	— W. Borner introduces °TcO_4 salivary gland scanning.	[1954]	MW
	— D. Hadden finds fault with °I tags of Human Gro Hormone.	[1963]	JHHB
	— Amersham introduces I-125 insulin in RIA kit form.	[1960]	
	— D. Sodee introduces new pancreas scan agent: Cs-131.	[1943]	Nuc
	— F. Pircher: first antitumor antibodies (glioma) scan, °I.	[1963]	JAMA

Radiation Hysteria and Health Physics * Obituaries *

27. Hyst	G. Andrews documents fifth intrauterine thyroid ablation.	[1956]	AEC
	— "Smoking is Bad" slogan goes on all cigarette packs.	[1964]	AP
28. React	— B. Modan finds 10% of PVA pts (no P-32 Rx) die with leukemia.	[1959]	JAMA
	— K. Halnan: no survival diff in PVA pts on °P-32 or not.	[1960]	La
	— L. Bustad notes fewer abnormalities in lo-dose rad mice.	[1963]	RR
29. Respo	— First Los Alamos accident victim (200 R) dies after 19y.	[1946]	AP

* * *

30. Obits	— R. Newell (1892–1965) Am Physician; radiol, nuc medicine.		RAD

CHRONOLOGY OF NUCLEAR MEDICINE — 1966

	Scientific and Technical Background		Ref.
1. Basic	— Nuc Data Group begins Nuc Data Sheets (Academic Press).	[1965]	Bk
2. Obser	— JAMA publishes US Adopted Names of °drugs (e.g., NaI I-131).		JAMA
	— AEC develops Pu-238 fueled cardiac pacemaker.	[1959]	AEC
4. # Med	— Union Carbide opens fifth °pharmaceutical co (Neisler).	[1964]	IRT
	— Stanford survey (USPHS) shows 2510 physicians used °nuclides.		
	526,476 pts got °nuclide test in 1966.	[1963]	
	409,461 pts were scanned; 33,743 got °Rx.	[1951]	
	1,919,948 pts got Co-60 teletherapy.	[1951]	PHR

	Organizations and Internal Politics		
5. Pol	— ORINS changes name to ORAU (OR Assoc Universit) Jan 1.	[1949]	AP
6. Socs	— M. Brucer begins pub of "Vignettes In Nuc Med" (Mallinckrodt).		V01
	— History of first 20y °isotope production published.	[1954]	IRT
	— Euratom Conf on labeled proteins in biochem at U Pisa.	[1958]	AP
	— A. Remenchik summarizes 3 Whole Body Counter symposia.	[1961]	JAMA
	— Am Board of Radiology has certified 7500 radiologists.	[1951]	ACR
7. Event	— AEC DISMANTLES "OLD GRANDMA," FIRST WORKING NUCLEAR REACTOR.	[1943]	AEC
	— P. Harper initiates use of "stop time" films.	[1964]	JNM

	Instruments, Units of Measurement, and Drugs		
8. Instr	— N. Horwitz designs "Spintharicon" (spark discharge cam).	[1964]	Rad
	— D. Kuhl adds a perforated tape digital scan recorder.	[1964]	JNM
	— J. McAfee uses a commercial 8" dia scanning crystal.	[1964]	JNM
9. Units	— E. Smith calculates elec capture and int convers dose.	[1964]	JNM
	— R. Fink calculates gamma atomic fluorescent yields.	[1964]	RMP
10. Concp	— D. Kuhl introduces transmiss scans for anatomic localization.	[1962]	JNM
	— D. Lockner notes diurnal variation in °Fe turnover.	[1965]	BJH
	— J. Dupois does activ analy of infant's needle biopsies.	[1955]	JNM
11. Drugs	— M. Blau finds Hg-197 poor -203 substitute in scanning.	[1963]	ANM
	— D. Taylor measures metab of Sc-47 (daughter of Ca-47).	[1959]	BJR
	— I. Grotenhuis develops lo-density plastic microspheres.	[1962]	AEC
	— D. Goodwin prepares a 1.6h In-113m cow.	[1965]	Nuc

	Radioiodine, P-32, and Radioactive Therapy		
12. I-Res	— C. Welch says wide range of ca statistics is confusion.	[1965]	JAMA
	— F. Clements cures endemic Tasmanian goiter (I-127 bread).	[1959]	La
	— G. Freund finds 1 mg/L (swim pool I-127) cuts °I uptake.	[1960]	JCEn
	— D. Weaver: 1915 vs 1950 slides say I causes Hashimotos?	[1964]	AS
	— R. Reed disagrees: thyroid cells in neck nodes are mets.	[1965]	JAMA
13. I-Dx	— H. Greenberg: low uptake, high PBI says hemorr in adenoma.	[1981]	JNM
	— Editorial marks end of PB°I; now use T3 in vitro uptake.	[1961]	JAMA
	— K. Hardy: 15.5% ca in all Melbourne solitary adenomas.	[1965]	MJA
	— M. Hays says gut °I recycles in first 3h of clearance.	[1962]	JCI
14. I-Rx	— F. Bauer finds °I Rx decreases Prog Malig Exophthalmos.	[1961]	AE
	— J. Einhorn proves °I Rx hypo is permanent by TSH stim.	[1964]	JCEn
	— T. Reeve: partial thyroidectomy result is hypothyroidism.	[1962]	AJR
	— J. Hamburger stimulates mets uptake with TSH, I def diet.	[1962]	M
15. P-Rx	— M. Overton injects Cr°PO_4 into cystic brain tumors.	[1956]	JNM
16. Tele	— In 1952 US shipped Co source to Canada for irradiation; in 1966 US ships 475 kCi Co-60 to Canada for it to sell.	[1952]	V14
	— In 1966 US produces 2.5 MCi Co-60 for sales program.	[1961]	IRT
	— Co-60 now produced at sp act up to 700 curies/gram.	[1963]	IRT
17. Other	— T. Everson documents spontaneous regression of tumors.	[1966]	Bk

Scans and Other Tests of Function in Various Organs

18.	Brain	— J. Mack describes normal anatomy of °TcO_4 brain scan.	[1965]	JNM
		— C. Maynard finds choroid plexus a normal scan feature.	[1964]	JNM
		— L. Levy shows short scan delay time misses lesions.	[1965]	JNM
		— J. Williams can visualize infarcts 1–2 weeks after CVA.	[1965]	N
		— D. Beiler: scan now part of routine workup in children.	[1964]	AJDC
		— R. Bell sets 6 probes to time carotid, sag sinus, jugular arrival.	[1964]	JNM
		— C. Fieschi says °IHSA transit time is index of cer flow.	[1964]	TANA
		— L. ROSENTHALL INTRODUCES °TcO_4 BRAIN PERFUSION AFTER BOLUS IV.		Rad
19.	Heart	— J. KRISS USES FAST FRAMES TO SEE PASS OF °TcO_4 THRU HEART.		JNM
		— J. Quinn injects coronary (°IMAA) to display capillary bed.	[1962]	JNM
20.	Liver	— T. Magita: regeneration after 85% removal of dog's liver.	[1977]	JNM
		— M. Hollenberg verifies 80%–20% portal-hepatic artery flow.	[1964]	AJPh
		— G. Burke uses camera to see °I-Rose Bengal hepatogram.	[1964]	JAMA
		— A. Gottschalk says °TcSC is a liver/spleen scan agent.	[1965]	JNM
		— G. Henegar notes °TcSC "shift" to spleen in cirrhosis.	[1965]	JNM
		— L. Caplan warns: defects only "Space Occupying Lesions."	[1963]	AJR
21.	Lung	— J. Quinn makes the posterior projection routine.	[1961]	JNM
		— V. Lopez-Majano says anterior projection must be added.	[1961]	AJR
		— M. Gwyther says 4 projections required on most scans.	[1961]	IJAR
		— C. Dollery follows Xe-133 buildup & washout by computer.	[1965]	CS
		— J. Quinn measures regional vent after °Xe inhalation,	[1965]	JNM
		calculates °IMAA blocks $1/10^4$ of 3×10^{11} sites.	[1964]	JNM
		— G. Taplin detects COPD after inhalation of °IHSA aerosol.	[1950]	JNM
		— W. Tauxe notes gravity effect on °IMAA deposition.	[1964]	JAP
		— F. DeLand: 3 phase washout of °IMAA: 0.9, 7.5, & 55 days.	[1957]	JNM
		— W. Gold notes no unsafe pulmonary response to °IMAA scan.	[1963]	JAMA
		— H. Dworkin notes first °IMAA fatality, a gross vasc defect.	[1963]	NEJM
22.	Bone	— H. Dworkin: F-18 uptake at fracture site persists >½y.	[1962]	RPh
		— L. Schaer notes supraorbital fibrous dysplasia (F-18).	[1962]	Rad
		— G. Andrews sees active marrow on °AuCol whole body scan.	[1964]	JNM
23.	Kidney	— M. Powell introduces triple renal: perfuse, scan, renogram.	[1965]	.JNM
		— G. BURKE BEGINS NEW SPLIT SCREEN DYNAMIC °I-HIPP STUDIES.		JAMA
		— B. Stract estimates Cr-51 EDTA GFR; an inulin type agent.	[1965]	Sc
		— H. Deckart measures vesiculo-ureteral reflux (children).	[1964]	KP
		— 12 articles (e.g., R. Earlam) evaluate & modify renograms.	[1965]	BJU
24.	Gut	— E. Anderson quantifies gut bleeding in °CrRBC stools.	[1963]	JNM
		— L. Hershenson measures steatorrhea, surface °fat counts.	[1965]	JNM
		— L. Wasserman assays serum VB_{12} with charcoal comp bind.	[1957]	BI
25	Blood	— F. Gardner says °P, °S, °Se, °C, KO's platelets, use °Cr.	[1965]	T
		— L. Schiffer finds °CrRBC survival down after irradiation.	[1962]	BI
		— R. Kinlough uses °CrRBC surv to select splenectomy pts.	[1962]	MJA
26.	Other	— E. Kaplan subtracts °AuCol liver from °Se pancreas.	[1965]	JNM
		— B. Hibbard changes to °TcHSA placental scans.	[1963]	COG
		— P. Klopper sees parathyroids with °Se-meth in dogs.	[1964]	S
		— R. McCardle sees tumors after fibrinogen °I-antibody.	[1965]	JNM

Radiation Hysteria and Health Physics * Obituaries *

27.	Hyst	— J. Rall: increased PBI in Marshallese fallout victims.	[1958]	AIM
		— J. Rall starts myth: fallout rad causes thyroid nodules.	[1966]	NEJM
28.	React	— J. Lawrence finds no hint of danger in I-131 or P-32 Rx.	[1969]	IRT

* * *

30.	Obits	— G. Hevesy (1885–1966) Hun chem; radioisotopes.	Bio
		— U. Portman (1887–1966) Am physician; radiotherapy, roentgen.	Rad
		— R. Stone (1895–1966) Am physician; starts Health Physics.	Rad

CHRONOLOGY OF NUCLEAR MEDICINE — 1967

	Scientific and Technical Background		Ref.
2. Obser	— Brit Inst Radiol adopts "Nuclide" for "Isotope."	[1947]	BJR
	"NUCLIDE" HAS REPLACED THE INCORRECT USE OF "ISOTOPE"		V22
3. # Nuc	— 42 naturally occurring radioactive species exist.	[1961]	GSA
	— S. Glasstone: how long must it last to be a "species"?	[1959]	GSA
4. # Med	— J. Hidalgo finds 25% of labs are considering °Tc-cow.	[1964]	PL
	Organizations and Internal Politics		
5. AEC +	— Stanford publishes its criteria for "Isotope Committee."	[1956]	JNM
	— Australian AEC is producing °nuc to supply Aust & Asia.	[1960]	SN
6. Socs	— Nuclear Medicine Soc of Great Britain formed in London.	[1964]	JAMA
	— McGraw-Hill pubs final issue of Nucleonics (first Nuc J).	[1947]	Nuc
7. Event	— Dual probe rectilinear scanner is introduced in Japan.	[1961]	SN
	Instruments, Units of Measurement, and Drugs		
8. Instr	— M. Bender shows clinical studies by "Autofluoroscopy."	[1964]	JNM
	— P. Richards devises a 1045 hole lo-energy collimator.	[1964]	JNM
	— G. Hines devises a "line source phantom" for cameras.	[1964]	JNM
	— M. Ter-Pogossian devises a 3 × 5 mm crystal for esophag count.	[1966]	Cir
	— F. Pircher develops small solid state eye counter.	[1961]	JNM
9. Units	— Thirteenth CGPM redefines second as periods in rad of Cs-133.	[1960]	NBS
	— CGPM adopts the kelvin (K) as unit thermodynamic temp;	[1954]	NBS
	the celsius unit of temperature change is permitted.		NBS
10. Concp	— J. Tyson describes non-linear curve fitting methods.	[1965]	JNM
	— J. Kennedy says °Tc adsorption on glass is serious error.	[1960]	JNM
	— P. Johnson: no false + scans, just false + interpretation.	[1963]	JNM
	— N. Simon scans bremsstrahlung from Y-90 (Rx dose).	[1934]	Rad
11. Drugs	— S. Yeh introduces °Tc-citrate as a kidney scan agent.	[1965]	JNM
	— R. Hayes develops °Ga colloids as particulate agents.	[1965]	JNM
	— J. Christie tries 3.2d Au-199 158 keV for scans — costly.	[1961]	Rad
	Radioiodine, P-32, and Radioactive Therapy		
12. I-Res	— Consumer Reports: fast food hamburgers at 30 × I-127 RDA.	[1928]	
	— IAEA finds goiter in entire pop of Himalayan village.	[1966]	IAEA
	— A. Costa describes acute hot nodule epidemic in Turin.	[1965]	La
	— J. Quinn notes thyroids on routine °TcO_4 brain scans.	[1964]	JNM
	— F. Seif finds LATS in 1/2 of 32 hyperthyroids; antibodies?	[1955]	DMW
	— H. Wagner starts clin use of I-123, production problems.	[1949]	IRT
	— T. Evans measures °I uptake in 36 fetal thyroids.	[1962]	JNM
13. I-Dx	— S. Yoshida: 1/2 of ca, 1/5 of sol nodules are asymptomatic.	[1966]	CJS
	— I. Jackson: 6% of 152 solitary nodules found malignant.	[1966]	BJS
	— G. Burke finds 10 of 19 hot nodules are autonomous.	[1965]	AnIM
	— V. Bockner: lo-PB°I in 300 women on oral contraceptives.	[1966]	MJA
14. I-Rx	— I. Hales treats auton nodules with °I under T4 suppress.	[1965]	MJA
	— R. Hamilton: ophthalmopathy not related to any Rx.	[1966]	MCP
	— A. Hayles' 30y followup of subtot-ectomy notes 38% myx.	[1966]	MCP
	— W. Beierwaltes notes 43% hypo 10y post-surg for hyper.	[1966]	JAMA
	— E. Chapman's 2y followup favors low dose Rx (80 µCi/g).	[1964]	NEJM
	— JAMA EDITORIAL SAYS I-131 Rx HAS REPLACED 37y OF SURGERY.		JAMA
15. P-Rx	— E. Tong gives first parathormone in P-32 Rx prost mets.	[1965]	AJR
	— W. Maxfield relates success of °P Rx to Sr-85 uptake.	[1965]	JNM
	— L. Morin says Rx of prostate mets is palliation only.	[1965]	JU
17. Other	— I. Ariel tries IL Y-90 microsphs & Cr°PO_4 in melanoma;	[1965]	SGO
	— I. Ariel tries intra art °nuclides + chemoRx in liver ca.	[1965]	Ca
	— N. SIMON: "BRACHYTHERAPY" IS NO LONGER PART OF NUC MED.	[1937]	NYMJ

Scans and Other Tests of Function in Various Organs

18. Brain	— C. Maynard blocks choroid plexus °Tc uptake with $KClO_4$.	[1966]	JNM
	— R. Witcofski's 1000 scans show 7.5% malig SOL, 6.2% non.	[1959]	JNM
	— M. Budabin: 3h scan delay time helps detect A-V malforms.	[1966]	JNM
	— F. Pircher finds cer infarcts seen best in second–third week.	[1966]	N
	— L. Rosenthall does Cerebral Perfusion with 5 sec frames.	[1966]	Rad
	— M. Pollycove does first perfusions with 1.5 sec frames.	[1966]	JNM
	— G. Burke confirms Rosenthall with 1 sec frames.	[1966]	JNM
	— Cerebral blood flow is measured by:	[1929]	ANP
	V. Kak with °IHSA in subarach hemorrhage.	[1966]	La
	S. Crunquist with Xe-133 in CVA.	[1965]	BJR
	M. Loken with Xe-133 by carotid injection.	[1964]	JNM
	W. Christ with Xe-133.	[1965]	CirR
	— C. Tator locates block in hydroceph with cisternography.	[1965]	CMAJ
19. Heart	— R. Gorlin starts "regional" flow with myocard °Kr inject.	[1961]	JCI
	— T. Malek locates °I-tetracyc only in damaged myocardium.	[1961]	Na
	— S. Knoebel measures cor flow (bolus Rb-84 in 33 normals).	[1966]	Cir
	— S. Knoebel adds leg exercise to show stress change in flow.	[1965]	JAP
	— R. Phibbs proves microsphere flow same as blood (freeze).	[1962]	Na
20. Liver	— W. MacIntyre: °Au 411 keV is unsatisfactory for cameras.	[1965]	Rad
	— R. Maas introduces °Tc-tin complex for faster scans.	[1964]	IJAR
	— P. Johnson's 1000+ scans: 7–12% false neg, 3–12% false +.	[1963]	JNM
	— J. Kuba does splenoportograms with large particle °TcSC.	[1961]	FGR
	— M. Magalotti: spleen uptake of °AuCol says portal hypert.	[1966]	JNM
	— P. Farrer uses liver/spleen ratio to show portal hypertension.	[1966]	JNM
	— T. Verdon: 2% of °Au shifts to spleen are myeloprolif dis.	[1966]	JNM
21. Lung	— W. Tauxe shows variable nature of scans in asthma pts.	[1966]	SMJ
	— L. Bennett warns of "shine through," use oblique views.	[1966]	JNM
	— M. Loken introduces °Xe-in-saline for injection scan.	[1965]	JNM
22. Bone	— D. Sklaroff has bone-scanned 1000 + patients with Sr-85.	[1964]	JAMA
	— L. Rosenthall introduces °TcSC as a bone marrow agent.	[1966]	JCAR
	— J. Kriss introduces °Tc-Fe-Colloid as bone marrow agent.	[1966]	JNM
23. Kidney	— C. Elwood gets same GFR with °I-iothalamate and inulin.	[1966]	BJR
	— M. Blaufox follows PAH with °I-Hipp clearance, exter cpm.	[1966]	JNM
	— G. Burke perfuses kidneys (°I-Hipp), records fast snaps.	[1966]	AJR
	— 10 articles (e.g., G. Burke) evaluate renogram in diseases.	[1966]	AJR
	— 6 articles (e.g., A. Graham) evaluate kidney scan technics.	[1965]	BJU
24. Gut	— K. Setala draws 3-D display of °Tc, °I, °Sr, stomach uptake.	[1964]	AR
	— F. Curtis compares arm/fecal counts as Ca-47 absorption.	[1959]	JLCM
	— A. Skyring: °Y-RBC for GI bld loss; aspirin adds 3.5 ml/d.	[1966]	MJA
25. Blood	— R. Cavalieri finds °Se gets into WBC by active process.	[1965]	Na
	— 21 articles (e.g., M. Takasugi) discuss ferrokinetics.	[1965]	AJMS
26. Other	— W. Beierwaltes notes C-14 dopamine's hi-adrenal uptake.	[1961]	JNM
	— S. Wax measures testicle blood flow with Xe-133.	[1961]	SF

Radiation Hysteria and Health Physics   * Obituaries *

27. Hyst	— E. Albright finds 5 thyroid ca adults who had neck irradiation.	[1986]	JAMA
	— O. Bizzozero describes rad leuk in Hiroshima, Nagasaki.	[1955]	AnIM
28. React	— M. Eisenbud studies KI block of thyroid °I vs dose time.	[1960]	JAMA
	— R. Maas finds no histologic damage to lung after °IMAA.	[1966]	AJCP
	— S. Dahlgren: 2 sarcomas/1000 pts 25y post Thorotrast.	[1960]	NYAS

* * *

30. Obits	— H. Muller (1890–1967) Am genetics; rad damage in fruit fly.		Sc
	— J. Cockroft (1897–1967) Eng physics; high energy partic accel.		AP
	— R. Oppenheimer (1904–1967) Am physics; A-Bomb project.		PAPS
	— R. Van de Graaff (1905–1967) Am physics; electrostatic gener.		Sc
	— P. Aebersold (1910–1967) Am physics; Isotopes Div AEC.	[1958]	AP

CHRONOLOGY OF NUCLEAR MEDICINE — 1968

Scientific and Technical Background

			Ref.
2. Obser	— AEC °nuclide production capacity is at planned peak.	[1963]	AEC
3. # Nuc	— M. Brucer up-dates Sullivan's Trilin Chart to 1447 nucs.	[1961]	Bk

Organizations and Internal Politics

5. AEC +	— M. Blau catches AEC in deliberate lie on Hg-203 hazard.	[1961]	JNM
	— K. Williams: Gov't tries to control Med by safety rules.	[1962]	JNM
6. Socs	— U. Mexico initiates 2y post-grad course in Nuc Science.	[1962]	PL
	— NAS holds symposium, Body Composition in Animals & Men.	[1955]	NAS
	— F. Spiers' "Radioisotopes in Human Body" pub (Academic Pr).	[1956]	Bk
7. Event	— First medical paper from new Thailand AEC (on Mn tox).	[1962]	JNM
	— R. Lewis starts emergency room scanning idea (cardiac).	[1966]	JAMA
	— Coronary bypass surg started, requires ischemia test.	[1966]	SA

Instruments, Units of Measurement, and Drugs

8. Instr	— P. Ronai: montage of camera snaps is a whole body scan.	[1964]	JNM
	— P. Hoffer makes device for thyroid I fluorescent scans.	[1964]	Rad
	— H. Anger scans 6 planes of focus on tomographic device.	[1963]	Bk
	— Japanese firm advertises dual probe rectilin scanner.	[1961]	JJN
	— W. Ashburn builds Cardiac Perf inst, stops 60 frames/sec.	[1966]	JNM
9. Units	— G. Brownell's absorbed dose calcula is first MIRD report.	[1964]	JNM
10. Concp	— E. Gregg proposes modulation transfer function.	[1960]	JNM
	— W. Nelp states feasibility of in vivo neut activ analys.	[1966]	PMB
	— M. Quinian follows one °microsphere in mucociliary flow.	[1966]	FP
11. Drugs	— P. Richards prepares °Tc-EDTA citrate.	[1967]	PJR
	— J. Britten finds thallium toxicity at 20 mg/kg level.	[1983]	BBA
	— E. Pochin introduces cow-produced 1.5h 393 keV In-113m.	[1966]	JAMA
	— W. Myers introduces Sr-87m for bone scans.	[1939]	JNM
	— J. Kriss introduces ultra short-lived nuclides ($T_{1/2}$ = sec).	[1974]	JNM
	— G. Andrews reintroduces I-130 (keV too high for camera).	[1941]	JNM
	— H. Wellman uses I-123 clinically in spite of cost.	[1967]	JNM

Radioiodine, P-32, and Radioactive Therapy

12. I-Res	— T. Oddie says US daily I-127 (240–740 μg) affects uptake.	[1967]	JCEn
	— C. Bowers synthesizes TRH, causes prompt TSH release.	[1966]	JCEM
	— V. Sodd bombards Te-122, 2h Xe-123, decays to 13h I-123.	[1967]	JNM
	— T. Shepard says organic I binding begins 73rd day gestation.	[1962]	Bk
	— J. Vander follows 5127 nontox nodules for 15y, no malig.	[1967]	AnIM
	— L. Hemplemann asks if nodules are caused by radiation?	[1967]	Sc
13. I-Dx	— R. Young finds 12% malig in 97 solitary cold nodules.	[1967]	JNM
	— D. Winikoff: estrogen in contraceptive changes PBI & T3.	[1967]	MJA
	— P. Richards scans trapping of °TcO_4 at 10m scan delay.	[1967]	JNM
	— D. Enrich measures PBI at 2–6h & 24–48h to find hypos.	[1967]	DMW
	— P. Harper quantifies perchlorate washout of °I.	[1967]	JNM
	— J. Miller does the suppression tests on I-131 scans.	[1967]	AS
	— V. Bay: autonomous hot nodules have rapid uptake & loss.	[1967]	FM
	— Abbott Labs introduces an I-125 T4 in vitro kit.	[1962]	
14. I-Rx	— E. Saenger: same leukemia incidence after all thyroid Rx.	[1963]	JAMA
	— M. Tubiana: pts with °I uptake in mets survive longer.	[1966]	PrM
	— G. Hagan finds 30–70% hypo 10–20y after I-131 Rx.	[1966]	MCNA
	— J. Philip gets poor results in Co-60 Rx of hyperthyroid.	[1927]	La
	— O. Beahrs gets myxedema in 43% of 337 thyroidectomies.	[1967]	AS
	— H. Zellman details long-term success in °I Rx of hypers.	[1967]	LCB
15. P-Rx	— B. Stoll: circadian rhythm in °P counts over breast tumors.	[1966]	ca

16. Tele — M. Schulz lists many 250 keV, 1700 Co-60 units, 43 V de Graaffs, 27 betatrons and 35 linear accelerators operating. [1951] AJR
17. Other — Ford Hosp (Detroit) reviews its Rx of malig effusions. [1962] PL
— I. Ariel gets palliation by °I-ethiodol in 75 lymphomas. [1964] JNM

Scans and Other Tests of Function in Various Organs

18. Brain — J. Clements introduces Yb-169 as a new brain scan agent. [1964] AJR
— A. Rhoton says scan delay should be 3–5h post-injection. [1967] JNM
— 13 articles (e.g., G. Burke) detail perfusion technics. [1966] JAMA
— D. Patton shows cisternography in norm press hydrocephalus. [1967] JNM
— W. Ashburn detects CSF rhinorrhea in 14 pts with camera. [1967] JNM
19. Heart — C. MULLINS INTRODUCES AUTOMATIC ECG-GATED BLOOD POOL SCANS. [1962] AJCr
— A. Maseri demolishes myth that bld mixes in heart chambers. [1963] JCI
20. Liver — J. Stover describes °Tc-Sb-sulfide as a new scan agent. [1967] JNM
— A. Townsend separates hepatic from portal flow on scan. [1966] JNM
— N. Riccioni introduces dual agent liver scans: °Au & °I. [1965] JNBM
— F. DeLand shows liver regen after partial hepatectomy. [1966] JNM
— J. Morris studies liver/sacral ratios in cirrhosis. [1967] ARa
— Y. Bahk says bld clearance of °AuCol differs in abscess. [1966] BJR
21. Lung — H. Wellman gives reasons for oblique projections. [1967] JNM
— N. Poe compares inhale & perfusion scans in emphysema. [1965] AJR
— A. GILSON COMBINES VENTILATION & PERFUSION SCANS. [1965] JNM
— E. Suprenant: bronchograms & angios cause perfusion defects. [1966] JNM
— G. Duffy notes hot spot artifact on °IMAA scans. [1964] JNM
22. Bone — N. Charkes says mets are most common Sr-85 abnormality. [1967] JAMA
— W. Ashburn: scans see early Hodgkin's bone involvement. [1967] ca
— J. Cameron measures mineral density with ext I-125 source. [1963] IR
— R. Affram sees °Sr uptake from 5d to 19mo after injury. [1966] JBJS
23. Kidney — 10 articles (e.g., H. Warembourgh) on renogram techniques. [1967] PrM
— 8 articles (e.g., K. Schmidt) evaluate kidney scan agents. [1967] MM
— 6 articles (e.g., H. Favre) describe measurement of GFR. [1967] BMJ
— L. Reese uses Hg-203 scan to locate biopsy site. [1967] CMAJ
— L. Timmermans uses camera to see vesicoureteral reflux. [1966] JUN
24. Gut — S. Kaihara uses C-14 tag fats to measure malabsorption. [1967] JLCM
25. Blood — S. Albert develops "Unitag" bag for ease & sterility. [1966] JNM
— J. Adamson finds Ht a poor index of bld loss or deficit. [1964] JAMA
— R. Oberfield finds 8.6% less bld vol in immobilized pts. [1965] Aero
— B. Hulme finds °IPVP whole body count mol wt dependent. [1963] JNM
26. Other — R. Hayes does first Ga-68 lymph node scan in Hodgkin's pt. [1965] AEC
— G. DeChiro says salivary glands seen during brain scan. [1966] AJR
— R. Hardon notes salivary gland inhibition after $KClO_4$. [1967] QJP
— F. Mishkin does placenta scan with In-113m for low dose. [1966] JNM
— H. Glass does placenta scans with inhaled C-11 monoxide. [1966] JNM
— P. Atkins finds Deep Venous Thrombo with °I-fibrinogen. [1966] BJS

Radiation Hysteria and Health Physics * Obituaries *

27. Hyst — Does fallout cause thyroid nodules? Yes, L. Hemplemann. [1913] Sc
— J. Barron reports accidental fatal dose, 200 mCi °AuCol. [1964] IAEA
A. Casarett postulates hormesis can't be true rad stimulation. [1965] Bk
28. React — A. Dekaban lists timetable of 26 rad birth defects. [1963] JNM
I. Chaikoff gets °I thyroid ca only in genetic sens mice. [1963] APa
— W. Mills measures population exposure in Kerala, India. [1965] HP
29. Respo — AEC list all (very few) radiation accidents & exposures. [1964] AEC

* * *

30. Obits — L. Meitner (1878–1968) Aus physics; nuclear fission. Bio
— O. Hahn (1879–1968) Ger physics; radioisotopes, fission Bio
— W. Sullivan (1914–1968) Am phys chem; trilinear chart. NBS

CHRONOLOGY OF NUCLEAR MEDICINE — 1969

Scientific and Technical Background			Ref.
1. Basic	— First polyatomic molecule (formaldehyde) detected in space.	[1925]	Sc
2. Obser	— Astronauts see pinpoint light flashes (cosmic rays ?).	[1925]	AP
	— M. Tefft finds Pediatric Nuclear Med again respectable.	[1959]	JAMA
3. # Nuc	— G. Goles lists elements cosmic abund in Hndbk Geochem.	[1967]	Bk
4. # Med	— G. Seaborg says about 8 million Nuc Med procedures/y. 50% Co-60, 33% °I Dx & Rx, 7% °Tc Dx.	[1966]	AEC

Organizations and Internal Politics			
6. Soc's	— J. Hubbell revises attenuation coef from 10 keV — 100 GeV	[1952]	NBS
	— L. Badash pubs Rutherford–Boltwood letters (Hopkins).	[1907]	Bk
	— Third IAEA Symposium on Scanning published.	[1964]	IAEA
	— M. Born's "Physics in My Generation" pub (Springr-Verl).	[1926]	Bk
7. Event	— Quebec Coll Physicians & Surg Name Nuc Med a specialty (1987		JNM)

Instruments, Units of Measurement, and Drugs			
8. Instr	— S. Cohn describes BNL 54 crystal whole body counter.	[1966]	PMB
	— Polaroid film is pulled for fast frame exposures.	[1968]	JNM
	— C. Muelbaecher develops a div-con collimator for camera.	[1967]	JNM
	— J. Zimmerman invents supersensitive human magnetism sensor.		SN
	— D. Cohen develops magnet shield for human mag sensor.	[1985]	SN
9. Units	— CIPM suggests adoption of seventh basic SI unit, the mole.	[1967]	NBS
10. Concp	— W. Oldendorf finds I-125 worthless in scanning, Pb fluor.	[1962]	JNM
	— A. Petushkov measures elements by fingernail act analysis.	[1968]	JNM
11. Drugs	— H. Stern labels Hum Ser Alb microspheres with Tc-99m.	[1968]	JNM
	— G. SUBRAMANIAN BEGINS MANY NEW °Tc LABELING PROCEDURES.	[1968]	JNM
	— E. Potchen describes new 2d Sn-113 — 1.65h In-113m cow.	[1968]	JNM
	— T. Jones describes a 4.58h Rb-81 — 13s Kr-81m cow.	[1968]	BJR
	— M. Larsen notes pos uses for imidodiphosphate relatives.	[1959]	Sc
	— J. Burdine lists attempts to push In-113m as universal agent.		Rad

Radioiodine, P-32, and Radioactive Therapy			
12. I-Res	— J. Shimmins finds no organic Tc binding after 3h.	[1964]	JNM
	— R. Fierro-B finds 50% I-def goiter in hi-Andes Village.	[1966]	NEJM
	— P. Hoffer does thyroid scans with fluorescent radiation.	[1968]	AJR
	— D. Gitlin finds embryo thyroglob immune react on 29th d.	[1968]	JCE
13. I-Dx	— J. PITTMAN SAYS °I UPTAKES LOWER FROM WHITE BREAD I-127.	[1968]	JAMA
	— R. Caplan (others) re-evaluate uptakes in I-127 excess.	[1968]	JAMA
	— C. Thomas finds 29% cold nodules malignant on histology.	[1968]	AS
	— L. Kendall finds 21% sol cold nodules malignant on histology.	[1968]	La
	— C. Vergiani measures T4-binding prealb by immunochem.	[1963]	CC
	— H. Higgins finds 10 min thyroid uptake satisfactory.	[1968]	JCEn
14. I-Rx	— W. Grieg tries to reduce hypos with I-125 toxicosis Rx.	[1974]	La
	— G. Burke says may be 70% hypos years after I-131 Rx.	[1968]	JAMA
17. Other	— G. Sheline calculates Stone's 1939 n dose (no unit then).	[1942]	ICR

Scans and Other Tests of Function in Various Organs			
18. Brain	— S. Kanafani shows intra-carotid °IMAA is safe for scans.	[1967]	AJR
	— D. Gilay introduces 31.8d Yb-169 DTPA as scan agent.	[1968]	Rad
	— J. Handa says scans improve with increased scan delay.	[1967]	AJR
	— G. Alker summarizes value of cistern- & ventril-ography.	[1967]	AR
	— J. Goodman reveals unique perfusion pic of "Brain Death."	[1983]	JAMA
	— 8 authors (e.g., R. Palvolgi) on techniques for blood flow.	[1967]	JNs
	— R. Sephton says scan delay of min diff from hours scan.	[1967]	AuR

19. Heart	— E. Braunwald confirms cardiac perfusion clinically.	[1966]	Cir
	— G. Burke takes first 1 frame/sec cardiac perfusion pics.	[1966]	JNM
	— G. Burke eyeballs chamber-to-chamber transit times.	[1968]	JNM
	— R. Ross says more left heart coronary flow than right.	[1964]	CdR
	— R. Gorlin says left myocardial blood flow same as right.	[1964]	JCI
	— L. Lamb: mild exercise inadequate in trained animals.	[1967]	Aero
	— H. GARCIA ESTIMATES MUSCLE BLOOD FLOW WITH °Xe WASHOUT.	[1967]	JCS
	— P. Cannon combines perf & °Xe washout to test myocard.	[1967]	Cir
	— J. Friedman measures single pass Rb-86 muscle bld flow.	[1967]	AJPh
	— G. Oliver measures digitoxin by RIA technique.	[1963]	JCI
20. Liver	— E. Seymour describes the bowel barium meal artifact.	[1967]	AJR
	— D. Brown describes °AuCol scans following transplant.	[1964]	Rad
	— P. Richards makes a true °Tc colloid (°TcSC is microagg).	[1968]	JNM
	— V. McCready: °TcSC worthless in lymphoma, back to °CrRBC.	[1966]	IAEA
	— M. Loken introduces °Hg-MHP (propane) for spleen scans.	[1966]	JNM
	— J. Burdine prefers °Tc-heat damaged RBC for spleen scan.	[1966]	Rad
21. Lung	— J. Dahlen finds pulmonary embolism in >25% of autopsies.	[1964]	V70
	— M. Webber shows hot spots on °IMMA scan (macro-macroagg).	[1968]	Rad
	— G. Miorner studies regional radiospirometry with Xe-133.	[1966]	SJCL
	— J. Mack finds post oblique projec necessary to find PE.	[1966]	JNM
	— J. Mack says some pts require 8 projections to find PE.	[1966]	Rad
	— H. Waldman: angiography is NOT "gold standard" in PE.	[1968]	V70
	— E. Varpela says serial scans (days) are often required.	[1966]	ACG
	— 3M Company has albumin microspheres in 7 to 65 nm size.	[1968]	JNM
	— S. Golman notes weak perfusion scan after radiotherapy.	[1961]	Rad
	— M. Croll introduces "cardiopulmogram" to detect shunts.	[1955]	BJR
22. Bone	— Many compare F-18, Sr-85, and Sr-87m at Symposium.	[1966]	IAEA
	— N. Charkes finds scan delay (to 48h) important in Sr-87m.	[1967]	JNM
	— C. Bassett's myo ossif DDP Rx success suggests °agent.	[1974]	La
	— Bauer's scintimetry in bone; Maxfield's in joint fluid.	[1969]	JNM
	— E. Rand: scan bone first then do X-Rays, prior to surgery.	[1968]	JNM
	— E. Bell recognizes import of photopenic areas on scan.	[1964]	Rad
	— R. DeGowin shows irradiation effect on bone marrow scan.	[1961]	ArIM
23. Kidney	— O. Charamaza prepares °Tc-Sn complex for renal scanning.	[1968]	NMG
	— R. Nordyke: renograms & scans are screens for unilat dis.	[1968]	JAMA
	— F. Hosain sees kidney and glomerular func with Yb-169.	[1966]	Rad
	— 10 authors (e.g., A. Barns) show scans in various diseases.	[1968]	La
	— 8 authors (e.g., M. Ram) run GFR with various techniques.	[1968]	La
24. Gut	— M. Layrisse tags foods by biosynth °Fe for absorption.	[1968]	Bl
	— W. Meier-Ruge: °Tc uptake in parietal, °I in chief cells.	[1967]	His
	— J. McAfee says not so, mixed cell pop with both.	[1967]	JNM
25. Blood	— R. Berger devises method for labeling RBC with Tc-99m.	[1967]	WZN
	— W. Crosby reviews ferrokinetic physiology since 1958.	[1967]	JAMA
26. Other	— W. Beierwaltes: hi-adrenal cortex uptake of °I cholest.	[1967]	JNM
	— C. EDWARDS SAYS °Ga IS A TUMOR, NOT A BONE, AGENT.	[1968]	V81
	— S. Kazeto scans ovaries (dogs) with °I-chorion gonadotrop.	[1967]	AJOG

Radiation Hysteria and Health Physics * Obituaries *

27. Hyst	— USPHS says ALL I-131 scans are bad. (Rumor states that I-123 money changed hands to get this stupidity in the Fed Reg.)		
	— E. Bland: I-125 in mother's milk caused hypo baby (Wrong).	[1965]	La
	— C. Neil worries about Doc's hand exposure by syringe °Tc	[1968]	JNM
	— DDT is ostracized because of immoderate overuse.	[1962]	SN
	— FDA removes cyclamates from market on poor evidence.	[1965]	FDA
28. React	— R. Sampson: more thyroid ca in non-bomb exposed Japanese.	[1964]	JAMA
	— R. Miller finds no genetic effect of atom bomb exposure.	[1955]	ABCC
29. Respo	— M. Tefft: Pediatric Nuc Med has removed age restrictions.	[1968]	JNM

* * *

30. Obits —

POWELL RICHARDS INTRODUCES °Tc-99m

- In 1938 there was no technetium.
- In 1948 Tc was an exotic element.
- In **1958** one man said °Tc has med use.
- In 1968 °Tc is part of Nuclear Med.
- In 1978 °Tc dominates Nuclear Med.

Four major changes in Nuclear Medicine terminology occurred in the 1960s:

1. In 1960 "*short* half-life" meant shorter than 8d I-131. After °Tc it meant a few hours $T_{1/2}$ or less.
2. "Low energy" meant <364 keV of I-131. After °Tc it meant <140 keV.
3. In 1960 "millicurie" was a therapeutic unit. After °Tc it became diagnostic level radioactivity.
4. The word "cow" became Nuclear Med lab language. (Wimps say "generator.")

Physicians who worked with °isotopes before Cassen's 1950 scanner were first generation Nuclear Medics. Those who can remember working without °Tc are properly called second generation.

A 6-hour $T_{1/2}$ was too short for °isotope shipping logistics, but not if it could be milked from a cow. (G. Failla's descriptive terms for "milking" short-lived radon from long-lived radium. [Vig1915 .Cow]) The "Hot Lab" division of Brookhaven National Laboratory set up a project to make short-lived °nuclides available. L. Stang, leader of the group, developed a molybdenum-technetium cow system in 1957. Shortly thereafter P. Richards joined the team to adapt the Mo-Tc system for medical use, but an ESSO research group purchased the first practical cow in 1961 to solve mixing problems in large vats.

In 1960, while flying to a European Nuc Med Conference, Richards convinced P. Harper (U of Chicago) that a 6 hour $T_{1/2}$ °Tc-99m was long enough for most tests:

- Its shortness minimizes contamination.
- 140 keV is ideal for external counts.
- High cpm output maximizes sensitivity.
- °Tc is chemically friendly to tagging.
- °Tc shows little toxicity.
- The cow system makes it available.
- Health Physicists love it.

By the end of the flight Harper was converted. The first "medical" °Tc-99m cow was shipped to Argonne Research Hospital in 1961. Harper and C. Lathrop milked the cow, injected the $°TcO_4$ into a mouse, and scanned it. To their surprise they saw high uptake of pertechnetate in thyroid, salivary glands, and stomach. After a year's investigation of thyroid distribution a 1962 publication caused little comment.

°Tc Plus the Gamma Camera is a Hit

In Dec 1962 C. Kellershon in the French Atomic Energy group at Orsay received the second medical °Tc cow. No outstanding papers emerged. At the 1963 Montreal meeting of the SNM, Harper announced a new liver scanning agent, a °Tc-thiocyanate-fat emulsion — it caused no comment. But he heard that pertechnetate had extra-cellular-space localization in the brain and might be useful in brain scanning. He already had done one disappointing pertechnetate brain scan, but decided to try it with a new thin crystal gamma camera. The result was outstanding.

At about the same time P. Richards had developed a new liver-spleen scanning agent, °Tc-Sulfur Colloid. It resulted in remarkable scans. Thyroid scans gave remarkable fast-trapping pictures. J. McAfee substituted °Tc for °I in the best °IHSA brain scanning agent. At a January 1964 Bad Gastein Conference, Harper and R. Beck read a paper on "The Optimization of Scanning." It documented Richards' arguments on Tc-99m. Within weeks °Tc cows were shipped to Oak Ridge, Berkeley, and Johns Hopkins.

Two years earlier Nuclear Chicago, Inc, had installed its first Anger camera. By 1965 sufficient cameras had been sold for H. Anger to preside at a gamma camera symposium. The thin crystal camera was hostile to scanning 364–411 keV energies of °I and °Au. It was perfect for the 140 keV emission of °Tc. Further, millicurie doses of °Tc allowed perfusions to be imaged in seconds. A new class of dynamic function studies, impossible on the linear scanner, was born.

From 1965 on, °Tc, the gamma camera, and dynamic function studies expanded in parallel growth to dominate Nuclear Medicine.

[See Vig1949 .Phr; Vig1961 .Pan]

THE FIRST RADIOACTIVE ISOTOPE INJURY

Radioisotopes were stereotyped by newspapers in 1946 as "deadly monsters." This carry-over from the radium-dial painters scandal of 1926 was exploited by newspapermen and a school of Health Physicists who saw federal funds emanating from "Danger." Radiologists had been imprinted with "X-ray danger" (for good reason), but knew nothing about the new °isotopes. AEC released pictures of workers using mechanical hands over thick walls to manipulate "incredibly small doses." The whole panoply of licensure was justified "to protect the public." The AEC unknowingly manufactured radiation hysteria during its first 10 years.

An Advisory Field Service was set up by AEC's Isotopes Division in 1947 for on site review of laboratory design, safe handling, equipment, instrumentation, and measuring techniques. They had authority to stop unsafe use, but emphasis was on education and information. But in 1966, 20 years after the first shipment, only one injury had been reported from 1.3 megacuries of °isotopes shipped:

On 29 March 1960 a 33-year-old male graduate student at U of Wisconsin was accidentally exposed to a 200 curie Co-60 source. A total body dose of 250–300 R was estimated and he developed an acute radiation syndrome. He made a satisfactory recovery without any specific therapy. (25 years later "no specific therapy" turns out to be the best therapy at this level of dose.)

A few misadministrations of wrong dose or wrong °nuclide had occurred; but these were not health physics problems. Most of us who were pushing °isotopes complained about overblown safety precautions imposed on every °isotope licensee. Lawrence's successful P-32 therapy of chronic leukemias was dropped by hematologists because less successful chemotherapy did not require AEC license. Intracavitary °AuColloid was dropped because of AEC licensure hassles. At the 1984 Sixth Int Colloquium on Radioimmunology, Lyons, France, the search for a non-radioactive substitute was justified by time consuming and insulting °nuclide licensure.

[See Vig1964 .ARS, Acute Rad Syn]

AN ALMOST SUCCESSFUL PANCREAS SCAN AGENT

(From a Story Told by J.L. Quinn)

The pancreas has always been hidden from radiologists. J.L. Quinn's introduction to Nuclear Medicine as a resident in radiology at Bowman Gray was an attempt to visualize the pancreas. His group was using manganese and zinc compounds to find a localizing agent. Their scans were always highly unsuccessful.

Monte Blau at Roswell Park had long been interested in the same problem. In 1960 he noticed an article showing the distribution of amino acids in tumors and in normal tissues: amino acid concentration in the pancreas was an order of magnitude higher than in other organs. He labeled a few amino acids with °iodine and tried scanning the upper abdomen. It didn't work. But the sulfur in methionine lent itself to good labeling. S-35 is not a scan agent. However, selenium-75 could be scanned and might substitute for sulfur.

Selenomethionine cannot be made by chemical synthesis. It was necessary to make it by culturing yeasts in a sulfur-poor selenium-rich medium. Ordinarily not a particularly difficult procedure, it was time consuming to get the high specific activity of a scan agent. But Se-75 had a 120 day half-life, hence *relatively* few gammas/gram. It had a mixed bag of 21 gamma energies, 15 – 822 keV. A good nuclide for wet chemistry counting, it was not a good scanning agent.

Blau presented some pancreas scans at the 1961 Pittsburg Soc Nuc Med meeting. They were greeted with enthusiasm, and most labs took it up. But too much was expected of pancreas scans. A pancreas scan required great technical patience, and was never very clear. Within 10 years only 20% of labs scanned the pancreas on a routine basis. By then, the cost of Se-75 selenomethionine had tripled (biological labeling never comes cheap). A dual-agent liver-subtraction procedure had a brief fling, but Se-75 died out as a clinical °nuclide. Other uses for Se-75 were confined to the laboratory. Pancreas scanning must be considered one of nuclear medicine's noble failures.

[cf Vig1955 .Liv, Liver Scan]

SMALL PARTICLE HEMODYNAMICS AND THE LUNG SCAN
(After Stories by J. Quinn and G. Taplin)

Trapping small particles in capillaries or Kupffer's cells had been investigated back in 1952. Most studies were directed towards liver, spleen, and RES uptakes. Prinzmetal in Los Angeles used °labeled glass beads to quantify coronary flow. The beads were superseded by 3M's development of ceramic microspheres. In 1953 B. Benacerraf's group in Paris heated °IHSA to get a "physiologically acceptable" particulate, but they were thinking of RES uptake, primarily in liver.

Ever since liver scanning with °particulates started (about 1955) we have been plagued with "how to get rid of lung background." J. Muller's 1953 suggestion that particles over 50 microns were filtered out of blood by lung capillaries had not been forgotten. In 1960 M. Loken's group (U of Minnesota) attempted lung therapy with 60-micron ceramic microspheres — large enough to be mini-lung emboli. But diagnostic scanning was not attempted. T. Haynie (U of Michigan) took Loken's therapy attempt and changed it to diagnostic visualization of the lungs. Hg-293 labeled microspheres gave beautiful lung pictures in the frog. On a few attempts in humans, infarcts on X-Ray were also seen on lung scans. [JLCM, 1962] I. Ariel (NY surgeon) used °I labeled ceramic microspheres in lung cancer therapy. He was first to demonstrate pulmonary embolism on a lung scan and believe it despite a negative X-Ray. [JAMA, 1963]

For almost three years G. Taplin's group at UCLA had been fussing with °IHSA. By simple manipulation of pH, heat, and mild agitation, they could adjust particle size to either micro- or macroaggregated °I-albumin. They noted that macroaggregate produced temporary arteriolar blockade in the lungs with a 50-fold margin of safety. Taplin thought the controlled particle size aspect worth reporting.

Taplin (unknowingly) Lights a Fuse

At the June 1963 Montreal meeting of the Society of Nuc Med, Taplin presented a paper on "Gastric Photoscans with Colloidal Aggregates." At the end he sneaked in a few slides of his first °IMAA lung scans in dogs. But even more important, because more people saw it, was a picture of a dog lung scan in his exhibit at the same meeting. His beautiful gastric scans (a technical triumph) went unnoticed and nobody was more surprised than Taplin at the boiling interest in his lung scans.

Some people left the meeting, went home to cook up a batch of °IMAA and started scanning patients.

Is Producing Multiple Small Emboli Safe?

Taplin's UCLA group were hesitant to induce pulmonary embolism in order to detect pulmonary embolism. At Bowman Gray, Quinn could not use °IMAA in humans until somebody else said it was safe. Henry Wagner in Baltimore, however, did the ultimate test. He cooked up a batch of °IMAA, injected it into himself, and did the first human lung scan.

G. Hevesy drank the first dose of D_2O. J. Hamilton injected the first dose of °Na into himself. C. Finch gave himself the first dose of °iron. M. Brucer took the first dose of °Co-60 VB_{12}. These were not mock-heroics but simple belief in scientific evidence of safety. However, a nasty publicity followed J. Hamilton's death from radiation exposure (from an entirely different, and massive, source). It caused AEC Health Physicists (all unbelievers in science) to make self-administration of °nuclides illegal, immoral, and non-compliance (a capital crime).

J. Quinn presented a works-in-progress paper at the December 1963 Radiology meeting: the first report of successful lung scans for pulmonary embolism. An interesting sidelight occurred at the Bowman Gray Nuc Med symposium in January 1964. H. Wagner (Johns Hopkins) learned of Quinn's report and demanded that its publication be delayed until the JAMA announced Wagner's first lung scan. Quinn's retort was unpublishable.

In practically every Nuc Med meeting in 1964 someone presented a new set of °IMAA lung scans. During 1965 more than 70 papers were published on lung scanning. By 1970 it was estimated that over a million lung scans had been done — all stemming from a paper on the distribution of small °particles in the stomach.

[cf Vig1960 .°Tc, Intro of °Tc]

THE ACUTE RADIATION SYNDROME

The effect on various species in various states of health to different energies of different kinds of radiation exposed for various time periods to low or high doses is complex biology. A simplified model had to be invented — say X-rays suddenly exposing a whole body. By 1905 H. Heinke gave the first description of such an acute radiation disease — leukopenia, thymus and spleen sensitivity in rabbits, based upon an acute whole body exposure.

In 1913 A. Fernau first described the hemorrhagic phase of overexposure. In 1917 K. Franz described a gastrointestinal death pattern after high-dose therapy, and in 1926 M. Tsuzuki began the first systematic study of high-dose exposure. But few instruments before World War II could produce the high-dose-rate required for the neurological phase. After his Manhattan Project experiences, R. Stone named the Acute Radiation Syndrome (ARS) in a seminal 1949 JAMA article.

The Paradigm Acute Radiation Syndrome

The syndrome describes clinical signs and symptoms following a short burst of moderate energy X or gamma rays to expose the whole body. An infinite variety of modifications of kinds of exposure are also Acute Radiation Syndromes, but the R. Stone paradigm is basic.

"Short" means seconds to many hours (up to three days at Chernobyl). When exposure is prolonged or fractionated, as in the pre-1920 radiologists, response to high-dose is different than in the ARS. When less than the whole body is involved dosage and response depend as much upon what is shielded as upon which organs are irradiated. Most radiation accidents, partial body exposures of hands, are in a separate class. Neutron, heavy particle, and low (<100 keV) or high energy gamma rays (>1250 keV), modify the typical ARS considerably. However the Acute Radiation Syndrome is the basic model from which the modifications are described.

Peripheral Blood Signs of ARS

Lymphocytes: decreased lymphocytes may be the only sign of non-lethal exposure. Lymphopenia begins within an hour post exposure at relatively low dose (<100 rads), reaches a low point in 5 to 10 days and begins a slow recovery in 3–4 weeks. After lethal exposure the count may plunge below 500/ml^3 within a few days.

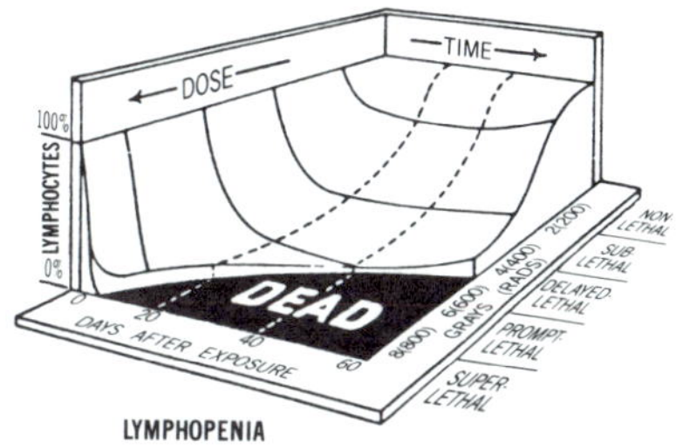

LYMPHOPENIA

Leukocytes: Mobilization of leukocytes from bone marrow is followed by a rapid decrease to a temporary plateau for about a week. Then a steady decrease to as low as 1000/ml^3 (in sublethal exposures). Slow recovery begins after 6–7 weeks of profound immunosuppression.

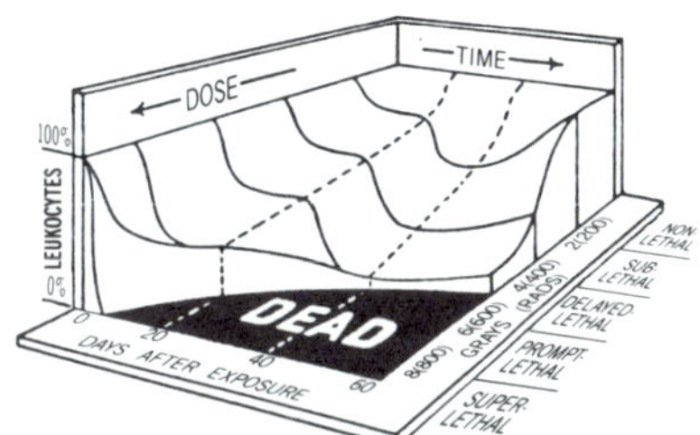

LEUKOPENIA

Platelets fall to half-normal in 5–6 weeks, or a third of normal in 6–7 weeks even in sublethal exposures (100+ rads). Patients are subject to bleeding until recovery, which may require months.

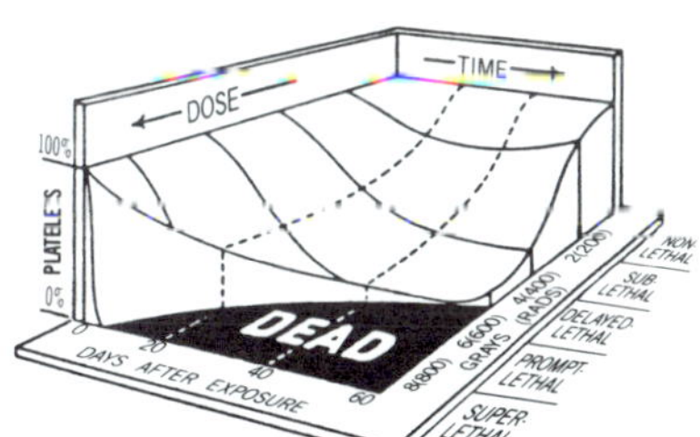

PLATELET COUNT

Three Signs of High Exposure

Vomiting. Nausea (in sublethal) and vomiting (common in lethal range) may be delayed for days; absence is a good sign of low dose. Early severe vomiting indicates high dose. Bloody diarrhea is sign of intestinal radioactive contamination.

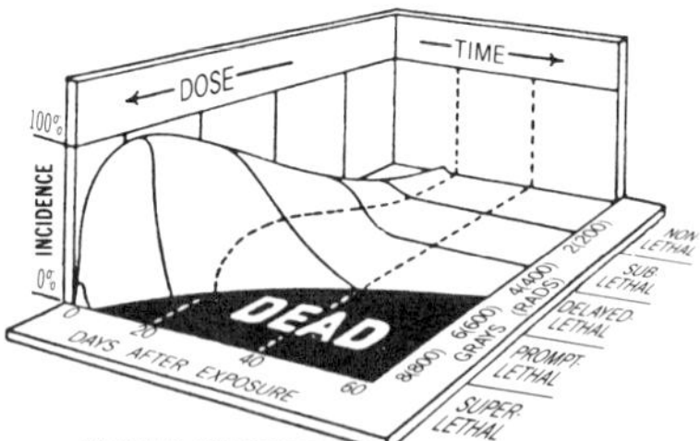

VOMITING AND NAUSEA

Fatigue or vague asthenia cannot be quantified but always occurs in sublethal exposures. The higher the dose the earlier it appears. Waves of "washed-out-feeling" may last for days. Recovery may take many months.

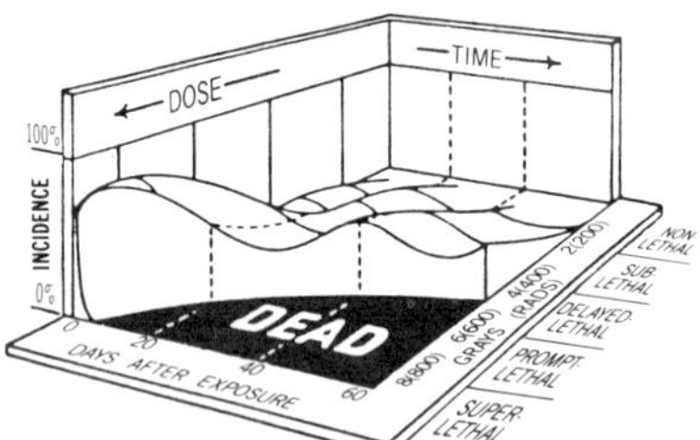

FATIGUE AND ASTHENIA

Erythema is most common with beta contamination or low energy radiation. The higher the dose the earlier it appears. Superlethal exposures produce immediate erythema. Unpredictable variation occurs among patients.

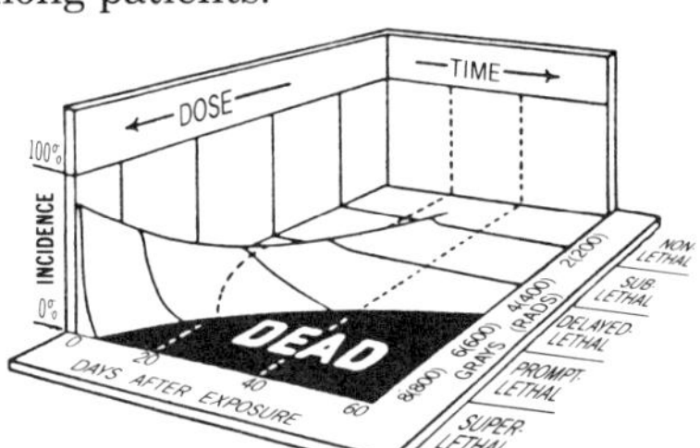

ERYTHEMA

Three Delayed Signs of Exposure

Epilation occurs on the 17th to 21st day in patients who have received much over 200 rads (delayed in sublethal range). Regrowth occurs within several months. (Permanent epilation occurs after very high dose partial body exposures.)

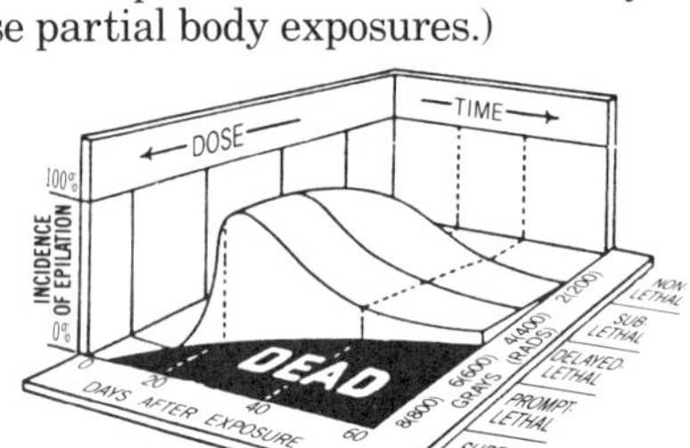

EPILATION

Bleeding: During the weeks of thrombocytopenia, petechia, easy bruising, and mild GI bleeding is expected and not serious. Massive trauma or surgery may require clotting aids. The only aspect of clotting dysfunction is platelet paucity.

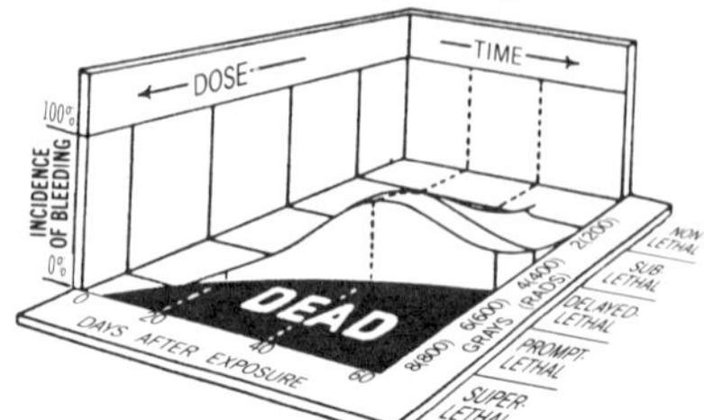

BLEEDING

Fever develops immediately in very high (krad) exposures. At 500 rads fever may develop after a few weeks but is not a common sign. Usually it is a response to superimposed infection to which patients are inordinately susceptible.

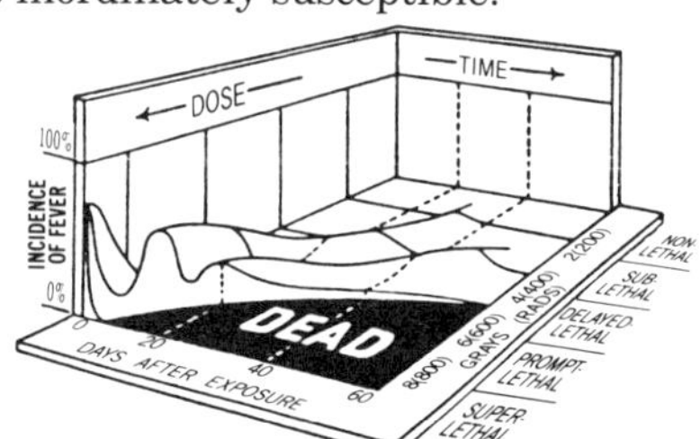

FEVER

Dose-Time-Lethal Effect of Radiation

<200 rads — Non-lethal dose-range. Symptom-free victims, do not hospitalize.
200–400 rads — Hematological dose-range. Mild nausea, precipitate leukopenia. Few deaths, if any, at 4–6 weeks from infection, great immunosuppression.
400–600 rads — Gastrointestinal dose-range. Marked asthenia, leukopenia, vomiting, 50% lethality, profound immunosuppression.
600–800 rads — Neurologic dose-range. Hyperactivity at 600, to coma at 800 rads. Rare survivors get massive GI and blood defects and profound immunosuppression.
>800 rads — Super-lethal dose range. Victims dead within minutes to hours.

The first "nuclear" accident survivor (192 n + gamma) died of heart disease after 19 years. (Time 6 Aug 1965) He proved that recovery from ARS, if it occurs, is complete. In 1975 K. Hubner demonstrated that irradiated mice were immunosuppressed. 30 years of data immediately fell into place: ARS is an immunosuppression disease. Long term cffects are rare.

[See Vig1985 .Rum]

ACCURACY OF NUCLEAR DATA IS AN AVERAGE WEIGHTED BY A COMMITTEE OF PEERS

[S. Reynolds had been an analytical chemist at ORNL in 1944. He was also a long time member of the Nat Rad Council's °Measurements & Standards subcommittee. In 1966 he summarized 20 years' development of nuclear data. I have condensed his version of how people can mistake precision for accuracy, updated some facts and added a few stories.]

When the Oak Ridge National Laboratory (ORNL) began its °isotope "business" in 1946 there were no accepted °nuclide standards. Indeed the knowledge of the characteristics that defined a °nuclide was rudimentary. [See Vig1953 .RPK] Some simple decay schemes were known and were adequate for their early purpose: to account for the complete change in energy levels. But the schemes became more complex with each re-investigation. Ce-144, for example, was considered to have no gamma emission in 1946, several gammas in 1966 and seven by 1980.

The "Curie" Unit is Defined to Death

The commonly used millicurie unit of radioactive decay was a carry-over from the Berkeley cyclotron days. The "curie" unit was defined as the number of disintegrations/second (dps) of a gram of a complex radium decay scheme in equilibrium with all of its 9 (or 12, still incompletely known) daughters. [See Vig1910 .Ci] But radium mCi standards were not measured in dps; gamma rays emitted were counted. The first °nuclide, P-32, emitted no gammas, hence could not be measured in "curies," but the 3.7×10^{10} dps became a "curie." Most of the other °nuclides did emit gammas and a "radium-equivalent-curie" was adopted. The "radium-equivalent" was soon forgotten. By 1946 few workers realized that no unit of °activity existed.

Even the curie symbol "c" was unstable. In 1946 we all used "curies (c)," "millicuries (mc)," and millimillicuries (mmc). But some mathematician confused "c" with speed-of-light, and some female equal righter said it was named after Marie (wrong, after Pierre), so we went through confusing transitions to "C" and then "Ci." The "kilo" prefix was well known and by 1950 we had mega (M) and micro (μ) units. Brucer coined a "hecto" curie Co-60 machine before he learned the 1960 11th CGPM (Com Gen Poids et Mesures) had all prefixes under discussion and would go from Exa (10^{18}) to atto (10^{-18}) by 1971. In 1975 they threw out the curie for the becquerel (Bq).

Basic Data is Compiled with Difficulty

In 1946 the isotope abundances of C-14 were calculated from specific activities based upon a half-life of 5100 years. In a few years the accepted $T_{1/2}$ was 5568 years, then in 1953 became 5800 ± 100 years. In 1966 we accepted 5730 ± 400 years. which is still 5730y in 1986. Cs-167 had an accepted $T_{1/2}$ of 33 or 37 years in 1948, depending upon who you believed. Published values then dropped as low as 26 years. The weighted mean was 29.82 years in 1965. Reynolds had been following the decay of 4 Cs-137 sources for 7 years and had a tentative $T_{1/2}$ of 30.12 years in 1966; 30.17y in 1980.

In 1946 W.H. Sullivan at ORNL codified nuclear data and published it as a *Trilinear Chart of Nuclides* in 1949. He attempted to keep the data up to date by issuing gummed stamps periodically. However, the mass of data soon outgrew space on a hexagonal stamp. Brucer's revisions of the Trilinear Chart in 1968 and 1979 included only medically useful data.

Katherine Way organized Sullivan's Nuclear Data Group and moved it to the National Academy of Sciences in 1949 (now back to ORNL). The Nuclear Data Group publishes a continuous review of the sometimes conflicting accumulation of an ever more complex mass of measurements. [Nuclear Data Sheets (Academic Press).]

Each isobar of the Trilinear Chart is periodically reviewed. Generally the procedure is to assess all published articles, attempt to weight the probable accuracy on the basis of method of measurement, and "assign" a best weighted average value. It took a few centuries to achieve the accuracy of the basic SI units. Nuclear Data Committee decisions are only about 25 years old.

Accuracy of Nuclear Data in Medical Use

High precision scientists suspect any claim for accuracy greater than about 1%. 2% or 3% is a realistic goal; 20% error is not unheard of. Biology, when making measurements in living subjects, is low precision science. Nuclear characteristics *measured* in *clinical science* are suspect when claims of accuracy exceed about 5%. 10% or 20% accuracy is realistic as a goal. Order-of-magnitude error is not unusual.

Thyroid °iodine uptake measurements furnish a good example of clinical alledged and real accuracy. [See Vig1956 .°Rx] Carl Braestrup and Edith Quimby were two outstanding medical radiation physicists when I-131 was first released in 1946. Thyroid uptake was the major °isotope test in their New York hospitals across the street from each other. They each used hand-made equipment, but intercalibrated each week on point sources of fresh I-131. They were distressed at intercalibration errors >1%.

In 1953 Oak Ridge's mock-iodine manikins emitted an °I scatter spectrum similar to a human neck with a hyperactive thyroid. Braestrup's measurement of the manikin was over 10% low, Quimby's was about 20% high. Their point sources had little scatter; manikins (and patients) emitted mostly scatter. Their *precision* was very high, but their accuracy was a good clinical routine. [See Vig1953 .M°I]

Because it was a mixture of 10.5 year Ba-133 and 30 year Cs-137, the mock-iodine spectrum had no significant change for over 10 years. Twelve manikins with various uptakes of mock-iodine were sent to about 300 clinical labs. No matter what the true uptake, each lab should have measured the same uptake. 20% to 40% error was the rule, 50% to 80% error was not uncommon, and 100% error occurred quite often. One lab repeated measurements 100 times and demonstrated precision of about ±2%. Unfortunately their accuracy (from a chemically determined "true" uptake) was 15% off. When applied to a moving human patient with an ever changing uptake, a variety of body backgrounds, gland sizes, and instruments, the error would at least double.

Industrial Laboratories are No Better

About the time we in Oak Ridge were sending out the thyroid manikins, we were also dealing with industrial laboratories (GE, Westinghouse, Picker, etc.) on Co-60 teletherapy machine design. Some of the physicists laughed at my (MB) stories of thyroid manikin measurements. I asked if they could do any better and they claimed standard 1% accuracy in physical measurements. I had our machine shop turn a half inch piece of Heavymet (a W-Pb pressed alloy) into an irregular shape. It was sent to about 10 major industrial labs. They were asked to return it with one simple answer: its density in g/cc.

Density is the oldest combined unit in history and requires no special tools. No records were kept and the results were never published, but at the next meeting I told the physicists to go back to school. Nobody had come within 5% of the manufacturer's stated density, or each other.

Accuracy in measurement is defined as deviation from the "true" amount; precision is deviation of replications. A "true amount" is known only for 7 basic SI units, and these are "true" by definition. A better word than "true" is "exact." Practical calibrations of these units are comparisons with standards that are reasonably "exact" representations of the definition.

The 1914 definition of the curie unit of amount-of-°activity was amended twice to make it a precise definition, but its measurement was stochastic (i.e., in-exact). In 1948 the National Bureau of Standards began to develop radioactivity standards of commonly used °isotopes (they would not be called °nuclides for another 15 years). The first standards, carefully prepared liquid samples of I-131, were distributed in 1948. George Manov, in charge of the program, summarized the results: "*. . . we sent out 75 samples, got back 82 answers, and nobody got our measurement.*"

The half-life of I-131 is undoubtedly very close to 8.04 days, but for medical purposes it is just as accurate to say 8 days." For calculation of Health Physics fudge factor dosimetry, the essential $T_{1/2}$ (biological) is unknown. A health physicist made up the bio $T_{1/2}$ now in use.

[See Vig1977 .SI, SI units]

HOW NUCLEAR CARDIOLOGY GOT SOME BAD NAMES

M. Prinzmetal started nuclear cardiography in 1948 with a juicy new word, "Radiocardiography." Commonly used titles, "shunt detection," "pulmonary dilution curves," "cardiac blood pools," had become somewhat jargonish and were understandable only to limited audiences. When Hal Anger adopted "blood flow visualization" he was technically correct, because "blood flow measurement" had a specific ml/min physiological meaning. He changed his camera's visualizing to "Imaging" around 1965 because his new instrument did not "scan" a linear pattern the way Cassen's instrument did. However, the word "scan" is now (1987) specified as nuclear, SPECT, PET, CAT, NMR or ultrasound. "Imaging" appears to be gaining popularity as generic.

At the 1966 Society of Nuc Med meeting both J. Kriss and R. Polcyn carelessly described a "radioisotope angiography," and nuclear medicine terminology went to pot. "Angiography" then had a confusing ambiguity for perfusion through the chambers rather than vessels of the heart. Further, neither investigator used a radio*isotope*. (Tc-99m is an isomer.)

The word "perfusion" (which means "to pour through") is widely misused in nuclear medicine. When °IMAA is trapped in the lung arterioles it does not pass through the lungs. We scan the dispersion of trapped particles. When °TcO_4 is viewed on first pass through the heart, 9 to 15 seconds is insufficient to see details so we "stop the time" by storing it in computer memory and displaying small progressive segments. These are "stop-time" frames. In Chicago and California they were called "time-lapse," a term coined for watching flowers grow.

The most confusing obfuscation is misuse of "cardiac," "coronary," and "myocardium." Intravenous °TcRBC will perfuse cardiac chambers, but only 4% of the dose will perfuse coronary vessels; none will perfuse the extravascular myocardial space. Intracoronary injection of °IHSA will perfuse the coronary system; on first pass there is almost no perfusion of myocardial space. Tenth pass will show perfusion of the cardiac chambers.

The "Bolus Injection"

The misuse of "bolus injection" has caused confusion. The length of an 0.1 ml bolus is about 1 cm long (when measured as time to pass a point). As it enters the heart the same bolus has been stretched to 4 cm long. It streams out of the lungs stretched out to enter the left heart at 1.5 meters long (if in only one vessel). It is stretched again to re-enter the heart for second pass at >4 meters. After 10–15 passes the "bolus" is fairly uniformly mixed in circulating blood.

When we tried to quantify arterial, capillary, and venous phases in cerebral perfusion studies we saw another limitation. No matter how small the bolus, in patients with slow circulation time (i.e., arteriosclerotics) bolus length greatly increased. "Bolus injection" should not be used without verification.

Half-life and Half-time

"Half-life" has an exact definition. Short-lived (months) °decays can be measured with high precision, but never exact accuracy. A gigaBq of °activity will have an almost exact $T_{1/2}$. But the time of each disintegration varies. Therefore, by definition, low level dose measurements must always be suspect.

Biological sequences do not occur in half-lives. The proper term in biology is "half-time." Usually the second half-time is longer than the first as determined by curve stripping — an experimental procedure with built-in errors. The "biological half-lives" listed in health physics tables of Maximum Permissible Doses are order-of-magnitude one-mouse estimates.

The Units of Radiation Protection

The roentgen unit has an exact definition and can be measured with high precision in SI units of J/kg. The SI gray (100 of the old rad unit) is defined exactly and can be precisely measured in the laboratory, but with only very low precision in human bodies. Dose equivalents, sieverts, the rem, quality factors, are mathematical manipulations of the gray unit with unmeasurable phantasies. As used by social workers, they have no place in scientific discourse.

[See Vig1928 .R, The Roentgen]

THE CANDELA IS A TRIPLE PHASE UNIT

(The Sixth Basic SI Unit)

The *candela* (Cd) specifies intensity of the source of light. As light travels in space from a source its intensity is measured in *lumens* (lm). When lumens shine on the surface of something the intensity is measured in *lux* (lx). The lumens in a beam of light (called its "luminance") that illuminate a surface (called its "illuminance") depends upon both distance (the radius of the sphere around the candle) and the area covered by the beam. Both lumen and lux are geometry dependent.

Ancient geometers devised a method to overcome this problem. If an arc is 1 radius long, a 57° angle between its ends is called a *radian*. Rotate the circle in a 3-D sphere. At 1 radian of rotation the arc covers an area of 1 radius^2 and its solid angle is called a *steradian* (sr). Every radius within a steradian (important in defining a candela) is perpendicular to the surface. A point of light emits rays in every direction. The number of rays in any direction = the candela (cd) in the source and the solid angle steradians (sr) being illuminated; this cd • sr is called a *lumen*. In physics the number of particles crossing a surface per second is called a flux; hence, the number of light rays striking a surface per second is called a light-flux or lux (lx):

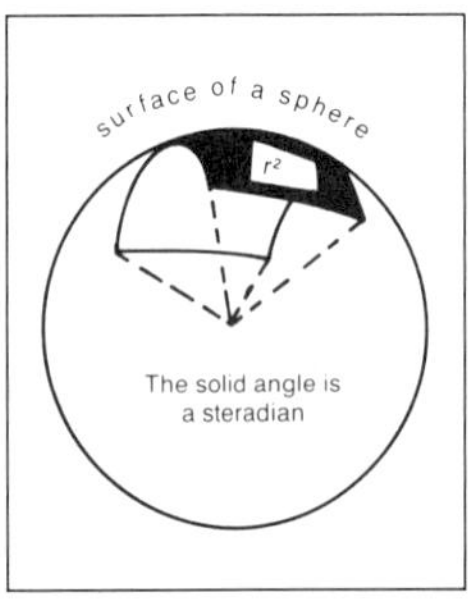

lm = cd • sr; lx = cd • sr/m^2.

The Definition of the Candela

Christian Huygens in 1690 said sunlight could be considered as wavelike rays traveling in straight lines until deflected by something. Observe the sunlight pouring through a window pane. Some of the rays bounce off the glass (called reflected light), but some get through the glass into the room (called transmitted light). You can easily demonstrate a third kind of light. Paint half of the glass pane with a thin layer of black paint. More rays are now reflected than get through, but feel the warmth of the darkened glass. Some light rays are absorbed and deposit energy in the glass.

Now imagine a perfect black paint from which no light is reflected, through which no light is transmitted, but which absorbs all light rays. Physicists call this a perfect "black body."

Heat a black body by passing an electric current through it. It will suddenly glow a dull then a bright red. As the black body gets hotter it emits blue and finally intense white light. It had been emitting heat all along, but the sudden glow occurred because our eyeball light detector is insensitive to long heat wave lengths. As soon as the black body's emission reached a wavelength of 0.76 μm (micrometers) we can see it as red light. Our eyes are sensitive to the spectrum of red through blue to 0.38 μm (called violet color). The 0.76 to 0.38 range is visible light. At longer wavelengths we "see" light, but with radiosets not eyeballs; at shorter wavelength we "see" light with GM tubes.

White light, a combination of all wave lengths, is a universal source from which the basic light unit is defined. Because "whiteness" depends upon temperature, we specify a handy standard: melting platinum (1769°C) at 760 mmHg. The number of light rays from any source depends upon its size, so we specify a pin head (1/60th of a cm^2). The rays must be measured perpendicular to their line of flight; hence, the candela SI unit is:

The Luminous Intensity
(which means light that we can see)
In the Perpendicular Direction
(means we use steradian geometry)
Of a Surface of 1/600,000 Square Meter
(the pin head size)
Of a Black body
(the universal radiator)
At the Temperature of Freezing Platinum
(1769°C)
Under a Pressure of 101,325 Newtons/m^2
(sea level at 45° latitude).

The SI candela is not a new ball game. It is just a more precise measure of the same intensity as the 1948 "new candle," which was the same as the 1939 "international candle" which was the same as the 1909 "candle," which was the same as the 1860 spermacetti "candle power." The CGPM (Commission on Weights & Measures) had to change names in 1967 because they were no longer allowed to kill sperm whales. [See Vig1860 .Cd; Catch a Whale]

PREVENTION OF GOITER WITH IODINE LEADS TO A NEW DISEASE

David Marine proved in 1907 that colloid goiters in sheep caused a variable potency in Armour's *Desiccated Thyroid*. The goiter, in turn, was caused by iodine deficiency in the diet. [See Vig1907 .Mar] Armour & Co. had the word spread quickly to veterinarians: *we will buy no more thick-necked animals — put iodine in the diet*. Lambs and sheep were a cash crop in Michigan, and goiter disappeared in a few years — in animals, that is.

Marine had turned his attention to the human problem in Ohio, but nobody in Michigan paid much attention until World War I. In 1918 the Feds instituted a draft and insulted the state of Michigan: 30% of Michigan's draftees were disqualified because of goiter. Marine's large scale experiment in Akron, Ohio, showed that goiter was preventable. [ArIM 25:661, 1920] But Michigan's Dept of Public Health trusted neither Dock's 1895, nor Marine's 1907, work. They measured iodine in well-water and resurveyed many school children for goiter. They discovered that iodine in well-water varied inversely with incidence of goiter, just as Dock guessed in 1895 and Marine said in 1907. [JAMA 82:1328, 192–4]

A Simple, but Objectionable, Cure

At the instigation of the pediatric section of the Michigan State Medical Society, iodized salt was made available on a voluntary basis. Naturally there was an uproar of disapproval by the Federal authorities who, being illiterate, considered the food additive unsubstantiated. They were joined wholeheartedly by fundamentalist Christians who demanded to see one mention of iodine in the Bible. If God had meant iodine to be in salt he would have put it in. That pithy argument was answered by pointing out that God had put iodine in salt; the Salt Company Trust took it out.

A more difficult argument came from anti-iodine-adulteration kooks about ten years later. Goiter prevalence in school children had been cut to remarkably low levels, they admitted, but only half the salt consumed in Michigan was iodized. A veterinarian physician scotched that argument by pointing out that vets had been adding iodine to sheep, cattle, and poultry feeds since about 1910, and some Michigan kids ate lots of chicken.

Physicians in Michigan were highly impressed by the statistic that thyroidectomies for non-toxic goiter had fallen from 3.2% of all operations in 1927 to 1.0% in 1954. But then the reduction ceased — or was there more surgery for toxic nodular goiter? Was iodine doing more than preventing goiter?

From Iodine-Deficiency to Iodine-Excess

Marine's success in Ohio, confirmed in Michigan, took time to get around. In 1963 the Nutrition Institute of Brazil surveyed 886,217 school children and found up to 90% goiter in some areas. [JAMA, 1963] In Phortse, a village on the road to Everest, almost every inhabitant had goiter. [IAEA Bull. 1967] In Andean villages in Ecuador, 54% had goiter. [NEJM, 1969] 23% of Idjwi island in the Congo had goiter in 1971. [AJCN]

In 1949 a noteworthy iodine deficiency occurred in Tasmania. Iodized salt was impractical in salt rich Tasmania. Instead they gave each child 10 mg KI tablets and told them to take 1 each day. The tablets tasted bad and the kids did what should have been expected. 16 years and many goiters later, they admitted failure and started a new system: 2 ppm of potassium iodide was baked into all bread. Within three years (1960) the incidence of new goiter was the same in Tasmania as in 1969 Ohio — and Tasmanian bread didn't get stale for weeks.

The remarkable success in preventing goiter was reported by F. Clements (School of Public Health, U of Sydney). Eleven pages later in the same issue of Lancet, R. Connolly, from a hospital in Tasmania, confirmed the absence of colloid goiter. But he reported more than double the incidence of toxic nodular goiter — exactly what happened in 1954 Michigan.

To prove the point, a pathologist at the U of Michigan, D.K. Weaver, surveyed his department's surgical path slides. He pulled all the thyroid tissue slides from 1915–1920 (before iodine prophylaxis) and compared them with sections five, ten, and fifteen years after the introduction of iodine. Five to twenty slides from each of

2,642 thyroid glands were histologically reclassified to modern terminology.

> *"The salient histopathological feature ... before iodine prophylaxis (1915–1920) was the **paucity** of lymphocytes in parenchyma and, more important, the absence of thyroiditis in any form."*
>
> [AS 98:183, 1969]

After the introduction of therapeutic and prophylactic iodine, a steadily increasing incidence of "lymphocytic goiters" occurred.

White Bread Never Gets Stale

Around 1968 J.A. Pittman in Birmingham, Alabama, noticed that his "normal" thyroid uptakes seemed lower. He checked back ten years when he had used exactly the same technique. Upon statistical comparison an uptake of 29% in 1959 was the same as an uptake of 15% in 1968. He compared some carefully detailed patient histories to find what was suppressing their thyroid uptake. Only one thing stood out, most patients ate white bread. Pittman brought a slice from home the next day. It contained 150 micrograms of I-127, enough to suppress any thyroid gland. By careful inquiries (bakers did not know the substance added "to prolong freshness" was iodine) he determined that all batch-baked white bread in his area contained iodine. The doses would have been called "therapeutic" 10 years earlier. His 1969 "normal" thyroid scans were called "iodine suppression scans" in 1959. [NEJM 280:1431, 1969]

The first confirmation came from B.A. Sacks in New York. His patients, from the kosher Bronx, showed no decrease in thyroid °iodine uptake; they ate bagels. A companion study in Columbia, MO — few kosher bakeries, showed a 5–15% decrease in uptake. [BMJ 1:79, 1972] A study by N.P. Alazraki in San Diego, among Mexican-Americans who ate tacos, confirmed the Bronx study. [Rad 105:611, 1972] By 1976 Consumers Union noted "unusually high concentrations of iodine" in hamburgers (now a ubiquitous fast food). If Weaver's 1969 thesis is true, most American children, who devour hamburgers, will have nodular lymphocytic goiters. Many oncologists and health physicists said that the 1969 thyroid nodules were cancer precursors. If true, then thyroid cancer must now be USA's prime cause of death.

Anti-Radiation Pays Off

Toward the end of the 1960s a non-causal association was detected between neck irradiation in infants and later development of thyroid cancer in adolescence. It was a typical money-making hysteria: many adolescents who had the rare thyroid cancer had received neck irradiation, but of millions of children who received neck irradiation only a very few developed thyroid cancer. Following the usual scare headlines, Federal funds were distributed to study, assess, pass laws, appoint committees, and milk thousands of patients for unnecessary thyroid tests. By 1972 a more serious radiation scam was building up. In this one "victims" might make money (after lawyer's fees, of course).

From Nevada, according to Ban-The-Bomb dissidents, waves of lethal fallout were deposited on children's playgrounds in Utah. A New Mexico study reported to the newspapers that fallout went straight to the thyroid and caused nodularity-that-may-cause-cancer. A statistically controlled comparison in Arizona (out of the fallout wind pattern) with Nevada and Utah school children, showed no difference in incidence of thyroid nodularity. But all states showed much thyroiditis. [JAMA 233:1069, 1972] Therefore, concluded the study, we must look harder and search for cancer-please-send-another-grant. (And they got it from AEC.)

It was not coincidental that the increase in nodular thyroiditis occurred shortly after the introduction of iodine into bread. In 1963 E. Aston found that 51% of autopsies (in Boston) showed thyroid nodules. In 1965 W. London found bread the major source of I-127 in the diet. In 1967 the hot autonomous nodule was noted. In 1968 T. Oddie found 240–740 μg I-127 in US daily diet (compared to Marine's 40–80 μg/day in 1920). In 1975 Consumer Reports noted a >30× Recommended Daily Allowance of I-127 in fast foods. In 1977 R. Bubenhofer noted an increase in papillary thyroid cancer since I-127 prophylaxis. By 1978 the evidence was piling up that I-131 in high dose prevented the later development of thyroid cancer. But I-127 in high dose promoted nodules. The DOE had inherited AEC's excreta but no longer attempted scientific reasoning in Health Physics. [See Vig1985 .Rum]

THE NEW SI ROENTGEN

In 1969 the CIPM [See Vig1971 .7U] had to adjust the roentgen unit to fit SI requirements. They also acceded blindly to the disparagement of all ionizing radiation by the Oak Ridge covey of health physicists in the ICRP (Int Com Rad Protect). With inquisitorial zeal they dropped the "bad" name "roentgen." In order to protect all mankind from evil they called their adjusted roentgen an "X" unit, then disguised it in unmeasurable sieverts and political working levels. By 1984 a US District Court declared the honcho anti-radiation health physicist a liar and the "roentgen" again became respectable. But the old esu/cm^3 air still had to be converted to coherent SI C/kg. Its conversion depends upon IUPAC (Int Union Pure & Appl Chem) conversion factors. Using 1981 IUPAC tables, the "roentgen" in C/kg is by definition:

1 roentgen (r) = 1 esu/cm^3 of air

but an ion pair = $4.803 \ldots \times 10^{-10}$ esu

Hence,

$$1\ \text{r} = 2.082 \ldots \times 10^{9}\ \text{ion-pairs/cm}^3\ \text{of air}$$

but 1 cm^3 air = $1.293 \ldots \times 10^{-3}$ gram air

Hence,

$$1\ \text{r} = 1.610 \ldots \times 10^{12}\ \text{ion-pairs/gram of air}$$

Charge = 1.602 ... coulombs/ion pair

Hence,

$$1\ \text{r} = 2.579 \ldots\ \text{C/g air}$$

In 1957 the symbol "r" was changed to "R." In order to convert to SI units the gram had to be changed to kilogram, the coulomb was already a special SI name for the ampere•second unit charge. The "R" was changed back to "r" by SI rules.

Hence,

$$\begin{array}{l} 1\ \text{r} = 1.61025 \times 10^{12}\ \text{ion-pairs/g (air)} \\ \quad \times\ 1.60209 \times 10^{-19}\ \text{coloumbs/ion pair} \\ \hline \quad 2.57976 \times 10^{-7}\ \text{C/g (air)} \end{array}$$

But the fluctuations in IUPAC physical constants causes uncertainty in the second decimal place. There is no natural standard against which the roentgen must be compared. And, of course, kilograms must be used.

Hence, in 1975 the CGPM made the new roentgen unit *exact by definition:*

(They tend to unuse the word "roentgen.")

$$1\ \text{SI roentgen} = 2.58 \times 10^{-4}\ \text{old (1928) roentgens}$$

Hence,

$$1\ \text{roentgen} = 2.58 \times 10^{-4}\ \text{C/kg}$$

or 0.000 258 C/kg

or 0.258 mC/kg (millicoulombs/kg)

or 258 μC/kg (microcoulombs/kg)

Say it any way you like, the roentgen is still Paul Villard's 1908 measure of quantity of ionizing radiation, and it is still the only *measurable* unit.

CHRONOLOGY OF NUCLEAR MEDICINE — 1970

Scientific and Technical Background

			Ref.
1. Basic	— J. Bistirlich discovers H-4 in Los Alamos pion beam.	[1934]	PR
2. Obser	— D. Kuhl explains axial section emission scanning.	[1966]	JNM
	— F. Mishkin gives ??? advantages to minified scan images.	[1969]	AJR

Organizations and Internal Politics

5. AEC +	— Nuclear backward states sign Nuc Nonproliferation Treaty.	[1959]	AP
	— FRC is dissolved; Environ Protect Agency (EPA) formed.	[1959]	FR
	— ICRU Report #16 introduces concept of microdosimetry.	[1959]	
	— ICRU gives pro & con of Linear Energy Transfer (LET).	[1942]	ICRU
6. Socs	— R. Cloutier chairs Symposium on Rad Dose and Effects.	[1968]	AEC
7. Event	— Medi+Physics makes F-18 commercially available.	[1966]	

Instruments, Units of Measurement, and Drugs

8. Instr	— D. Goodwin attaches dual spectral gates for °nuc scans.	[1968]	JNM
	— G. DeNardo enhances scan display by computer techniques.	[1964]	JNM
	— E. Kaplan devises whole body scanning table for camera.	[1963]	JNM
	— M. Hayes supports validity of div-con collimator.	[1969]	Rad
	— M. Satterfield describes new solid-state med spectrometer.	[1965]	JNM
10. Concp	— M. Dixon: fast camera replaces precordial probe in RCG.	[1969]	JNM
	— M. Farmelant adapts dual reg-of-interest to renograms.	[1968]	JNM
11. Drugs	— G. Taplin achieves °TcHSA to replace °IHSA.	[1969]	JNM
	— J. Cooper proposes high sp act °TcHSA kit for CSF scans.	[1969]	Rad
	— S. Lorber tries 13.8h Zn-69m prostate & pancreas scans.	[1959]	JNM
	— M. Croll has instant label method for °TcMAA & °TcCuAA.	[1964]	JNM

Radioiodine, P-32, and Radioactive Therapy

12. I-Res	— T. Oddie says daily I-127 intake highly variable in US.	[1968]	JCEn
	— R. Connolly: toxicosis double with KI in Tasmania bread.	[1966]	La
	— N. Fleischer: plasma TSH up after injecting synth TRF.	[1968]	JCEM
	— P. Hoffer uses Am-241 as source for I fluorescent scans.	[1969]	JAMA
	— K. Sterling defines T3 toxicosis as separate dis entity.	[1967]	JAMA
13. I-Dx	— J. Bernard says lower uptake normal due to I-127 excess.	[1969]	JNM
	— H. Strauss scans hypos with 1 mCi °TcO_4 at 30m scan delay.	[1969]	Rad
	— W. Hung: irregular uptake in child's Hashimotos on scan.	[1964]	JP
	— C. Derghazarian finds 20% malig in 35 sol cold nodules.	[1969]	UMC
	— I. Murray uses Cs-131 to evaluate malignancy in nodules.	[1969]	BMJ
	— E. Voelkel devises calcitonin test for medullary ca.	[1963]	JCEn
14. I-Rx	— B. Hetzel controls I deficiency in Papua for 5y by IM "I-oil."	[1969]	MJA
	— J. Franco uses propanolol for Rx of 18 hyperthyroid pts.	[1969]	JNM
	— W. BEIERWALTES: LOWER DEATH RATE IN ca PTS GIVEN °I Rx.	[1968]	JAMA
	— S. Werner notes failures in I-125 Rx of hyperthyroids.	[1969]	La
15. P-Rx	— S. Corwin uses testosterone primer in prostate mets Rx.	[1967]	JU
17. Other	— R. Sellwood: Y-90 implants better than hypophysectomy.	[1965]	Bk

Scans and Other Tests of Function in Various Organs

18. Brain	— L. Zeigler notes hi-beta dose to chord in cisternograms.	[1969]	AEC
	— E. Heinz finds pattern in sympt occult hydrocephalus.	[1969]	Rad
	— A. James describes anatomy of cisternogram image of CSF.	[1969]	AJR
	— A. Das finds R transverse sinus dominant, most cerebral perfus.	[1969]	JNs
	— W. Hauser introduces °TcDTPA as new brain scan agent.	[1969]	Rad
	— H. Rosler: only 45% scan + in early CVA; 80% after 3wks	[1968]	SMW
	— R. Cowan finds subdur detection related to lesion's age.	[1969]	JNs
	— W. Obrish measures cer blood flow with carotid Xe-133.	[1969]	N
	— F. Simeone measures cer blood flow by Kr-85 washout.	[1969]	JAMA
	— S. Halpern sees scan pattern in herpes simplex encephalitis.	[1978]	JNM

19. Heart — M. Quaife finds Cs-131 cold spot scan + in some trauma. [1967] JNM
— Y. Yano shows good myocard uptake of 1.33d hi-E Cs-129. [1963] JNM
— R. Smith introduces 22.3h K-43 for hi-E myocard scan. [1963] SMJ
— P. Harper suggests thallium-199 but E poor for camera crystal. [1968] JNM
— M. Endo finds Quinn's coronary °IMAA perfectly safe. [1966] AHJ
ENDO INTRODUCES THE MYOCARDIAL CAPILLARY DISPERSION SCAN
— J. Conway pulls Polaroid snaps fast for perfus sequence. [1969] AJR
— B. Zaret shows clinical use, Braunwald's gated bld pools. [1962] NEJM
20. Liver — A. Cuaron finishes 2500 pt °AuCol amoebic abscess scans. [1964] JNM
83% detected on Ap; 95% detected on Ap & RLp;
97% detected on Ap & Pp; 99% detected on Ap, Pp, & RLp. [1967] JNM
— L. Samuels makes °I-RB scan part DDx children's abdom mass. [1966] SGO
— L. Williams says Dx is choledochal cyst from °I-RB scan. [1966] NEJM
One of few absolute diagnoses possible in Nuc Med. [1959] YB
— B. Sauerbrunn measures 220–800 nm particles in °TcSC kits. [1967] JNM
— M. Cohen finds >1 μm particles in °TcSC kits. [1967] JNM
— R. O'Mara: need many projections in Emerg Rm spleen scan. [1969] SGO
— C. McCARTHY COMPARES NUC SCANS WITH ULTRASOUND. BJR
21. Lung — R. Holmes sees diffuse pulm calcification on Sr-85 bone scan. [1967] JNM
— D. Preston: hot spot artifact due to aggregated °IMAA. [1969] JNM
— D. Cook nebulizes $°TcO_4$ for inhalation bronchography. [1968] JNM
— J. Miller measures °Xe regional func in normal breathing. [1969] ARRD
— G. DeNARDO BEGINS Xe-133 VENTILATION SCANS
IN Dx OF PE. [1968] NEJM
— Y. Yano uses 13 sec Kr-81m for lung function scan. [1969] JNM
22. Bone — L. Samuels sees extraosseous Sr-87m in child malignancy. [1969] AJR
— L. DuSauct: long (but not flat) bone lesions show °TcSC. [1969] Rad
— R. Polcyn interprets $°TcO_4$ scans in arthritic diseases. [1969] A&R
23. Kidney — M. Short uses camera for renogram. [1968] JNM
— W. Maxfield does camera scan & renogram in 104 neonates. [1966] AJDC
— W. Hauser introduces °TcDTPA for kidney and brain scans. [1969] Rad
— A. Rodrigues-A detects transplant reject on °I-Hipp clearance. [1969] JU
24. Gut — T. Jewett tries $°TcO_4$ gut scans as surgical aid. [1962] S
— R. Harvey measures stomach transit time with °meals. [1969] La
— A. Musso studies malabsorp with both $°VB_{12}$ & °folic acid. [1969] JNM
25. Blood — P. Benjamin gives new fast labeling method for °TcHSA. [1966] JNM
— L. Rubin proves central venous press bld vol method is wrong. [1968] AS
— D. Funk finds no diurnal variation of PIT in 45 normals. [1969] JNM
— S. Seidl measures platelet surviv time, 59 purpura pts. [1965] DMW
26. Other — D. Brown scans placentae with 5 pCi In-113m & ultrasound. [1968] JNM
— J. Siefert tries lymph node scans in known breast ca. [1963] FGR
— L. Rosenthall tries leg vein inject, °TcMAA for DVThrombosis. [1965] Rad
— C. Edwards uses Ga-67 scans to stage lymphomas. [1969] JAMA
— S. Vaidya confirms Ga-67 usefulness in abdominal tumors. [1969] La

Radiation Hysteria and Health Physics * Obituaries *

27. Hyst — J. Lima reports fifth case of ca after °I Rx for hyperthyrodism. [1968] JNM
— B. Dobyns finds 3 malig, 21 thyr atrophy in 67 Marshallese. [1966] JAMA
— L. Pauling proves that hi-dose Vit C cures anything. [1965] AP
28. React — R. Sampson finds 16% occult thy ca in lym nodes autopsy; [1963] ABCC
1 victim died with thy ca, others unaware of dis. [1969] Ca
— S. Jablon finds no increase in ca after in utero rad. [1926] La
— D. Grahn notes increased survival of mice after lo-dose. [1965] RR
29. Respo — J. Stanbury: no danger in a few rads of whole body rad. [1966] JNM

* * *

30. Obits M. Born (1882–1970) Ger math physics; nuclear theory. Bio

CHRONOLOGY OF NUCLEAR MEDICINE — 1971

Scientific and Technical Background

			Ref.
1. Basic	— L. Spencer studies "energy deposition in cavities" theory.	[1970]	AR
2. Obser	— J. Beaver can make °Tc-99m on cyclotron (but expensive).	[1954]	JNM
	— W. Burch detects Cerenkov light from P-32 in eyes.	[1969]	Na
	— M. Adatepe notes changed distribution with pH changes.	[1937]	IJAR
4. # Med	— E. Grigg estimates 5000 Nuclear Medics (most part time),	[1958]	
	4000 rectilinear scanners, 1300 cameras.	[1969]	JNM

Organizations and Internal Politics

5. AEC +	— G. Seaborg retires as AEC chairman; J. Schlesinger in.	[1947]	AEC
	— FDA requires I in salt in spite of nutritional excess.	[1970]	FDA
	— ICRU Report #9 defines terms in microdosimetry.	[1970]	ICRU
6. Soc's	— "Seminars in Nuclear Medicine" begins publication.	[1967]	Snm

Instruments, Units of Measurement, and Drugs

8. Instr	— J. Laughlin says Sloan-Kettering med cyclotron on.	[1965]	AP
	— M. Hayes develops 11 1/2" dia crystal camera.	[1962]	JNM
	— D. Kuhl shows scans on transverse section emiss scanner.	[1964]	Rad
	— P. Lauterbur finds way to visualize NMR spatially.	[1974]	ApR
9. Units	— FOURTEENTH CGPM ADOPTS "MOLE" AS SEVENTH BASIC UNIT.	[1965]	CGPM
	— CGPM allows "special name" coherent units (J, C, Hz, etc).	[1963]	NBS
	— I. Syed calculates 28.7h 268 keV Ba-135m dose constants.	[1966]	Rad
10. Concp	— P. Braunstein miniaturizes to maximize scan resolution.	[1970]	JNM
	— J. Keany finds large °Xe dose errors: adsorp on syringes.	[1970]	JNM
	— G. Freedman measures °TcSC loss in disposable syringes.	[1960]	Rad
	— S. Cohn gets total body Ca, Ba, Cl by in vivo neutron act anal.	[1969]	JNM
11. Drugs	— H. Winchell evaluates tin binder in °TcHSA preparation.	[1969]	JNM
	— J. Bassingthwaighte: I-125 antipyrine = body water agent.	[1963]	JNM
	— Y. Yano warns that aluminum from °cow agglutinates RBC.	[1969]	JNM

Radioiodine, P-32, and Radioactive Therapy

12. I-Res	— JAMA editorial recognizes T3 autonomous goiter as a disease.	[1968]	JAMA
	— F. Ashkar sees °TcO_4 trap time increase in hypothyroid patients.	[1968]	JAMA
	— M. Blum measures 2–32 mg I-127/slice of NY white bread.	[1970]	JNM
13. I-Dx	— G. Ghahremani changes "normal" uptake, 15–45% to 7–33%.	[1970]	JAMA
	— T. Mitsuma describes new RIA technique for serum T3.	[1963]	JCI
	— I. Chopra now measures serum [T3] by RIA method.	[1963]	JCI
	— W. Baxley now measures serum [TSH] by RIA method.	[1968]	AnIM
	— W. Hauser: °TcO_4 uptakes higher in Hashimoto than nod gland.	[1970]	AJR
	— M. Usher notes °I and °Tc scans do not always match.	[1969]	JNM
14. I-Rx	— N. Thallassinos: 63% relapse rate in drug Rx for hypers.	[1970]	La
16. Tele	— V. Abazov uses proton beams in teleRx in Dubna, USSR.	[1965]	AP
17. Other	— G. Sheline reviews Stone's 1948 fast neutron results.	[1982]	AJR

Scans and Other Tests of Function in Various Organs

18. Brain	— G. Taplin finds optimum scan delay time is 3 or 4 hours.	[1969]	JAMA
	— D. Kuhl shows samples of 1536 axial (emission) tomograms.	[1964]	Rad
	— D. Moody sees carotids in extended neck perfus position.	[1968]	JNM
	— F. DeLand sums Yb-169 DTPA cisternography on 125 pts.	[1970]	JNM
	— M. Mamau uses suboccip inject for cerebelopontine angle.	[1970]	PrM
	— D. Goodwin suggests 279 keV In-111 for cisternography.	[1970]	JNM
	— T. Milhorat does injection ventriculography with °IHSA.	[1969]	AN

19. Heart	— W. MacIntyre: tape of perfus gives Reg-of-Int playback.	[1966]	JNM
	— F. Wilcox: first card bl pool transmiss + emission scans.	[1968]	JNM
	— J. Goodrich measures chamber-to-chamber transit times.	[1969]	SF
	— H. STRAUSS INTRODUCES CARDIAC EJECTION FRACTION CALCULATIONS.		AJCr
	— E. Braunwald scans °IMAA in R cor, °TcMAA in L, sees both.	[1970]	Cir
	— N. Fortuin uses 15 nm spheres to see coron sinus filling.	[1969]	V89
	— W. Asburn uses 30–100 nm spheres to measure dispersion.	[1969]	V89
	— R. Gorlin shows uptake in ischemic areas in Kr-85 ARGs.	[1967]	Cir
	— J. Clausen: exercised ant tib muscle clears Xe-133 in 1m.	[1969]	CvR
20. Liver	— L. Rosenthall begins 4.5/1.5 min clearance ratio (°TcSC).	[1968]	Rad
	— P. Dovey checks cold spots on 48 °TcSC scans:	[1950]	
	25 patients had cirrhosis; 9 had hepatoma; 14 had no apparent cause.	[1970]	PRSM
	— A. Kagan diagnoses hemangioma with °AuCol + °IHSA.	[1968]	JNM
	— J. Hingran: scan better than Alk Phos & BSP in ca mets.	[1964]	JNM
	— H. Mundschenk says °AuCol and °TcSC yield different scans.	[1970]	JNM
	— J. Maksoud: stool counts more reliable than hepatogram.	[1964]	P
	— P. Mehnert displays obst jaund with °TcSC, °I-RB, & °IHSA.	[1970]	JNM
	— S. Jhingram compares BSP, Alk P, and scans in ca mets.	[1964]	JNM
	— R. Spencer: liver/spleen °TcSC ratio fails to Dx portal hyperten.	[1968]	Rad
21. Lung	— J. Burdine finds °TcHAM scans safe in 115 patients.	[1969]	JNM
	— M. Farmelant says °gas ventilation resolves PE problems.	[1970]	JNM
	— M. Arborelius: multi-seg-bronchial block affects perfus.	[1969]	SJR
	— T. Isawa shows perfusion loss in bronchial obstruction.	[1968]	Rad
	— K. Moser: combined ventilation/perfusion scans helpful.	[1968]	AnIM
22. Bone	— T. Chaudhuri: extraoss lesions need hours scan delay.	[1969]	JNM
	— G. Husby finds excess °TcO$_4$ uptake in inflamed joints.	[1970]	TNL
	— K. Collins notes corticoster effect on °TcO$_4$ hand scans.	[1970]	ARD
	— D. Van Dyke sees increased blood flow in myelofibrosis.	[1965]	JNM
23. Kidney	— F. Maher says I-125 iothalamate (Conray) is inulin type.	[1967]	MCP
	— G. Buckberg notes errors measuring bld flow with °HAM.	[1969]	JAP
	— W. Hauser introduces °Tc-Fe-ascorbic acid (kidney agent).	[1970]	Rad
	— L. Rosenthall does renogram study with °TcO$_4$ on camera.	[1970]	CMAJ
	— J. Sziklas estimates GFR with °Yb- & °In-DTPA & °C-Inulin.	[1970]	JNB
24. Gut	— D. Duszynski finds enough °TcO$_4$ in Meckel's to scan.	[1970]	AJR
25. Blood	— W. Tauxe sets $T_{1/2}$ for urine excr of °Cr-RBC @ 43–63 days.	[1966]	AJCP
	— P. Richards gives method for labeling RBC with °Tc.	[1969]	Rad
	— R. Wilson finds Cen Venous Press unrelated to blood vol.	[1968]	SGO
26. Other	— R. O'Mara sees uptake of Ga-67 in non-malignant lesions.	[1969]	JNM
	— J. LAVENDER SEES Ga-67 IN INFLAMMATORY & NEOPLASTIC LESIONS		BJR
	— Y. Ito sees °Ga in affected lymph nodes of 58 lung pts.	[1970]	Rad
	— R. Hayes sees Ga-67 in lysosomes by electron-micro-ARGs.	[1970]	JNCI
	— W. Beierwaltes scans adrenals (°I-choles) of Cushing pt.	[1969]	JAMA
	— F. Ashkar stimulates parathyroids (glucagon) for °Se scan.	[1964]	JNM
	— D. Alarcon-E scans 28 Sjogren's syndrome pts (°TcO$_4$).	[1965]	AJR
	— G. Schall does sequential scans in duct obst, Sjogren's.	[1968]	JAMA
	— S. Wax measures testicle blood flow with percut Xe-133.	[1967]	IU
	— M. Brucer survey: 80% of labs stop pancreas scanning.	[1970]	PL

Radiation Hysteria and Health Physics * Obituaries *

27. Hyst	— Many satisfied arthritis pts sit in Montana mines;	[1952]	AP
	state restricts pts to 90 min or 10–20 mr/d.	[1904]	AP
	— Cigarette advertising prohibited on radio & TV.	[1964]	AP
28. React	— E. Epstein tells of children who did NOT get rad ca.	[1970]	JAMA
29. Respo	— T. Hoshina: no F_1 leukemia in 22,442 children in Hiroshima.	[1969]	AJE

* * *

30. Obits	— F. Dessauer (1881–1971) Ger physics; first depth dose, point heat.		Str

CHRONOLOGY OF NUCLEAR MEDICINE — 1972

Scientific and Technical Background

			Ref.
2. Obser	— G. Brownell says thin crystal a serious camera handicap.	[1971]	IEE
	— B. Lagras finds some forms of data manipulation valid.	[1970]	JNM
	— J. Morales transmits scan display by phone.	[1970]	JNM
4. # Med	— J. McAfee notes 80 of 97 med schools have nuc med depts;	[1964]	
	4500 physicians in nuc med, 1200 full time;	[1960]	
	others 42% radiol, 33% intern, 15% pathol.	[1966]	SNM
	— F. Mettler: 3.3 million/y, US in vivo nuc med exams.	[1982](1985	JNM)

Organizations and Internal Politics

6. Soc's	— Am Bd Nuc Med certifies specialists in Nuc Med.	(1974	JNM)
	— British Nuclear Medicine Society organized.	[1962]	EJNM
7. Event	— J. AMBROSE INTRODUCES COMPUT AXIAL TOMOG (CAT SCANS).	[1971]	JAMA

Instruments, Units of Measurement, and Drugs

8. Instr	— E. Kaplan builds a whole body 3-strip bone scan table.	[1970]	JNM
	— W. Blahd finds scanner superior to camera (for F-18).	[1970]	Rad
	— T. Higasi builds semiconductor for multi °nuclide detect.	[1970]	JNM
9. Units	— ICRU updates "Radiation Quantities and Units," Rep #19.	[1971]	ICRU
	— B. Doust finds use of mg/kg invalid in angio & bld volumes.	[1959]	Rad
10. Concp	— S. Lane devises 3-way stopcock bolus inj (no BP cuff).	[1962]	JNM
	— F. DeLand extends "gating" concept to breathing.	[1968]	JNM
11. Drugs	— H. Winchell develops a kit for °Tc-tin-colloids.	[1971]	JNM
	— P. Richards develops a very high sp act °TcHSA prep.	[1970]	Rad
	— M. Staum: °TcSC flocculates with Al-ion in cow eluate.	[1971]	JNM

Radioiodine, P-32, and Radioactive Therapy

12. I-Res	— C. Thilly finds 32% goiter endemic in Congo, hi-uptake.	[1969]	AJCN
	— B. Sacks: Jews in Bronx eat bagels have normal °I uptake;	[1970]	
	gentiles in MO eat white bread have low °I uptake.	[1971]	BMJ
	— N. Alazraki says same for taco eating Mexican-Americans.	[1971]	Rad
	— A. Vagenakis sees Jod-Basedow in goiter pts fed KI.	[1970]	NEJM
13. I-Dx	— W. Gray devises 20 min Perchlorate Washout Test.	[1968]	JCEn
	— IAEA recommends <30min & 24h uptakes with thyr shield.	[1969]	IJAR
	— E. Mincey introduces Effective Thyroid Ratio (ETR) test.	[1971]	JNM
	— A. Ferraz sees auton hot nodules in 6.4% of 1643 scans.	[1971]	JNM
	— W. Van't Hoff sees 4h °I uptake about same as 20m °TcO$_4$.	[1971]	BMJ
	— M. Brucer requires 3 projections on thyroid scans.	[1970]	Bk
14. I-Rx	— W. Blahd: no relation between total dose and later hypo.	[1969]	ArIM
	— G. Krishnamurthy: remnants develop >5y after total surg.	[1971]	JNM
	— W. Mitchi notes 49% hypos 7y post partial thyroidectomy.	[1968]	BMJ
15. P-Rx	— C. Merrin: P-32 relieves pain in 7/8 prostate mets pts.	[1970]	JSO
17. Other	— J. Edwards tries °P-lipiodol in malig melanoma & skin ca.	[1963]	JNM

Scans and Other Tests of Function in Various Organs

18. Brain	— J. Quinn wants perfusion, first static, & 3h delay scans.	[1971]	JNM
	— A. Scleif notes vertex proj artifact: stomach (in child).	[1965]	JNM
	— D. Gilday sees perfusion & scan pattern in cereb inflam.	[1968]	AJR
	— G. Krishnamurthy correlates autopsy-2258 scans: 75% acc.	[1969]	JNM
	— E. Burrows finds 56% skull-floor lesions missed on scan.	[1971]	BMJ
	— F. Hosain suggests In-111 DTPA ideal in cisternography.	[1971]	BJR
	— A. Waltz describes methods for carotid °Xe blood flow.	[1970]	JNM
	— A. Bligh notes pattern on scan in herpes simplex enceph.	[1970]	JNN

19.	Heart	— D. Van Dyke resurrects precordial probe for portable EF.	[1954]	JNM
		— J. Parker develops new °TcHSA Ejection Fraction tech.	[1971]	JNM
		— L. Schwartz: narrow coronaries unrelated to °Xe washout.	[1970]	AJCd
		— K. Bennett sees exercise stress with K-43 serial scans.	[1971]	AHJ
		— C. Jansen shows L & R coronary fields with °Tc & °IMAA.	[1971]	JNM
20.	Liver	— 6 articles (e.g., J. Joyner) note °TcSC hot spot as real.	[1966]	JNM
		— M. Coel notes °Tc hot spot does not show on °I-RB scan.	[1970]	JNM
		— T. Chaudhuri: sm liver/lrg spleen/high BM is Budd-Chiari.	[1971]	JAMA
		— 8 articles (e.g., J. Christie) show A vs V kinetics.	[1967]	SNM
		— H. Neibling requires 24-48h °I-RB scan for obstruct Dx.	[1971]	AJSr
		— L. Gould sees "flying bat" pattern in Congest Heart Fail.	[1967]	JAMA
		— U. Scheffel uses °TcHAM to evaluate RES function (0.6 μm).	[1971]	JNM
		— M. Tubis describes cholegraphic agent: °Tc-penicillamine.	[1968]	JNM
		— J. Christie explains physiology of scan agents:	[1964]	
		A °AuCol void means a Kupffer's cell blockade,	[1967]	
		A °I-RB void means a polygonal cell blockade,	[1965]	
		A °TcSC void means perisinusoidal space block.	[1969]	SNM
		— °TcSC is perisinusoidal space, NOT Kupffer's cell agent.	[1969]	V33
21.	Lung	— H. Steinback: lung uptake of °TcSc can be Al contaminate.	[1971]	TM
		— R. Spencer: lung °IMAA retention $T_{1/2}$ is 7 to 31h in 20 pts.	[1970]	Tho
		— J. Burdine starts vent (°Xe) followed by perf (°Tc) scans.	[1971]	JNM
22.	Bone	— R. MARTY: sees bone mets (breast ca) on °Sr scans in February.		AJSr
		GETS IMPRESSIVE BONE SCANS WITH FIRST °TcPP IN MARCH.		JNM
		G. Subramanian shows °TcPP (PolyPhosphate) is safe in March.		Rad
		R. Marty learns in July that R. Perez used °TcPP in January.		(no pub)
		JAMA gives major publicity to a new bone scan in September.		JAMA
		G. Subramanian says °TcEHDP is an improved bone agent.		JNM
		F. Castronovo says °TcHEDSPA (diphosphonate) is better.		JNM
		Y. Yano says a new °TcEHDP is still better.		JNM
		A. Tofe says his (Proctor & Gamble) °TcEHDP is even better.		JNM
		— J. Quinn says kidney uptake of F-18 has no significance.	[1969]	JNM
		— J. Burdine measures bone absorption with I-125, Am-241.	[1968]	Rad
		— D. Lilien says °InCl is an ideal bone marrow agent.	[1969]	JNM
		— R. Knisley says there is no satisfactory b-marrow agent.	[1969]	Sem
23.	Kidney	— M. Dewanjee labels °Tc-tetracycline for kidney scan.	[1968]	JNM
		— S. Halpern labels °Tc-penicillamine as kidney agent.	[1971]	JNM
		— L. Chervu makes angiotensin RIA kit for renin activity.	[1965]	JNM
		— J. Conway: °TcO_4 in bladder shows vesicoureteral reflux.	[1968]	AJR
24.	Gut	— K. Lathrop finds 25% of IV °TcO_4 localizes in stomach.	[1971]	PNM
		— L. Rosenthall: 4 scans + for Meckel's vs 8 + on surgery.	[1971]	Rad
		— R. Shafer: °triolein absorption doesn't require pure fat.	[1968]	JNM
25.	Blood	— L. Sanchez-Medal: theory & math basis for °RBC survival.	[1966]	JNM
		— H. Atkins labels RBC in vitro (°Tc) for spleen sequest.	[1971]	JNM
26.	Other	— V. Chan: urine RIA for T3 & T4 is clinically acceptable.	[1971]	La
		— F. DeLand suggests hepatitis assoc antigen (HAA) for RIA.	[1965]	JNM
		— J. Nouel labels bleomycin with Co-57 as tumor agent.	[1983]	PrM
		— J. Pokoria finds symmetry of nodes by retrostern °AuCol.	[1970]	BLL
		— Z. Szendroi fails to scan prostate with °I-estradiols.	[1970]	La
		— H. Rossomondo describes lachrimal scintillography.	[1961]	AJO
		— R. Barnes takes rapid frames to see vein distribution.	[1978]	SF
		— R. Hayes details distribution of carrier-free Ga-67.	[1971]	JNM

Radiation Hysteria and Health Physics * Obituaries *

28.	React	— W. Sy measures °Hg in 18 week fetus, dose given mother.	[1969]	Rad
		— D. Grahn: lifetime lo-dose decreases leukemia in mice	[1970]	RR
		— S. Coan uses 50 Ci Pu-238 sources for tot body act analysis.	[1971]	JNM

* * *

30.	Obits	— B. Cassen (1902–1972) Am med physics; the scanner.	JNM
		— S. Berson (1919–1972) Am physician, radioimmunoassay.	AP

CHRONOLOGY OF NUCLEAR MEDICINE — 1973

Scientific and Technical Background

			Ref.
2. Obser	— A. Waxman calc relative economic value of Nuc Med procs.	[1966]	JNM
	— R. Hayes runs Diff Absorp Ratios on Einsteinium No. 99.	[1937]	Na

Organizations and Internal Politics

5. AEC +	— PRES NIXON ORDERS AEC SPLIT INTO REGULATION & PRODUCTION.	[1970]	AEC
	— AEC & FDA sponsor I-123 production, force use in med.	[1968]	JAMA
	— Dixie Lee Ray (Marine Biol) succeeds pol as AEC Chairman.	[1971]	AEC
	— FDA approves perchlorate after 6y use in brain scans.	[1967]	JNM
6. Socs	— Pakistan AEC establishes its Fourth Nuclear Med Center.	[1968]	JAMA
	— Harvard Med Sch offers course in Pediatric Nuc Med.	[1969]	JAMA
	— Brit J Rad (75th Anniversary) pubs hist of UK Nuc Med.	[1967]	BJR
7. Event	— "WET" NUC MED PROCEDURES HAVE LEFT NUC MED (EXCEPT T3 & T4).		PL
	— G. Hounsfield introduces the CAT scanner.	[1972]	BJR
	— EMI installs a CAT scanner in MGH; changes Radiology.	[1972]	AP

Instruments, Units of Measurement, and Drugs

8. Instr	— C. Lim: new positron detector: multiwire proport chamber.	[1972]	IEE
	— M. Ter-Pogossian compares semiconduct vs GM vs NaI(Tl).	[1972]	Rad
	— W. Ashburn adds a tape storage/playback on camera.	[1971]	JNM
	— P. Lauterbur pubs NMR pictures of 2 test tubes of H_2O.	[1974]	ApR
9. Units	— MIRD pubs method & dose from Se-75 meth & °Ga doses.	[1968]	JNM
10. Concp	— D. Watson devises rapid bolus injection of some °nucs.	[1965]	Rad
	— J. Muller states method of measuring instr dead time.	[1968]	NIM
	— S. Lynch shows circadian variation in rat plasma Fe-59.	[1968]	CS
	— P. Dewalde measures K-40 in 750 patients as a routine.	[1963]	JNM
11. Drugs	— F. Castronovo prepares 2.55m Ba-137 EDTA in closed syst.	[1960]	JNM
	— P. Raban: how to label Fe-free albumin microspheres.	[1969]	JNM

Radioiodine, P-32, and Radioactive Therapy

12. I-Res	— A. Keys remeasures BMRs after 20y, questions age effect.	[1963]	M
	— V. Caride finds rectal absorp of °TcO_4 diff than °I (dog).	[1964]	JNM
	— H. Atkins compares I-123 to I-131 on 100 thyroid scans.	[1968]	AJR
	— G. Vidor notes thyrotox epidemic after I added to bread.	[1972]	V91
	— B. Catz: 40% of thyroidectomies show lymphocytosis (Hash).	[1966]	SGO
	— C. Kirkegaard: nonlinear relation of °TcO_4 & °I uptakes.	[1971]	AE
13. I-Dx	— J. Mahlstedt sees °Tc scan wipeout from I-contrast-media.	[1970]	DMW
	— D. Koutras notes fast °Tc washout of autonom hot nodules.	[1972]	CE
	— R. Kirkland says 40% ca in 30 childhood sol cold nods.	[1970]	P
	— M. Brucer: 15m °TcO_4 and 24h °I scans have different uses.	[1971]	V91
14. I-Rx	— P. Bricout wants mCi °I dose scans post surg in thyroid ca.	[1966]	JCAR
15. P-Rx	— J. Gumpel reviews synovial effusion Rx, 77% success.	[1962]	ARD
16. Tele	— M. Schulz lists few 250 keV, 2500 Co-60 teletherapy machines, 50 22MeV betatrons, 250 linear accelerators.	[1968]	AJR

Scans and Other Tests of Function in Various Organs

18. Brain	— I. Meschan says °TcO_4 perfusion part of routine scan.	[1972]	Rad
	— D. Watson warns, minor valsalva blocks thoracic bld flow.	[1971]	Rad
	— S. Nordlander determines "brain death" with perfusion.	[1969]	JNM
	— P. Braunstein judges "brain death" from perfusion study.	[1969]	JNM
	— P. Alderson: 2 aseptic meningitis after cisternograms.	[1972]	JNM
	— T. Rudd finds clearance $T_{1/2}$ measures shunt function.	[1970]	JNM

19. Heart	— E. LEBOWITZ: 3.1d 167 keV Tl-201 IS MYOCARDIAL AGENT.	[1956]	JNM
	— H. Strauss introduces exercise modified myocardial scan.	[1972]	Rad
	— B. Holman localizes dog infarct with °Tc-tetracycline.	[1970]	JNM
	— F. Bonte says °Tc-oleic acid shows promise (but unstable).	[1970]	Rad
	— R. Chandra says cyclotr 3h Cs-134m is myocardial agent.	[1970]	JNM
	— H. Park adapts R-heart-only perfus to shunt detection.	[1971]	JNM
	— T. Miyamao sees sup vena cava obst with °TcO_4 perfusion.	[1970]	Rad
	— C. Jansen reports on 400 coronary dispersion scans.	[1971]	Rad
20. Liver	— G. Subramanian introdu °Tc-phytate as °AuCol substitute.	[1972]	JNM
	— J. Siemsen devises a thick crystal scanner to see °I-RB.	[1972]	JNM
	— T. Evans: °TcSC is a perisinusoidal space agent by ARG.	[1972]	Rad
	— W. Klingensmith evaluates lung uptake of °TcSC.	[1972]	JNM
	— 5 authors (e.g., Morita) report hot spots on liver scans.	[1972]	JNM
	— G. Evans reports on liver scan in abdominal trauma.	[1968]	JAMA
21. Lung	— L. Harding: about 0.15% vessels are blocked with °TcHAM.	[1971]	JNM
	— S. Inkley checks spirometry by °Xe over lung field sites.	[1969]	JNM
	— P. Hoffer says 36d Xe-127 superior to Xe-133 on camera.	[1970]	JNM
22. Bone	— N. Charkes: every clinical facet of bone scan seen on °Sr.	[1967]	Rad
	— R. Tilden locates °TcPP sites with microautoradiography.	[1967]	JNM
	— F. Hosain compares F-18, Sr-87m, and 3 °Tc agents.	[1969]	JNM
	— G. Berg notes °TcDP uptake in primary breast ca.	[1972]	Rad
	— D. Weber says °TcPYP requires 3h scan delay time.	[1971]	Rad
	— Y. Yano introduces the diphosphonate °TcDP agent.	[1969]	JNM
	— M. Blaufox devises °Tc-Sr-F (Fluorotec) to get F metab.	[1966]	Rad
	— Mallinckrodt introduces °Tc stannous pyrophosphate: °TcPYP.	[1972]	
23. Kidney	— A. Israelit sees GFR with subQ °I iothalamate (inulin).	[1971]	KI
	— R. Boyd starts using °Tc-glucoheptonate for kidney scan.	[1972]	BJR
	— 10 articles (e.g., Antoniades) scan various diseases.	[1969]	JU
	— M. Short uses gamma camera for a "quantified" renogram.	[1971]	BJR
	— C. Park says kidney image on °TcPP bone scan is valid.	[1972]	JNM
24. Gut	— T. Chaudhuri: do not use °TcO_4 to assess gastric acid.	[1972]	JNM
	— T. Berquist sees first adult with Meckel's on °TcO_4 scan.	[1972]	MCP
	— T. Berquist sees Barrett's esophagus on °TcO_4 scan.	[1972]	MCP
	— M. Fish rates plasma over stool assays for dual °VB_{12}.	[1970]	JNM
25. Blood	— D. Briedis introduces dual Co-57, -58 VB_{12} tests.	[1970]	JNM
	— G. Gillespie gives method for °Tc labeling of WBC.	[1969]	JNM
26. Other	— W. Carlton evaluates lachrimal drain dacryocystography.	[1972]	JNM
	— G. Dunson uses 0.1 μm minicol °TcSC for lymph node scans.	[1972]	Rad
	— W. Moore measures °Xe skin flow to fix amputation level.	[1970]	AS
	— J. Hartsuck adds lung scan to Deep Ven Thromb leg scans.	[1972]	BMJ
	— B. Rhodes follows distribution of °Tc-microsph in legs.	[1971]	AJR
	— J. Quinn injects °TcMAA (dual foot vein syst) to see DVT	[1970]	JNM
	— G. Duffy adds exercise to Deep Ven Thromb leg scans.	[1972]	BMJ
	— R. Cloutier finds whole body Ga-67 $T_{1/2}$ is 29d.	[1972]	JNM
	— R. Burleson locates abscesses with °Ga label leukocytes.	[1972]	AnS
	— G. Johnston gets Ga-67 scan + in 60% of 770 tumor pts.	[1971]	JSO
	— 7 articles (e.g., R. Blair) note Ga-67 uptake in infections.	[1971]	JNM
	— T. Maeda finds °Co-bleomycin uptake in liver tumor.	[1972]	Ri
	— Medi + Physics says °In-bleomycin uptake in 70% of tumors.	[1972]	

Radiation Hysteria and Health Physics * Obituaries *

27. Hyst	— L. DeGroot: 20 of 50 thyroid ca had childhood neck rad.	[1967]	JAMA
	— L. Zeitz measures S-35 uptake in human hair.	[1964]	IJNM
	— E. Kreps notes ninth proved case of thyroid ca post-I-131.	[1970]	JAMA
28. React	— D. Reinwein finds no risk of ca or leuk in 300,000 °I Rx.	[1970]	DMW
	— D. Bottino: lo-dose irrad yields increased plant growth.	[1972]	RBo

* * *

30. Obits —

CHRONOLOGY OF NUCLEAR MEDICINE — 1974

		Scientific and Technical Background		Ref.
2.	Obser	— R. Yaes: High Energy Physics is sterile from Gov't help.	[1970]	NS
3.	# Nuc	— COMMERCIAL NUCLEAR PHARMACIES BEGIN OPERATING.	[1954]	PL
4.	# Med	— M. Brucer estimates >10 million scans done in US:	[1963]	
		3.8M brain (decreasing), 2.0M liver, 1.6M thyroid,		
		1.3M bone (increasing), 1.2M lung, 0.1M kidney.	[1969]	PL
		Organizations and Internal Politics		
5.	AEC +	— Az Pharm Board demands a °pharmacist in every Nuc Med Lab.		PL
6.	Soc's	— Oak Ridge Nuclear Res Hosp (first in much) closed by AEC.	[1947]	AEC
		— Am Coll Nuc Physicians organized, incorp in Illinois.	[1970]	ACNP
7.	Event	— India becomes sixth power with peaceful nuc explosion.	[1967]	AP
		— J. Mallard (Aberdeen) decides to build NMR scanner.	(Smith 1980	BMJ)
		Instruments, Units of Measurement, and Drugs		
8.	Instr	— R. Cesareo builds 10 mCi Pu-238 biol trace nuc analyzer.	[1971]	MP
		— P. Steele builds a bedside Ejection Fraction instrument.	[1971]	BHJ
9.	Units	— W. Ney (Sec ICRU) redefines bolixed "special curies" units.	[1972]	Rad
10.	Concp	— J. Ehrhardt measures effect of scattering media on scan.	[1969]	JNM
11.	Drugs	— L. Colombetti produces 13s Kr-81m from °Rb cow.	[1969]	JNM
		— 12 articles (e.g., A. Romhilt) suggest ultrashort °nuclides.	[1968]	Cir
		— M. Davis uses Milli, Nuclepore filters to size °colloids.	[1969]	JNM
		— J. McRAE: °TcO_4 DISTRIB CHANGES AFTER STANNOUS INJECTION.	[1972]	JNM
		Radioiodine, P-32, and Radioactive Therapy		
12.	I-Res	— US FDA compiles I-127 in diet foods: most = 1–50 ng.		
		sea water = 50 ng/ml, sea food = 300–3000 ng/g,		
		I-table salt = 76 μg/g, kelp meal = 1.2 mg/g.	[1970]	FDA
		— D. Wood says 40 mg KI is optimal thyroid block (in ±6h).	[1970]	JCAR
13.	I-Dx	— J. Karelitz: oblique projections required for nodules.	[1972]	JNM
		— G. Shambaugh gets hot °TcO_4 but cold °I nod in 7/204 pts.	[1972]	JAMA
		— W. Kaplan finds 7/19 sol cold nodules malig; 3 are °Ga +.	[1973]	JNM
14.	I-Rx	— K. Burman: 1 of 54 auton hot nodules toxic, no Rx in 53.	[1973]	ArIM
		— W. Beierwaltes: thyroidectomy + °I is effective in 333 ca.	[1973]	AS
		— J. Siemsen notes I-125 Rx for hyper does not stop hypo.	[1970]	JNM
		— B. Dobyns finds °I Rx of hyper prevents later thyroid ca.	[1970]	PHR
		— Age restriction on °I Rx for hyper reduced, 40 to 25y.	[1969]	PL
15.	P-Rx	— C. Merrin gets P-32 palliation in 7 of 8 prostate mets.	[1972]	JSO
17.	Other	— I. Ariel reports ± results on 1000 Y-90 microspher pts.	[1967]	MO
		— R. Pozderac reports IV °IHSA no help in synovial effus.	[1964]	JNM
		Scans and Other Tests of Function in Various Organs		
18.	Brain	— R. Spencer compares perfusions and scans in 200 pts.	[1972]	JNM
		— G. Krishnamurthy evaluates EEG vs scans for false ±.	[1972]	ArIM
		— H. Wagner suspects reflux in neck veins in some perfus.	[1971]	JNM
		— R. Morin describes distribution and dose in cisternogram.	[1973]	JNM
		— R. Paxton compares 650 nuc scans on EMI-CAT scanner.	[1973]	Rad
19.	Heart	— P. Eldh modifies LAO (30° up-tilt) to see all chambers.	[1972]	Cir
		— F. Bonte says °TC-PYP deposits in infarct during first wk.	[1974]	Cir
		— B. Holman announces °Tc-tetracyc as myocardial agent.	[1970]	NEJM
		— D. Van Dyke measures Ejection Fraction on bedside instr.	[1972]	BHJ
		— L. Greenfield explains RCG hemodynamics with °Xe & °TcSC.	[1957]	Rad
		— F. Mishkin: InfVenaCava perfusion reflux is valve defect.	[1971]	BHJ

20. Liver	— F. DeLand notes at least 8 °I-Rose Bengal substitutes.	[1973]	JNM
	— R. Beihn subtracts °TcSC from °Ga scan to detect abscess.	[1973]	JNM
	— G. DeNardo snaps fast frame buildup of °TcSC trapping.	[1973]	Rad
	— A. Paraf injects °TcHSA into spleen for splenoportogram.	[1967]	SHP
	— M. Steinberg gives rectal I-131 for portal supply scan.	[1964]	SJG
	— D. McCauley documents pendulous breast artifact.	[1969]	JNM
	— J. Carey observes Xe-133 buildup on lung ventilation scan.	[1973]	JNM
	— H. Handmaker:slow bile flow causes °I-RB kidney uptake.	[1971]	JAMA
21. Lung	— R. Secker-Walker supps bronchoscopy with vent/perf scan.	[1972]	JP
	— 4 ARTICLES (e.g., J. Jacobstein) DESCRIBE VENT/PERFUSION SCANS.		JNM
	— M. Lin uses ultrasonic °TcCol nebulizer for inhalation scan.	[1970]	Rad
	— L. Heck: proper dose is about 60,000 particles injected.	[1973]	JNM
	— B. McNeil says normal perfusion scan rules out embolism.	[1970]	JAMA
22. Bone	— D. Weber repeats scan delay is most significant factor.	[1973]	AJR
	— M. Brucer repeats: X-Rays can also be false pos & neg.	[1967]	JAMA
	— J. Thrall describes normal variants on °TcPP bone scans.	[1967]	AJR
	— R. Frankel sees false norm °TcPP scan (uniform hi-uptake).	[1967]	Rad
	— G. Grames notes Diffuse Interstit Pulm Calcific on scan.	[1970]	JAMA
	— Y. Suzuki sees myosit ossific on °TcPYP scan, but not on X-Ray.	[1969]	Rad
	— T. Goergen says cold lesions are important on bone scans.	[1969]	JNM
	— R. Hattner says kidney picture is meaningful with °TcPYP.	[1972]	JNM
	— S. Miller: Paget's display with °TcDP same as for °F, °Sr.	[1973]	AJR
	— A. Tofe introduces Procter & Gamble's °Tc-Sn-EKDP.	[1973]	JNM
23. Kidney	— T. Lin compares 7 organomercurial kidney agents.	[1972]	JNM
	— O. Salvatierra studies °I-Hipp graph on 500 transplants.	[1970]	AnS
	— U. Meldoleski: °I-Hipp (clearance) & °YbDTPA(GFR), 3000 pts.	[1970]	NMS
	— P. Peters compares °I-Hipp & °Xe (washout) for blood flow.	[1970]	MMW
24. Gut	— W. Kirwan measures transit times with I-131 capsule.	[1970]	SJG
	— C. Wine says 14 proved Meckel's seen on $°TcO_4$ scans.	[1973]	JPSr
	— J. Chanard measures Ca-47 absorption by plasma level.	[1967]	JNM
	— A. Doscherholmen simplifies serum $°VB_{12}$ assay, 140 pts.	[1973]	JNM
25. Blood	— A. Ferrant says °Tc-tin RBC label is valid for volumes.	[1970]	JCPa
	— J. McRAE SAYS TIN IN °Tc-PYP CAUSES A 7 DAY RBC LABEL (RATS).		JNM
	— C. Ries studies °Cr-platelet survival in thrombocytopenia.	[1970]	AnIM
26. Other	— H. Denffer introduces dacryocystography on °Tc camera.	[1973]	AKO
	— D. WHITE: ULTRASOUND HAS REPLACED NUCLEAR PLACENTOGRAPHY.	[1970]	Bk
	— E. Norman scans parathyroids with °I-toluidine blue.	[1971]	ACSd
	— P. Eberstadt's HTO total body water gives H_2O/body wt.	[1952]	IJNM
	— W. Millar proposes °Tc-urokinase to see Dp Vein Thromb.	[1973]	La
	J. Silva notes Ga-67 detects 21 of 28 deep infections.	[1973]	JID
	— R. Greenlaw locates 78% of proved lymphomas with Ga 67.	[1973]	JNM
	— G. Johnston locates 90% of proved Hodgkin's with Ga-67.	[1973]	JNM
	— R. Villareal notes 6/30 false positive $°TcO_4$ mammograms.	[1973]	Rad
	— L. Goranson injec paraxiphoid °TcSC for lymphnode scans.	[1973]	AR

Radiation Hysteria and Health Physics * Obituaries *

27. Hyst	— B. Modan finds thyroid ca after childhood scalp irradiation.	[1973]	La
	— F. Becker notes 15 thyroid ca pts,necks irrad as child.	[1968]	AnIM
	— T. Hashizume says Jap genetic X-ray dose = 86.5 mRad/year.	[1972]	NIR
	— Ozone depletion in upper atmosphere is new media crisis.	[1971]	Sc
28. React	— D. Dobyns: 9 malig (50 expected) after 34,681 I-131 Rx.	[1973]	JCEM
	— L. Parker says 74 thyroid ca in Hiroshima, barely signif.	[1969]	AnIM
	— Bibliography of ABCC scientific papers 1947–74 published.		NAS
	— A. James first txtbk, Pediatric Nuc Med. (forbid 10y ago).	[1969]	Bk

* * *

30. Obits	— K. Fajans (1883–1974) Pol-Am p chem; isotopes.	V4
	— D. Tabern (1900–1974) Am chem; salesman of radioisotopes.	PL

CHRONOLOGY OF NUCLEAR MEDICINE — 1975

Scientific and Technical Background

			Ref.
1. Basic	— K. HUBNER SAYS IRRAD MICE ARE IMMUNOSUPPRESSED.	[1960]	IJRB
	— G. Kohler develops hybridoma monoclonal antibodies.	[1957]	Na
2. Obser	— M. Phelps measures Attenuation Coefficients for tissues.	[1969]	Rad
	— J. Jones questions validity of equiv point assumption.	[-1972]	PMB
	— G. Lugmair measures first Sm/Nd ratio in moon rocks.	[1980]	SN
4. # Med	— USSR Acad Med Sci calls for more Nuc Med res centers.	[-1972]	JAMA
	— 4473 °I Rx for hyperthy (1957–1975) at Karolinska.	[1974]	JNM

Organizations and Internal Politics

5. AEC +	— PRES FORD KILLS AEC WITHOUT CEREMONY (27y 18d OLD). ERDA & Nuc Reg Comm start with the same AEC people.	[1946]	SN
5. Pols	— ABCC disbanded with AEC, Rad Effects Res Found starts.	[1948]	RERF
	— IAEA has 110 member states, $40 mill budget, 1200 employ.	[1969]	IAEA
	— FDA Bur Rad Health attempts to force med use of I-123.	[1973]	FDA
	— FDA wants to regulate the new nuclear pharmacies.	[1984]	FR
	— FDA terminates "Kefauver" exemption of °pharmaceuticals.	[1963]	FDA
6. Socs	— S. Albert's textbk on "Blood Volume" pub (C.C Thomas).	[1959]	Bk
7. Event	— 150 power, 350 research reactors now in operation.	[1963]	IAEA

Instruments, Units of Measurement, and Drugs

8. Instr	— D. Kuhl adds computerized scanning to axial tomography.	[1973]	JNM
	— M. Ter-Pogossian introduces β^+ Emis Transaxial Tomogra.	[1973]	Rad
9. Units	— MIRD calcs rad dose from 7 °I, °Au, & 4 cardiac agents.	[1973]	JNM
	— CGPM (100th anniv) adopts Bq(s^{-1}), Gy(J/kg), X (the R,C/kg) says abandon Ci, Rad, R by 1985. (Wyckoff 1976	[1889]	NBS Rad)
10. Concp	— R. Bing ranks coinci & non-coin counting, Rb-81 vs K-43.	[1955]	JNM
	— M. Brucer explains Field-of-Vision in moving fields.	[1949]	V49
	— A. Kurisu notes Co-58 inhal accident; bio $T_{1/2}$ 11 & 78d.	[1967]	NIR
	— C. Christiansen measures bone minerals by photon absorp.	[1969]	SJCL
11. Drugs	— M. Lamson calculates amount of Tc in °TcO_4 from cow.	[1972]	JNM
	— P. Grant announces 1.25m β^+ Rb-82 from 25d Sr-82 cow.	[1969]	JNM

Radioiodine, P-32, and Radioactive Therapy

12. I-Res	— Consumer Reports notes >30× RDA iodine in fast foods.	[1974]	
	— B. Dobyns notes increase in pre-nodular thyroiditis.	[1970]	JAMA
13. I-Dx	— B. Paull finds °Tc trap in 51 Hashimoto cold nodules.	[1971]	Rad
	— K. Britton outlines strategy for using thyroid tests.	[1973]	BMJ
	— A. Burrows describes function tests in geriatric pts.	[1974]	BMJ
14. I-Rx	— R. Shafer notes a rare "thyroid crisis" after I-131 Rx.	[1942]	JNM
	— A. Safa uses hi-dose I-131 because all get hypo anyway.	[1972]	ArIM
	— A. Taft sees 42% pts euthyroid 15y after low dose I-131.	[1972]	La
15. P-Rx	— W. Ashburn says abd loculation is °P contraindication.	[1968]	JNM
17. Other	— J. Topp: 70% pts improved 2y after °AuCol knee effusion Rx.	[1974]	CMAJ

Scans and Other Tests of Function in Various Organs

18. Brain	— I. Jenkinson prefers °TcDTPA for brain scanning.	[1970]	INM
	— T. Irino finds scan + in CVA pts scanned within 24h.	[1971]	St
	— J. Sheldon sees only some tumors fill in arterial phase.	[1973]	Rad
	— J. Korein says no perfusion of IV bolus is "Brain Death."	[1973]	Cir
	— M. Heilbrin measures carotid °Xe region bld flow in TIA.	[1970]	Ns
	— W. Obrist measures inhaled °Xe regional blood flow.	[1972]	St
	— B. Rhodes: 3 aseptic meningitis pts after °InDTPA cistern.	[1972]	Rad
19. Heart	— B. Holman times infarct pick up of °Tc-Tetracycline.	[1974]	JNM
	— H. Strauss introduces °Tc-Glucoheptenate hot spot agent.	[1973]	JNM
	— E. LEBOWITZ INTRODUCES 3d 135–167 keV THALLIUM-201 AGENT.	[1953]	JNM

19. Heart	— M. Brucer: fast frames of IV bolus have replaced graphs.	[1970]	V78
	— P. Rigo combines myocard scan with bolus K-43 bld pool.	[1972]	Rad
	— D. Berman uses gated °TcHSA pools for Ejection Fraction.	[1974]	JNM
	— P. Cannon's cor bld flow is second phase slope °Xe washout.	[1973]	Cir
	— R. Pozderac injects °Xe in muscle, washout is bld flow.	[1971]	Rad
20. Liver	— H. Wellman explains bowel artifact over lower Rt liver.	[1974]	JAMA
	— T. Chaudhuri warns: surgery can't call scan false +.	[1972]	JAMA
	— I. Vido finds laparoscopy less accurate than °TcSC scan.	[1971]	DMW
	— 4 Japan articles (e.g., M. Abe) study °Tc-phytate scans.	[1973]	Ri
	— A. Gilson describes improved I-123 hepatobiliary agent.	[1974]	JNM
	— R. Baker announces °TcPyridox-Glut (°TcPG) as bile agent.	[1974]	JNM
	— E. Harvey describes °TcHIDA as a new bile agent.	[1974]	JNM
	— E. Eikman injects cholecystokinin to see patent duct.	[1974]	AnIM
	— P. Ell uses °CrRBC spleen scan to stage Hodgkin's dis.	[1974]	BJR
21. Lung	— 5 articles (e.g., D. Tow) compare angiog with scan for embolism.		PCD
	— G. DeNardo reviews 8 Xe & 3 Kr °nucs for ventilation.	[1946]	JNM
	— M. Siegel finds °TcDP collects in malig pleural effus.	[1968]	JNM
	— P. Johnson: dual liver-lung scan doesn't rule out lesion.	[1965]	Rad
22. Bone	— M. Majd recommends scans (not X-Rays) in child bone dis.	[1974]	AP
	— G. Subramanian introduces °Tc-Sn-MethyleneDP (°TcMDP) scan.	[1974]	JNM
	— G. Subramanian introduces °Tc-imidoDP as a new bone scan agent.	[1974]	JNM
	— D. Gilday uses early & 2hrs °TcMDP scans to see osteo.	[1970]	Rad
	— R. Letts: °Tc scan + before X-Ray in child osteomyelitis.	[1974]	SGO
	— D. Pistenma gets 17% false neg X-Ray, only 2% on scan.	[1974]	JAMA
	— W. Sy does °TcPP scans on 14 patients on renal dialysis.	[1970]	BJR
	— W. Sy reviews neglected "cold" lesions on °TcPP scans.	[1974]	BJR
	— A. Watkins does °TcHSA joint scans for popliteal cysts.	[1971]	BMJ
23. Kidney	— R. Arnold compares 17 agents used in kidney scanning.	[1974]	JNM
	— R. Kenny uses I-123 Hipp to derive a tubule trans time.	[1974]	BJR
	— R. Rohloff modifies °I-Hipp blood clearance method.	[1974]	NMS
	— B. Evans studies °I-Hipp vesicouret reflux on 136 pts.	[1968]	JU
24. Gut	— T. Berquist says $°TcO_4$ unlike °I in Barrett's esophagus.	[1973]	AJR
	— J. Ho uses $°TcO_4$ to find GI bleeding site (also Meckel's).	[1974]	Rad
	— M. Hyman monitors chronic g.leuk with $°VB_{12}$ serum levels.	[1974]	AJCP
25. Blood	— Mallinckrodt's °TcPYP tin content binds °Tc onto RBC.	[1974]	
	— 5 articles (e.g., A. Bardy) on in vivo °TcPYP RBC label.	[1974]	JNM
	— C. Bowring measures spleen °CrRBC destruction externally.	[1972]	JCP
26. Other	— N. Datta sees 23 intrascrot lesions by fast frame $°TcO_4$.	[1971]	JAMA
	— D. Stephens finds CEA (embryo antigen) poor in 956 pts.	[1972]	BJC
	— T. Ghose: °I-antibodies to mouse tumor localize on tumor.	[1972]	Rad
	— H. Brizel sees $°TcO_4$ on cornea in lacrimal flow (pinhole).	[1973]	Rad
	— R. Ghanadian sees prostate with °I-oestradiol in 4 pts.	[1972]	IJAR

Radiation Hysteria and Health Physics * Obituaries *

27. Hyst	— R. Conard notes 1 Marshallese myel leuk (175 rads @ 1y).	[1970]	JAMA
	— L. Hempleman's fourth survey: 5% rad induced thyroid ca.	[1974]	JNCI
	— S. Refetoff sees 6.8% thyroid ca post-neck irrad.	[1974]	NEJM
	— J. Arnold finds 3% thyroid ca in 1452 post-neck irrad.	[1974]	Rad
28. React	— RERF reports no excess brain tumors after Hiroshima.	[1974]	RERF
	— M. Rallison finds no "fallout" nodularity in 5179 children.	[1968]	JAMA
29. Respo	— A. Safa reviews °I Rx in children, says no age restrict.	[1974]	NEJM
	— P. Durbin: 4/16 pts given Pu-239, alive at 30y.	[1958] (1965	HP)

* * *

30. Obits	— W. Coolidge (1877–1975) Am phys; X-ray tubes.	Rad
	— C. Dunham (1907–1975) Am physician; dir AEC Biomed Div.	JNM
	— T. Evans (1917–1975) Am. radiobiol; med use of °nuclides.	JNM

CHRONOLOGY OF NUCLEAR MEDICINE — 1976

	Scientific and Technical Background		Ref.
1. Basic	— G. Seaborg redefines "element"; decay pattern is proof.	[1913]	Sc
2. Obser	— T. Hiraoka develops new tissue equivalent material.	[1975]	NIR
	Organizations and Internal Politics		
5. Pols	— FDA ADOPTS POLICY: NO DOSE OF RADIATION IS THE ONLY SAFE DOSE.	[1947]	FDA
	— FDA will regulate nuc pharmacies to stop new °drugs.	[1974]	JNM
	— Chinese Bomb fallout detected @ 500 pCi/L milk by ERDA.	[1974]	AP
	— FDA, ERDA, State AECs warn: "wash vegetables of fallout."	[1962]	AP
	— Medi+Phys says I-123 is available @ 10× cost of I-131.	[1975]	
6. Soc's	— European J Nuc Med starts publication.	[1971]	EJN
	— Clinical Nuc Med (Lippincott) starts publication.	[1971]	CNM
	— J. Krohmer: Am Assoc of Physicists in Med (AAPM) over 1100 members.	[1972]	Rad
	Instruments, Units of Measurement, and Drugs		
8. Instr	— H. Wagner converts VanDyke Instr into "Nuc Stethoscope."	[1974]	JNM
	— D. Ashby compares 15" with 10" camera screens in 20 pts.	[1970]	CNM
	— G. Cohen corrects field uniformity with flood source.	[1966]	Rad
	— H. Anger devises 80-lens camera for fast frame perfus.	[1970]	JNM
9. Units	— MIRD calculates °TcO_4 radiation dosimetry, Report #8.	[1975]	JNM
10. Concp	— M. Bruchez evaluates >500 keV Whole Body Scan response.	[1975]	EJN
	— M. Lye notes lower exchangeable °K in older (+65) adults.	[1973]	EJN
	— R. Bigler studies osteoporosis, changes to Ar-37 by nAA.	[1971]	INM
	— A. Guey proposes partial body (hand) neut Act Analysis.	[1971]	EJN
11. Drugs	— E. Aulbert localizes °Ga in lysosomes of rat liver cells.	[1974]	JNM
	— M. Loberg has new imindiacetic acid agents for °Tc tag.	[1972]	JNM
	Radioiodine, P-32, and Radioactive Therapy		
12. I-Res	— T. Gimlette: 5 methods of assessing function — no diff.	[1975]	JNB
13. I-Dx	— B. Schober: normal uptakes now @ 3–13% (4h), 7–26% (24h).	[1972]	CMAJ
	— T. Lemarchand analyzes TSH, T3, T4 in 50,000 patients.	[1972]	EJN
	— S. Berens finds °I & °TcO_4 mismatched in 8% of 237 scans.	[1973]	CNM
	— P. Alderson notes 17% ca in solitary cold nodules.	[1974]	Ch
14. I-Rx	— K. McCowen: no diff at y between low and high dose Rx.	[1975]	AJM
16. Tele	— J. Lawrence sums 17y good results in heavy particle Rx.	[1971]	JAMA
17. Other	— J. Cassar says 6/8 normals after pituitary °Au implants.	[1970]	BMJ
	— I. Bahous has success in 396 intra-articular injections.	[1975]	SMW
	Scans and Other Tests of Function in Various Organs		
18. Brain	— J. Burdine follows "luxury" perfus to normal, 3 CVA pts.	[1975]	Rad
	— H. Baltaxe says valsalva can obstruct sup vena cava.	[1974]	Rad
	— E. Yeh notes jugular reflux (arm down) in 6 pts.	[1974]	Rad
	— D. Hayt notes jugular reflux in 3.5% of 371 perfusions.	[1974]	JNM
	— W. Sy reappraises "doughnut & rim" signs in perfusions.	[1967]	CNM
	— M. MIKHEAL MARKS END OF STATIC NUCLEAR BRAIN SCANNING.	[1974]	RAD
	— A. Passalaqua: both °Tc & CAT scans better than either.	[1974]	CNM
19. Heart	— W. Walsh compares N-13 ammonia scan with °microspheres.	[1974]	Cir
	— B. Holman finds °TcPYP positive in hours post-infarct.	[1974]	JNM
	— K. Lyons finds °TcPYP fades 4–6 days post-infarct.	[1974]	CNM
	— H. Strauss modifies Tl-201 myocar distrib with exercise.	[1973]	JNM
	— F. Wackers finds Tl-201 positive 6 hours post-infarct.	[1975]	NEJM
	— J. Ritchie compares EKG with rest & stress Tl-201 scans.	[1973]	AJC

19. Heart	— H. Schelbert studies serial EF in 63 post-MI pts.	[1975]	AJC
	— M. Kan finds things on °TcO_4 perfusion not seen on scan.	[1974]	CNM
20. Liver	— S. Rosenthal scans 1688 (°TcSC); 21% false −, 23% false +.	[1975]	DD
	— U. Ryo: false defect on Ap is due to kidney impression.	[1975]	CNM
	— W. Klingensmith explains lung & renal °TcSC uptake (rats).	[1974]	JNM
	— M. LORBERG: NEW BILIARY AGENT, IMINODIACETIC ACID, °TCIDA.	[1975]	JNM
	— G. DeNardo: new bile agent, pyridoxylideneglutamate, °TcPG.	[1975]	Rad
	— H. Kubota compares °TcPG with °I-RB as biliary agents.	[1975]	JNM
	— A. Syrota does splenoportograms; injects °TcHAM, °TcRBC.	[1974]	G
21. Lung	— A. Maseri measures pulmonary bld vol @ 10% of total vol.	[1974]	AJC
	— A. Gottschalk finds POblique projections better than Pp.	[1969]	Rad
	— B. McNeil develops ventilat/perfusion strategy for PE.	[1974]	JNM
	— M. Lin describes °TcColloid inhalation scans in COPD.	[1974]	Rad
	— A. Bertrand sees mucocilliary transport with °Tc-aerosol.	[1974]	EJN
22. Bone	— R. Spencer develops °Tc-imidodiphosphate as bone agent.	[1975]	BJR
	— G. Methlin finds 17% of pre-op breast ca scans positive.	[1973]	EJN
	— G. Geslein: 200 stress fractures (°TcPP) not seen on X-Ray.	[1975]	Rad
	— J. Alexander displays scans in the maxillofacial region.	[1973]	JOS
	— J. Sebes displays 108 scans of the shoulder region.	[1970]	Rad
	— C. Beckerman displays 40 normal hand & wrist scans.	[1971]	Rad
	— L. Rosenthall: scan neg 3-d post-trauma R/Out fracture.	[1968]	Rad
	— T. Ryerson: a 50y old fracture is still positive on scan.	[1968]	CNM
23. Kidney	— G. Subramanian introduces °Tc-Sn-acetylcystein for scan.	[1975]	EJN
	— N. Vanlic-R introduces °Tc-DMSA (dimercaptosuccinic acid).	[1974]	EJN
	— P. Johnson describes scans of kidney bed in first minutes.	[1974]	Rad
	— J. Conway compares direct/indir vesicoureteral reflux.	[1972]	JNM
	— J. Kuikka does card output & renal bl flow with °I-Hipp.	[1975]	EJN
	— J. Kolfnska studies static & dynamic °I-Hipp in newborns.	[1975]	EJN
24. Gut	— J. Meyer uses °TcSC chicken liver meal for Gast Emp Time.	[1974]	AJD
	— A. Doscherholman: eggs in meal inhibit VB_{12} absorption.	[1975]	BJH
	— 3 articles (e.g., T. Berquist) use °TcO_4 to see Meckel's.	[1975]	JNM
25. Blood	— P. Richards prepares a °TcRBC labeling kit.	[1975]	JNM
	— A. Segal gives method for labeling leukocytes with °In.	[1969]	La
	— H. Glenn gives method for labeling leukocytes with °Tc.	[1983]	INM
26. Other	— B. Lentle notes salivary gland °Ga uptake after radioRx.	[1971]	JCAR
	— Y. Kim sees °Ga uptake in 12% of normal breasts.	[1974]	Rad
	— T. Chaudhuri shows °TcO_4 dacryocystograms in 50 pts.	[1974]	CNM
	— G. Edge injects °AuCol, °TcSb subQ, sees mamm lymph nodes.	[1973]	IJO
	— D. Hayt injects °TcMAA in feet, follows on moving bed.	[1973]	Rad
	— A. MacDonald follows foot vein °TcMAA with lung scan.	[1973]	BJR

Radiation Hysteria and Health Physics * Obituaries *

27. Hyst	— EPA: MPD for Rn in water is 5 μCi/L; outlaws Maine.	[1971]	JAMA
	— N. Kochupklai: backgnd is 1.5–3.0 r/y in Kerala, India.	[1976]	Na
	— Ill rad health unit spots Ra dial watch in bank vault.	[1959]	JAMA
	— M. Favos finds 5.7% thyroid ca in necks irrad in childhood.	[1975]	NEJM
	— FDA mandates shielded syringes in spite of evidence.	[1976]	FDA
28. React	— D. Piers: I-131 Rx protects against later thyroid ca.	[1970]	La
	C. Lushbaugh can't find any malformed infant from irrrad parents.		ca
	— E. Hahn notes radiation aspermia is transient & reversible	[1964]	Rad
	— S. Sarkar finds no genetic effects in hi-dose °I Rx pts.	[1969]	JNM
	— N. Berlin finds no cancer from any medical irradiation.	[1973]	JNM
	— H. Planel notes lo-dose increases paramecium population.	[1973]	IAEA

* * *

30. Obits	— G. Whipple (1878–1976) Am physician; first use of °Fe in hematol.		JAMA
	— F. Bauer (1917–1976) Am physician; first scan interpretations.		JNM

CHRONOLOGY OF NUCLEAR MEDICINE — 1977

	Scientific and Technical Background		Ref.
4. # Med —	R. Hayes estimates 250,000 Ga-67 scans done this year.	[1968]	PL

Organizations and Internal Politics

5. Pols —	ERDA (Ener Res Devel Admin) changes name after 2y 8mon.	[1975]	AP
—	New Dept of Energy (DOE) absorbs ERDA & Nuc Reg Comm (NRC).		AP
6. Socs —	European Society of Nuclear Medicine organized.	[1972]	EJNM
7. Event —	Many articles compare nuclear, CAT, & ultrasound.	(e.g., 1976	Rad)
—	RADIOIMMUNOASSAY IS CLIN PATH; NO LONGER CONSIDERED NUCLEAR MEDICINE.		
—	Nuc Med declared official med specialty in W Germany.	[1972]	JAMA

Instruments, Units of Measurement, and Drugs

8. Instr —	W. Hinshaw shows a human wrist by Nuclear Mag Resonance.	[1974]	Rad
—	Z. Cho develops a $Bi-Ge_3O_{12}$ crystal for B^+ detection.	[1975]	JNM
—	An Emission Cat Scanner (ECAT) announced by CLEON.	[1975]	
—	N. Lassen ties 254 crys-phototubes to computer bld flow.	[1963]	JNM
—	B. Legras modifies isocount lines to present scan image.	[1948]	ENM
9. Units —	ICRP & ICRU propose unmeasurable sievert (Sv) unit.	[1962]	ICRP
—	Am Environ Soc recommends using "rad" not "rem" unit.	[1962]	HPN
—	V. Krishnaswany measures dose around I-125 (0.8 nm) source.	[1973]	Rad
—	L. Berklet calculates °Zn nuclides dosimetry in man.	[1973]	HP
10. Concp —	P. Murphy: hi-count rate camera electronics are emerging.	[1976]	JNM
—	P. Hoffer sees very large field cameras emerging.	[1976]	JNM
—	K. Krohn sees very short-lived °pharmaceuticals emerging.	[1974]	IJAR
—	Y. Najean notes circadian rhythm in plasma °Fe turnover.	[1973]	ENM
—	A. Warbick shows errors in particle sizes below 100 nm.	[1974]	JNM
11. Drugs —	H. Susskind measures body Xe-133 retention after inhale.	[1973]	JNM
—	Y. Yano develops a new 25d Sr-82 to 1.25h Rb-82 B^+ cow.	[1975]	JNM
—	J. Dunnick has lipid-protein vesicles, contain °nuclides.	[1976]	JNM
—	C. Beckerman notes end of °Bleomycin, °Ga is better.	[1973]	Rad
—	H. ATKINS DETAILS Tl-201 CHARACTERISTICS IN HUMAN BODY.	[1976]	JHHB

Radioiodine, P-32, and Radioactive Therapy

12. I-Res —	M. Hochstein sees a hypo (Hashimoto's?) pt become hyper.	[1975]	JAMA
—	S. Strand finds diff geometric, optic & spectrometric depths.		ENM
—	R. Bubenhofer finds more pap ca since I-127 prophylaxis.	[1972]	SMW
13. I-Dx —	P. Hooper sets new normal 24h uptake at 0–24% in Wisconsin.	[1976]	JAMA
—	P. Hooper finds Wisc I-127 ingestion at 0.2–1.5 mgl/day.	[1974]	JAMA
—	E. Wong says Minn uptakes up again with less dietary I.	[1969]	JAMA
—	S. Wu describes a new RIA for T2 blood concentration.	[1965]	JCEn
—	S. Shukla: °TcO_4 uptake decreased with 4 mg/cm^3 Al contam.	[1972]	ENM
14. I-Rx —	R. Caplan: excess dietary I-127 prevents I-131 ablation.	[1942]	JNM
—	T. McEwan calcs 0.59 rads/mCi to bone-marrow after I-131.	[1976]	BJR
15. P-Rx —	S. Alderman notes prophylactic success of intracav P-32.	[1973]	OG
—	G. Mathe says P-32 PVA Rx as good as chemoRx on trials.	[1961]	NEJM
17. Other —	O. Metz gives prophylac intrathecal °Au to 26 leuk children.	[1966]	DMW

Scans and Other Tests of Function in Various Organs

18. Brain —	NIH confirms Dx of cerebral "brain death" by perfusion.	[1975]	JAMA
—	K. Mettinger: °I-fibrinogen detects carotid sclerosis.	[1968]	La
—	F. Hahn details scan in hyperostosis frontalis interna.	[1973]	Rad
—	J. Wittes says scan not useful in lung ca mets to brain.	[1959]	JAMA
—	E. Silberstein says Wittes methods were inadequate.	[1969]	JAMA
19. Heart —	J. Downsy: °TcPYP hot in exper contused myocardium (dogs).	[1976]	JNM
—	R. Prasquier sees diffuse °TcPYP in 14% of non-cardiacs.	[1976]	Cir
—	J. Soin sees diffuse °TcPYP in 9% of pts after bone scan.	[1976]	Rad

19.	Heart	— P. McLaughlin tests reproducibility of 25 Tl-201 scans.	[1976]	Cir
		— R. Burrow sets automatic edge detection for Ejec Fract.	[1976]	JNM
		— S. Bacharach builds blood pool gated image by computer.	[1975]	JNM
		— J. Idoine injects 4h Rb-81 as internal cow to get 10^5y Kr-81, washout of Kr-81 is proportionate to bld flow.	[1975]	JNM
		— D. Hantowich milks 5s Ir-191m from Os-191 for first pass.	[1974]	Rad
20.	Liver	— M. Davis uses °Tc-phytate for true Kupffer's cell scan.	[1975]	IJAR
		— G. Subramanian prepares °Tc-pyridoxals as °I-RB substit.	[1976]	INM
		— M. Kato makes 2 new hepatobiliary agents (amines).	[1976]	JJN
		— B. Wistow compares IminoDiacetic Acid (IDA) bile agents.	[1976]	JNM
		— A. Salvo finds 35 pts with focal nod hyperplas (°TcSC).	[1973]	Rad
		— M. Ahmad finds Xe-133 in fatty livers of 15 patients.	[1974]	JNM
		— M. Brucer publishes history of Nuclear Hepatology.	[1954]	Bk
21.	Lung	— H. Dworkin says true dose is "number of particles."	[1974]	JNM
		— H. Simon gets vent/perf mismatch without pulm embolism.	[1976]	CNM
		— G. Taplin develops aerosols for inhalation scans.	[1976]	JNM
		— Smoke inhalation leaves X-Rays neg but °Xe scans +.	[1965]	JAMA
		— M. Rubin finds 40% of lung scans for PE not diagnostic.	[1974]	JAMA
		— H. Atkins says 36d Xe-127 scans better than 5.3d Xe-133.	[1973]	JNM
22.	Bone	— F. Mishkin says bone scans are NOT a screen for mets.	[1976]	JAMA
		— Z. Chayes says bone scans ARE a screen for metastases.	[1975]	JAMA
		— R. Shafer chooses scans over X-Ray, bld chem in prost ca.	[1964]	CNM
		— W. Sy scans hands of 463 pts referred for bone diseases.	[1976]	JNM
		— M. Gelfand finds °TcEDTA pos in 16/19 child with osteo.	[1975]	JAMA
		— M. Madsen measures bone minerals by photon absorption.	[1975]	IR
23.	Kidney	— D. Rothwell: renogram field sees vesicoureteric reflux.	[1976]	La
		— J. McAFEE COMBINES °Tc-GLUCOHEP SCAN & °I-HIPP RENOGRAM.	[1975]	JNM
		— A. Taylor uses °Tc-penicillamine for cortical scans.	[1972]	JU
		— R. Hattner's serial °I-Hipp scans separate ischem & fail.	[1974]	JNM
		— A. Piepsz measures GFR from °TcDTPA kid & heart washout.	[1974]	ENM
24.	Gut	— T. Chaudhuri: °TcO_4 in mucosal, not pariet & chief cells.	[1973]	Rad
		— J. Miskowiak locates gut bleed site with plasma °TcHSA.	[1975]	La
		— D. Loebl measures relative blood loss after aspirin.	[1975]	JAMA
25.	Blood	— M. Welch prepares Ga-68 labeled RBC and platelets.	[1976]	JNM
		— D. PAVEL FOLLOWS COLD Sn-PYP WITH °TcO_4 FOR IN VIVO RBC LABEL.		JNM
26.	Other	— N. Tonami introduces Tl-201 as gen malig tumor agent.	[1976]	CNM
		— G. Johnston finds °Ga scans 88% positive in Hodgkin's.	[1976]	JNM
		— R. Hayes describes uptake mechanism of °Ga.	[1971]	JNM
		23 articles (e.g., A. Niden) on °Ga scans in various dis.	[1973]	JAMA
		— P. Eberstadt gives established body water distrib value.	[1974]	INM
		— G. Morris can't fit °I-fib DVT scans to autopsy finding.	[1968]	BMJ
		— J. Christianson tests arterial flow (legs) with Tl-201.	[1973]	ENM
		— F. Mishkin gives method for °TcO_4 scrotal scans.	[1975]	AJR
		— T. Pertynski shows oviduct patency with Xe-133 in NaCl.	[1967]	ENM

Radiation Hysteria and Health Physics * Obituaries *

27.	Hyst	— E. Paloyan says 20 pts irrad for acne, 12 get thyroid ca.	[1975]	AD
		— Worker awarded $75,000 by court because he "feared" rad.	[1961]	FR
		— ICRP adopts ALARA principle in praise of ignorance.	[1959]	
		— H. Simpkins calculates danger to pathologists in °autopsy.	[1952]	NEJM
28.	React	— 29 letters protest Simpkins' miscalculation; he retracts.		NEJM
		— H. Schwartz: risk/benefit ratios cannot be calculated.	[1982]	RAD
		— Drinking 10,000 liters water/d gives ICRP H-3 limit.	[1959]	IAEA
		— R. Evans sums 1930s Ra dial & IV Ra Rx story: bioeffects were some maligs, few leuks, ~50% hormesis.		(TransAmClinClimatolAs)

* * *

30.	Obits	— H. Blumgart (1895–1977) Am physician; first Nuc Med procedure.		NEJM

CHRONOLOGY OF NUCLEAR MEDICINE — 1978

Scientific and Technical Background			Ref.
2. Obser	— R. Mahon explains fluid dynamics of angiographic inject.	[1973]	Rad
4. # Med	— B. Rogers estim 10% of hosp pediatric pts get °nuc test.	[1975]	ApR
Organizations and Internal Politics			
5. Pols	— FDA use of °Tc, I-131, I-123 goes against expert advice.	[1973]	JNM
	— S. Larson explains red tape for FDA phase I, II, III.	[1956]	JNM
7. Event	— K. Hetzel: NM, X-ray, CAT, ultrasound converging to one.	[1977]	PL
	— Symposium on Natural Radiation Environment in Brazil.	[1980]	Bk
	WE BEGIN TO REALIZE THAT NORMAL LIFE IS RADIATION "HOT."	[1905]	
Instruments, Units of Measurement, and Drugs			
8. Instr	— T. Hill scans 6 pts with Cleon ECAT instrument.	[1977]	Rad
	— D. Kuhl pushes positron ECAT instrument for scanning.	[1977]	JNM
	— G. Brownell scans C-11 on MGH positron camera.	[1975]	JNM
	— M. Ter-Pogossian makes fourth positron emission (PET) instr.	[1975]	RAD
9. Units	— S. Bushong calculates doses in pediatric Nuc Med.	[1975]	HP
	— H. Wyckoff reports ICRU meeting on new units.	[1977]	Rad
	— H. Adler proposes a *de minimus* dose, a legal trifle.	[1977]	HP
	— C. Parmentier measures dose to lymphs with °Tc label.	[1987]	JNM
10. Concp	— C. Metz's ROC analysis defines sensitivity & specificity.	[1977]	Sem
11. Drugs	— P. Grant asks:is Sr- to Rb-82 cow influenced by carrier?	[1975]	JNM
	— B. Holman uses 21.7d W-178 to 9.3m Ta-178 cow system.	[1977]	JNM
	— G. Ehrhardt uses 288d Ge-68 cow for pure 68m Ga-68 B^+.	[1967]	JNM
	— Y. Suzuki discusses preparation and use of pure I-123.	[1973]	NIR
	— W. Pettit finds 2 particle sizes in °TcHSA tin colloids.	[1975]	JNM
Radioiodine, P-32, and Radioactive Therapy			
12. I-Res	— M. Rukuchi finds Tl-201 uptake in goiter and cold nods.	[1977]	JJN
	— J. Patton compares fluorescent with emission scans.	[1970]	JNM
	— D. Baldwin: thyroid disease incidence in Conn is 5.8%.	[1968]	JAMA
	— H. Kammer sees hyper nodule disappear after TSH stimula.	[1966]	JNM
	— K. Ohara measures °I in perspiration (Rx pts) @ 12 mCi/h.	[1963]	JJN
13. I-Dx	— S. Sostre notes changing uptake values from 1967–76.	[1977]	JAMA
	— H. Dige-Peterson: 16% mismatch in °TcO_4 and I-123 scans.	[1973]	ENM
	— A. Isman develops fully automated RIA for serum T4.	[1977]	CC
14. I-Rx	— A. Hayek: only 5 child cases of post-°I "storm" known.	[1975]	JP
	— A. Toft reports 20% hypos after subtotal thyroidectomy.	[1972]	NEJM
	— H. Lessig reports 77–89% success in °I Rx of cardiac pts.	[1960]	AR
	— C. Gorman restricts °I to over age 40 pts to prevent ca.	[1945]	AnIM
	POST-°I Rx CANCER HAS BEEN PROVED FALSE FOR >10 YEARS		
	— S. Von Hofe asks: does °I Rx or diet I-127 cause hypo?	[1977]	JNM
15. P-Rx	— M. Potsaid: 20% pts with prost bone pain relieved by °P.	[1977]	JNM
17. Other	— R. Pezner reviews intracav °AuCol Rx for ovarian ca.	[1968]	ca
	— I. Ariel cures a rhabdomyosarc by inj Y-90 intralymph.	[1968]	INM
	— J. Kutzner treats bone pain from prost mets with Sr-89.	[1942]	INM
Scans and Other Tests of Function in Various Organs			
18. Brain	— G. Gergans adds cereb perfusion dynamics to all statics.	[1976]	JAMA
	— B. Bok notes jugular reflux caused by arm position.	[1976]	ENM
	— T. Sargent introduces °I-catecholamine as new scan agent.	[1975]	JNM
	— E. Breitschuh: acoustic tumor not seen on CAT, EEG, sonic.	[1976]	Nr
	— C. Karlin sees herpes simplex enceph over temporal lobe.	[1972]	Rad
19. Heart	— 25 articles (e.g., J. Ritchie) discuss various Tl-201 scans.	[1977]	AJCr
	— O. Blood does °Tl in exercise, then after redistribution.	[1976]	Cir
	— 13 articles (e.g., D. Kelly) discuss various °TcPYP scans.	[1977]	ANZM

19. Heart	— K. Barth examines °TcPYP in graded myocard injury (dogs).	[1975]	Rad
	— 13 articles (e.g., P. Ell) try other ways to see myocard.	[1975]	BHJ
	— J. Thrall notes Tl-201 replacements (e.g., fatty acids).	[1973]	JNM
	— 17 articles (e.g., W. Ashburn) discuss Ejection Fraction.	[1977]	PCD
	— J. Berger measures right ventriclular ejection fraction.	[1976]	AJCr
	— H. Hecht measures EF and wall motion on first pass.	[1977]	JNM
	— U. Raiker measures 12 normal inf vena cava transit time.	[1974]	ENM
20. Liver	— L. ROSENTHALL REPLACES °I-RB WITH °Tc-HIDA (BETTER IMAGE).	[1977]	CJS
	— B. Wistow compares 6 new HIDA derived biliary agents.	[1977]	Rad
	— M. Friedman compares CAT with more sensitive °TcSC scans.	[1978]	CNM
	— U. Scherer prefers °Tc-phytate to CAT in diffuse dis.	[1977]	ENM
	— C. Henke notes hot spots in sup vena cava obstruction.	[1977]	CNM
	— J. Sutherland notes Xe-133 uptake in 15 fatty livers.	[1977]	JCAR
21. Lung	— G. Coates says perfusion followed by Xe-127 is best.	[1977]	JNM
	— D. George: lower dose from 36d Xe-127 than 5d Xe-133.	[1977]	JNM
	— D. Allen: microsph toxicity related to no of particles.	[1977]	JNM
	— G. McIlmoyle devises portable °Xe trap for exhaled °Xe.	[1977]	Rad
	— G. Schall finds long °Xe retention in 67 burn patients.	[1976]	JAMA
	— E. Turbiner sees *Pneumocystis Carinii* on °Ga scan (AIDS).	[1985]	Rad
22. Bone	— B. Lund scans fracture healing for 24h with °TcPYP.	[1976]	AOS
	— C. Aprile: °TcPYP in pleural effusions needs calcium ion.	[1974]	ENM
	— N. Hammond says °TcPYP scan + in 28% of pre-op breast ca.	[1976]	CA
	— Brit Breast Group says scans + in 10% of breast ca.	[1976]	BMJ
	— M. O'Connell says bone scan + in 34% pre-op breast ca.	[1976]	MCP
	— D. Tow scans jaws of 25 pts with dental diseases (°TcDP).	[1975]	JNM
23. Kidney	— 6 articles (e.g., R. Fleay) push °TcEDTA for renal scans.	[1977]	AuR
	— W. Jakubowsici compares 12 kidney agents, likes °TcGluc.	[1977]	ENM
	— R. Johanson compares °InDTPA with I-125 iothalamate GFR.	[1977]	ENM
	— P. Belitsky locates renal ca with °I-antitumor antibody.	[1975]	Rad
24. Gut	— B. Cooper: serious problems with serum $°VB_{12}$ measures.	[1975]	NEJM
	— V. Jovanovich measures gut absorp with oral °Ca & IV °Sr.	[1974]	ENM
25. Blood	— C. Ricketts reviews clinical status of °ferrokinetics.	[1969]	CNM
	— F. HEGGE ANNOUNCES °TcPYP IN VIVO & IN VITRO RBC LABELS.	[1977]	JNM
	— A. Segal finds rad damage in In-111 labeled leukocytes.	[1976]	JNM
26. Other	— 32 articles (e.g., P. Hoffer) on Ga-67 use and uptakes.	[1975]	JNM
	— R. Chavis times lachrymal flow with °TcSC in saline.	[1976]	AO
	— A. Alavi uses °Tc-Sn-Phytate subQ for lymph node scans.	[1976]	JNM
	— C. Tountas uses $°TcO_4$ to scan bld flow to hands & wrists.	[1977]	MnM
	— N. Tonami finds Tl-201 an effective malig tumor agent.	[1977]	CNM
	— D. Goldenberg uses °CEA & gonadotropin to locate tumors	[1975]	Sc

Radiation Hysteria and Health Physics * Obituaries *

27. Hyst	— J. McKillop reports laryngeal ca 8y after 60 mCi I 125.	[1974]	La
	— E. Browning sees hi-contam from liquid I-131 Rx doses.	[1954]	JNM
	— J. Cerletty finds 3% "rad induced" thyroid ca (evidence?).	[1977]	AS
28. React	— ABCC SUMS 110,000 BOMB VICTIMS: LEUK IS ONLY BIOEFFECT.	[1975]	RERF
	— D. Hoffman finds no evidence that I-131 causes cancer.	[1977]	NEJM
	— W. Beierwaltes follows 22,000 °I Rx pts; no leuk, less ca.	[1976]	Sem
	— G. Raulston notes kidney damage only in hi-dose monkeys.	[1976]	Rad
	— C. Gorman (Mayo) says no age restriction on I-131 use.	[1975]	JAMA
	— J. Cerletty scans 1825 childhood neck irrads, neg result.	[1976]	AS
29. Respo	— Peking China group finds no cancer in 10y after °I Rx.	[1976]	CMJ
	— H. Schwartz finds no bioeffects in pregnancy <50 rads.	[1976]	JAMA
	— G. Andrews: no histo damage to liver with 395 mCi °AuCol.	[1971]	Rad

* * *

30. Obits —

CHRONOLOGY OF NUCLEAR MEDICINE — 1979

	Scientific and Technical Background		Ref.
3. # Nuc	— G. Seaborg devises superheavy element Table: to Z = 168.	[1976]	Sc
	— M. Brucer revises Trilinear Chart to include 2452 nucs.	[1968]	Bk
	Organizations and Internal Politics		
5. Pols	— NRC accepts 500 hrs training for Cardic Nuc Med License.	[1955]	NRC
	— Pres Carter's mandatory hospital cost control defeated.	[1984]	AP
	— NRC finds lo-level waste has become a public phobia.	[1965]	AP
6. Socs	— Nuc Med sixth labor dispute: Brachy, Tele, Thy, RIA, Chemo, Heart.	[1956]	SNM
	— SNM pubs "Heritage of Nuc Med" (31 historic articles).	[1978]	SNM
	— ICRP pub #30 changes from crit-organ to whole-body risk.	[1959]	ICRP
7. Event	— H. Pendergrass tells polite History Of West Rad Soc.	[1976]	Rad
	Instruments, Units of Measurement, and Drugs		
8. Instr	— First ECAT scanner to UCLA, second to ORNL, third to Orsey France.	[1978]	AP
	— R. JASZCZAR INTRODUCES SPECT (SINGLE PHOTON EMIS COMP TOMOG).		SNM
	— M. Frick compares Emis CAT & X-ray CAT (favors ECAT).	[1978]	JNM
	— W. White (Searle): 10" camera has peak sensit & resolu.	[1976]	Rad
	— R. Vogel builds 7-pinhole collimator for cardiac tomog.	[1976]	AJCr
9. Units	— 16th CGPM defines candela unit of luminous intensity.	[1960]	NBS
	— J. McAfee does °TcDTPA distrib for MIRD dose studies.	[1976]	JNM
	— S. Turner calcs °TcSC: 0.5 rem/mCi (liver), 1.0 (spleen).	[1978]	Rad
11. Drugs	— M. Osborne labels liposomes (°Tc) for lymph node scans.	[1978]	INM
	— B. Holman uses 27d W-178 — 9.3m Ta-178 cow, for first pass.	[1973]	Rad
	— R. Neirincks tags MAA with 65 keV Ta-178 for lung scans.	[1978]	JNM
	— T. Ku suggests 8.3h Fe-52 to 21m Mn-52m cow for B^+ scan.	[1977]	Rad
	Radioiodine, P-32, and Radioactive Therapy		
12. I-Res	— I. Flickinger says no uptake change of hypers 1965–1977.	[1978]	JAMA
	— J. Oppenheimer finds T3 major cell functional hormone.	[1976]	Sc
	— J. Weiner gives natural history of Plummer's disease.	[1913]	CNM
13. I-Dx	— S. Halpern says dose must be high to detect thyroid met.	[1973]	JNM
	— C. Sawin asks, does TSH level increase with age? (Yes).	[1976]	JAMA
	— A. Lipson finds T3, T4 higher in 209 older women.	[1976]	JNM
	— Y. Kim finds T3, T4, TSH subnormal after neck irradiation.	[1969]	Rad
	— M. Fukuchi notes high Tl-201 uptake in 37 of 37 goiters.	[1978]	JNM
14. I-Rx	— L. Reynolds reports few successful medical Rx in Graves.	[1971]	ArIM
	— D. Slingerland reports 76% antithyroid drug remissions.	[1971]	JAMA
	— J. Freitas: I-131 Rx choice in children on 20y followup.	[1978]	JNM
15. P-Rx	— D. Roberts: 34/46 good, 6/46 poor results in Rx of mets.	[1974]	CNM
	— R. Lanning reports °P Rx in choroid hemang & mal melano.	[1972]	AJO
	Scans and Other Tests of Function in Various Organs		
18. Brain	— D. Tanasescue finds °TcGluc best scan agent in 859 pts.	[1978]	Rad
	— J. Keyes soaks skulls in °TcSC to make scan models.	[1961]	Rad
19. Heart	— C. Morehouse studies image degradation by heart motion.	[1968]	Rad
	— B. Holman reports sequential perfusions with Ta-178.	[1976]	Rad
	— M. Quaife: °TcPYP in pericard fluid of 3 breast ca pts.	[1964]	JNM
	— R. Sonnemaker finds Tl-201 good as ECG for angio screen.	[1977]	Rad
	— J. Beck devises a Tl-201 myocard bkgnd correction (dog).	[1977]	JNM
	— Denver Group (P. Steele) popularizes stress Ejec Fract.	[1977]	AHJ
	— J. Ritchie begins "exercise followed by redistribution."	[1978]	JNM
	— R. Slutsky measures LV vol on a gated blood pool.	[1977]	Cir

20. Liver	— J. Snow prefers °TcSC over CAT and Ultrasonics for ca.	[1978]	AJR
	— M. Kan attempts to calc liver vol from °TcSC ECAT scans.	[1978]	JNM
	— W. Klingensmith finds °TcIDA better than °TcPIPIDA scans.	[1978]	Rad
	— J. Blackwell uses °I-Ioglycamic acid for biliary scans.	[1978]	ENM
	— R. Shafer evaluates Xe-133 uptake in livers (fatty).	[1978]	JNM
	— M. Ahmad notes hi-Xe-133 in 45 biopsied fatty livers.	[1978]	JNM
	— R. Armas scans spleen only with heat-denatured °TcRBC.	[1975]	Rad
21. Lung	— D. BIELLO GIVES PE HIGH, INDETERMINATE, LOW PROBABILITY.	[1977]	AJR
	— R. Kelly: in lung ca pts: 5% liver, 7% brain, 14% bone mets.	[1977]	JAMA
	— G. Tisi says scans replace regional bronchospirometry.	[1974]	ARD
	— M. Short prefers °Tc-aerosol over Kr-81m for function.	[1977]	JNM
	— J. Shepard: pulm vasodilator has no affect PE scan (dogs).	[1977]	JNM
22. Bone	— P. Matin finds fractures scan + in 72h; 90% clear in 2y.	[1978]	JNM
	— I. Khalkhali notes °TcPYP uptake in heel & tarsal joints.	[1976]	JNM
	— N. Charkes sums up the mechanisms for skeletal uptake.	[1973]	JNM
	— J. Hunt sees muscle damage with °TcPYP in electric burns.	[1974]	JT
	— D. Front: 35% pre-op breast ca pts have pos °TcMDP scan.	[1978]	JAMA
	— R. Komnki: 40% pre-op breast ca pts have pos °TcPYP scan.	[1978]	AJR
	— M. Nakama uses Tl-201 to distinguish malignant lesions.	[1978]	JJN
23. Kidney	— J. Clorius assesses 50 renal grafts with °TcO_4 & °I-Hipp.	[1974]	JNM
	— C. Alberts does I-125 absorptions in 38 pts under dialysis.		ENM
	— I. Arlat shows °I-Hipp, °In-EDTA, °TcDTPA in renal hyperten.	[1967]	CR
	— J. Leonard prefers °Tc-Glu over IVP to see renal SOL.	[1978]	JNM
	— H. Kohn stresses value of lateral proj in kidney scans.	[1976]	ENM
	— C. Hotte measures °I-Hipp in vitro stability, 92% in 28d.	[1977]	JNM
24. Gut	— T. Rudd shows esoph reflux of °TcSC milk in 20/25 child.	[1976]	Rad
	— S. Heyman localizes gut bleeding site with °TcRBC scan.	[1977]	S
	— A. Newcomer has C-14 triolein breath test for malabsorp.	[1968]	G
25. Blood	— J. Konet detects no effect on suvival after tin RBC tag.	[1975]	JNM
	— P. Chisholm notes cell damage after hi-dose °In WBC tag.	[1976]	JNM
26. Other	— 24 articles (e.g., S. Sarkar) on varieties of Ga-67 scans.	[1977]	JNM
	— J. Robertson: dacyro scans give 0.1–0.4 mRads/μCi °TcO_4.	[1978]	Rad
	— R. Boedecker diagnoses 23 swollen scrotas with °TcO_4.	[1977]	JP
	— S. Kogan finds a false negative scrotal torsion scan.	[1977]	JU
	— P. Bently prefers X-Ray to °TcMAA venography.	[1976]	BJR
	— K. Hubner scans C-11 amino acids for B^+ ECAT pancreas.	[1971]	JNM
	— L. Berger says ultrasnd replaces °nuclide pancreas scans.	[1971]	La
	— W. Kaplan prefers °Tc-Sb-sulfide to °Tc-Sn-sulf for lymph.	[1978]	JNM
	— G. Ege compares °Tc-Sb-sulf to °Tc-phytate lymphography.	[1978]	BJR

Radiation Hysteria and Health Physics * Obituaries *

27. Hyst	— THREE MILE ISLAND BECOMES DISASTER BY NRC & NEWSMEDIA GOOFS.		PL
	Windscale discharged 20,000 Ci I-131 — nobody hurt!	[1957]	AP
	TMI discharged 17 Ci I-131, unmeasurable in people,	[1977]	PL
	Gov evacuates town, J. Califano (HEW) orders KI cure.	[1977]	HP
	— Pres Carter fires expert, adds $50 million & anti-nukes to NRC.		AP
	— Col State pols prohibit ALL °active waste disposal, until they learn they can't legislate against nature.	[1978]	AtE
	— T. Warner says his pt's ca caused by 30 mCi °I 18y ago.	[1978]	La
	— H. Maxon says use I-123 because I-131 is dangerous.	[1978]	JAMA
	— I. Bross. leukemic damage at 1 rad (bkgd) expos level	[1978]	AIP
28. React	— RERF: excess mult myeloma only in exposures $\gg$ 100 rads.	[1970]	RERF
	— RERF: aging is myth, survival effects only $\gg$100 rads.	[1957]	RERF
	— Adm. Rickover finds less ca in rad workers than expect.	[1976]	SN
	— B. Tribukait: no breast feeding dose, after 2 mCi °TcMAA.	[1972]	AR
29. Respo	— B. Cohen finds rad is low in public's "Catalog of Risks."	[1960]	HP

* * *

30. Obits	— G. Taplin (1910–1979) Am physician; lung scanning, °colloids.		JNM

HOW INTERNATIONAL UNITS ARE DETERMINED

(Le Systéme International D'Unités is Designated SI in All Languages)

Whether you like it or not, in a few years you will use only SI units. The last body to change will be US Congress. That doesn't matter because they authorized a metric system in 1866 — but did not make it mandatory. The marketplace is rapidly mandating SI units. The units on a bottle of wine were the first to "go metric" (c1980). Then sales of metric wrenches increased. Then the popular caliber of handguns and most cosmetics went metric. By 1985 practically every scientific journal in the field of Nuclear Medicine had begun changeover to SI units. However, the system is not yet fully metric. If you think our generation's change of units is difficult, think of and pity the generation that attempts to convert the 360° circle or duodecimal clock face. Because you will be talking in SI units for the rest of your life you should know how the decisions are made.

Reform of Units of Measurement Begins

Around 1789 a new United States started reform of units by adopting a metric coinage. In 1795 the Paris Academy of Sciences devised a metric system of measurement based on the meter. They realized that such a system had to be universal to be fully useful and began a long period of selling the idea. The effort culminated in 1875 with a diplomatic meeting in Paris. The Treaty of the Metric Convention was signed by 17 nations (including the US) and a *Bureau International des Poids et Mesures* (BIPM) was set up in Paris as a scientific laboratory.

The diplomats also began the task of organizing a *Conférence Générale des Poids et Mesures* (CGPM) to give political clout to the BIPM's standards. The first CGPM was held in 1889 and defined the meter and kilogram with prototype standards made by the BIPM of a new platinum-iridium alloy. They also defined the "second" as a fraction of the mean solar day, and the centigrade temperature scale. That is all any CGPM does. It defines units. The BIPM makes standards. Individual governments are responsible for the use of these standards.

During the golden age of science (1820–1940) defining units was not simple. Every technology multiplied its units into a glorious confusion. Each sub-unit in this hodgepodge could be derived from some combination of length, mass, time, current, temperature, and light intensity. During World War II many scientists had time to think about the confusion of units. After the explosion of atomic energy, with another load of new units, it seemed important to clear up the whole mess.

Decisions Are Not Democratic Compromise

Historically the most important decision of the first *Conférence Générale des Poids et Mesures* (CGPM) in 1889 had been that their conclusions were incomplete and might be flawed. [See Vig1889 .CGP] The third CGPM (1901) corrected the first CGPM's "weight vs mass" terminology error. The seventh CGPM (1927) modified the definition of the meter and considered electrical standards. The eighth (1933) took up photometry standards.

After a lapse of 15 years during World War II, the ninth CGPM (1948) made a fundamental decision that would change the language of all sciences and much commerce. They instructed their scientific arm, the *Committee International des Poids et Measures* (CIPM), to study the feasibility of a new *coherent* "System of Units." ("Coherent" in metrology means all derived units are multiples of basic units without numerical adjustment.)

In 1950 the tenth CGPM announced a coherent 6 basic unit system that encompassed all measurements and invited comment. The eleventh (1960) CGPM formally adopted the six basic unit *Systéme International d'Unités* — abbreviated *SI* in all languages. The chemists soon objected: no combination of 6 basic units could express "the *amount* of a chemical substance." At the 1971 fourteenth CGPM a seventh basic unit, the mole, was added.

From the beginning the diplomatic conferees realized that no small group of persons could be expert in all sciences. They would need consultants. After World War II, determination of internationally acceptable "Weights and Measures" had become an interlocking hierarchy from individual scientists to national laboratories to governments:

72 GOVERNMENTS. Each member nation of the CGPM appoints delegates to meetings. It may or may not make a Unit of Measurement the law for its people.

CONFÉRENCE GÉNÉRALE DES POIDS ET MESURES (CGPM). Delegates from 72 member nations meet every six years and may recommend the adoption of Units to their governments. They approve or reject reports from the CIPM. They make the final decisions on Units of Measurement. (But only governments can make units legally binding.)

COMMITTEE INTERNATIONAL DES POIDS ET MESURES (CIPM). The technical arm of the CGPM meets èvery two years and has 18 delegates from 18 different member nations. They make no decisions but advise the CGPM and supervise the BIPM. They may appoint ad hoc Consultative Committees for expert advice.

CONSULTATIVE COMMITTEES in various specific scientific fields (meter, time, electricity, radiation, etc) meet at irregular intervals. The chairman of each ad hoc committee is a member of the CIPM. They make no decisions but advise the CIPM.

BUREAU INTERNATIONAL DES POIDS ET MESURES (BIPM). The scientific laboratory of the CIPM is located near Paris on international territory (ceded by the French government). It is funded by the CGPM and is responsible for:
— establishing primary standards & scales
— comparing international standards
— determining physical constants
— coordinating measurement techniques.

NATIONAL LABORATORIES (National Institute of Standards & Technology, formerly National Bureau of Standards, in the US) maintain each country's secondary standards. They provide standardization and calibration services for commerce, feed data to the CIPM, and do research in metrology.

VARIOUS NATIONAL AND INTERNATIONAL SCIENTIFIC SOCIETIES. The International Union of Pure and Applied Chemistry (IUPAC), Internat Com on Rad Units (ICRU), Standardization in Hematology (ICSH), etc, any scientific body that relates to measurements, may and does feed data and its needs into the system.

THE INTERNATIONAL MECHANISM
FOR MAKING DECISIONS
ON WEIGHTS AND MEASURES
("Poids et mesures" in a local dialect)

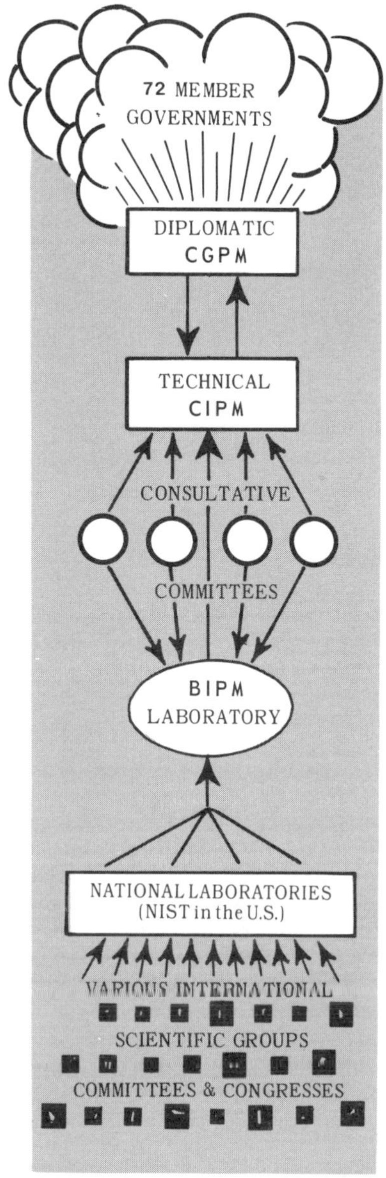

The SI system is not perfect. (Look at a clock.) The CGPM has made and will continue to make mistakes; but it is set up so that eventually it corrects its own mistakes. The CGPM is not impervious to stupidity (witness the immeasurable fads in radiation safety). But the CGPM is the only organization we have for determining universal Units of Measurement.

[See Vig.1977 .SI, SI Units]

PREFIXES BECOME ACCEPTABLE

(They Adapt SI Units to Every Science)

Prefixes from the Latin, *milli, centi, deci,* represent a thousandth, hundredth, and tenth of any unit; those from the Greek, *deca, hecto,* and *kilo* represent ten, hundred, and a thousand. With adoption of SI units at the Eleventh Conférence Générale des Poids et Mesures (CGPM), prefixes from *pico* to *tera* became part of the system. At the twelfth CGPM in 1964, *atto* and *femto* were added. At the fourteenth in 1971, prefixes were felt to be complete for "practical" measurements:

deca	da	10^1	deci	d	10^{-1}
hecto	h	10^2	centi	c	10^{-2}
kilo	k	10^3	milli	m	10^{-3}
mega	M	10^6	micro	f	10^{-6}
giga	G	10^9	nano	n	10^{-9}
tera	T	10^{12}	pico	p	10^{-12}
peta	P	10^{15}	femto	f	10^{-15}
exa	E	10^{18}	atto	a	10^{-18}

Remember: The CGPM was set up as an international **diplomatic** body to meet needs of **practical** commerce. Scientists are only technicians who screw up the works by demanding consistency merely to be sensible. Witness: the successful substitution in about two years of *liters* for *quarts,* without any explanation by the USA liquor industry. Compare this with substituting *km/hr* for *miles per hour* by strident bureaucrats. Over the age of twenty, the human mind is seldom changed, especially over something as ingrained as pounds and mph. Fortunately, the old ducks eventually die off and minds under age 20 are imprinted with a new dogma which, in another lifetime, might be just as silly as the old.

An unfortunate and confusing exception to uniform terminology of prefixes in SI units occurs in the unit of mass. The unit is "*kilo*gram," not "gram." The kilogram appears to be a non-coherent unit derived from the gram, but it isn't. The kilogram (kg) is the original basic; the gram is really a millikilogram, but multiple prefixes are forbidden. Since the *milli* and *kilo* cancel each other, $10^{-3} \cdot 10^3 = 10^0 = 1$. To avoid the *kilo* a new name would have had to be introduced. The popularity of "kilogram" made any substitution unwise, and the CGPM chose to go along with the "inconsistency."

MARTY BEGINS °TcPYP BONE SCANNING

(°TcPYP Becomes the Most Popular °Nuclide)

Raymond Marty's first paper on bone scans came from a talk to surgeons in Feb 1972. He had described a 30% incidence of metastases to bone seen on Sr-87m bone scans immediately following mastectomy. Thin skinned surgeons smelled an accusation not intended. All Marty had said was, "We should scan before surgery."

An abstract had already been prepared for the July SNM meeting in Boston. It mentioned only Sr-87m but, in March, Marty began to use a °Tc labeled pyrophosphate (first called °TcPP, later °TcPYP). The first °TcPYP scans were shown to an SNM chapter meeting in Vancouver, BC, in May, 1972. They were technically outstanding, and simpler than the old °Sr scans. The incidence of pre-mastectomy metastases to bone was startling. The substance of Marty's talk was disseminated by word of mouth long before publication.

At the July 1972 SNM meeting in Boston, Marty's talk hardly mentioned Sr-87m as printed in his abstract; he talked only of °TcPYP. At the meeting he met R. Perez from Paris who was also giving a talk on °TcPYP. Perez revealed that he had started °TcPYP bone scanning 3 months before Marty, but his first publication would not be out until the next October (1972).

At the May Vancouver meeting the long standing argument among oncologists — simple versus radical — focused on a new point. Surgeons already knew the odds on metastases and a premastectomy bone scan would only confuse the issue. But did it? J. Allen Miller (pathologist, then in Helena, Mont) went home from the meeting and persuaded his surgeons to make a simple prediction before cutting into the breast — benign or malignant? To his surprise (and theirs) the first 100 predictions were 92% correct. He didn't believe it, and repeated the test. It stood up. This unpublished observation convinced Miller that no matter which side of a question — simple vs radical, pre vs post irradiation, early vs late chemotherapy — bone scans would be used to support the decision.

[See Vig1959 .BoS, Early Bone Scans]

THE AEC: IN WITH A BANG, OUT WITH A WHIMPER

The Atomic Bombs were dropped on Japan in August 1945. During this year there had been debate among scientists, and during 1946 much acrimonious debate in Congress, on how to wrest control of atomic energy from the military. Civilian control won. (Of course, a few hidden clauses kept the bulk of the budget under military control.)

Much of the civilian victory was due to overblown cures for cancer and "°isotopes were the 'key-to-life-itself'." (Radiation science would not be relieved from this stigma until the DNA hype came along in the 1960s.) The military Manhattan Engineering District (MED) gave way to a civilian Atomic Energy Commission (AEC) on 1 January 1947.

The AEC also Inherited a Flaw

For the next 15 years practically all "radioisotopes" came from the AEC. Almost every advance in Nuclear Medicine came about with major AEC funding (including many of the foreign advances). A large portion of all nuclear, and much non-nuclear science, received its financial support from the AEC. But the AEC also inherited an ultimately fatal flaw from the Manhattan Engineering District — an Oak Ridge anti-radiation health physics cabal.

No industrial safety statistics have ever matched the AEC radiation safety record. (The corset makers industry came second.) Atom-Bomb fallout started the trend toward radiation hysteria. Some of the more vocal AEC Health Physicists remembered a 1935 theoretical explanation of genetic change. One ionizing event can break a chromosome. By extrapolation they devised the linear hypothesis: If 1000 rem could kill 1000 fruit flies, then 1 rem can kill 1 man. Many geneticists and the Oak Ridge school of health physics annually predicted 300,000 dead babies per year, killed by fallout from AEC bomb testing.

In 1954 AEC published a brochure introducing "The Peaceful Atom." A full page color photo of the first nuclear submarine said, "Look! We can produce useful power." Admiral Strauss, chairman of AEC, didn't think the public would notice that a submarine was not a very peaceful toy.

As "peaceful use" became equated with nuclear power in the 1960s, hysteria shifted to reactors. Safety standards were piled upon impossible 100% safety standards. Once competitive with fossil fuels in price, and without their danger, nuclear power was priced out of business and the AEC was savaged as "Judge and Jury" on safety. President Nixon's response was to break off a segment of AEC to become an independent Nuclear Regulatory Commission (NRC). The staff was the same group of file clerks who had caused the trouble in the first place. They became judge, jury, inspector, and hangman by their own rules.

A New Beginning and a *New* New Beginning

After the Watergate scandal the new president Ford signed an executive order putting the AEC out of business on 19 January 1975. After 27 years, 5 months, and 18 days, the impact of its demise was less than earth shaking. Most AEC money went into bombs; this secret remained under military control. Nobody noticed a difference. A new letterhead and signs on the buildings now read ERDA (Energy Research and Development Administration). After 2 years, 6 months, and 16 days, on 4 August 1977, a *new* new letterhead and all the signs on buildings were again replaced to proclaim President Carter's new cabinet Department of Energy (DOE).

The bulk of old AEC bomb making was still controlled by the military. The same coterie of social workers was still licensing radioisotopes, but power production and surveillance was under NRC control. Insofar as the great 1955 "Peaceful Atom" was concerned, radioisotope research and development was forgotten. "Radionuclides" had become a thriving private business.

Postscript to the End of the AEC

During a 1980 talk to medical students on the subject of Nuclear Medicine I mentioned the great contributions of AEC. One of the students asked, "Who was this man A. Eecee?" What many people considered the greatest organized effort in history, and after a quarter century of public relations hype, the AEC was forgotten in less than 5 years.

[See Vig1905 .Rum]

THE Rem, A DIVINE REVELATION
(Health Physics is Born-Again Religion)

S.A. Russ, an English radium therapist, proposed in 1918 that a biological unit of radiation effect should reflect its purpose, e.g., a "rad" of therapeutic irradiation would be the amount lethal to a standardized mouse cancer. (The name "rad" was from "*rad*iation"). (ARE, 23:226, 1918) But this "unit" was impossible to calibrate exactly. Various "biological" units proposed during the 1920s, e.g., 50% death of bean sprouts or drosophila eggs, were considered irrelevant to therapy.

In 1918 the German radiotherapist L. Seitz had defined a dose related to a minimal blush of the skin. He called it an "erythema" dose. G. Failla adopted the unit and calculated "threshold erythema" in calories/g tissue. It achieved a world popularity when calibrated against older physical dosimeters. But with the 1928 "roentgen" O. Glasser found no correlation between radiation effect and roentgens. G. Failla stated flatly, *"There is no unit of biological dose!"* [GSR, Rad, 1933]

Soon after its organization in 1928, the ICRU (Int Comm Rad Units) recognized that an equal number of roentgens did not produce the same bioeffect in different animals, or in different tissues of the same animal, or even in different cells of the same tissue. A **r**adiation **a**bsorbed **d**ose (rad), though not yet recognized as such, was one of the first requirements of radiobiology. By mid-1930 neutrons and protons were added to the alphas and betas that required measurement.

The "Roentgen" Becomes a "Rad"

The roentgen began (1928) as a measured e.s.u. of charge in a cc of air. In 1929 W. Mayneord added a correction factor to make it a unit of "dose" or energy absorbed in a *gram of tissue:* the gram-roentgen. L. Gray preferred *ions/cc air* corrected to read in ergs/cc of air; by 1939 he had measured it at 93 *ergs/gram* of water. L. Marinelli adapted the r to fit beta absorption with an energy unit (eu), and H. Parker measured this at 83 *ergs/gram* of tissue equivalent. He called it a **r**oentgen **e**quivalent **p**hysical (rep). The 83 (or was it 93?) ergs per gram (or was it cc?) of air (or water or tissue?) caused considerable confusion.

In 1953 the ICRU solved the confusion by replacing smelly biology with undefiled mathematics: a new **R**oentgen **a**bsorbed **d**ose (Rad) would be equal to 100 ergs absorbed per gram of whatever it was absorbed in. Under laboratory conditions this rad was measurable. But gamma ray absorption from about 100 to 1000 keV was almost the same; hence, in clinical situations, a roentgen could easily be converted to a rad by multiplying by "1." It is hard to describe the great satisfaction some physicists got in converting to "dose" by multiplying by 1.

The "rep" Becomes a "rem"

However, alpha rays produce more ionizing events per unit tissue than beta rays which produce more than gamma rays. It would seem that biological reaction must follow suit. Grossly it does, but it depends upon the end-point of bioeffect. When lethal dose in mice (50% in 30 days) is the end-point, alphas were 2, 5, 10, or 20 times more dangerous than betas. When a less exact end-point was used (50% drop in WBC in 24 hours) the biologic response became even more variable. But, if standardized, this simple correction factor, a **R**elative **B**iological **E**ffect, RBE as measured by radiobiologists, could convert a "rep" to a "dose" unit. Parker proclaimed Rep • RBE = **r**oentgen **e**quivalent **m**ammal (rem). Public relations expertise converted this to a **r**oentgen **e**quivalent **m**an.

The "rem" Becomes a Political Unit

After the atom bombs, money gushed into health physics and radiogenetics in proportion to the hysteria generated by AEC bomb testing in Nevada. So many RBEs served so many different rems, both for and against atomic bombs, that Health Physics became known as a numbers game. A new rem (**r**oentgen **e**quivalent **m**oney) became the only visible means of support for health physics, radiobiology and for much research in genetics.

In 1952 the ICRP issued hysterical warnings on possible genetic effects of radiation. In 1953 L. Russell pleaded that women's diagnostic X-Rays be restricted to the first 10 days post-menstruation. In 1954 ABCC revealed 65 cases of leukemia in 76,891 atom bomb survivors (almost 100%?). In 1955 H. Muller predicted genetic catastrophe from A-bombs. In 1956

K.Z. Morgan declared 5 rem/year the Maximum Permissible Dose. (He admitted the "rem" couldn't be measured but considered that irrelevant.) In 1957 Congress published 2064 pages of hearings on "Fallout" radiation. (Most of the expert witnesses proved radiation a non-problem but all requested more money for research; I admit that I was one of the leeches.) In 1958 United Artists showed *On the Beach* in which Gregory Peck proved beyond doubt that nuclear bombs killed all life on earth. In 1959 the Great Cranberry Crisis taught bureaucrats the monetary value of "crisis." [See Vig1959 .GCC] In 1962 Rachel Carson's *Silent Spring* set the population up for two decades of crises.

Health Physics Abrogates Science

In 1960 a new Federal Radiation Council (composed of health physicists and geneticists) had declared 0.1 r/year the Maximum Permissible Dose (thus outlawing Denver). R. Sievert then disclosed that people got more radiation from medical X-Rays than from natural background. In 1962 the ICRU accepted the unmeasurable "rem" as a unit of measurement. (It was required professional courtesy, because charter member Sievert chaired the ICRP.)

To fake "measurements" of rem you had to be a liar. In 1965 the licensing branch of AEC forbade °IHSA as a cysternographic agent based upon a *rumor* of a death. When his action was questioned *by phone* the health physicist said one case didn't matter because physicians hid many deaths from the AEC. Three years later M. Blau caught the AEC in a lie *in print* on hazards of Hg-203. [JNM 9:206, 1968] By 1971 ICRU began to manipulate "dose" with undefined factors in unmeasurable rems. In order to get SI coherence, ICRP proposed converting the rem with a Q factor to a new "sievert" unit.

Because no RBE measurement ever agreed with any other RBE, the ICRP solved the problem by inventing *quality factors*. In ICRP's own words "Q" is "... *based on judgmental extrapolation of experimental information involving RBE data not directly applicable to the protection situation.*" Even this fudge factor could not match the fuzzy results of RBE data, so fudge factor number two was added. Called N (for nonsense) it was *"the product of all other factors used in weighting the absorbed dose."* [Quoted from ICRU report 33, page 18, 1980] This weighted extrapolation from a floating assumption could not be measured by instruments used in science, but would be cast as a horoscope and, hence, designated "H": H = DQN.

This dose equivalent was given the special name, sievert ($v). (R. Seivert, the original 1928 Swedish member of the ICRU and long time chairman of the ICRP, died in 1966.)

$$1\ \$v = 1\ \mathrm{Jkg^{-1}} = 100\ \mathrm{rem} = 100\ \mathrm{rad\ (adjusted)}$$

The unit needs no instruments and is calibrated by the toothfairy.

Health Physics Becomes a Religious Cult

By 1979 the NCRP (a local breeding ground for the ICRP) dropped all pretense at science and assumed there was a risk in every radiation exposure. Exposures must be kept *"As low as practicable (referred to as ALARA) below the recommended permissible dose equivalent."* The Arizona Atomic Energy Commission expected all its licensees *"to be committed (and dedicated) to the ALARA concept..."* In 1980 Arizona you could not get a license to use radionuclides unless you worshiped the ALARA religion in public.

[Arizona AEC letter to all medical licensees, 31 Dec, 1979]

The Arizona AEC was reflecting the actions of a politically troubled Federal Nuclear Regulatory Commission that had botched the 1979 Three Mile Island accident. With trivial measured contamination they proclaimed ALARA with evangelical fervor. Their clones in Arizona's AEC had also been caught faking dangers from an unmeasurable "pollution" with tritium by a Tucson luminous dial plant. Within 5 months the Arizona AEC was fired and replaced by a new politicized Radiation Regulatory Commission.

The Units of Radiation

The units of amount-of-radioactivity and energy-of-radiation and physical exposure to radiation are measurable with sufficient precision to fall within "science." But I quote G. Failla in 1929, *"There is no unit of biological dose."* There has been no change since then, nor is there now even the slightest milliwhisper of research to find such a unit.

THE SI UNITS OF MEASUREMENT
(from NBS special pub 330, 1977 ed)

In 1971 the fourteenth *Conférence Générale des Poids et Measures* (CGPM) completed, to date (it will never be complete), its modern revision of the *Systéme International d'Unités* — abbreviated SI in all languages. This system may look French but it isn't. (Even when written in a cyrillic alphabet it has no ethnicity, even during a war.)

SI units apply only to a restricted intellectual domain: measurement of any and all physical phenomena. (Religion, politics, gossip, and kind thoughts are played under different rules — not necessarily better or worse, but different rules.) All measurements can be made with one, or some combination of seven basic units. Any quantity is a physical phenomena that can be measured in terms of a specific number of units. Each unit, precisely defined in terms of a reference sample, called a standard, is available to all scientists. It is designed to be exceedingly stable in our space and time.

For example: the meter (1981 definition) was 1,650,763.73 wavelengths, in a vacuum, of the orange-red radiation of krypton-86. Any trained person with a few million dollars worth of equipment can measure this for himself. However, the high precision requirements are so demanding that we leave the measurement to some country's National Bureau of Standards.

The Old Standards Are Dated But Not Dead

For many years "the meter" was the distance between two lines scratched on a Pt-Ir bar in a vault in Paris. This bar is still a fairly good standard for the unit of length envisioned as:

- the distance primitive man could reach,
- the Roman legionnaire's pace,
- Huygen's one-second-beating pendulum,
- or the English yard, or many other local units.

The CGPM has defined the unit of length more precisely.

The kilogram is the mass of a chunk of platinum-iridium in a Paris vault. Any scientist can look, but few may touch it because greasy hot fingers change its mass. In 1790 James Watt suggested the standard: a decimeter cubic container filled with sea water. The variables were too great, even in 1800 technology, for this mass to define a unit, but it did become a unit of volume — the liter. The mass of one liter of water is too sloppy for a standard, so they solidified it in platinum-iridium. In 1989 NBS scientists approached a pure crystal natural unit of mass.

The Seven Basic Units

Seven basic quantities of the SI system of units can be used to measure every "thing" in existence. (A "thing" is defined as an entity that takes up space in your time.)

Basic Quantity	Basic Unit	Symbol
Length	meter	m
Mass	kilogram	kg
Time	second	s
Electric Current	ampere	A
Temperature	kelvin	K
Luminous Intensity	candela	cd
Amount of Substance	mole	mol

Derived Units

Most practical units are simply some combination of these basic units and are called derived units:

Derived Quantity	Basic Units	Symbols
Area	square meters	m^2
Volume	cubic meters	m^3
Speed	meters per second	m/s
Acceleration	speed per second	m/s^2
Force	newtons	$kg\ m/s^2$
Energy	joules	$kg\ m^2/s^2$
Power	watts	$kg\ m^2/s^3$
ElecMotForce	volts	$kg\ m^2/s^3A$

Any number of derived units are acceptable provided they are coherent with the seven basic units. "Coherent" means they are derived by multiplication or division of basic units without any numerical factor. For example, the Rad unit of absorbed radiation dose equals 0.01 J/kg. The 0.01 numerical factor made it non-coherent in SI units and a new unit had to be introduced as the "gray," which equals 1 J/kg. The curie unit of radioactivity is 3.7×10^{10} disintegrations per second; hence, it is non-coherent. A new unit, the becquerel, had to be defined as 1 disintegration per second.

[See Vig1910 .Ci; Vig1928 .R]

Special Names for Some Coherent Units

A large number of "special names" have been given to coherent units that have especially widespread use: coulomb, joule, hertz, newton, etc. These are acceptable in SI. Another group are deeply imbedded in some sciences but are not coherent and should be slowly phased out of our language: mmHg, roentgen, acre, BTU, erg, foot, gallon, etc.

The liter was adopted as unit volume. We all used "cubic centimeters" (cc) to measure blood, oil, water, any fluid, before 1948, but it fit only water at 4°C. We changed "cc" to "ml" after World War II. The 1000 cc liter was then abrogated by 1964s twelfth CGPM because it is not coherent; one cubic meter must, in a coherent system, be the unit. But it is much too large for commercial, meaning household, use. The "liter," a milli-m^3, was reluctantly accepted as a special name because of its widespread use as a unit of capacity. It is in such widespread use that it could not be disregarded.

Supplementary Units

The CGPM was not certain whether the "radian" (plane angle) and "steradian" (solid angle) were units of space or a part of the language. They called them supplements and put off the decision until tomorrow.

Prefixes and Exceptions

An astrophysicist measures in billions of meters, a nuclear physicist in billionths. The SI system provides for this wide range with a set of prefixes.

exa	E	10^{18}	deci	d	10^{-1}
peta	P	10^{15}	centi	c	10^{-2}
tera	T	10^{12}	milli	m	10^{-3}
giga	G	10^{9}	micro	f	10^{-6}
mega	M	10^{6}	nano	n	10^{-9}
kilo	k	10^{3}	pico	p	10^{-12}
hecto	h	10^{2}	femto	f	10^{-15}
deka	da	10^{1}	atto	a	10^{-18}

The SI unit of time is the second and all of its multiples are non-metric. Although hours to years are inconsistent with the system, the Conférence Générale was scared to touch it. But they limited its multiples to four defined names:

minute	m	=	60s
hour	h	=	3,600s
day	d	=	86,400s
year	y	=	31,556,925.9747s exactly!

(The year is not a constant time span, but may be used when an error of many seconds is of no consequence. The "exactly" is a convenient average for use in computer simulations of long-term studies.)

Grammatical Rules for SI Units

Many publications have their own style sheets, e.g., *The New York Times Style Book*. If any of these publications say you must capitalize the joule unit because Joule is a man's name, they are wrong. When referring to the SI unit "joule" in text, the name is not capitalized. In written SI, the CGPM takes precedence over any style sheet because the CGPM wrote the language.

Capitalization: names of units in a text are always lower case, but symbols from proper names are always capitals (e.g., joule [J], meter [m]).

Plurals: symbols have no plurals and less than 1 unit is singular. (e.g., 1 meter and 10 meters are 1 m and 10 m; 0.1 meter is 0.1 m)

Punctuation: symbols are not abbreviations; they are not followed by a period (except at end of sentence).

Multiplication of units: a mid-line period or space indicates a product. The familiar × is sometimes ambiguous (e.g., a newton meter is Nm or N • m, not N × m).

Division of units: is indicated by a line (——) or a solidus (/) or a negative exponent (x^{-1}). The negative exponent is preferred.

Large numbers: figures are grouped in threes around a decimal point (e.g., 425 000 000.0 and 0.000 000 425). [This no comma usage is not easily accepted.]

Prefixes: these may not be combined (e.g., 0.000 000 002 m is 2 nanometers or 2 nm, not 2 millimicrometers or 2 mμm). Beyond 20 places exponents must be used.

SI Units are Inherently Incoherent, Inconsistant, Incomplete, etc.

CGPM decisions must be ratified by at least 72 political bodies. If they move too fast Weights & Measures go back to chaos. The system is closer to perfect than chaos. It has now been accepted by everybody except US congressmen.

[See Vig1889 .CGP]

BACKGROUND RADIATION IS FINALLY MEASURED

Since Elster & Geitel's world-wide look at background radiation before World War I, this source has been of concern to persons who measure small amounts of radiation. For 50 years spot measurements of background were common technical data. The first "public" (as opposed to scientific) estimate of total background from all sources occurred at the Indianapolis AAAS symposium in December 1957. [AAAS #59, 1959]

AAAS Tries to Educate the Public

At least 50 scientific articles tried to quantify background before 1953. Then, atom bomb fallout began to make the subject a public affair. By 1957 fallout Sr-90 was being calibrated daily in the newspapers with "millymikes," and "micromikes." The AAAS tried to put "background" and "fallout" in their proper perspective. MIT physicist R.A. Dudley estimated radiation dose to each person in the population as:

Cosmic rays	30 mrad/y
Terrestrial rays	45 mrad/y
Internal body emitters	32 mrem/y

Dudley used an RBE to change rad to rem for alphas, and added two new sources,

Medical diagnostic rays	75 mrad/y
Cs-137, Sr-90, I-131 fallout	15 mrad/y
TOTAL	**197 mrad/y**

In his 1956 presidential address to the British Institute of Radiology, F.W. Spiers had pointed out, *"[background] radiation is an inevitable accompaniment to life and has been so throughout man's evolution."*

[BJR 29:409, 1956]

After almost 20 years of measurements, in 1968 he put his estimate of man's whole body dose rate at:

Cosmic rays	30 mrad/y
Terrestrial rays	50 mrad/y
Internal K-40 etc.	19 mrad/y
All others (Ra, etc.)	1.5mrad/y
TOTAL	**100 mrad/y**

But Spiers stressed the great variation between individuals. If low level radiation is to be considered hazardous, the level at which hazard begins must be orders of magnitude beyond background variations. But what is the range of variation in background radiation?

Background Radiation is Measured

A page 1 squib in the New York Times on Monday 3 Dec 1961 stated that the New Hampshire Conway granite (used in many public buildings) could be a substantial energy source in a thorium breeder reactor. The statement had come from a group at Rice University who had been studying the geochemistry of 3 primary radiators, Th, U, and K, for years. It led to convening the first International symposium on the Natural Radiation Environment in Houston in 1963.

A second symposium in 1972 reinforced the collection of world-wide reports on highly variable backgrounds. In June 1975 a symposium on the very high background region of Brazil looked at the effect of low radiation exposure. At a hundred times the 100 mrad/y rate no demonstrable effect on humans was observed.

In April 1978 a third symposium, held in Brazil, detailed many areas in the rads/y level in highly populated regions with sophisticated demographic histories (Finland, Colorado, India, etc.). No health hazard, but a hint of radiation *hormesis,* was found. (Hormesis = low dose is beneficial.) The published proceedings of this symposium in 1980 is a good milestone to mark a reversal of American radiation phobia. The next year T. Luckey's "Radiation Hormesis" was published. Although growth of hysteria was reversed, cure of the existing phobia will require death of an entire generation of bureaucrats and newspaper editors. Their mindsets will never change. A new generation will take over.

[T.F. Gessel, TIC Conf 780422, 1980]

How Much Background Radiation?

Uranium miners spend much time in a very high radiation environment; ocean sailors have low exposure. Disregard a few such exceptions. Most people are exposed to radiations over which they have no control. Controllable background is too small to be worth controlling. (Unless, of course, you are paid to stop the tides.) In England in the 1950s an attempt was made to ban importation of the single largest source of radioactivity: Brazil nuts. It was calculated that the population's genetic overexposure to radium and its daughters was reached with only a ton/day eaten. Why take a chance?

How Much Radiation Do You Get Each Year?

	mRad/year exposure min	max
If you live under the sky		
at sea level near the equator	25	
on a mountain near the poles		60
If you live on earth with		
little uranium-thorium content	30	
lots of uranium-thorium		1000
If your natural K-40 is in		
a skinny fashion-model body	40	
a 250 lb football hulk		100
If you work for a living		
in an office or school	10	
underground or in an airplane		300
If you live in a house of		
canvas (tent) or snow (igloo)	10	
brick or concrete		140
If you get medical X-Rays		
a single film snapshot	5	
a complex series or CAT scan		400
In order to be alive		
Your minimum milliRads/year is	**120**	
or maximum might go up to		**2000**

You will also receive some radiation exposure that is more or less preventable depending upon your lifestyle:

	mRad/y
• cook your meals over gas	10
• eat 2 eggs for breakfast daily	9
• are a vegetarian	8
• drink 2 beers each day	7
• 1 day vacation at Carlsbad Cavern	6
• take a few airplane trips	5
• 2 packs cigarettes each day	4
• live near coal-fired power plant	3
• attend school with 30 other kids	2
• sleep with spouse most nights	1
• sleep with non-spouse many nights	0.7
• watch few hours TV most nights	0.5
• shower every Saturday night	0.2
• read daily New York Times	0.1
• There is no end to this list	0.+
Total unnecessary dose =	**10 to 100**

Thus, no matter what your lifestyle, you can't possibly absorb less than 100 mRad/y. Optimum for human life is a hormetic level around 1 rad/year. A small group of ancient health physicists and radiobiologists whose income derives from radiation hysteria dispute this. (They first manufactured a contagious hysteria in the 1950s and were good salesmen.)

What Evidence Supports Low-Level Dangers?

In 1942 Robert Stone was asked to set up radiation safety procedures for a new atom bomb project. He was the only radiologist with experience in handling small diagnostic and large therapeutic doses of X, gamma, alpha, beta, and *neutron* radiation. Realizing that unheard of amounts of many °isotopes might be involved, he established an As-Low-As-Possible exposure policy with an upper limit Maximum-Permissible-Dose of 0.1 r/day. He had *NO* evidence that 0.1 r/day was hazardous and he didn't think it was. But this level was so far below the X-ray danger level that his "health physicist" policemen could monitor *all* workers in safety.

The radiobiology dogma of the day said that in theory one gamma ray could nick one chromosome, hence might cause one cancer; *NO* evidence, but 100% of cancer patients had been exposed to radiation (background, but still ionizing).

> [The following is a direct quote from JAMA 5 Sep 1986, "When we know anything is carcinogenic we have to consider that even a low dose may be hazardous."]

Within a few years "aging" was added to the list because everybody exposed to radiation tends to get older.

What Evidence For Radiation Hormesis?

1985–Lower cancer rates found after TMI.
1984–US Dist Court calls Hlth Phys "liar."
1983–No risk found in neonate °I scans.
1982–Windscale (1957) had no bioeffect.
1981–>1200 papers on radiation hormesis.
1980–No leukemia found after Dx X-Ray.
1979–A-Bomb cancer only after >200 rads.
1971–No genetic effect after Hiroshima.
1970 Thyroid I-131 prevents later cancer.

> [35 such references in the Chronology of Nuclear Medicine go back to Sievert in 1950.]

In 1950 Sievert asked and answered two questions that define rad safety:

1. At what level does a radiation worker *feel* safe? This is a psychologically manipulatable level.
2. At what level is the worker actually safe? At the total accumulated dose of the oldest healthy worker.

After 1981 health physicists began a slow return to Seivert's ideas of safety.

[See Vig1926 .bkg]

THREE MILE ISLAND PEAKS RADIATION PHOBIA

(A Newspaper Farce Shows its True Face)

Early Wednesday 28 March 1979 the Dauphin County Office of Emergency Preparedness (OEP) was ordered by Pennsylvania's Emergency Management Agency (PEMA, Harrisburg, PA) to prepare for a 5 mile radius evacuation of 25,000 residents: Three Mile Island's nuclear plant was about to explode! Television newscasts verified the disaster with Red Alerts to surrounding states. [JAMA 245:1656, 1981]

Dauphin and three other counties went into near panic. By Friday 1308 hospital patients and 2400 nursing home patients (ambulatory to comatose) were ready for evacuation. Four hospitals in Harrisburg and the nearby Hershey Medical Center had cancelled all but emergency surgery and reduced patient census to a minimum.

A second teletype from PEMA on Friday raised the evacuation zone to a 10 mile radius with 200,000 people — maybe 20 miles. Governor Thornberg then advised all four counties in the area to prepare to evacuate 900,000 people. Nurses coded all patients as medical, surgical, obstetric, intensive care, neonatal; with subdivisions by truck or ambulances w/life support, monitors, respirators, Stryker frames. Color coded strips were attached to all patients' wrists.

After the dire warnings of the first day, Metropol Edison, who owned the plant, informed the public that everything was under control. Panic subsided to hysteria until special news bulletins from the Nuclear Regulatory Commission (NRC) declared a special emergency. Rescue squads from Brookhaven and Oak Ridge descended upon Three Mile Island (TMI). Walter Cronkite, TV's most popular news oracle, spoke of the horrors of a dreaded "meltdown" in Harrisburg. (Wrong place for TMI, but airplanes departing Harrisburg were sold out and the roads were jammed with fleeing traffic.) A Metro Edison spokesman told reporters "We are not in a China Syndrome situation" so the Governor issued bulletins requesting orderly evacuation of pregnant women and children. TV showed stock pictures of Health Physics technicians masked against the dreaded cancer-causing poison gas.

[Time 9 April 1979]

The Actual Accident (really an incident)

A minor mechanical malfunction occurred in Three Mile Island Unit 2 at 4 AM Wednesday morning, March 28, 1979. The 850 MW_e pressurized-water reactor automatically shut down. Feedwater pumps that supplied steam generators had been closed and residual heat from the core caused temperature and pressure of reactor coolant to rise. A relief valve on top of the pressurizer opened, as it was designed to do. But it did not close in seconds and produced a loss-of-coolant emergency.

Three emergency feedwater pumps automatically started 14 sec after the first shutdown. The operator did not notice two panel lights that said *valves closed* (lights hidden by a stupid NRC "safety-tag"). No water was getting to the reactor. The reactor safeguards automatically took over and 1000 gallons of water per minute flooded the reactor until, incredibly, 30 seconds later an operator shut off the flow. As a result, steam bubbles began to form in the coolant system and the operators misdiagnosed again; they opened a coolant letdown system to drain even more water from the reactor. The temperature rose to the point of fuel cladding failure and some fuel melted. This radioactive melt passed into cooling water, leaving the system via a relief valve into a basement specially built just for this purpose.

The core temperature rose to the point where failed zirconium cladding reacted with steam to produce hydrogen. By early afternoon an H_2 bubble appeared in the reactor's fuel container. At 3 PM two workers, trying to reroute plumbing circuits, opened a pipe full of radioactive gas. A puff escaped to register 1500 mrad on a film badge. The news media went into an orgiastic climax and predicted the end of the world. Twenty NRC advisors helicoptered to the site to devise some way to control future puffs, which continued to occur irregularly, to the delight of the press.

Metro Edison's chief technical spokesman told reporters that the H_2 bubble was "a different ball game than we expected." A more knowledgeable reporter asked why there was no valve in the reactor dome to let the gas escape. The answer was that the area was too "hot" for anyone to open. Another reporter asked how, if it was such a new ball game, there could be a built-in valve to take care of bubbles. At this point Met Edison refused further news conferences; the NRC would issue all news bulletins. [Science, 13 Apr 1979]

So long as the bubble maintained high pressure, the reactor would produce radioactive gas. A backup valve that could be operated manually was located between the pressurizer and the open relief valve. It was finally closed at 10:30 AM, 6½ hours after the first minor glitch. If the operators had kept hands off, the reactor would have shut itself down. After an incredible series of operator errors the core was now completely covered with water.

The Short Term Aftermath

Immediately after the accident, Access to Energy, a low-circulation monthly, said "safety" was a reactor whose automatic safe-guards work. In spite of operator stupidity and unconscionable NRC interference, no one was measurably irradiated. By July 5, the editor of the New England Journal of Medicine published complaints from six physicians for publishing lies about TMI. But the anti-nukes made news.

On 6 May 1979 65,000 people demonstrated against nuclear power on Washington, DC mall; 90% wanted all nuclear plants shut down. [Science 205:885, 1979] In this atmosphere the Smithsonian Magazine published part of a transcript of NRC meetings during the accident. It read, they said, like "a committee of plumbers discussing a faucet leak." President Carter, trained as a naval nuclear engineer, but never given command, had to, as president, support the nuclear navy. He responded to civilian nuclear power by appointing two anti-nuclear activists as commissioners on the NRC.

Immediately after TMI, Carter appointed a twelve member commission, headed by Dartmouth College president J. Kemeny, to excoriate nuclear power. In November the Kemeny Commission came up with the wrong answer. They cleared the reactor of any fault but recommended abolition of the NRC, which was primarily to blame. This was totally unexpected. Carter immediately appointed a panel of known anti-nukes to review the Kemeny review. Then he fired a nuclear engineer from the NRC chairmanship and appointed a mildly anti-nuke Washington attorney in his place.

The Long Term Aftermath

The credibility of the NRC, and of the entire regulatory process, was the primary casualty of TMI. Carcinogenesis was the big scare word. K.Z. Morgan predicted 50 excess cancers from the weak puff of TMI radiation. [New Eng Jr Med 4 Oct 1979] Instead of denouncing this as false, the anti-nuke editor allowed six scientists to respond with convoluted honesty. Many professional people noted the bias, and Morgan's school of anti-radiation health physics began to lose favor. It was reversed around 1980–1985.

On 16 May 1980 fallout of 1.5 cubic miles of Mount St. Helens deposited 40 *mega*curies of radon over the northwestern states. [Science 209:1116, 1980] *"Fortunately,"* said Time magazine, *"the gas has a short half-life (3.8 days) and quickly climbs high into the sky before it can affect people."* (Time 2 June 1980 was wrong; very heavy radon gas hugs the ground and daughters average 4 alphas in 30 years.)

Vicious lip-smacking descriptions of bloody gore that never occurred marked a peak American radiation phobia. Then:

1. in the first popular vote on the subject, (23 Sep 1980) Maine voted 2.3/1.6 to keep nuclear power;
2. "National Radiation Environment" was published;
3. Chinese scientists found no bioeffects in high background areas;
4. cancer occurred in only <2/1000 atomic bomb survivors;
5. "Radiation Hormesis" was published.

No minds were changed by the new outlook, but nuclear phobia began to evaporate as the generation of anti-technology flower children reached senility.

An Item of Interest: PEMA (the official emergency headquarters) had estimated it would take 4–8 hours to assemble the transportation to evacuate TMI area's hospitals. Local emergency offices estimated (in a review a year later) that trucks could not have been gathered, loaded and dispatched in less than 36 hours — the time it took to evacuate 45,000 people at Chernobyl in 1986.

[See Vig1986 Che]

THE MATURITY OF NUCLEAR MEDICINE AND THE DECLINE OF RADIOPHOBIA 1980 through 1989

- A remarkable symposium on the Natural Radiation Environment was convened in Brazil 74 years after the German gas mantle industry was caught stealing Brazil's monazite sands [1904]. The proceedings, published in 1980, confirmed measurements begun in a flower garden by Elster & Geitel in 1901: the earth exhales radioactivity at a rate far beyond that desired by the EPA.

- In 1980 the ICRU issued Report #33; an explanation of SI radiation units. The Roentgen, nuclear science's only measurement of "dose" (really a high precision measure of exposure) was discarded as of no value. The Commission decreed the Rad (an estimate) adjusted by a Quality Factor (a committee agreement) multiplied by N (a divine revelation) would be the Sievert "unit of dose." Health Physics had left science for religious divination. Four years later a Federal court would dismiss a high priest of Health Physics as dishonest.

- A reactor malfunction at TMI in Pennsylvania became a newsmedia distortion of astounding proportions. Nobody was irradiated beyond background levels because automatic controls overrode incredible human stupidity. The event marks the peak in radiation hysteria. After TMI the public began to realize what some scientists had been preaching for years: everything is a poison in improper dose.

- An ages-old principle of pharmacology says low-dose stimulates what high-dose destroys. It was resurrected by T. Luckey under the name "Radiation Hormesis," in a mass of evidence dating from the year radioactivity was discovered. Radiation is not only a ubiquitous necessity in life; in small doses it is good for you.

- Nuclear Medicine was "organized" (1954) partially in response to Radiology's offer to let anybody use °isotopes provided they were certified in Radiology. Nuclear Medicine achieved a similar maturity during its labor dispute with Cardiologists: anybody can do Nuclear Cardiology so long as they have the training of a Nuclear Medic.

- Around 1980 J. Lawrence's old P-32 therapy was being rediscovered. The age limits for I-131 for I-131 therapy had been reduced to zero. Radiotherapy was again permitted in non-terminal diseases. Multiple scanning modalities were taking over the old "Physical Diagnosis." W. Bale's old °antibodies were being hailed as the new "Magic Bullets" in cancer diagnosis and therapy. Radiation Phobia had run its course; no minds were changed by logical argument, but the phobiacs were dying off. A new generation of Health Physicists attempted to stem radiation phobia. The Chronology after 1980 becomes more political and social than scientific:

CNM1980 Background radiation unveiled.
CNM1981 Radiation hormesis resurrected.
CNM1982 SPECT, ECAT, PET, NMR, 3-D, etc.
CNM1983 Clinical °antibody tags used.
CNM1984 Is payment by DRGs a threat?
CNM1985 Radiation phobia is relaxing.
CNM1986 Low dose risk is thrown out.
CNM1987 Superconductivity over 77K.
CNM1988 "Metric System" (SI) wins out.
CNM1989 Linear hypothesis proved false.

CHRONOLOGY OF NUCLEAR MEDICINE — 1980

			Ref.
	Scientific and Technical Background		
1. Basic	— R. O'Nions confirms most earth's heat is from °K, Th, U.	[1925]	SA
2. Obser	— IUPAC will name all elements over #103 by number only.	[1979]	Sc
4. # Med	— RSNA estim 7.76 million Nuc Med studies/y in US hosp.	[1977]	Rad
	Organizations and Internal Politics		
5. Pols	— $125,000 rad emerg decontam unit built in local hosp.	[1979]	AJR
6. Socs	— ICRU issues Report #33 on new SI units rad dose.	[1978]	ICRU
7. Event	— Mt St Helens erupts 40 MCi Rn into US fallout pattern.	[1979]	HPN
	— Chinese find no bio effect in high rad bkgd region.	[1979]	Sc
	— T. Gessel & W. Lowder pub "Natural Radiation Environment."	[1978]	Bk
	RAD BACKGROUND IS 10 to 1000 TIMES GREATER THAN EXPECTED		
	— B. Cohen demolishes linear hypothesis of radiation risk.	[1977]	HP
	— RERF finds no excess ca in Bomb victims @ <200 rads.	[1979]	RERF
	THESE EVENTS MARK BEGINNING OF END OF CURRENT RAD PHOBIA		
	Instruments, Units of Measurement, and Drugs		
8. Instr	— J. Hutchison (Aberdeen) makes first Nuc Mag Reson images.	[1977]	BJR
	— F. Smith scans first pt with NMR, esophageal ca with mets.	[1977]	BMJ
	— R. Boyd gives method to evaluate °Tc cow performance.	[1975]	IJAR
	— C. Partain compares NMR and CAT images of thorax & abd.	[1977]	Rad
	— N. Watson says ECAT scanner does not justify its cost.	[1979]	JNM
9. Units	— I. Lockwood makes MIRD dose calc for N-13 ammonia.	[1974]	JNM
	— ICRU fakes biol dose with unmeasurable Q factor in Sv.	[1962]	NBS
	— B. Toombs sees dose to bladder from microsphere excreta.	[1979]	Rad
10. Concp	— J. McAfee: °TcDTPA has different distrib than °InDTPA.	[1979]	JNM
	— R. Hayes: Sc in plasma changes °Ga distribution in rats.	[1972]	JNM
	— D. Chen: Ga-67 in bowel (rats) is intestine secretion.	[1972]	JNM
11. Drugs	— T. Ruth builds automated 4.6h Rb-81 to 13s Kr-81m cow.	[1975]	IJAR
	— C. Loc'h describes a 27d Ge-68 to 1.1h Ga-68 B^+ cow.	[1978]	JNM
	— C. Cheng builds 15.4d Os-191 to 4.9s 129keV Ir-191m cow.	[1979]	JNM
	— B. Ballou scans °labeled monoclonal antibodies in mice.	[1978]	Sc
	— K. McElvany substitutes Br-77 for °I to label proteins.	[1973]	IJAR
	— R. Counsell incorps °I-choles into Hi Dens Lipoprotein.	[1971]	JNM
	Radioiodine, P-32, and Radioactive Therapy		
12. I-Res	— R. Shore: ca risk from child neck irrad = $3.8/10^6$ pt yrs.	[1977]	HP
	— I. McDougall finds 3 thyr ca after 4000 rad radiotherapy.	[1978]	ca
	— A. McGregor notes immunosuppres from antithyroid drugs.	[1979]	NEJM
13. I-Dx	— T. Nikolas finds lymphocytic dis = hi-T3, T4, lo °I uptake.	[1978]	ArIM
14. I-Rx	— J. Sawers notes transient hypo (weeks) in 17% I-131 Rx.	[1978]	JCEM
	— L. Dodson finds hi serum thyroglob in active thyroid ca.	[1979]	AJM
	— A. Pinchera correlates thyroglobulin & body scans in ca.	[1979]	CE
	— C. Kuni: low (30 mCi) doses worthless after thyroid ca surg.	[1976]	Rad
	— W. Horst discards I-125 Rx from data in 2000 hypers.	[1974]	CNM
15. P-Rx	— G. WETHERLEY-M ADVISES °P Rx FOR ASYMPTOMATIC THROMBOCYTHEMIA.	[1961]	CT
	Scans and Other Tests of Function in Various Organs		
18. Brain	— J. Marc-Vergnes sees accurate cer bld flow with Xe-133.	[1972]	AJPh
	— D. Aneri prefer Tl-201 over °Tc as agent for cereb mets.	[1979]	BJR
	— T. Rudd reviews 7y experience, °nuc scans of CSF shunts.	[1973]	P
	— Z. Oster suggests 2.9d Ru-97 replace °In cysternograms.	[1976]	JNM
	— J. Greenberg maps cereb glucose metab with °F deoxygluc.	[1970]	Sc
	D. Kuhl applies B^+ ECAT to see SOL with °FDGlucose.	[1979]	AnN

19. Heart	— G. Beller says stress washout time spots myo ischemia.	[1979]	Cir
	— A. Nielsen finds exercise °Tl uptake is a blood flow measuremt.	[1979]	Cir
	— J. Gerry notes °Tl redistrib independent of blood flow.	[1979]	AJCr
	— J. Turner runs °Tl exercise scans 3 weeks post infarct.	[1978]	Cir
	— H. Gutgesell runs °Tl scans in 16 infants for anomalies.	[1978]	Cir
	— S. Rerych studies training effects on L vent function.	[1978]	AJCr
	— R. Slutsky estim R ventricular EF with bicycle & °TcHSA.	[1978]	AJCr
	— S. Sorensen validates °TcRBC outputs and vols with Fick.	[1979]	Cir
	— M. Ter-Pogossian: myocard metab by C-11 palmitate on PET.	[1978]	Cir
20. Liver	— B. Collier prefers °I-RB for bile scan in neonates.	[1972]	Rad
	— R. Sarper uses fast frames; sees art vs ven flow in mets.	[1972]	JNM
	— R. Zeman compares °Tc-HIDA scans & ultrasnd in acute dis.	[1979]	AJSr
21. Lung	— B. McNEIL: PE IS DIAGNOSED AS "HIGH" OR "LOW" PROBABILITY.	[1979]	Rad
	— J. Rinderknecht uses aerosol delivery to see clearances.	[1979]	ARD
	— C. Campbell does V/P scan on first (1954) pulm art repair.	[1978]	AJCr
	— B. Line develops Xe-127 cinepneumography to stop motion.	[1978]	JNM
	— J. LeMoine scans legs & lungs (°TcFib) after hip surgery.	[1975]	JAMA
22. Bone	— Controversy building: bone scan value in uncommon ca.	[1979]	YB
	— R. Henkin finds long °TcPhos incubation time is required.	[1979]	Rad
	— A. Ali use many agents to chart hyper pulm osteoarthrop.	[1974]	AJR
	— K. Meurman finds stress fractures in foot with °TcMDP.	[1977]	Rad
	— D. Fink-Bennett sees deltoid tuberosity, looks like met.	[1987]	JNM
	— G. Ho discusses the sacroiliac joints on °TcMDP scans.	[1976]	ARh
23. Kidney	— J. Carlsen compares 4 °TcDTPA kits for GFR; finds differences.	[1979]	JNM
	— R. Sherman sees image failure of kidney on °I-Hipp.	[1979]	Np
	— G. Mendez: pyeloneph cannot be Dx from °Ga scans alone.	[1977]	AJR
24. Gut	— R. Szlabick pushes °Tc-iprofenin for acute cholecys Dx.	[1977]	AS
	— J. Blumhagen scans for gastoesoph reflux after °TcSC.	[1979]	AJR
	— P. Domstad measures gastric empty time with °Tc-oatmeal.	[1976]	JNM
25. Blood	— R. Coleman studies abscess localiz by In-111 leukocytes.	[1979]	AJSr
	— R. Hawker gives method to tag platelets with °In-oxime.	[1972]	CS
	— Int Comm Std Hematol recommends °RBC & °plasma vols.	[1974]	JNM
26. Other	— M. Daly injects ID °Xe to get capillary permeability.	[1978]	JNM
	— T. Simon says repeat °Ga scans at 48h for infec dis Dx.	[1979]	Rad
	— F. Deland detects °antibodies by scanning.	[1975]	CaR

Radiation Hysteria and Health Physics * Obituaries *

27. Hyst	— R. Chu says Xe-127 has low biol dose but high contamination;	[1978]	
	sales poor because NRC says protect the dosimeter.	[1968]	Rad
	— R. Shore finds 26 thyr ca 10y after 2650 thymus irrad.	[1976]	HP
	— L. Luckhett measures exposures to volatile liquid °I.	[1978]	JNM
	— L. Brateman: ultrasnd techs overexposed to Nuc Med pts.	[1978]	Rad
	— NRC does NOT compare St. Helen's 40 MCi Rn with TMI's 17 Ci °I.		
	Am Psych Assn: 150 mental dis, drops Freudian terminol.	[1895]	SN
	Still makes all Dx with no units of measurement.	[1968]	SN89
28. React	— J. Gray criticizes Fed safety regs as pure "news hype."	[1978]	ACR
	— M. Brucer says they are deliberate NRC misinformation.	[1968]	
	— J. Gray finds no leuk in Dx & Rx exposures from 1955–72.	[1947]	NEJM
	— H. Maille says Life Tables are "absolute" — all deaths over Life Table number MUST be caused by radiation.	[1977]	HP
	— A. Linus finds no leukemia in diagnostic rad exposures.	[1979]	NEJM
	P. Moore: special skin decontamination soaps unnecessary.	[1965]	JNM
	— H. Nishiyama finds minimal intern contam in °Tc handlers.	[1978]	Rad
	— RERF is studying 25,000 children of A-Bomb survivors.	[1970]	RERF
29. Respo	— R. Zelac finds no rad hazard in pediatric Nuc Medicine.	[1959]	HP
	— D. Taylor finds 10 day after menstruation rule unnecessary.	[1978]	BJR

* * *

30. Obits	— G. Andrews (1918–1980) Am physician; °nuclide Rx, emergency care.	JNM
	— J. Quinn (1933–1980) Am physician; Nuc Med, lung scan, ed of YB.	YB

CHRONOLOGY OF NUCLEAR MEDICINE — 1981

Scientific and Technical Background

				Ref.
1.	Basic	— W. Schull proves NO genetic effect in A-Bomb survivors.	[1955]	RERF
4.	# Med	— T. Parker surveys 10% of US hosp, finds 50% of thyroid scans are done with °Tc; uptakes on 78%; thyroid studies are 6.7% of all 7,760,000 scans done in the US.	[1978]	(1983 Rad)

Organizations and Internal Politics

5.	Pols	— Blue Cross-Shield questions payment for Nuc Med tests.	[1984]	SNM
6.	Socs	— Int conf at Banff, Canada, on clinical use of Ga-67.	[1980]	INM
7.	Event	— Int PVA group abandons chemo Rx, returns to P-32 Rx.	[1961]	NEJM

Instruments, Units of Measurement, and Drugs

8.	Instr	— P. Hoffer builds miniature CdTe semicond crystal probe.	[1977]	Rad
		— W. Harvey builds miniature NaI(Tl) crystal surgical probe.	[1956]	JNM
		— C. Partain describes the principles of NMR — CAT scan.	[1980]	Rad
		— R. Ordidge describes an NMR system for <60 sec images.	[1980]	BJR
		— J. DeLayre makes gated Na-23 NMR images of rat heart.	[1980]	Sc
		— H. Abrahamson says all photomult tubes drift off peak.	[1979]	JNM
9.	Units	— P. Brown calculates dose for °Tc-HIDA in disease states.	[1979]	JNM
11.	Drugs	— R. Tilbury tells how to make 7.6m B^+ K-38 for scanning.	[1977]	JNM
		— E. Garcia devises 1.7d Hg to 30s Au-195 cow system.	[1983]	JNM
		— G. Hinkle makes a kit for Hippuran labeling with I-123.	[1978]	JPm
		— R. Hayes studies mechanism of °Ga incorp into tissues.	[1977]	JNM
		— J. Dutcher studies °In-granulocytes migration to infect.	[1974]	NEJM
		— T. Wilbanks finds Fab IgG frags uptake in rat breast ca.	[1978]	Ca

Radioiodine, P-32, and Radioactive Therapy

12.	I-Res	— K. Tamura notes Graves' dis after thyroid hi-dose irrad.	[1979]	NYMJ
		— O. Khan find tenth ca in an autonomous hyperfunc nodule.	[1973]	PgM
13.	I-Dx	— B. Sayle: 10 of 24 whole body scans are + after ca Rx.	[1980]	CNM
		— T. Higashi notes high Ga-67 uptake in anaplastic ca.	[1980]	Rad
		— J. Massie scans, $°TcO_4$ & ultrasonic, bilat hemor cyst.	[1966]	CNM
		— U. Ryo says extrathyroid uptake masses are usually ca.	[1974]	JNM
		— W. Resinger finds tomograms superior to pin hole images.	[1974]	JNM
14.	I-Rx	— A. Siddiqui requires 150 mCi & TSH for post-surg ablate.	[1980]	CNM
		— H. Waxman says 10 mCi doses necessary to see ca mets.	[1980]	JNM

Scans and Other Tests of Function in Various Organs

18.	Brain	— B. Rao proves a jugular ven reflux caused by valsalva.	[1978]	CNM
		— Z. Oster: Ru-97 DTPA better than In-111 for cisternogram.	[1980]	JNM
		Fewer cisternograms are being done each year in US.	[1980]	PL
		— J. Greenberg sees brain metabolism of °FDGlucose on ECAT.	[1980]	Sc
		— M. Marcus: °Xe clearance doesn't measure cer blood flow.	[1975]	CirR
		— F. Bonte: SPECT Xe-133 scan measures regional bld flow.	[1979]	JNM
19.	Heart	— F. Knapp: fatty acid chain length affects myocard uptake.	[1978]	JNM
		— H. Coenen says 98m B^+ Br-75 has fast hi myocard uptake.	[1977]	JNM
		— S. Sorensen: R-o-I site affects Ejec Fraction in normals.	[1980]	JNM
		— G. Sutherland studies °TcRBC in blunt chest trauma.	[1978]	JT
		— G. Winzelberg studies R-vent on gated first-pass °TcRBC.	[1979]	C
		— M. Goldberg estimates R-vent first-pass °Xe Ejec Fract.	[1978]	AJCr
		— H. Berger estim pulm hypertens with first-pass studies.	[1978]	AJCr
		— F. Basilico compares echogram, syst timing, & first-pass.	[1978]	BHJ
		— W. Tauxe measures wall motion with gated blood pools.	[1978]	AJCr
		— B. Segal uses °Tl stress to clarify the inconclusive ECG.	[1980]	AJCr

19. Heart	—	R. Kline sees myocard in 2 min with I-123 B-guanethidine.	[1980]	AJCr
	—	R. Lerch sees myocard with C-11 palmitate on PET scan.	[1980]	Cir
	—	M. Sandler notes "hot spot" scan in tricusp valve insuff.	[1978]	CNM
20. Liver	—	W. Fajman finds art/port bld flow sensitive to met dis.	[1980]	JNM
	—	B. Kumar tries Ga-68 Fe-hydroxy colloid as a PET agent.	[1980]	AJR
	—	P. Zeman compares °Tc-HIDA with sonograms in 200 pts;	[1980]	AJSr
		delayed (hours) scans required to Dx acute dis.	[1971]	JNM
	—	G. Glazer questions °Tc-HIDA scans in pancreatitis pts.	[1979]	BJS
	—	G. Edlund questions °Tc-HIDA scans in pancreatitis pts.	[1979]	JNM
	—	G. Spencer scans for spleen after splenectomy (°TcRBC).	[1979]	BJS
	—	D. Ostfeld checks °TcSC scans on short interval autopsy.	[1977]	Rad
	—	S. Fritz does a ROC analysis of 7025 °TcSC liver scans.	[1978]	JNM
21. Lung	—	R. Cheely results on V/P scan vs angiogram questioned in		YB
	—	J. Wallace scans 80 normal 18y olds; finds some defects.	[1979]	ARD
	—	M. Lippmann: angio required in Dx of PE in severe COPD.	[1980]	C
	—	P. Alderson finds PE can be hi-probability on V/P scan.	[1980]	Rad
	—	J. Lavender assesses 5 years Kr-81m (& reverse mismatch).	[1979]	AJR
	—	H. Susskind: Xe-127 is superior to Kr-81m as scan agent.	[1879]	JNM
	—	D. Stanley finds PE mimics on scan (but no change in wk).	[1980]	SMJ
22. Bone	—	R. Shafer compares °TcPP and °Ga in maxillofacial dis.	[1976]	JNM
	—	H. Bergstedt discusses facial bone scans and tumors.	[1976]	AR
	—	K. Vyas tries quantified sacroilliac joint assessment.	[1980]	AJR
	—	R. LaMont shows tech to see vascularity of femoral head.	[1960]	JBJS
	—	T. Lahtinen measures blood flow (°Xe) in normal femurs.	[1976]	JNM
	—	S. Christensen finds °TcMDP in rat's epiphyseal plates.	[1980]	JNM
23. Kidney	—	L. Forstrom says °In-leuks predict transplant rejection.	[1979]	CNM
	—	J. Pollet uses IV °Tc-DTPA to detect vesicorenal reflux.	[1977]	JU
	—	C. Yee notes many physiol things change °TcDMSA uptake.	[1976]	JNM
24. Gut	—	J. Moore uses °In & solid °chicken liver test meals.	[1980]	DD
	—	P. Som finds heat treated °TcRBC lost slowly in GI bleed.	[1979]	Rad
	—	A. Alavi finds °TcSC superior to angiograms for GI bleed.	[1979]	AJR
	—	P. West: $C\text{-}14O_2$ breath test best for fat malabsorption.	[1979]	BMJ
25. Blood	—	M. Ezekowitz uses °In-platelets to detect L-vent thrombi.	[1980]	Cir
	—	M. Thakur gives improved method for °In label platelets.	[1980]	JNM
	—	M. Rovekamp: first results of °In-leuk scans in inflam dis.	[1980]	BJS
	—	M. Dewanjee introduces °In-tropolone as platelet label.	[1980]	JNM
26. Other	—	W. Moore gets amputa level by IC °Xe in saline washout.	[1975]	ASr
	—	E. Dunn describes $°TcO_4$ pattern in missed testic torsion.	[1979]	Rad
	—	T. Burt sees uterine uptake as false + on Meckel's scan.	[1975]	JNM
	—	R. Hull uses °I-fibrinogen to detect deep ven thrombo.	[1977]	AnIM
	—	A. Fenech uses autol In-111 platelets to see dp ven thr.	[1977]	BMJ

Radiation Hysteria and Health Physics * Obituaries *

27. Hyst	—	C. Williams worries about calibration of small °Mo leaks.	[1980]	Rad
	—	R. Waldron designs $125,000 hosp °decontamination unit.	[1979]	AJR
	—	H. Abrams tells lies to make nuclear war more horrible.	[1977]	NEJM
	—	R. Prinz finds parathyroid dis in pts with neck irrad.	[1977]	AJS
	—	P. Davis finds no danger in NMR but warns people anyway.	[1980]	AJR
28. React	—	R. Evans estimates risk from environmental Rn-222 +.	[1980]	Na
	—	J. Smith reviews 1979 TMI non-rad accident fiasco.	[1979]	JAMA
	—	A. Thomas tries hard but can find no dangers in NMR.	[1980]	BJR
29. Respo	—	H. Kaplan treats non-cancer (rheum arth) with radiation.	[1956]	NEJM
	—	T. LUCKEY LISTS >1200 ARTICLES DISPUTING LO-DOSE HAZARD.	[1980]	Bk
		REINTRODUCES PHARMACOLOGY'S HORMESIS, BUT IN RADIATION.		

* * *

30. Obits	—	H. Urey (1893–1981) Am chem, heavy water, H-2.		Sc

CHRONOLOGY OF NUCLEAR MEDICINE — 1982

Scientific and Technical Background

			Ref.
2. Obser	— D. Halliday reviews the use of stable isotopes.	[1975]	CS
4. # Med	— S. Fihn estimates >3 million bone scans/y in US.	[1981]	JAMA
	— F. Mettler est 7.5 million in vivo nuc med exams in US.	(1985	JNM)

Organizations and Internal Politics

5. Pols	— SNM vs cardiologists in labor dispute on FDA licenses.	[1966]	FR
6. Socs	— J Magnetic Resonance in Medicine begins publication.	[1980]	JMR
	— P. Richards writes history of medical Tc-99m.	[1979]	IJAR

Instruments, Units of Measurement, and Drugs

8. Instr	— R. Alfidi describes a whole body NMR scanner.	[1981]	Rad
	— O. Ratib describes a rotating slant-hole collimator.	[1979]	Rad
	— S. Huange makes double °nuc B^+ Comput Tomograms (PCT).	[1979]	JNM
	— M. Ter-Pogossian looks at cardiac motion prob on PET.	[1975]	JCA
	— M. LEWIS APPROACHES 3-D RECONSTRUCTIONS ON SPECT SCAN.	[1979]	JNM
9. Units	— MIRD reports 10 calc dose for °Tc-albumin microspheres.	[1980]	JNM
	— K. Kearfott estims dose: 22 organs with B^+ gases on PET.	[1980]	JNM
	— J. Johnson: fetal thyroid dose is about twice mother's.	[1972]	HP
	— P. Brown calculates dose from 5 °Tc-IDA biliary agents.	[1981]	JNM
10. Concp	— J. Keyes asks: "clinical" (not theoret) value of SPECT?	[1979]	JNM
11. Drugs	— R. Okada labels a long-chain fatty acid with Te-123m.	[1980]	Cir
	— D. Wong sees endocarditis with °Tc-S aureus antibody.	[1980]	JNM
	— F. Wackers uses 42h Hg-195m to 30.5s 262keV Au195m cow.	[1980]	AJCr

Radioiodine, P-32, and Radioactive Therapy

12. I-Res	— C. Gonzalez-V: 28% of child irrad glands devel nodules.	[1981]	AnIM
	— H. Peter says multiple processes make hot to cold nods.	[1981]	JCEM
	— H. Levy finds pyram lobes in 10% of eu, 43% of hyper pts.	[1977]	CNM
13. I-Dx	— O. Senga compares °TlCl vs °Ga cancer scans, wants both.	[1981]	JNM
	— S. Chervu details troubles in measuring I-123 uptake.	[1954]	JNM
14. I-Rx	— L. Holm counts 72% hypo 24 years after °I Rx for hyper.	[1980]	JNM
	— L. Degroot: 30 mCi less successful ablation than 50 mCi.	[1981]	AnIM
	— C. Ramatiotti pushs NIH 50 mCi ablation of remnants.	[1980]	JNM
	— W. Beierwaltes summarizes 1947–80 Rx of thyroid ca.	[1978]	JNM
17. Other	— I. Ariel treats 40 pts mets to liver, Y-90 microspheres.	[1978]	JSO
	— H. Grossman tries I-123 implants in 100 prostate ca pts.	[1976]	U
	— R. Levy: Rx with monocl antibodies to B-cell lymphoma.	[1986]	NEJM

Scans and Other Tests of Function in Various Organs

18. Brain	— G. Bydder shows 140 NMR images of the brain.	[1981]	AJR
	— T. Hill uses new I-123 isoprop-iodoamphetamine (IMP).	[1981]	JNM
	— D. Kuhl measures cer blood flow on SPECT with °I-IMP.	[1980]	JNM
	— Y. En-Lin blames some jugular reflux on Compton scatter.	[1981]	JNM
	— R. Lee compares I-123 IMP scans on camera and SPECT.	[1981]	JNM
	— D. Fink-Bennett finds no diff between 1h & 2h scans.	[1971]	JNM
	— W. Powers sees carotid art thrombi with °In-platelets.	[1977]	N
	— G. Gates measures child strokes; °TcDTPA cerebral perfusion.	[1975]	CNM
19. Heart	— J. Links estimates L-ventric vol from gated blood pool.	[1981]	Cir
	— R. Okada scans cardiac blood pool to see pulm blood vol.	[1980]	Cir
	— K. Korr measures R-vent Ejection Fraction in normals.	[1981]	AJCr
	— D. Dymond finds EF higher in RAO than LAO on first-pass,	[1981]	Cir
	but Pulm Trans Time is highly dependent on bolus.	[1971]	Cir
	— J. Lindsay studies exercise EF before & after by-pass.	[1949]	ATS
	— C. Maynard compares EF after cold-pressor vs bicycle.	[1981]	Cir

19. Heart	— R. Gibson notes increased Tl-201 uptake after exercise.	[1981]	AJCr
	— S. Bergmann finds perfusion isn't measured by washout.	[1980]	AJCr
	— W. Hutchins shows venous collaterals in v-cava obst.	[1978]	AJr
20. Liver	— F. Doyle shows some NMR images of the liver.	[1981]	AJR
	— G. Edlund: °TcHIDA not in acute pancreatitis G-bladder.	[1981]	JNM
	— W. Schuman notes false + °TcIDA scans in alcholism.	[1979]	AJR
	— D. Knopf compares slow contrast CT with fast °TcSC scans.	[1981]	AJR
	— J. Szymendera: plasma CEA & scans to Dx colorect mets.	[1981]	YB
	— Y. Yonekura notes °F-glucose uptake in mets from colon.	[1980]	JNM
	— S. Patel uses °Xe uptake to separate fat from SOLesions.	[1979]	AJR
	— J. Wagstaff finds (non-cirr) "hot spleens" have high IgM.	[1979]	ca
	— U. Ryo says dark breast band on Ap liver due to scatter.	[1978]	Rad
21. Lung	— E. Heidelberger has a new gas phase F-18 NMR vent scan.	[1981]	JMR
	— J. Wallace scans smoke & non-smokers, finds no lesions.	[1979]	ARD
	— G. Newman reviews 55 °TcMAA scans showing diffuse dis.	[1981]	Rad
	— H. Sostman discovers "stripe sign" means no PE.	[1980]	Rad
	— S. Yamazakin shows reduced bld flow in reexpanded lungs.	[1976]	C
	— H. Modell finds little Kr-81m mixture with lung gas.	[1981]	JNM
	— R. Johnson notes °TcSC in 1 lung after blunt chest inj.	[1981]	JNM
	— R. Johnson lists 11 possible causes for pulmonary °TcSC uptake.	[1972]	JNM
	— M. Vorne finds °Tc-glucohep uptake in 23 of 26 lung ca.	[1979]	JNM
22. Bone	— D. Kean discusses NMR imaging of the knee.	[1981]	JMR
	— J. McAfee tries °Tc-miniMAA (30–100 nm) bone marrow scans.	[1972]	JNM
	— R. Burt finds uptake in ascep nec only after steroid Rx.	[1981]	AJR
	— J. Greiff measures rate of bone callus form with °TcPYP.	[1979]	Inj
	— S. Kattapuram discusses asymp skull lesions and Paget's.	[1974]	SR
	— A. Goldman scans subtalar foot dis not seen on X-Ray.	[1980]	AJR
23. Kidney	— F. Smith scans kidneys with NMR.	[1981]	Rad
	— M. Barker labels renal stones in vivo with IV °TcMDP.	[1973]	BJR
	— J. Belis predicts salvageable bad kidney with °TcDTPA.	[1981]	JU
	— G. Gates estimates GFR on 6min °TcDTPA scan for each kidney.	[1977]	AJR
	— H. Handmaker reviews °scanning in acute pyelonephritis.	[1980]	Sem
24. Gut	— Y. Ichiya says °Ga scans better than X-Ray for lymphoma.	[1977]	Rad
	— W. Haladik: morphine and methadone inhibit bile into gut.	[1974]	Sem
25. Blood	— R. Callahan gives modified method for in vivo °TcRBC tag.	[1979]	JNM
	— M. Dewanjee introduces °In-tropolone platelet label.	[1955]	Rad
26. Other	— F. Smith scans pancreas with NMR.	[1981]	Rad
	— A. Syrota uses C-11 methionine PET scan to see pancreas.	[1981]	Rad
	— A. Gromes compares contrast X-Ray with °TcMAA venograms.	[1979]	Rad
	— H. Fanous confirms vasculogenic impotence with $°TcO_4$ penogram.		YB

Radiation Hysteria and Health Physics * Obituaries *

27. Hyst	— P. Larson says 14 of 86 hi-dose Marshallese hypothyroid.	[1975]	JAMA
	— J. Burks measures dose to nurses at few mrem/quarter.	[1981]	YB
	— R. Prinz says 11% of hyperparathyroids may have thyroid ca; 8 of series of 12 had prior neck irradiation.	[1981]	ca
	— A. Upton finds risk is 4–18 ca/y/10K persons at risk/Sv.	[1981]	SA
	— W. Straub: 0.7% ca in 553 thyroids had 300 R as child.	[1978]	CNM
	— K. Parthasarathy describes safe autopsy, pt with 50 mCi °I.	[1977]	JNM
28. React	— I. McDougall reviews all world's 26 cases of ca after °I Rx; by pure chance alone there would have been >60.	[1979]	CNM
	— B. Cohen: no excess ca at Hanford, states "risk" pitfalls.	[1979]	YJBM
29. Respo	— A. Thomas: no mutagenic effects in bacteria from NMR.	[1981]	BJR
	— M. Goldman: how to deal with mystics & "ALARA" nonsense.	[1980]	WJM
	— 1957 Windscale °I release had no biological effects.	[1978]	NCRP
	* * *		
30. Obits	— E. Quimby (1891–1982) Am rad phys; dosimetry, examiner ABR.		Rad
	— C. Braestrup (1897–1982) Am rad phys; film badge, rad protect.		Rad

CHRONOLOGY OF NUCLEAR MEDICINE — 1983

		Scientific and Technical Background		Ref.
4.	# Med	— H. Royal devises phone transfer of nuc cardiac studies.	[1963]	Rad
		Organizations and Internal Politics		
5.	Pols	— FDA rushes °Tc-Ant Trisul (Sb_2S_3) to phase III IND. Why?	[1979]	FDA
		— FDA finally (4 yrs) releases Taplin °TcDTPA as aerosol.	[1977]	FDA
6.	Socs	— ICRU issues Report #36 on Microdosimetry.	[1980]	ICRU
		Instruments, Units of Measurement, and Drugs		
8.	Instr	— N. Tamaki rotates camera for 3-D gated blood pool scans.	[1982]	Rad
		— R. Moore builds a variable angle slant-hole collimator.	[1982]	JNM
9.	Units	— 17th CGPM defines meter: a distance traversed by light.	[1960]	NBS
		— S. Thomas estim rad dose from Ga-67 scans in children.	[1982]	Rad
10.	Concp	— S. Jahangir: camera orient changes image (mag shield).	[1981]	JNM
		— S. Lukes: hydration of crytal causes °Tl (not Co-57) spots.	[1981]	Rad
		— W. Evanant succeeds: P in vivo NMR spectroscopy (mouse).	[1982]	PNAS
		— C. Harris warns: coincidence sum of Tc-99m looks like °I.	[1953]	Rad
		— F. Cavailoles: diff °Tl distribu in fasted and fed rats.	[1977]	ENM
11.	Drugs	— D. Hnatowich devises a simple °DTPA IgG labeling method.	[1981]	Sc
		— A. Ando studies chem mechanism of Ga-67 tissue labeling.	[1981]	INM
		— R. Proffitt incorporates In-111 into tumor liposomes.	[1979]	Sc
		Radioiodine, P-32, and Radioactive Therapy		
12.	I-Res	— E. Gaitan: resorcinol in H_2O, Colombia hi-goiter district.	[1972]	SN
14.	I-Rx	— J. Wiener finds °I Rx necessary (not surg) in Plummer's.	[1979]	CNM
		— J. Connell notes 5 trans & 19 perm hypos after 55 °I Rx.	[1982]	BJR
		— D. Ross rethinks Means' 1938 adjunctive KI after °I Rx.	[1942]	JCEM
15.	P-Rx	— R. Mantravadi: Cr°PO_4 Rx via sup mes art for liver mets.	[1982]	Rad
		— D. Sullivan shows IP distribution of Cr°PO_4 with °TcSC.	[1975]	Rad
		Scans and Other Tests of Function in Various Organs		
18.	Brain	— R. Ott tries dual °nuc (°Tc, °I-antibody) to scan tumors.	[1981]	BJR
		— H. Kumg tries a new I-123 HIPDM as agent for SPECT scan.	[1982]	JNM
		— N. Lassen compares °Xe with I-123-IMP cerebral blood flows.	[1982]	JNM
		— J. Schwartz detects "brain death" with portable scan.	[1977]	JAMA
		— J. Lynn: diff in Dx of intracranial vs cerebral death.	[1977]	JAMA
		— A. Nisbet: °nuc brain scan should be first in many pts.	[1978]	BJR
19.	Heart	— I. Mena uses 30.5s Au-195m for sequential first-passes.	[1981]	JNM
		— H. Roesler: °I-fatty acid (HDA) is homogen in good hearts.	[1981]	JNM
		— M. Seiderer studies effect of background on R-o-I count.	[1954]	BJR
		— C. Foster looks at exercise protocol's effect on tests.	[1982]	AJCr
		— C. Maynard compares L & R function, supine & sitting pts.	[1982]	AJCr
		— M. Osbakken finds end diastolic filling a factor in EF.	[1982]	AJCr
		— L. Jordan: cold press stim unreliable sub for exercise.	[1982]	AJCr
		— M. Ahmad: cold press stim sensitive in severe disease.	[1982]	AJCr
		— R. Patterson: °Tl scan cannot see 3-vessel dis (disputed).	[1982]	AJCr
		— B. Segal says °Tl scan helps predict result of bypass.	[1982]	AJCr
		— A. Maurer estimates "absolute" LV vol on gated bld pool.	[1982]	AJCr
		— R. Uren measures LV vol with 30° slant-hole collimator.	[1982]	Rad
		— D. Sugrue uses IV Kr-81m to evaluate RV function & anat.	[1982]	BJR
20.	Liver	— P. Alderson: °TcSC detects colon mets as well as CAT.	[1982]	Rad
		— A. Magrini studies hep art/port vein flow ratio °TcHSA.	[1981]	IJG
		— P. Wickremesinghe: °Tc-HIDA checks bile diversion surgery.	[1982]	G
		— A. Nunn analyzes 33 IDA derivatives, takes °Tc-Mebrofenin.	[1979]	JNM
		— W. Klingensmith takes fast moving °Tc-TriMethBrom-IDA.	[1979]	Rad
		— V. Kalff finds many false + °Yc-DIDA biliary scans.	[1982]	Rad

20. Liver	— YB Ed says fasting patient is common to many false + scans.		YB
	— R. Pace notes stenosis causes delayed °TcHIDA dumping.	[1981]	CJS
	— W. Al-Seikh discusses delayed °TcPIPIDA dumping in gut.	[1981]	AJR
	— J. Gerhold separates neonatal-J from B-atresia by °TcIDA.	[1980]	Rad
21. Lung	— D. Osborne compares angiog; questions SPECT scans in dog.	[1981]	Rad
	— L. Wesselives develops a °Ga uptake index of lung dis.	[1980]	ARD
	— O. Nieweg chooses Co-57 bleomycin over °Ga to see tumors.	[1977]	Tho
22. Bone	— M. Brown: 40% of solitary lesions in children metastatic.	[1982]	JNM
	— R. Kloiber uses scans to Dx hip effusions in children.	[1975]	AJR
	— L. Rosenthall sees pseudoarthroses with °Ga & °Tc-PP.	[1975]	CNM
	— T. Ries: H-sign on post sacrum scan indicates fracture.	[1981]	Rad
	— M. LaManna scans °Ga & °Tc to Dx painful arthroplasty.	[1975]	O
	— M. Bunyon: is high kidney uptake sign of hypercalcemia?	[1974]	BJR
	— J. Butler reports scans of subtrocanteric stress fract.	[1981]	AJSM
	— L. Greenwald: X-Ray missed rib fracts after open ht surg.	[1976]	Rad
	— J. Sty starts controversy on battered child synd scans.	[1975]	Rad
	— B. Ghelman localizes osteoid osteo at surg by °Tc-MPD.	[1977]	Rad
	— I. Fogelman says "hot patella" sign has no significance.	[1979]	JNM
23. Kidney	— J. Clorius introduces exercise renograms in hyperten.	[1973]	JNM
	— N. Alazraki: °Ga uptake in normal kidneys in liver dis.	[1980]	CNM
	— K. Ford can est renal blood flow from °TcDTPA renogram.	[1973]	Rad
	— J. Pullen evaluates uretral obstruction on bone scan.	[1975]	AJR
24. Gut	— D. Stein tries °In-leuk to locate Crohn & ulcer colitis.	[1981]	G
	— R. Holloway: °TcSc egg salad measures esoph emptying.	[1981]	G
	— S. Sagar: °Tc-bran meal measures gastric emptying time.	[1981]	CIR
	— S. Heyman: °TcSC in milk measures gastroesoph reflux.	[1981]	Rad
	— P. Christian discusses tech details for gastric scan.	[1977]	JNM
	— T. Vasquez notes sacral °Tc in gastric ulcers (rabbits).	[1972]	Rad
25. Blood	— H. Sugarman: platelets easier to harvest than leuks.	[1981]	AS
	— A. Peters: advantages of °In-tropolonate labeled leuks.	[1981]	JNM
	— V. Runge: °In label eosinophils detect parasitic inflam.	[1981]	Rad
26. Other	— D. Chen reports $°TcO_4$ accurate in 109 scrotal scans.	[1981]	JNM
	— W. Thomas reviews 80 scrotal scans to see Dx range.	[1981]	BJS
	— F. Vieras questions "rim" sign in missed testic torsion.	[1981]	Rad
	— R. Dhenke injects °Tc-HAM into both feet for venography.	[1976]	Rad
	— P. Bardfield detects deep venous thromb after IV °TcSC.	[1981]	Rad
	— P. Matin detects hard-exercise muscle damage with °TcSC.	[1981]	JNM
	— E. Silberstein: ICap °Xe washout finds amputation level.	[1981]	Rad
	— S. LARSON PRODUCES °I MONOCLONAL ANTIBODIES FOR MELANOMA.	[1980]	JNM
	— R. Wahl produces °I monoclonal $F(ab')_2$ for use in Dx.	[1980]	JNM
	— G. Ferlin subtracts $°TcO_4$ from °Tl scan, sees parathyroids.	[1974]	JNM
	— D. GOLDENBERG USES °ANTIBODY IgG PAP TO Dx PROSTATIC CA.	[1975]	JAMA

Radiation Hysteria and Health Physics * Obituaries *

27. Hyst	— Sci News (in ignorance) says NMR will replace CAT scan.	[1982]	SN
	— ABC TV screams, Az Nuc Power Plant has buried evils.	[1984]	AP
28. React	— R. Hickey sees beneficial effects of lo-level radiation.	[1981]	HP
	ORNL survey finds home Rn levels vary by orders of mag.	[1981]	HPN
	— R. Halnan finds °I Rx protects against later ca of thyr.	[1970]	BMJ
	— H. Beekhuis says neg risk of ca after neonate °I scans.	[1948]	ENM
29. [illegible]	— J. [illegible] finds [illegible] variability completely unknown	[1981]	NCRP
	— J. Auxier finds ALARA is used to feather the HP nest.	[1980]	HP

* * *

30. Obits	— M. Friedman (1906–1983) Am radiotherapist; supervoltage, Co-60.	Rad
	— N. Holter (1914–1983) Am biol physics; first SNM, heart monitor.	JNM

CHRONOLOGY OF NUCLEAR MEDICINE — 1984

Scientific and Technical Background

			Ref.
1. Basic	— ALL SIGNIFICANT A-BOMB EFFECTS REQUIRE >1 Gy OF DOSE.	[1980]	RERF
2. Obser	— Controversy erupts over β^+ glucose metab in PET scans.	[1982]	Sc
	— C. Crawley says "Apparent H-3 $T_{1/2}$ is 9 ± 2y in USA.	[1956]	HP
	— "De Minimis" (new HP term) = lower limit of rad of reg concern.		HP
3. # Nuc	— German physicists add element #108, name is #108.	[1980]	SN
4. # Med	— >200 NMR machines said to be operating in med research.	[1983]	PL

Organizations and Internal Politics

5. Pols	— MEDICARE WILL PAY HOSPITALS ONLY ON A DRG SYSTEM.	[1981]	AP
	— FDA delay is threatening production of biliary agents.	[1983]	JNM
	— FDA requires 100 × dose be non-toxic in lab animals.	[1976]	JNM
	— FDA pubs Guidelines for Nuclear Pharmacies.	[1975]	FR
	— 19 States (+ 9 pending) regulate Nuclear Pharmacies.	[1976]	JNM
	— D. Swanson explains FDA procedures for IND applications.	[1983]	JNM
	— EPA stops reg on airborne rad because no hazard exists.	[1981]	Sc
	— Clinch River Breeder Reactor voted out by Congress in spite.		SN
	Exper Breeder (EBR-2) operating safely for 20 years.	[1951]	SN
6. Socs	— Soc Nuc Med asks NRC require 6 mo trng to license cardiologists to use °nuclides, no cardiac trng asked of SNM.	[1982]	SNM
	— ICRU, Report #37, "Tables of Stopping Power. . . ."	[1924]	ICRU
	— Sixth Int Colloq °immunoassay, Lyons, Fr, says major fault is Gov't bureaucracy, "°assay requires special license."	[1948]	PL
7. Event	— J. White describes the COMPLETE nervous system of *C. Elegans*;		Sc
	302 neurons in 1 mm worm (1 × 10^{11} neurons in man).	[1861]	Sc
	— Shippingport Reactor decommissioned after 24 years.	[1966]	SN
	— Gene labeling tests for bacty & genetic dis on market.	[1925]	SN

Instruments, Units of Measurement, and Drugs

8. Instr	— NMR has't yet produced a "clinically" significant image.	[1982]	PL
	— B. Collier raises spectral window to sharpen resolution.	[1983]	Rad
	— C. Kelsey gives reason for film badge: legal requirement.	[1983]	HP
	— Hollerith punch-cards no longer being made.	[1890]	SN
	— SPECT scanner is now commercially available.	[1983]	AP
9. Units	— Health Physics Soc will adopt SI units, begin Jan 1985.	[1975]	HP
	— H. Beekhuis calculates MIRD dose for Co-57-55 bleomycin.	[1983]	JNM
	— P. Dimitriou estimates dose to bladder wall from °TcO_4.	[1982]	JNM
	— Neutron RBE in A-Bomb victims either 5 or >50.	[1956]	RERF
10. Concp	— F. Wolfs finds in/outdoor Rn depends on wind direction.	[1981]	HP
	— B. Cohen estim 10^{-7} probabil of injesting Rn particle.	[1981]	HP
11. Drugs	— M. Nakajo notes intense salivary gland uptake of °I-MIBG.	[1976]	JNM

Radioiodine, P-32, and Radioactive Therapy

12. I-Res	— Am Thyroid Assn says NO KI for reactor accidents <1 Gy.	[1974]	JAMA
14. I-Rx	— P. Allweiss: 11% of hi-dose °I ca pts get sialadenitis.	[1976]	JNM
	— D. Becker says °I Rx is current choice, few exceptions.	[1982]	NEJM
	— R. Utiger says °I Rx is choice but doesn't treat Graves.	[1982]	NEJM
17. Other	— J. Ferens tells prep of °I Rx-level monoclon antib frag.	[1983]	JNM
	— Thousands of pts say rad in mines good for arthritis;	[1971]	HP
	Health Physicists say their pain relief is inconsequential.		PL

Scans and Other Tests of Function in Various Organs

18. Brain	— S. Chervu shows method to measure cereb shunt patency.	[1980]	JNM
	— R. Brauner: hi-dose cranial irrad causes precoc puberty.	[1978]	NEJM

19. Heart	— D. Dymond tries first-pass °TcDTPA after pulm art inject.	[1982]	Rad
	— J. Siegel measures absolu LV vol from gated blood pools.	[1983]	Rad
	— M. Starling measures LV vol from °TcHSA equilib blood pools.	[1983]	JNM
20. Liver	— R. Pettigrew measures 5 normals with °TcSC on SPECT.	[1981]	Rad
	— L. Strauss devises measure of organ volume from SPECT.	[1979]	JNM
	— D. Choy introduces morphine to prove gallbladder fill.	[1982]	Rad
	— W. Williams measures bile flow, 5 agents in 115 normals.	[1982]	JNM
21. Lung	— D. Biello: no consensus interpretation, VP scans for PE.	[1982]	ApR
	— R. Crane sees a pattern on scan of tumor microembolism.	[1983]	JNM
22. Bone	— L. Holder sees shin splints on delayed 3-phase scans.	[1979]	JNM
	— P. Kirchner compares °TcPYP & °Ga in soft tissue sarcoma.	[1980]	JBJS
23. Kidney	— J. Garcia: °Ga uptake in 50% pts with no renal disease.	[1983]	JNM
	— G. Gates develops a computer prog for GFR from °TcDTPA.	[1982]	JNM
24. Gut	— J. Seibert tries °TcSC vs pH probe in gastroesoph reflux.	[1980]	AJR
25. Blood	— S. Kipper scans °In-leuks, locates infection in dialysis.	[1983]	Rad
	— D. Cunningham: °In-platelets locate platelet deposits.	[1983]	Rad
	— P. Cook evaluates °In-leuks in finding occult infection.	[1983]	Rad
26. Other	— A. Strashun finds °Tc & °Ga best Dx in malig ext otitus.	[1980]	Rad
	— I. Singer compares °TcRBC & X-Ray venograms in DVT.	[1982]	Rad
	— P. Lawrence: °TcPYP scan predicts healing of leg ulcers.	[1978]	AJSr

Radiation Hysteria and Health Physics * Obituaries *

27. Hyst	— Juarez, Mex. 450 Ci Co-60 source melted into scrap iron.	[1979]	HP
	— News media strive to see hazard in harmless microwaves.	[1983]	SN
	— Few of 5×10^6 known chemicals have been toxicity tested.	[1944]	NAS
	— ICRP #30 says Rn-232 (gas) & Po-218 (metal) have same	[1981]	
	metabolism. W. Dundulis says ICRP is stupid.	[1907]	HP
	— A. Ruttenber admits U tailings dose too low to cause ca.	[1982]	HP
	— Nuc Pwr insurers get claim/mo, but no exposure >3 Rem.	[1913]	HPN
	— Nuc Plant Contractor digs $300K hole to prove AEC lied.	[1983]	AP
	— NAS reports 60,000 chemicals in use, no toxicity data.	[1944]	SN
28. React	— S. Sarkar finds no effect on progeny from hi-dose °I Rx.	[1976]	NEJM
	— W. Wiatowski finds hosp °contam from Nuc Med trivial.	[1952]	HP
	— FDA DOWNPLAYS RAD TOXICITY TESTING BECAUSE IT IS SO RARE.		FDA
	— Controversy erupts on desirability & honesty of ALARA.	[1982]	HP
	— L. Holm finds °I Rx protects against later thyroid ca.	[1978]	NEJM
	— J. Ballou gives rats 10,000 × MPC of Kr-85, no bio effect.	[1982]	HP
	— G. Dagle finds no risk to dogs from paws injected w/Pu.	[1982]	HP
	— RERF finds no excess gastric ca in Bomb victims @ <200 rads;		
	no change in chromosomes of F_1 generation of survivors;		
	increased lung ca only in >2 Gy exposed survivors.	[1980]	RERF
	— Otake & Schull: 40% mental retard if rad 8–15 wks gestation.		RERF
	— H. Kohn finds no ca, doses <150 rads, in A-Bomb survivors.	[1980]	NEJM.
29. Respo	— US Dist Court finds K.Z. Morgan's Health Phy "dishonest."	[1980]	HPN
	— US Govt liable for rad deaths of 9 from Nevada fallout	[1962]	Sc
	— VA awards compensation for lymphoma from 3.4 mR expos.	[1913]	VA
	— ICRP notes lo-dose irrad risk is lower than reported.	[1968]	ICRP
	— J. Rust says no irrad burro ever developed cancer.	[1979]	PL
	— Nat ca Advis Bd finds NO criteria for carcinogen tests,	[1979]	
	SAYS BIOLOGICAL FACT IS *NOT* PROVED BY STATISTICS,		
	says *predictive* carcinogenesis has proved false.	[1982]	Sc
	— NCRP recognizes that background varies up to 2.8 rad/y.	[1983]	HP
	— Europe, USSR think nuc power reduces fos fuel pollution.	[1960]	AP
	— DOE gives grant to study radiation phobia as a disease,		
	. . . implying that the NRC is sick-sick-sick.		SN

* * *

30. Obits	— P. Kapitsa (1894–1984) Rus physics; solid state, lo-temp, hi-pres.	AP
	— G. Moore (1898–1984 Am Surgeon; fluorescent °dye, brain scan.	JAMA
	— P. Dirac (1902–1984) Eng theor physics; pair produc, anti-matter.	RR
	— H. Parker (1910–1984) Eng Am physics; first health physicist.	HP

CHRONOLOGY OF NUCLEAR MEDICINE — 1985

	Scientific and Technical Background		Ref.
1. Basic	— R. Kammrer: metal corrosion caused by deposited bacteria.	[1876]	SN
2. Obser	— c250 GW$_e$ elec power in world, 15% from 313 nuc reactors.	[1975]	IAEA
	— S. Goldsmith: attacks on "nuclear" are Orwellian Radiology.	[1984]	JNM
4. # Med	— European Nuc Med Conf has 3000 members, gets 1400 absts.	[1979]	EJNM

	Organizations and Internal Politics		
5. Pols	— Congress overrules FDA on saccharin prohibition, but aspartame has taken over much sweetener business.	[1958]	FR
	FIRST MAJOR FAILURE OF FED REGULATORS TO CAUSE HYSTERIA.	[1984]	AP
	— FDA approves use of 100 μCi °TcO$_4$ for dacyrocystography.	[1978]	JNM
	oral 300 μCi °TcSC for esophageal transit.	[1983]	JNM
	oral 500 mCi °TcSC for pulm aspiration study.	[1982]	JNM
	— EPA limits risk from air emissions to 1 cancer/10,000 years.		JAMA
	— NRC rules Cardiologists must have 4 months trng in Nuc Med.	[1984]	JNM
	— Hlth Care Finance Adm adds another uniform test name.	[1980]	JNM
	— At least 30 govt bureaucracies control Nuc Med.	[1947]	JNM
6. Socs	— SNM adopts the correct term Nuc Mag Resonance (NMR);	[1947]	
	Radiology uses meaningless Mag Res Imaging (MRI).	[1984]	JNM
	— First Int Conf on Rad Hormesis meets with overflow crowd.	[1981]	HPN
	— J. Mallard (Hevesy Award): Nuc Med must be more than scan.	[1949]	JNM
7. Event	— F. Culler: °release in reactor accidents is exaggerated.	[1980]	SN
	— F. Culler: Nuc Power Industry has massive public ed going.	[1980]	SN
	— Internat groups accept rad food processing (US holds back).	[1961]	IAEA
	— DOE finally makes "China Syndrome" in exper test reactor.	[1984]	Sc
	— USS Nautilus (first Atoms-for-Peace sub) is retired.	[1954]	AP

	Instruments, Units of Measurement, and Drugs		
8. Instr	— PET scanner commercially available.	[1981]	SN
	— N. Tamaki shows multislice whole body PCT (B$^+$ Comp Tomo).	[1982]	JNM
	— W. McLaughlin patents 0.1 mm dia liquid chem dosimeter.	[1981]	JNM
	— M. Kulkarni compares NMR & °nuc scans in 56 patients.	[1984]	JNM
	— MIT produces biomagnetic image of human biomag field.	[1969]	SN
9. Units	— NBS (TimeFreqDiv) has hydrogen clock, accuracy 266 ns/y.	[1929]	NBS
	— J. Harvey estims dose from 6-°fluoro-L-DTPA (2.6 rem/mCi).	[1983]	JNM
	— B. Breitenstein measures 25y retention of 1 nCi Am-241; autopsy of all tissues to check HP dose calculations.	[1975]	HP
10. Concp	— A. Keenan reviews status of monocl antibod in Nuc Med.	[1983]	JNM
11. Drugs	— R. Baldwin hooks monoclonal antibodies onto methtresate.	[1984]	SN
	— M. Thakup prepares kit for In-111 merc oxide leukocytes.	[1983]	JNM
	— J. Spicer reports rare reaction to °TcMPD (22nd case).	[1984]	JNM

	Radioiodine, P-32, and Radioactive Therapy		
12. I-Res	— T. Hiraoka: Mean lethal dose to in vitro cells is 66 Rad.	[1906]	RERF
	— W. McKitrick describes errors in pinhole imaging.	[1947]	JNM
	— K. Miller: Tinct iodine on skin blocks thyroid °I uptake.	[1932]	HP
13. I-Dx	— V. Teixeira shows T3, T4, Tg, THS, TRH in subac thyroiditis.	[1978]	JNM
	— J. Floyd replaces 24h I-131 with 4h I-123 uptake.	[1971]	JNM
14. I-Rx	— J. Hamburger uses 25–200 mCi Rx of toxic multinod goiter.	[1913]	JNM
	— W. Spiegel: sialadenitis in 30% °I Rx of ca in 20 years.	[1965]	JNM
17. Other	— S. Larson: good prelim, I-131 Fab Rx of malig melanoma.	[1984]	Rad
	— W. Beierwaltes describes M°IBG Rx and renewed P-32 Rx.	[1982]	JNM
	— E. Silberstein brings back Sr-89 for Rx of bone pain.	[1978]	JNM
	— A. Turner suppresses hepatic hematopoiesis with Au-198.	[1978]	JNM

Scans and Other Tests of Function in Various Organs

18.	Brain	— J. Curnes detects CSF fistula by °TcDTPA rhinorrhea.	[1968]	Rad
19.	Heart	— C. Bouched evaluates dipyridamole as stress in °Tl scan.	[1983]	NEJM
		— J. McMeekin compares first pass & gated °ventriculograms.	[1984]	ApR
		— J. Parker: multigate scans & wall motion do not jibe.	[1983]	Rad
		— A. Maurer corrects attenuation in LV peak & end sys vol.	[1983]	Rad
20.	Liver	— R. Lee detects Sphinct Oddi stenosis by GI dumping time.	[1974]	Rad
		— R. Sigar finds first 9 NMR hemangioma scans same as °scan.	[1984]	JNM
		— R. Stadalnik introduces °TcNGA hepatic binding ligand.	[1984]	JNM
21.	Lung	— M. Lee follows 69 low probability pts; finds Dx accurate.	[1981]	Rad
		— R. Lambert: °Ga has no uptake in asbestos worker pleura.	[1982]	JNM
		— T. Barron scans *pneumocyst carinii* pneumonia with °Ga.	[1983]	Rad
		— D. Coleman compares °Ga & broncoscope in AIDS *p. carinii*.	[1983]	ARD
22.	Bone	— F. Mettler says bone scan is now most common scan.	[1972]	JNM
		— C. Vellenga measures scan changes after Rx of Paget's.	[1974]	ENM
		— R. Campbell: scan not a screen for renal cell ca mets.	[1984]	JU
		— P. Davey: scan not a good screen for bladder ca mets.	[1984]	JU
		— N. Papanicolao uses °TcMDP in excised osteoid osteoma.	[1983]	Rad
		— L. Nilas compares 1 & 2 photon absorption in osteoporosis.	[1977]	JNM
		— H. Wahner tests Gd-153 bone mass measure in cadavers.	[1979]	Rad
23.	Kidney	— A. Tamkin notes delayed excretion on renogram after SCI.	[1977]	JU
		— J. Jacobs compares °TcDMSA & °TcGlucohep in function test.	[1981]	AJR
		— H. Lee studies mechanism of °TcGlucohep tubular uptake.	[1979]	JNM
		— G. Bower compares Nuc cyctography methods in 30 children.	[1982]	JNM
24.	Gut	— J. Cardarelli measures Co-57 VB_{12} absorption on camera.	[1978]	JNM
25.	Blood	— B. Gilbert locates renal abscess with °In labeled WBC.	[1984]	JNM
26.	Other	— L. Knight labels Frag E_1 with I-123 to detect DVT.	[1983]	Rad
		— S. Halpern: good prelim use of In-111 monocl antibodies.	[1983]	Rad
		— M. McCalley sees patent Fallopian tube with °TcHAM.	[1981]	JNM
		— G. Winzelberg subtracts °TcO_4 from °Tl for parathyroids.	[1983]	Rad
		— I. Fogelman subtracts °TcO_4 from °Tl for parathyroids.	[1983]	ENM

Radiation Hysteria and Health Physics * Obituaries *

27.	Hyst	— FDA whimsically declares food irrad a food additive!	[1958]	NEJM
		permits irrad of wheat (insects), potatoes (stop	[1925]	NEJM
		sprouting), spice (sterilization).	[1958]	NEJM
		— J. Rotblat: Acute Rad Synd LD_{50} is 6Gy (Eng), 4.5Gy (US),	[1970]	SN
		cites proposed reduction to 1.5Gy with no new data.	[1960]	SN
		— S. Sivak documents new popular newspaper hysteria: AIDS.	[1965]	NEJM
28.	React	— C. Wu: rats accum genetic change twice faster than man.	[1976]	PNAS
		— E. Harvey: twins irrad (<4 rad) in utero have lo-excess ca.	[1983]	NEJM
		— B. MacMahon: no evidence for assoc fetal irrad & cancer	[1982]	NEJM
		— P. Butler: ave "chest X-Ray" exposure now 20 mr (3–120 mr).	[1959]	Rad
		— Rn bkgd varies by orders of magnitude over land mass.	[1983]	HPN
		— J. Beyea reviews TMI dosimetry by NRC, DOE, EPA, FDA, PA & MD,		
		state and utility, finds their estimates political.	[1980]	HPN
		— F. Cross says 10 μCi Rn-222/L is "tolerance" for drinking.	[1981]	HP
		— C. Mays admits metabolism of U is not adequately known.	[1981]	HP
29.	Respo	— EPA limits water to 100 μg U/L(67 pCi/L) based on faith.	[1981]	HP
		— H. Checkoway finds rad hormesis in 8375 ORNL workers.	[1985]	BJIM
		— J. Acquavella: 7,616 men exposed (<91rem, 27yrs) live longer.		HP
		— Lo-dose effluent from Savannah River Pu reactors causes DOE		
		field mice to live longer with increased reproduction		
		through 10 generations of field study.	[1981]	DOE
		— H. Muller finds lower ca rates in PA 6y after TMI.	[1981]	JNM

* * *

30. Obits —

CHRONOLOGY OF NUCLEAR MEDICINE — 1986

Scientific and Technical Background

			Ref.
1. Basic	— 10×10^6 bacteria/g found at 850 feet below soil surface.	[1908]	SN
	— P. Diaconis questions current concept of "random" statistics. IF TRUE, ALL SMALL SAMPLE STATISTICS IS QUESTIONED	[1886]	Sc
2. Obser	— Greenwich Observatory (1675) to be moved again.	[1949]	Sc
3. # Nuc	— Dubna (USSR) reports, but can't confirm #110.	[1984]	SN
	— Darmstadt (W Ger) has confirmed existence of #109.	[1984]	SN
	— ORNL produces 300 hi-enrich, of all stable elements.	[1982]	HPN
	— ORNL produces 200 Ci/m of Gd-153, for osteoporosis inst.	[1985]	HPN
	— 57.7K engineers, 16K scientists, 50.4K technicians are employed in nuclear-related activities, down 10%.	[1971]	DOE
4. # Med	— Market for NM products is: 60% US & Canada, 20% Japan, 15% Europe, 5% Australia, <1% all others.	[1964]	JNM
	— $1.2 billion sales in W Europe of Dx image equipment.	[1951]	JNM
	— 191 residents in Nuclear Medicine in 91 programs in US.	[1971]	JAMA

Organizations and Internal Politics

5. Pols	— Congress cuts NRC budget, says "research" real problem.	[1985]	FR
	— Pres. Reagan says July 27–Aug 2 is national Nuc Med wk.	[1777]	JNM
	— DOE (ex AEC) still supports Nuc Med applications.	[1984]	JNM
	— Japan each year budgets c$10 million for RERF (ABCC).	[1984]	Sc
	— Draft of Revised 10 CFR 20 is totally unintelligible.	[1985]	HPN
	— NCRP & ICRP writes 10 CFR 20; adopted in FR 1/9/86.	[1959]	FR
	— FDA insane requirements designed to stop all Nuc Med.	[1985]	JNM
	— EPA drinking water rules have been "miserable failure."	[1985]	SN
6. Socs	— $890 3-day course given, "How to understand 10 CFR 20."	[1985]	JNM
	— HP Soc members declare new 10 CFR 20 is undecipherable.	[1968]	HPN
7. Event	— Voyager 2 reaches Uranus, powered by 3 °nuclide generators, each producing c160 watts or 30 Mwatts in 8 y.	[1985]	SN

Instruments, Units of Measurement, and Drugs

8. Instr	— $232 million sales Nuc Mag Res equipment in world in 1985.	[1977]	JNM
9. Units	— ICRU pubs report #40 on Quality Factor, old RBE,	[1980]	ICRU
	admits no firm scientific basis for rad protection.	[1968]	ICRU
	— NBS sells 6 standards for short lived Tl, Cr, In, Tc, I.	[1958]	HPN
10. Concp	— R. Shore studies Pediatric Nuc Med dosage adjustments.	[1980]	JNM
	— F. Edwards: Risk/Benefit dose models can't predict cause.	[1985]	Sem
11. Drugs	— C. Hoefnagel: °I-Meta-IodoBenzylGuanidine-norepineph.	[1984]	CNM
	— M. Berridge labels butanol with O-15 for CBF studies.	[1934]	JNM
	— C. Brihaye has a 15 day Os-191 to 5 sec Ir-191m cow.	[1980]	JNM

Radioiodine, P-32, and Radioactive Therapy

12. I-Res	— E. Gaitan: resorcinol & dihydroxybenzoic are goitrogenic.	[1983]	SN
	— R. Cooksey says millet contains goiterogenic flavinoid.	[1659]	SN
	— NCRP #80 finds no ca from I-131, °Tc, recommends caution.	[1974]	NCRP
	— I. Morimoto: no thyroid disease in 30y A-Bomb survivors exposed to <100 rads; 16/477 at >100 rads.	[1984]	RERF
13. I-Dx	— S. Amico: thyroid calcification seen on °TcHMDP bone scan.	[1981]	JNM
14. I-Rx	— D. Van Nostrand: bio effects from hi-dose Rx, no ARS.	[1947]	JNM
	— C. Hoefnagel says scan Tl-201 total body after ca Dx.	[1978]	JNM
	— M. Bohrer says hypo after any Rx is natural for hyperthyroidism.	[1983]	NEJM

17. Other	— J. Van Der Steen gives °I-MIGB Rx for neuroblastoma.	[1984]	HP
	— M. Eisenhut: bone mets pain relief in $<50\%$ with °I-BDP3.	[1968]	JNM
	— NIH says I-127 in DNA molecule enhances °sensitivity.	[1976]	SN
	— R. Levy: 4y cure of B-cell lymphoma with monocl antibody.	[1982]	JAMA
	Scans and Other Tests of Function in Various Organs		
18. Brain	— P. Sharp suggests routine Cer Bld Flows with °TcHMPAO.	[1982]	JNM
	— P. Rakic says human brain has more than 10^{14} synapses.	[1966]	Sc
19. Heart	— J. Tillisch uses °NH_3 PET scan to predict bypass result.	[1984]	NEJM
20. Liver	— H. Mok dates gallstones by using C-14 (from Bomb Test).	[1975]	NEJM
	— R. Lisbona reviews Xe-133 scans in 60 pts' fatty livers.	[1979]	CNM
	— S. Shinkichi shows RIA for liver fibrosis in alcoholism.	[1968]	JAMA
21. Lung	— W. Burch tries °Tc-pseudogas (0.12 μm size) for vent scan.	[1980]	JNM
	— N. Frankel: fewer angios in pts getting lung scan first.	[1969]	JNM
22. Bone	— D. Van Nostrand: 23 giant cell tumors, increased uptake.	[1985]	JNM
	— ORNL says Gd-153 osteoporosis device most common °test.	[1985]	HPN
	— P. Geusens measures density in 366 normals, 15–85 years.	[1985]	JNM
23. Kidney	— H. Abdel-Dayem sees uremic pleural effusion on renogram.	[1985]	CNM
	— A. Taylor tests °TcMAG to replace °I-Hipp in 10 normal men.	[1979]	JNM
24. Gut	— R. Sollitto sees *p. carinii* in AIDS with Ga-67.	[1985]	JNM
25. Blood	— N. Chonacky calculates plasma clearance by new formula.	[1946]	JNM
26. Other	— G. Hadley finds °I-MIBG uptake in 6/7 neuroblastomas.	[1979]	JNM
	— C. Hoefnagel: Dx & Rx of neural cres tumor with °I-MIBG.	[1979]	CNM
	— J. Anderson uses In-11 autologous leuks in pancreatitis.	[1982]	JNM
	Radiation Hysteria and Health Physics * Obituaries *		
27. Hyst	— S. Danall measures 4 Greek spas at kBq of Ra-226, K-40.	[1982]	HP
	— Irish Sea said to be "most °active" from English waste.	[1966]	Sc
	— 26 Apr – partial meltdown at Chernobyl, Ukraine, 31? dead.	[1979]	AP
	Fallout from Chernobyl picked up in most countries.	[1987]	Sc
	I-131 release said to be 30–40 MCi (doubted, too hi).	[1979]	HPN
	— S. Hoar: any carcinogen *must* be hazardous in lo-dose.	[1985]	JAMA
	— FDA says reduce Nuc Med dose to infants, no evidence.	[1985]	FDA
	— Surg Gen says 50% of cancer *caused* by cigarettes.	[1985]	AP
	— CDC (Atlanta) estimates: over 50% of males have smoked.	[1979]	JAMA
28. React	— Lung ca in males is in 10^{-4} range. Cause?	[1984]	JAMA
	— A. Jacobson: dose from 20 slice CT scan is c2–5 Rad.	[1985]	HP
	— "Quality Assessment" is now a Federal fake Q control.	[1956]	HPN
	— RERF studies relation between boiled fish & ca in ARCC.	[1985]	RERF
	— RERF finds fewer stroke deaths in A-Bomb survivors.	[1985]	RERF
	— Soc Nuc Med reports 3 adverse reactions/million doses.	[1960]	JNM
	— Houdini's ghost fails to show up for the 60th time.	[1849]	AP
29. Respo	— E. Zeighami: risk from $<$400 rad unknown in man & animal.	[1982]	HP
	NOT ENOUGH PEOPLE IN WORLD TO PROVE LO-DOSE RISK		
	— Information released on Loss-of-Fluid-Test reactor "China Syndrome" controlled "accident" in July 1985.		DOE
	— NRC has an Incident Investig Team (IIT) for Accidents.	[1968]	NRC
	— NRC issues operat licen to 99th–101st Nuc Power plants.	[1985]	HPN
	— E. Ritenour says no data exists showing rad causes ca.	[1985]	Sem
	— F. Ritenour says no bio effect ever shown below 15 rad.	[1985]	Sem
	— ICRP discards 10 day rule (X-Rays only after menstrual).	[1960]	DJR
	* * *		
30. Obits	— Henry D. Smyth (1898–1986) Am physics, 1945 Smyth report, ALC.		AP
	— Hyman Rickover (1900–1986) Am admiral USN; nuclear navy.		SN
	— James A. Victoreen (1902–1986) Am inst maker; Victoreen R meter.		HP
	— George E. Burch (1910–1986) Am cardiol; °Hg, °Na, metabolism, renog.		AP
	— Daniel R. Biello (1947–1986) Am radiol; lung scan V/P criteria.		Sem

CHRONOLOGY OF NUCLEAR MEDICINE — 1987

	Scientific and Technical Background		Ref.
1. Basic	— P. CHU FINDS SUPERCONDUCTIVITY ABOVE 77K LIQ NITROGEN.	[1911]	Sc
2. Obser	— NBS sees harmless amino acid in irradiated meat fibers.	[1985]	ScN
3. # Nuc	— Dubn (USSR) reports possible element #110, unconfirmed.	[1986]	ScN
	— Los Alamos Meson Facility major source for Be-7, Na-22, Cu-67, Ge-68, Br-82, Sr-82, Y-88, Rb-82,		
	— Brookhaven & Atom Ener Canada lead in Xe-127, Cd-109.	[1962]	JNM
4. # Med	— D. Pretschner finds 3500 gamma cameras, 14 PET units, in Europe.	[1979]	EJNM
	— F. Mettler notes 4.4×10^9 pop, 17×10^6 hosp beds, 3.7×10^6 docs on 408×10^3 Dx units do 1.24×10^9 Dx exams; estimated 315×10^6 dental exams; 18,000 Rx units do 4 million brachytherapy procedures; 22,300 scan units do 22.3×10^6 nuclear exams.	[1979]	HP
	Organizations and Internal Politics		
5. Pols	— NRC (NucRegComm) $100 Mill/y research produces no pubs.	[1984]	SN
	— 3 Day course given on how to read new NRC 10CFR20.	[1986]	AP
	— ORNL sets up Monitored Retrievable Storage for waste.	[1986]	DoE
	— Calif law says Gov must list carcinogens & sex toxins.	[1986]	Sc
	— Gen Account Office says NCI overstates cancer progress.	[1986]	AP
	— GAO finds improv in child leukemia Rx, none in chronic.	[1977]	Sc
	— Fed Court rules FDA must ban dye @ 10^{-19} Delaney risk.	[1986]	AP
6. Socs	— European Assoc Nuc Med formed (1986) from Soc Nuc Med Eur & Eur Soc Nuc Med; English to be official language.	[1967]	JNM
	— R. Wilbur questions survival of Nuc Med as specialty.	[1971]	JNM
	— Nat Acad Sc: USA Pu reactors, no accidents but unsafe.	[1984]	Sc
7. Event	— DOE shuts down 4 ORNL reactors in Chernobyl response.	[1986]	AP
	Instruments, Units of Measurement, and Drugs		
8. Instr	— SPECT (Siemens, Toshiba) now is top ranking scanner.	[1986]	CNM
	— 11 papers (e.g., M. Itoh) discuss clinical uses of NMR.	[1986]	JNM
	— 31 papers (e.g., D. Mankoff) discuss clinical uses of PET.	[1984]	JNM
	— 7 papers (e.g., M. Farlow) say NMR only c75% + in MS (etc).	[1986]	YB
	— Mfgr renews Thorius filter idea with erbium's K edge.	[1985]	Rad
9. Units	— *de minimus non curat lex,* law not concerned with trifles; after 7 years, still no agreement on de minimus dose.	[1957]	HP
	— 1 rem is now equated with 0.01 Sv; 1 Sv = 100 rem.	[1962]	HP
	— NRCP reduces cumulative exp from 5 (N•18 rem) to (N•1 rem).	[1984]	RRS
	— NRCP says Q (old RBE) should be 20 for neutrons.	[1984]	NCRP
10. Concp	— M. Frazier finds no typical rad change in oncogenes.	[1876]	HPN
	— Oncogenes are the current favorite "cause of cancer."	[1976]	SN
	— B. Romney lists legal breast milk manumission, °Tc, °I.	[1958]	ApR
11. Drugs	— R. Hayes: 30d Es-255 to 20h Fm-255 alpha cow described.	[1974]	ORAU
	— R. Hayes: must be used with monoclonal antibody tag.	[1986]	ORNL
	— M. Kilbourn compares protein labels, F-18, °I, °Tc, °Br, etc.	[1982]	JNM
	— H. Kung finds °I-PPA has brain scan agent requirements.	[1969]	JNM
	— A. Packard improves 15d Os-191 — 5s Ir-191m cow system.	[1986]	JNM
	Radioiodine, P-32, and Radioactive Therapy		
12. I-Res	— K. Endo reports 19/19 + °Tc-DMSA scans of meduallary ca.	[1970]	JNM
	— J. Chen measures thyroid volume with SPECT with I-123.	[1953]	JNM
	— P. Mountford: perchlorate suppresses °Tc & °I lactation.	[1955]	JNM
13. I-Dx	— E. Avalos uses serum free T_3 concentr to Dx questable thyrotox.	[1970]	JNM

13. I-Dx	— W. Szpunar says TBG assay test is superior in 2819 pts.	[1985]	JNM
	— H. Wasserman corrects uptake from °Tc coincidence sum.	[1979]	HP
	— W. Hedrick finds 3 × increase in uptake dose to newborns.	[1975]	JNM
14. I-Rx	— H. Creutzig sees 172/516 metastases 10 y after Rx.	[1968]	JNM
	— E. Watson recalcs I-131 dose in hyperthyroid patients.	[1963]	JNM
	— Z. Yoosufani finds second leuk after 820 mCi I-131 ca Rx.	[1973]	JNM
	— O. Schober finds minor cytopenia 5yrs after hi-dose °I.	[1942]	JNM
17. Other	— Rheumatoid spondylitis Rx with Ra-224 is reviewed.	[1983]	EJNM
	— W. Goeckeler considers Sm-153-EDTMP in Rx of bone malig.	[1983]	JNM
	— R. Atcher renews use of alphas with monoclon antibodies.	[1985]	JNM
	— A. Brendal finds °I-MIBG disappointing in neuroblastoma.	[1986]	JNM

Scans and Other Tests of Function in Various Organs

18. Brain	— W. Kaplan scans with °Tl, for highest path correlation.	[1987]	JNM
	— V. Lee sees sup sag sinus hint in 26/53 brain dead pts.	[1983]	JNM
19. Heart	— B. Holman finds second °Tl substitute, °Tc-CPI; first is out.	[1987]	JNM
	— K. Vyska measure °fatty acid uptake in 10 normals.	[1983]	JNM
	— K. Mossberg measures skel muscle blood flow with Rb-82.	[1975]	JNM
20. Liver	— 4 Authors (e.g., A. Mehta) study morphine in biliary scans.	[1984]	JNM
	— R. Wells says °Tc-IDA biliary scans best Dx in neonates.	[1987]	ApR
	— J. Hunter sees first(?) breast ca met in a "delta" sign.	[1980]	JNM
21. Lung	— A. Palla injects segmental pul arteriols (°Tc) for anat.	[1986]	JNM
	— J. Bitran finds a Ga-67 pattern in lungs of AIDS pts.	[1986]	JNM
22. Bone	— M. Adatepe: normal °TcMDP & °Ga means NO hemat pyogenic osteomyelitis.	[1936]	JNM
	— ORNL sees decreased demand for Gd-153 for densitometry.	[1985]	ORNL
23. Kidney	— D. Waller compares °Tc GFR with plasma clearance tech.	[1985]	JNM
	— J. Bomanji evaluates °TcDTPA transit after lithotripsy.	[1973]	JNM
24. Gut	— C. Divgi: Dx of protein-losing enteropathy with °TcHSA.	[1965]	JNM
	— G. Conrad measures gastric emptying in 8 fasting normals.	[1982]	JNM
25. Blood	— S. Vallabhajosula: 10.7d °In-tropolone platelet life-span.	[1982]	JNM
	— M. Meignan: no defects but warns of °Tc lympho toxicity.	[1978]	JNM
26. Other	— W. Nelp does lymphoscintography of malig melanoma antiB.	[1985]	JNM
	— S. Zwas combines °I-toluidine & $°TcO_4$ for parathyroids.	[1985]	JNM

Radiation Hysteria and Health Physics * Obituaries *

27. Hyst	— Rx of childhood benign bone dis with Ra-224 in 1950s caused >50% ca. How story found false is told at Eur SNM.	[1903]	JNM
	— AliMed Inc sells total body lead shield for surgeons.	[1953]	AP
	— 300 Spiritualist churches in USA, 100 y after hoax.	[1872]	AP
	— EPA mounts major anti-radon hysteria, MPC is 4 pCi/L.	[1986]	JNM
	IRCP says MPC is 8 pCi/L, UK says 20 pCi/L is MPC.	[1932]	JNM
	— Arizona newspaper finds 5.2 pCi Rn in homes, starts hysteria.	[1986]	AzDS
	— NRCP says *De Minimis* is 0.001 rem/y (Neg Individ Risk).	[1981]	NCRP
	— N. Newell says increase in CO_2 due to human exhalations.	[1940]	SN
28. React	— B. Cohen: ABCC results show BEIR risk much too high.	[1981]	HP
	— Chernobyl radiation deaths at 29 on first anniversary.	[1986]	JAMA
	— I. Morimoto: no thyroid A-Bomb damage under IGy in 30y.	[1986]	RERF
	— R. Gries sees *less* lung ca in cig smokers exposed to Rn.	[1983]	HP
	— D. Preston: irradiation does not produce excess cancer risk.		RERF
	— B. Specker calcs negligible risk in 2,000 lung scan pts.	[1986]	JNM
29. Respo	J. Forbes: potential litigation is reason for H Physics.	[1981]	HPN
	— L. Stoloff finds NO human carcinogens in aflatoxin.	[1984]	Sc
	— Center Disease Cont finds no damage from Agent Orange.	[1984]	Sc

* * *

30. Obits	— M. von Laue (1898–1987) Aust physics; wavelength of X-rays.	WoA
	— Milo Harris (1904–1987) Am physician; third Pres, Soc Nuc Med.	JAMA
	— M. Prinzmetal (1909–1987) Am physician; RadioCardioGraphy.	JAMA
	— Gerald J. Hine (1916–1987) Am rad physics; internal dosimetry.	JNM
	— Phil C. Johnson (1925–1987) Am physician; Xe ventilation scan.	JAMA

CHRONOLOGY OF NUCLEAR MEDICINE — 1988

	Scientific and Technical Background		Ref.
1. Basic	— D. Faust finds psychology & -iatry invalid as science.	[1903]	Sc
	— M. Moe: is it nutrinoless double β decay in Se→Br→Kr-82?	[1987]	SN
2. Obser	— Nat Geographic Mag (May) describes people in Kerala as India's healthiest, no mention of radon. (A hormesis example?)	[1985]	
3. # Nuc	— USA research isotope prod in trouble. Brkhaven & Los A cyclos are research funded for non-med, costs escalating.	[1965]	JNM
	Sr-82 = 800 mCi/mo; Ge-68 = >600 mCi/mo; Xe-127 = 7 Ci/mo; Cu-67 = 1 Ci/mo; about 32 cyclo isotopes now in demand.	[1987]	JNM
4. # Med	— Over 600 MRI (NMR) instruments in USA; 100 in Europe.	[1986]	Sc
	Organizations and Internal Politics		
5. Pols	— R. Alexander (HP Soc): Rad Protect is bureaucratic overkill.		HPSN
	— R. Alexander proposes to NRC, 15 mrem is *B*elow *R*egul *C*oncern.		HPSN
	— J. Campbell: EPA & NRC waste disposal regs impossible.	[1984]	Sc
	— 1957 Windscale reactor accident was censored by Brit.	(1988	Sc)
	— H of Rep subcom says ca death in fallout area should get $50K.		AP
	— USA life expect up 0.1y to 75.4y, blacks down 0.3 to 69.4.	[1980]	AP
6. Socs	— Soc of Digital Imaging Manag and Com (SDIMC), first meet.	[1987]	JNM
	— NCRP rep #93 says 1 mrem/y exposure is negligible, 360 mrem/y is average — 200 is from Rn.	[1985]	NCRP
	— NCRP proposes 10–20 mrem exposure is Below Reg Concern.	[1984]	HPN
	— NBS is NIST (Nat Inst of Standards & Technol) 8/23/88.	[1901]	HPN
	— A. Nero says EPA grossly misreps its own radon data.	[1987]	Sc
	— Antibody, Immuno & °pharmaceuticals; new quarterly pub.	[1987]	
7. Event	— Pop USA = 244.4 Mil; 74.9y expt. 3,829,000 births, 2,127,000 deaths last year in USA; 13,000 AIDS deaths (15th rank).	[1960]	SAb
	Instruments, Units of Measurement, and Drugs		
8. Instr	— R. Swaja: intercalib of 8018 neutron badges highly variable (605) for estimating doses in mSv levels.	[1984]	ORNL
9. Units	— J. Morton measures Am-241 & Ir-192 brachytherapy RBEs.	[1984]	RRS
	— NBS: new standard for voltage; frequency via Josephson junc.		Sc
	— J. Fabrikant: Working-level month (WLM) for radon = exposure to 3.7 Bq (100 pCi) of radon for 170 hours/month.	[1943]	Bk
	4.0 pCi/L Rn in air is USA EPA "action level."	[1976]	
	10.0 pCi/L is British, 15 pCi/L is ICRP level.	[1950]	Sc
	— D. Shearer notes Mo-99m $T_{B1/2}$ of 11–19 days in 16 pts.	[1949]	JNM
	— Pres Reagan signs Trade Act making Metric Units (SI) official; all federal agencies must comply by 1992.	[1980]	Sc
	— R. Leggett models kinetic biodose for 75sec Rb-82.	[1955]	HP
10. Concp	— J. Hardwick finds gene alteration in Ra dial painter.	[1931]	RRS
	— R. Dobson: no rad mutations to immature oocytes (hi-dose).	[1960]	RRS
	— W. Ellett: BEIR IV error in calc lung ca-from-Rn program increases smoking danger by 25%; other errors?	[1969]	Sc
	— H. Dunster says ALARA is article of faith & unworkable.	[1984]	HP
11. Drugs	— M. Sclar describes a gene (human) that gives rad resistance.		RRS
	— J. Lacy optimises 21.7d W-178 → 9.3m Ta-178 °cow.	[1978]	JNM
	— A. Bertrand: will °Tc-MIBI or Borinate replace Tl-201?	[1977]	JNM
	Radioiodine, P-32, and Radioactive Therapy		
12. I-Res	— F. Datz finds °Tl scans worthless in thyroid ca (comp to °I).		JNM
13. I-Dx	— S. Clarke: °TcDMSA, °TcMIBG, & °TcMDP compared in medullary carcinoma	[1987]	JNM

	— A. Brendel cannot recommend Tl-201 to DDx undif thyr ca.	[1970]	JNM
14. I-Rx	— R. Höschl finds °I in inflam lung after thyroid ca Rx.	[1985]	JNM
	— J. Malamitsi tries intracav Rx with °I-mono, antibod in 19 pts (breast & ovarian effusions), good in 13/14.	[1968]	JNM
17. Other	— G. Blake gets 850 rad/mCi Sr-89 in 10 prostate ca pts.	[1942]	JNM
	— J. Turner treats bone mets with 25–50 mCi Sm-153 EDTMP.	[1968]	JNM

Scans and Other Tests of Function in Various Organs

18. Brain	— N. Andreasen compares clinical CT, NMR, PET & SPECT scans.	[1979]	Sc
	— A. Keyeux finds low rCBF (°Xe inhal) in int carotid occ.	[1980]	JNM
19. Heart	— G. Segall questions dipyridamole quant in Tl-201 scans.	[1973]	JNM
20. Liver	— F. Hahn finds liver ca in 15/59 dogs inhaling hi-dose Ce-144.		RRS
	— M. O'Connor measures art vs portal bld flow, 4 methods.	[1981]	JNM
21. Lung	— B. Marshall uses C-14 urea breath test (bacty gastritus);	[1932]	
	— OK with C-11, but C-14 is a dirty contamination.	[1932]	
22. Bone	— A. Kwai: 76% of single sternal lesions are mets in breast ca.		JNM
23. Kidney	— O. Carlsen: °I-Hipp rads lower than °Tc-DTPA or X-renog.	[1978]	JNM
	— A. Taylor substitutes °TcMAG$_3$ (MercapAcetGly) for °I-Hipp.	[1986]	JNM
24. Gut	— B. Esses sees hi-dose damage (and repair) of taste buds.	[1914]	RRS
	— W. Murphy uses heparin to see °TcRBC bleeding in gut.	[1983]	JNM
25. Blood	— D. Schauwe compares °In granulo with mixed leuko effect.	[1982]	JNM
26. Other	— J. Seabold: 24h delay cuts errors in °platelet DVT scans.	[1985]	JNM
	— M. Cohen detects malig melanoma with °I-amphetamine.	[1951]	JNM

Radiation Hysteria and Health Physics * Obituaries *

27. Hyst	— HP's say ICRP 1987 recommendations hard to apply & use.	[1986]	HP
	— DOE puts Hanford "N" reactor on hold after Chernobyl.	[1986]	SN
	— J. Wang: Chinese radiologists have more ca (dose ???) (This 0 measurement study is NCI repeat of 1950s anti-rad fiasco)	[1958]	SN
	— R. Kerr (Sc Edit) *assumes* 5–20,000/y dead from indoor Rn.	[1984]	Sc
	— L. Anspaugh: ~15 PBq Cs-137 released from Chernobyl accident. 0 to negligible 50y risk of ca; no genetic effects.	[1987]	Sc
	— A. Konradi invents new hysteria: orbital debris will soon cause signif interact with hi-energy Van Allen Belt protons.		Sc
28. React	— R. Alexander: hormesis in ABCC leukemias under 50 rad.	[1985]	HPSN
	— R. Miller: 12/78 fetuses in utero got ≥10 rad are retarded.	[1984]	HP
	— K. Kopecky: A-Bomb exp no increase in lung ca by smoking.	[1982]	RERF
	Heavy smokers showed fewer lung ca than light smokers.	[1986]	RERF
	— C. Mays: 347 liver ca deaths in 1964 Thorotrast pts;	[1933]	HP
	— C. Mays: 16 osteosarc pts in world Thorotrast literature.	[1967]	HP
	— C. Mays: No increase in lung ca in German Thorotrast pts.	[1984]	HP
	— S. Tokuoka finds 77 ovarian ca in 70,000 ABCC women; (vs 74 ovarian ca in nonexposed women) in 40 year.	[1974]	RERF
29. Respo	— D. Preston recalculates risk estimates for RERF (ABBC).	[1986]	RRS
	— R. Johnson describes US Justice Dept Rad Litigation Team.	[1986]	RRS
	— J. Fabrikant: (BEIR IV) no evidence, lo-dose radon effect.	[1987]	Bk
	— V. Plaĉek reviews U, Fe, clay miners' Rn damage, barely sig.	[1953]	HP
	— L. Kinlan: Leuk clusters related to virus not radiation.	[1982]	La

* * *

30. Obits	I. Rabi (1899–1988) Am physics; Nuclear Magnetic Resonance.	AP
	— W. Mayneord (1902–1988) Eng physics, roentgen dosimetry, isodose surfaces.	BJR
	— L. Meyer (1906–1988) Am hematol; °vit B$_{12}$, °CO, °Cr, RBC.	JAMA
	— W. Myers (1908–1988) Am chemist; introduced Sr-87m.	AP
	— L. Alvarez (1911–1988) Am physics; H bub chamber, CT extinction.	Sc
	— G. Baylin (1911–1988) Am radiol; °gut physiology tests.	JAMA
	— R. Hayes (1923–1988) Am chem; Ga-67, scanning °pharmaceuticals.	AP

CHRONOLOGY OF NUCLEAR MEDICINE — 1989

Scientific and Technical Background

			Ref.
1. Basic	— B. Cohen proves Linear Hypothesis false; average Rn-222 level in highest lung cancer counties is half that in lowest lung ca counties.	[1988]	HP
2. Obser	— B. Kimler does MRI (formerly NMR) with metalloporphyrin agent (rats).	[1988]	RRS
	— M. Comforth fails in test of genetic "one hit" theory.	[1958]	RRS
	— W. Sweet: finds it possible that second Chernobyl explosion was nuclear.	[1987]	TR
	— USSR: 1957 "nuc" accident was chem waste, 2×10^6 Ci Sr-90+.		
	— T. Luckey puts 100 mrem – 20 rem acute whole-body exposure, or chronic exposure <800 mrem/day as hermetic radiation.	[1981]	HPN

Organizations and Internal Politics

5. Pols	— D. Kennedy: government "moved from reasonable regul [of nuclear energy] to something close to chaotic strangulation."	[1981]	AAAS
	— Life expect ('86) = 75.4y (white) up 0.1, 69.4y (black) dn 0.1.	[1988]	PHS
	— EPA guideline is 25 mrem/y w/body, 75 mrem/y thyroid; below background variation & does not fit statistics on thyroid ca.	[1986]	EPA
	— FDA: 1969 ban on cyclamate was "mistake," does not correct it.	[1969]	AP
	— NRC has **B**elow **R**eg **C**oncern policy under development.	[1986]	NRC
	— J. Walker (NRC) reviews history of Rad Safety Controversy (an attempt to back NRC out of extreme anti-nukery).	[1987]	JAMA
	— S. Tilyou: 1×10^{-6} risk = smoke 1.4 cigs in lifetime (NO evidence).	[1986]	JNM
6. Socs	— B. Kramer edits "Art of Measurement" (history of German PTR).	[1906]	Bk
	— Materials Research Soc: Internat symposium on °waste disposal recommends sphene ($CaTiSiO_2$) in granite over perovskite.	[1984]	SN
	— L. Taylor reminisces on history of rad units & standards.	[1913]	ICRU
	— R. Hewlett pubs AEC hist, "Atoms-for-Peace & War, 1953–61."	[1975]	Bk
7. Event	— Shippingport decommiss reactor buried (at Hanford) w/o event.	[1957]	AP
	— 3,913,000 births in USA, (birth rate of 15.9/1000) in 1988; 2,171,000 deaths in USA, (death rate of 8.8/1000) in 1988.	[1960]	AP

Instruments, Units of Measurement, and Drugs

8. Instr	— NIST (old NBC) Cs atomic clock off 1 sec in 3×10^6 yrs on 40 annivers.	[1949]	NIST
	— A PET scan extension of EEG relates "thought" to chemistry.	[1987]	JAMA
	— A. Katzir writes history of fiber optics in medicine.	[1957]	SA
9. Units	— NRC accepts 3 mSv [300 mrad] as US average natural bkgd.	[1988]	HPN
	— J. Feula measures RBE of fast neutrons at 1.37 – 1.91.	[1987]	RRS
	— ORNL opens Rad Calibration Lab, supplies many °sources.	[1986]	HPN
	— ICRU pubs #44, Tissue Substit: compos, rad absorb, density.	[1944]	ICRU
	— Bancroft uses kg/cm^2s^{-1} & Ringwood uses g/n^2day^{-1} for °leach rates; after much argument, find their diff units give same results.	[1984]	SN
	— D. Strom pleads for use of SI units in Health Physics.	[1984]	HP
10. Concp	— D. Strom: ARS epilation on sigmoid curve, ~75 to ~250 rad.	[1985]	RERF
	— M. Crane: Genetic abnormalities associated with lifestyle events, but non-lymphocytic leuk occurs only in the genetically prepared.	[1987]	JAMA
	— E. Morrel uses AutoRadioGrams to get quant In-111 distrib.	[1987]	JNM
11. Drugs	— IAEA: Goiânia showed Prussian Blue speeds Cs-137 excretion.	[1988]	HPN
	— G. Gerber: toxicity from 2×10^6y Tc-99 is probably impossible.	[1985]	HP
	— A. Sinusas: uses °Tc-methoxyisobutyl igonitrile(MIBI) as Tl-201.	[1987]	JNM
	— H. Coenen studies brain metabolism of L-[2-F-18] fluorotyrosine.	[1987]	JNM
	— Y. Fugibayashi makes 9.2h Zn-62→9.8m Cu-62 cow for PET.	[1979]	JNM

Radioiodine, P-32, and Radioactive Therapy

12. I-Res	— E. Yeo: antithyroid med changes micro morphology of gland.	[1945]	JNM
13. I-Rx	— C. Kim trys to quantify 24h uptake in mets from thyroid ca.	[1972]	JNM

15. P-Rx — R. Robinson palliates bone mets (from breast ca) with Sr-89. [1940] SN
— H. Maxon uses rhenium-186 & 2 others to revive bone ca Rx. [1985] SN

Scans and Other Tests of Function in Various Organs

18. Brain — T. Pellmar sees physiologic damage of rat brain cells @ 40 Gy. [1960] RRS
— A. Brunetti sees effect of AZT on brain defects with PET. [1986] JNM
— S. Vallabhajosula studies °TC-DADT agents in normal men. [1983] JNM
— F. Fazekas compares CT, MRI, & PET in Alzheimer's dementia. [1982] JNM
19. Heart — H. Kiat compares °TC-MIBG with Tl-201 in coron heart disease. [1987] AHJ
— S. Yamamoto compares Tl-201, °Tc, & Ga-67 in card transplts. [1979] JNM
— K. Hicks uses Rb-82 for quant automat 3D cardiac PET scan. [1987] JNM
— M. Walsh estimates myocard O_2 consumption; C-11 PET scan. [1987] JNM
20. Liver — E. Camponovo compares 5 agents in choledocal cyst scans. [1981] JNM
— H. Itoh finds reflux sign very sensitive of biliary disfunction. [1987] JNM
— S. Gambhir quantifies liver function with °Tc-DISIDA. [1985] JNM
— S-Y Yeh gives index for Xe-133 retention in fatty liver. [1977] JNM
21. Lung — H. Otsuki attempts to see lung vessels with °In-antibodies. [1985] JNM
22. Bone — D. Boxer studies the solitary metastasis in breast ca. [1988] JNM
— C. Palestro says rad Rx initially results in increased WBC uptake. [1985] JNM
23. Kidney — M. Tobes: changed distribution of °I-MIBG in anephric pt. [1987] JNM
24. Gut — W. Drane: gastric reflux °Tc-DISIDA is sign of duodenal path. [1984] JNM
25. Blood — J. Stratton: measures autol °In platelet clearance post splenect. [1981] JNM
26. Other — A. Catafau tries In-111 platelets n pancreas transplants. [1981] JNM
— K. Kubota sums 10 year search for pancreas °C, °I scan agents. [1982] JNM
— D. Giuliani gives fast (2 day) platelet-survival-time method. [1971] JNM

Radiation Hysteria and Health Physics * Obituaries *

27. Hyst — 3 Salvadorans override 3 safety locks, expos to 3–8 Gy Co-60. [1984] HPN
— S. Preston-Martin sees parotid tumors after rad Rx for acne. [1982] AD
— L. Sagan & Science try to sabotage Radiation Hormesis. [1988] S
— EPA blocks Ra waste disposal site in Colorado river branch. [1984] AP
— EPA says 10K–40K lung ca deaths caused by radon. (Cigs out of style.) [1988] EPA
— "NO Nukes Anywhere" graffiti smears Boston subway. [1988] AP
— DOE says Y-12 @ Oak Ridge is rad threat, NO evidence needed! [1988] AP
28. React — R. Alexander: "If protection required for rad were required for other hazards, human progress would come to a halt." [1987] HPN
— R. Buchli: mean Swiss house Rn is 4.8 – 20 pCi/L (178–724 Bqm^{-3}), human Rn-222 dose is ~0.53 rad/y. [1987] HP
— IAEA lists, only 59 pure rad deaths (17 accidents) since 1945. [1986] IAEA
— H. Cember repeats, no one can fix "cause" of any specific ca. [1988] S
— S. Weart: nuc phobia can't be fought with facts or reason. [1980] JAMA
— P. Abelson tries to stop "hazard" of electro mag fields, Office of Technology finds NO evidence, only v weak statistical assoc. [1988] Sc
— C. Kang: Cs-137 dose (in S Eng) from fallout <1% of bkgd. [1959] HP
— IAEA reveals 1957 USSR rad accident at Kyshtyn chem waste, no bioeffect noticed. [1982] HPN
29. Respo — NRC commissioner Carr: "forget de minimis, give me BRC number." (BRC – Below Regulatory Concern.) [1988] NRC
— Smoking down ~6% in USA, lung ca up by 0.8/100,000; ACS [1986] SN
wrong??? About 29% of adults smoke (vs 43% in 1960). [1960] AP
— R. Roscoe: 14 lung ca (1 expected) in 516 non-smok U miners. [1986] JAMA
— IAEA: 250 deaths in Chernobyl pop (450 expected). Hormesis? [1986] HPN
— BEIR finds no data linking any disease with lo dose radiation. [1988] HP
— J. Lubin: half of all studies show NO indoor Rn – lung ca link. [1988] HP
— H. Peterson: 0.03 mrem has same risk as living 1 story high. [1988] NRC
— D. Dickson: USSR admits explosion of °waste tank in 1957; released 2 MCi over 375 sq miles, near Kyshtym. [1988] SC

* * *

30. Obits — Wm. G. Pollard (1911–1989), Am physics; founded ORINS in 1946. ORAU

RADIATION UNITS OF MEASUREMENT

(Six Units to Measure Ionizing Radiation)

Units for the measurement of ionizing radiation fall into four successful classes and one series of failures: Measurements of:

Amount of Substance	(Bq/kg & s^{-1})
Energy of Radiation	(eV & R/Bq•h)
Amount of Radiation	(C/kg)
Physical Dose	(J/kg)
Biological Dose has flawed units.	

The need for units of measurement was felt almost immediately after Roentgen's announcement. Becquerel's discovery of radioactivity a few months later wasn't widely accepted until the Curies astounded science with radium:

1 Roentgen discovers X-rays 1895
[See Vig1895 .X-R]
2 Curies discover radium 1898
[See Vig1898 .Ci]
3 Rutherford discovers "decay" 1899
[See Vig1898 .ER1]

By 1910 so many physicians used radium without any accepted unit of amount that reporting of bioeffects was chaotic. Most physicians purchased radium by the milligram, but mg of what? The Manhattan District (MED) converted the curie unit to more easily measured disintegrations per second (dps). The Conf Gen des Poids et Mesures (CGPM) formalized a new unit:

4 Brussels conf accepts "curie" 1910
[See Vig1910 .Ci]
5 MED adapts curie to dps 1945
[See Vig1928 .G-M]
6 CGPM adopts Bq as 1 dps 1969
[See Vig1985 .C-B]
7 Specific activity is Bq/kg 1969
[See Vig1954 .rad]

The first radiation unit came from measurements of X-ray penetration. Half-Value-Layer, the only practical measure of X-ray energy for years, was replaced by NaI(Tl) crystal spectrometry in 1953. But the electron volt (eV) was accepted by the CGPM as a "special name" in 1971.

8 HVL measures x-ray energy 1901
9 Spectrometry measures eV 1953
[See Vig1953 .°MI]
10 CGPM accepts eV unit 1971
[See Vig1977 .SI]

Attenuation constants began as absorption coefficients by applying Rutherford's 1898 half-value idea to measuring penetration. HVL was an energy measure. During the 1920s radium therapy dosage was built around mg•hours exposure. Then the roentgen was defined and the r/mCi•h followed as a specific physical dose for radium.

After 1946 the many new radioisotopes inspired a simple roentgens per hour at a meter (rhm). When "rhm" specified gamma ray output of a point source it was a "specific gamma ray constant." With knowledge of its decay scheme, the rhm could be calculated for each nuclide:

11 Attenuation coefficients 1903
[See Vig1954 .Rad]
12 Radium therapy uses R/mCi•h 1919
[See Vig1910 .Ci]
13 Evans' rhm is measurable 1947
14 Specific gamma ray constant 1953

A unit "amount of radiation" had been suggested by Villard in 1908. His coulomb of charge in a cc of air was not accepted until a clinical measuring instrument, a thimble chamber, was invented. After three years delay the International Congress of Radiology (ICR) agreed to the "Roentgen" unit (r) in 1925 "with reservations," then adopted it in 1928.

The "r" was restricted to gamma and X-rays in air, so a roentgen equivalent physical (rep) was defined to accommodate particle radiation. A series of equivalents led to the adoption of a Radiation Absorbed Dose (rad) by a group of experts appointed by the 1925 ICR meeting to an International Commission on Radiological Units & Measurements (ICRU):

15 The roentgen accepted by ICR 1928
[See Vig1928 .r]
16 Many roentgen equivalents 1930s
[See Vig1954 .Rad]
17 The rep is defined 1937
[See Vig1976 .Rem]
18 ICRU adopts the rad 1953
[See CNM Appendix 5]
19 ICRP adopts unmeasurable rem1956
[See Vig1976 .Rem]
20 CIPM adjusts to Bq, Gy, C/kg 1969
[See CNM Appendix]

Pierre Curie's 1898 notation of a skin reaction to radium was verified many

Development of the Units

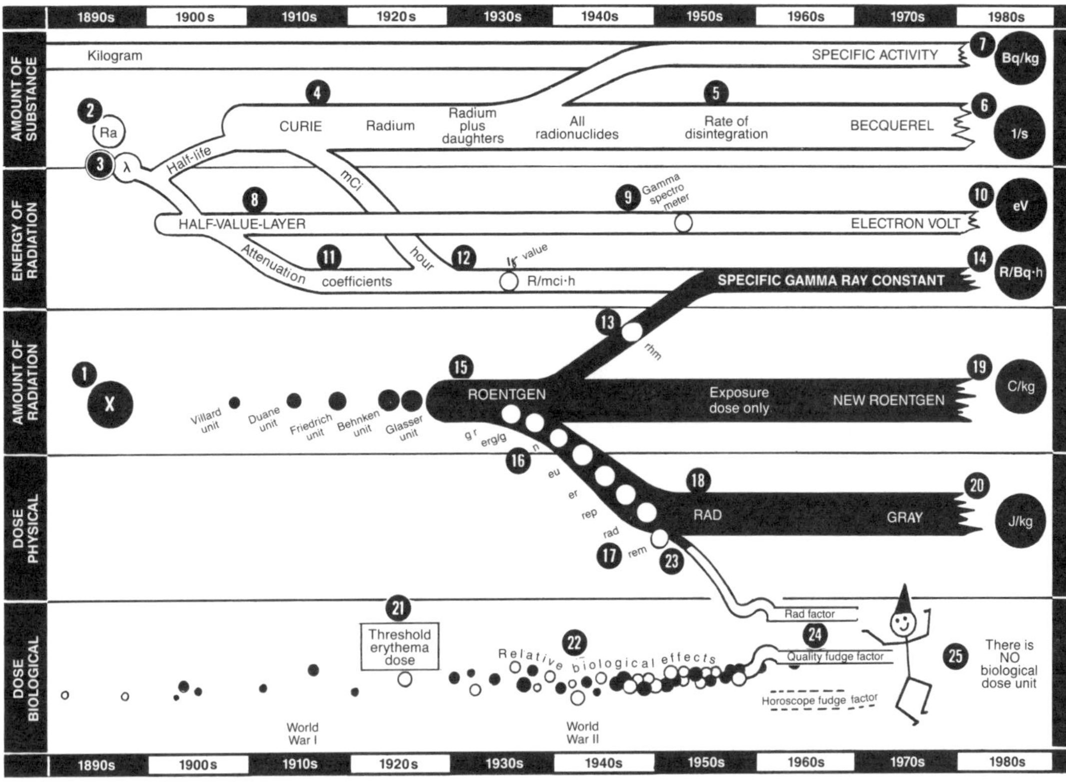

times, then quantified as a biological dose measure related to Holzknecht's chemical dosimeter: 3H = minimal skin reaction. Many biological dosimeters were devised (e.g., death of ascaris eggs or grasshopper larvae) because clinicians could see a lack of correlation between their Sabouraud-Noire 1902 exposure meters and wild variations in therapeutic results. In 1918 a Threshold Erythema Dose was adopted at Memorial Hospital in New York. After careful definition, this biological unit achieved widespread use:

21 Threshold Erythema defined 1918
[See Vig1954 .Rad]
22 Relative Biological effects 1931
[See Vig1976 .Rem]

But Threshold Erythoma was not well correlated with clinical results, and as soon as the highly accurate roentgen unit was adopted, erythema was proved to be an unsatisfactory end-point for a unit of biological radiation effect.

In 1931 with a dependable roentgen exposure unit, it was possible to subject a wide variety of tissues and animals to alpha, beta and soft and hard gamma rays with consistent results (under laboratory conditions). The concept of a Relative Biological Effect was defined and became the foundation of a science of radiobiology. In 1952 a small cult of radiation protection zealots split off from the ICRU, and from all falsifiable science, to form a mystic ICRP (Int Com Rad Protect):

23 Unmeasurable rem proposed 1953
24 Meaningless Quality Factors 1960s
25 Sievert is a religious unit 1980
[See Vig1976 .Rem]

Since 1931 the RBE and in 1955 the rad was declared unmeasurable in humans. Therefore, in 1956 the ICRP joined the two as the rem (or *r*oentgen *e*quivalent *m*ickey mouse). There is *no* biological dose unit.

[See Vig1928, 1953, 1969, 1976, ι units]

RADIATION HORMESIS AFTER 85 YEARS
(Background Radiation is Good For You)

Why does your pancreas secrete only when food has passed through the stomach? In 1902 an English physiologist, E. Starling, discovered that an acid extract of duodenum contained "secretin" that, when discharged into blood, stimulated the pancreas to secrete. By 1904 he coined "hormone" to designate any substance produced in small amounts but carried in blood to influence some other organ. It is from the Greek *hormo*, to excite.

A pharmaceutical principle practiced by the ancients was: a weak stimulus might stimulate what the same, but strong, stimulus inhibits. No medieval poisoner would dare kill somebody without first tasting the poison. Alchemists all knew that a poison in small dose was not poison. A few generations ago physicians carried strychnine in their bags for aged 50-year-old patients. Only in high dose was it a poison; prescriptions were for a stimulating tonic.

Toxicity is a Matter of Dose

No substance is without toxic effects at improper dose. Consider the most dangerous substance known to man: oxygen. It adversely affects the body at 5% too low a concentration. Moderate O_2 deficiency, however, stimulates RBC production. Most common drugs, alcohol, nicotine, caffeine, even water, are stimulants at low dose but deadly in high dose.

For a hundred years pharmacologists gave groups of animals various doses and plotted the percent killed, against dose. The amount of drug that killed 50% of the animals became the drug's LD_{50} (Lethal Dose for 50%). The complete curve was sigmoid, but an LD_{90} could be "statistically significant" in a very small population. With few dead at LD_{10} it took many animals and lots of time to find "significance." Hence, the low end of the curve was often "approximated." Few pharmacologists paid attention to very low-dose effects.

The Word "Hormesis" is Introduced

However, physiological chemistry (biochemistry's proper name during the 1920s) blossomed around vitamins and hormones, both low-dose materials. C. Southam and J. Ehrlich found that concentrations of oak bark extract *inhibited* fungal growth, but in low dose it *stimulated* fungal growth. Publishing in Phytopathology 33:517, 1943, they modified Starling's word to "hormesis" which described stimulation by low-doses of agents that are harmful, even lethal, at high-dose.

After World War II antibiotics were released to agricultural chemists. During the 1950s T. Luckey and colleagues were feeding antibiotics to livestock, expecting that the suppression of intestinal flora would decrease growth. Instead they discovered that low-dose dietary antibiotics caused a surge in growth. Since then feeding antibiotics has become standard practice for poultry, pigs, and cattle. Experiments in germ-free birds demonstrated a true chemical hormesis. In surveying the literature, T. Luckey found that hormesis was common, particularly when the "dose" was ionizing radiation.

One of the first studies in radiobiology (1898) found that X-irradiated algae grew faster than unirradiated controls. Stimulated growth was noted in trees (1908) and increased life span in invertebrates (1918) and insects (1919). X-rays stimulated seedlings (1927), plant growth (1937), guinea pigs, rabbits, and mice (1940s). Increased life span was the rule in low dose irradiated rats, dogs, and even house flies (1950s). In a 1981 monograph (CRC Press), T. Luckey revived the term "hormesis," but this time with ionizing radiation, and backed it up with a review of over 1250 articles from 85 years of experimental radiobiology.

Radiation "Danger" Takes the Spotlight

Before 1900 about 10 articles mentioned a probable hormetic response to X-rays, then 2 or 3 articles each year, until the death in 1906 of an English radiotherapist from overexposure caused the first radiation hysteria. [ArRR, 1906–1910] Skin damage to a number of German and French radiotherapists led to a new emphasis on protection from damage. Before World War I, into the 1930s, about ten articles a year mentioned a hormetic effect, but the idea did not grow.

Why Didn't Hormesis Take Hold?

A Russian histologist, Alexander Gurwitsch, had discovered in 1923 that living cells gave off a form of radiant energy that stimulated other growing tissues. [RA 100:11, 1923] "Gurwitsch" rays were confirmed outside of Russia, then denied. During the 1930s major WPA radiobiology programs studied these "mitogenetic rays," but with World War II geneticists and biologists dismissed the idea with shame. The rays had taught radiobiologists only how to juggle numbers and live off a government dole.

In 1925 H. Martland described 18 girl radium dial painters. After tipping brushes with their lips for five years they developed necrosis of the jaw bones and profound anemia. Other high dose patients, including possible osteosarcomas were, and are still, described in Sunday Supplement scandals. No newspaper ever featured the 30 year followup of 1155 low dose radium dial painters who had fewer cancers than the general population and lived longer.

[See Vig1926 .Ra]

In 1926 H. Muller published his work on genetic damage from irradiation of fruit flies. X-rays soon became standard for producing fruit fly mutations. In the 1930s "radiation" became synonymous, among geneticists, with chromosome damage. Chromosome defects of unknown significance occur in man after high dose, but postulated mutations after low dose are all mathematical extrapolations from data on fruit flies and mice.

Health Physics is Invented

The Manhattan Project expected large amounts of radioisotopes. Robert Stone gathered a new group he called Health Physicists to monitor this largely unknown danger. Their first experiment, raising mice in an atmosphere of uranium dust, showed exposed mice living longer than controls. They set up an arbitrary Maximum Permissible Dose (MPD) after proving that mice in radiation fields ten times the MPD lived longer than controls. Thus Health Physics began with a high MPD, and ended the war with record safety.

After World War II about 20 articles/year mentioned a hormetic effect in spite of a budding fallout hysteria. Health Physicists soon learned that their livelihood depended upon scaring the pants off Congress. H. Muller predicted genetic catastrophe from A-bomb exposure in a 1955 flurry of headline publicity. (No publicity was given the disproof 35 years later.) This was (for newspapers) scientific proof that radiation caused two-headed babies. In 1957 a fire in a power reactor at Windscale, England, released 20 curies of I-131 into the atmosphere. Newspapers predicted thousands of thyroid cancers in end-of-the-world headlines (but failed to mention, 25 years later, that *no* biologic effect had ever been detected).

Health Physics is Self-Perpetuating

Health Physics and Genetics were supported lavishly by radiation hysteria, and Radiation Biology was the most intensely researched science in history. At the 1955 Atoms-for-Peace conference an English geneticist uttered heresy at the opening session. Background radiation, he said, was probably the cause of most mutations throughout evolution, and the human race had not done too bad. He was almost read out of science for this heresy. Every Genetics budget meeting, 1955–1981, opened its request for funds with an antinuclear litany.

In spite of this atmosphere, during the 1960s and 1970s about 40 articles/year described hormesis. In 1963 the AEC repeatedly confirmed lower mortality in guinea pigs, rats and mice irradiated at low dose. In 1964 the cows exposed to about 150 rads after the Trinity A-bomb in 1946 were quietly euthenized because of extreme old age.

A Little Radiation is Good For You

In 1981 T. Luckey revived a very obvious radiation hormesis. *No* experimental evidence of damage at low-dose existed; self-serving extrapolations from high-dose data dominated health physics. One New York health physics bureaucrat passed off hormesis as a "theory" similar to evolution. But in 1983 M. Brucer published an article in the Health Physics Newsletter entitled "Radiation is Good For You," and over 200 reprint requests indicated agreement with his position.

In August 1985 a Conference on Radiation Hormesis in Oakland, CA, recognized the reversal in concepts of radiation effects. Its Proceedings, published in the Health Physics journal in 1987, finally recognized that low dose radiation is not only good for you, it is essential to life.

FROM THE CURIE UNIT TO THE BECQUEREL

Physicists in 1910 knew that disintegration-rate for each radioactive "species" was a constant. They were sure that Rutherford's lambda (λ), called half-value-period, was a fingerprint for each species. But everybody used his own unit of amount-of-activity. Ernest Rutherford in Manchester and Stefan Meyer in Vienna set up a committee to organize a world congress to define a "unit of radioactivity."

[See Vig1910 .Ci]

All committee members had experience in all known radioactivities. To them the true meaning of "radioactivity" was "rate-of-disintegration." The majority of attendees used only radium and some said the only "standard" of a substance was the kilogram in Paris. To compromise, the committee defined the "unit" as the rate-of-disintegration of a gram of radium — to be called a "curie." (Radium was expensive and they worked with milligrams, hence called them millicuries.)

The curie was adopted by most workers immediately — but applied only to radium. "Waddaya say?" replied everybody who used daughters of radium. And so in 1930 a new International Radium Standard Commission redefined the "curie" to include daughters of radium. "The hell you say" said the cyclotron drivers after 1934. The unit was the only one available to measure hundreds, then thousands of the new "radioisotopes."

Many attempts were made to measure the disintegrations per second (dps) of radium. The results ranged from 3.40 to 3.72 $\times$ 10^{10} dps. In 1959 the ICRU (Int Comm Rad Units) said drop the no longer useful radium tie-in; the curie is exactly 3.7 $\times$ 10^{10} dps of whatever. A year later The CGPM (Conf Gen Poids et Mesures), mother authority for all units, adopted SI units. A unit, they said, was "one dps," not 3.7 $\times$ anything. After 1985 the coherent SI unit of activity:

1 becquerel (Bq) = 1 dps.

CURIE TO BECQUEREL CONVERSION

1 Ci = 37 $\times$ 10^9 Bq [disints per sec] (or dps) — how many disintegrations?

1 femtocurie	=	37	microbecquerel	1 dis/7.5 hour
10 fCi	=	370	µBq	1 dis/45 min
100 fCi	=	3.7	millibecquerel	1 dis/4.5 min
1 picocurie	=	37	mBq	1 dis/27 sec
10 pCi	=	370	mBq	1 dis/2.7 sec
27.027 pCi	=	1	Bq	1 dis/1 sec
100 pCi	=	3.7	Becquerel	3.7 dis/1 sec
1 nanocurie	=	37	Bq	37 dps
10 nCi	=	370	Bq	370 dps
100 nCi	=	3.7	kilobecquerel	3,700 dps
1 microcurie	=	37	kBq	37,000 dps
10 µCi	=	370	kBq	370,000 dps
100 µCi	=	3.7	Megabecquerel	3,700,000 dps
1 millicurie	=	37	MBq	37,000,000 dps
10 mCi	=	370	MBq	370,000,000 dps
100 mCi	=	3.7	Gigabecquerel	3,700,000,000 dps
1 curie	=	37	GBq	37,000,000,000 dps
10 Ci	=	370	GBq	370,000,000,000 dps
100 Ci	=	3.7	Terabecquerel	3,700,000,000,000 dps

A RUMOR THAT WILL TAKE ANOTHER FIFTY YEARS TO SQUELCH

In 1950 I. Doniach discovered benign and malignant tumors in rats treated with I-131. [BJC 1950] It was confirmed by I. Chaikoff in rats given 400 μCi I-131. [PSEB 1951] Thyroid surgeons pointed with glee to the end of a threat to their lucrative business. But I-131 was getting so much publicity in hyperthyroidism therapy that Doniach repeated his study [BJC 1955]. He could not confirm his first study and neither could many others who tried ever larger doses.

An Explanation and a Retraction

By 1957 Chaikoff had an explanation for the tumors [CaR 1957]. A third of his *CONTROL* rats also developed thyroid cancer spontaneously. With low doses of I-131 ($<$100 μCi) the incidence of tumors was the same as in controls. High doses ($>$100 μCi) actually caused a decrease in thyroid ca. This hint was the first indication that I-131 therapy might prevent the later development of thyroid ca.

Established Dogma Triumphs

But the rumor was already established radiobiological dogma: I-131 causes thyroid cancer. Anti I-131 surgeons and many health physicists chose to ignore Chaikoff's retraction. The thyroids of 84 Marshallese exposed to fallout in 1954 were examined in intimate detail. Each nodule became an impending cancer. In the 1970s the thyroid glands of some New Mexico school children exposed to Nevada bomb test fallout were found to have nodules, *"which MAY become cancer."* Arizona school children *not* exposed had the same incidence of nodules. When Chinese Bomb fallout passed over the USA in 1976 every health physicist palpated his neck.

Leukemia is Added to the Dogma

Around 1950 the ABCC began reporting leukemia deaths in Hiroshima survivors — a massive dose ($>$100 rad) effect. At an Argonne Radioiodine Conference in 1956 many experts had an isolated example of leukemia following I-131 therapy. However, S. Feitelberg could remember no leukemia in the Mt. Sinai, NY, series of 3000 therapies for Graves disease. D. Clark reported none in the U. of Chicago series. K. Corrigan reported no leukemia in a Detroit series with blood workups. E. Pochin said the 4/100,000 incidence of spontaneous leukemia could account for the sporadic cases following I-131. [Ref in Vig1956 .°Rx]

The Established Dogma is Disproved

Twenty years later isolated leukemia and thyroid ca was still reported after I-131 therapy — usually with glee and raised eyebrows. In 1976 D. Piers answered one such report with a letter to Lancet. In the Netherlands hundreds of thousands of patients had been treated with I-131. Expected cancer incidence was 16; the actual number was 11.

B. Dobyns had found only 9 cancers in 35,000 I-131 therapy patients where 50 were expected. [JCEM 1974] By 1978 D. Hoffman could find no evidence that I-131 caused any cancer. [NEJM 1978] If anything, I-131 therapy for hyperthyroidism prevents later thyroid cancer. W. Beierwaltes found no leukemia and decreased cancer in a 20-year followup of 20,000 I-131 patients. [Sem 1978] In Peking, China, no thyroid ca was found on 10-year followup. [CMJ 1978] By 1980 even the NCRP admitted (but in very small type) that I-131 therapy did prevent later development of cancer.

Then why, in the face of such overwhelming evidence, did the FDA attempt to abolish the use of I-131 in 1975? Why, after Three Mile Island in 1979, did the Governor order evacuation of a town to prevent cancer? Why did HEW order KI for all residents? Why do health physics and medical textbooks, and FDA package inserts, still list thyroid cancer as a potential complication of I-131 therapy? The only answer is that radiation phobia serves the monetary needs of the bureaucracy and Health Physics.

How to Create a New Hysteria

Back in 1958 Bently Glass (Johns Hopkins) learned how to start a hysteria. He had given a television talk to explain to the public the minimal radiation danger from fallout. To put the problem in perspective, he compared fallout dose to the miniscule dose one gets from a radium dial wristwatch. The newspaper reaction was not what he had expected. He had ignited the great luminous dial wristwatch hysteria of 1958.

Now reconsider another fantasy: who proved that radon causes lung cancer?

[See Vig1981 .Hor]

THE CHERNOBYL (USSR) ACCIDENT
(USSR Demonstrates Proper Press Handling)

On 28 April 1986 routine background counts at the Forsmark nuclear power station outside Stockholm began to climb. The Swedes quickly traced the increase to an event outside Sweden, probably in Russia. By 29 April, nuclide analysis suggested a reactor fuel core accident. After world publicity, the USSR confirmed that an explosion had occurred in reactor unit No. 4 at Chernobyl, 80 miles north of Kiev. Two workers had been killed, 25 were in critical condition, 200 had been hospitalized, and 49,000 evacuated from the area.

The American television press reported the accident with great glee: 30,000 deaths on a gore littered site, 100,000 deaths from cancer about to happen. (The ABC news anchorman, Peter Jennings, later editorialized that they had *not* treated the matter with glee, which shows how ashamed he was of their performance.)

The Accident

At 1:00 AM on 25 April 1986 operators of Unit No. 4 began a planned shut-down from normal 3200 $\text{MegaWatts}_{(\text{therm})}$. In order to test a safety system, they wanted to disconnect from their grid and see how long the reactor produced power from its own thermal inertia. At 1:05 PM power output had dropped to 1600 MW and one generator was disconnected. With power down to 700 MW at 2:00 PM on the second generator, operators shut off the emergency cooling system to avoid any possibility of the system being activated during the test. (This step was a serious violation of safety regulations.)

It was now difficult to stabilize the reactor, and power dropped to 30 MW. In the meantime the normal buildup of xenon was poisoning the chain reaction, and to compensate, the reactor's control rods were withdrawn. When power reached 200 MW shortly after 1:00 AM on 26 April, more water pumps were connected to support the experiment; they supplied too much cooling water for the lower-than-expected power output. The low output caused the water level in the steam separators to drop. In order to prevent automatic shutdown the operators blocked safety signals from water-level sensors. (Another serious violation.)

At 1:23:04 the reactor seemed to be stabilized. The operators reduced the flow of feed-water in order to maintain steam pressure. Now there was too little cooling water: boiling increased, power started to climb sharply. At 1:23:40 the shift manager gave the emergency command to plunge the control rods into the reactor, but their almost complete withdrawal had slowed their response, and power surged. Intense steam generation around the fuel elements produced so much heat that fuel rods disintegrated and a steam explosion blew the reactor apart. Superheated steam reacted with zirconium cladding to ignite the graphite moderator which, in turn, produced a second hydrogen – carbon monoxide explosion. Flaming radioactive debris showered the reactor site and started about 30 fires, including a roof fire on the turbine room of Unit No. 3, still operating at full power.

It took 90 minutes for fire trucks from Pripyat and Chernobyl to reach the disaster, but by 5:00 AM most secondary fires were under control and all four reactors in the complex were shut down. Unit No. 4's burning graphite was beyond control; it was feeding itself. 5000 tons of boron, sand, clay, and lead were dropped by helicopter to encase the unit, and by 6 May its temperature started to drop. [data from W. Blair, HPN 15:5, 1987]

The Radioactive Fallout

Radioactivity was gushing out of the damaged reactor. After the reaction was under control, on 28 May 1986 (a month later) the International Atomic Energy Agency was informed of the accident. An estimated 100 megacuries of the core's fission products — about 7 MCi was I-131 — had been released. About 14 Ci were deposited within a 30 km zone around Chernobyl. A plume of radioactive smoke rose to a height of 1200 ft and moved west and then north. Close-in fallout radiation levels measured over 100 mR/hr about 1 km from the plant. The level decreased from 14 R/hr down to 1 R/hr in the nearby (2 km) town of Pripyat, and to as much as 0.8 mR/hr in Kiev to the south. Radiation near the damaged reactor must have been >1000 R/hr immediately after the blast, decaying to about 100 R/h after four or five hours. Most instruments initially read scale.

After 36 hours, 1000 buses moved into Pripyat and 45,000 people were evacuated. Their dose was estimated at up to 5 rads gamma with 20 rad beta to skin. 90,000 people and thousands of cattle were evacuated from a 30 km zone around Chernobyl. Cloud seeding was employed to minimize rainfall in the area. 400 wells were dug in the Kiev area to assure a source of drinking water. Kiev was thoroughly washed down. Central Ukraine's estimated 1986 dose (not to exceed about 150 mRad) was considered trivial.

Beyond the central Ukraine the average dose from fallout would be calculated at 30 mrem/year in neighboring Poland, to 15 mrem/year in most of Europe. In Italy about 7.5 mrem/year was an average calculation. In Poland a few health physicists scared the authorities into giving I-127 as a preventive measure against goblins. Swedish health physics cultists managed to overcome rationality and destroyed all of Lapland's reindeer meat with >300 Bq Cs-137/kg "contamination." The Lappish culture was probably destroyed in order to prevent ingestion of about 100 Bq/yr of Cs-137. This "Health Physics safety" precaution was the equivalent of saving K-40 exposure by eating one less egg for breakfast. In West Germany 10,000 anti-nuclear demonstrators smashed windows and threw rocks at police. Maybe it was effective, because the rise in background subsided.

The Medical Story

Explosion and fire at 1:23 AM 26 Apr 1986 — 2:30 AM, fire under control — 176 operational staff on duty at plant — 268 construction workers nearby. 29 victims were sent to the hospital in first half hour by medical staff. Within 3 hours blood and urine samples from 3 victims were found not to contain Na-24. By 6:00 AM 108 persons were hospitalized with nausea and vomiting (Acute Radiation Syndrome, ARS), another 24 were admitted during the day. One person died of severe burns (not radiation), at 6:00 AM (one had died immediately from the blast but could not be removed from hot reactor debris).

Twelve hours after the accident a team of medical specialists arrived, screened 350 persons, and took blood samples. Dosimetry was based upon clinical symptoms, blood profiles, and chromosome abberations in lymphocytes. (Hence, dose estimates were biased by Acute Radiation Syndrome (ARS) clinical literature.) 203 patients were diagnosed ARS, and hospitalized in Kiev or Moscow:

600–1600 rads, >60% thermal skin burns — 21 of 22 patients died within 4 to 50 days;
400–600 rads — 7 of 23 died within 2 to 7 weeks (6 had skin burns);
200–400 rads, no thermal burns, 1 of 53 died later;
<200 rads — treated, after body survey and wash up of contamination, as nonradiation related patients. (The 200 rad level was justified by the number of persons involved. <100 rads is usually considered trivial.)

Radiation plus thermal burns were considered major factors in 19 of 31 deaths. Cardiac and respiratory insufficiency appeared before death in patients who had received >800 rads. Bone marrow transplants were attempted in 13 patients in >600 rad group. Seven of the transplant patients died 9 to 19 days later, the other six had failed transplants; two of these had severe reactions that probably contributed to death. The Soviets considered marrow transplants over-publicized, but its total failure (under these emergency conditions) was never mentioned in the American press. Primary therapy was parenteral feeding for patients in the gastrointestinal phase, and fresh platelets with antibiotics for the <400 rad hemorrhagic phase. There was no evidence of ANY radiation sickness in persons away from the reactor site.

(HPN 15:6, 1987)

Predictions

If Hiroshima figures hold up, a predicted 100,000 cancers will become <20 leukemias in 10 years. The American press again predicted doom for nuclear power. A year after Chernobyl the IAEA summed up: 388 nuclear power units in 32 countries, also 144 units under construction. 12 plutonium breeders (dubbed sinful by the American press) were in operation in 7 countries. They estimated that 25% of electricity (95% in some countries) would be nuclear by the year 2000. The American press had again exaggerated nuclear power's death.

[See Vig1964 .ARS; Vig1979 .TMI]

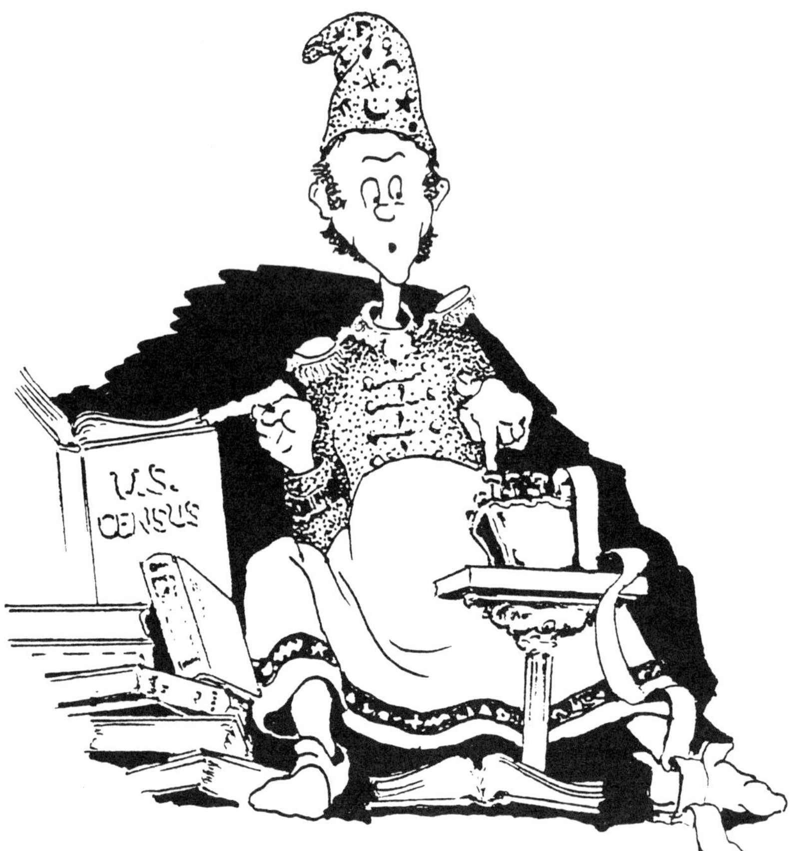

THE PRESIDENT'S WIZARD CANCER ADVISOR DISCOVERS THAT THERE ARE MORE CAUSES OF CANCER THAN THERE ARE PEOPLE.

Appendix

to

A Chronology of Nuclear Medicine

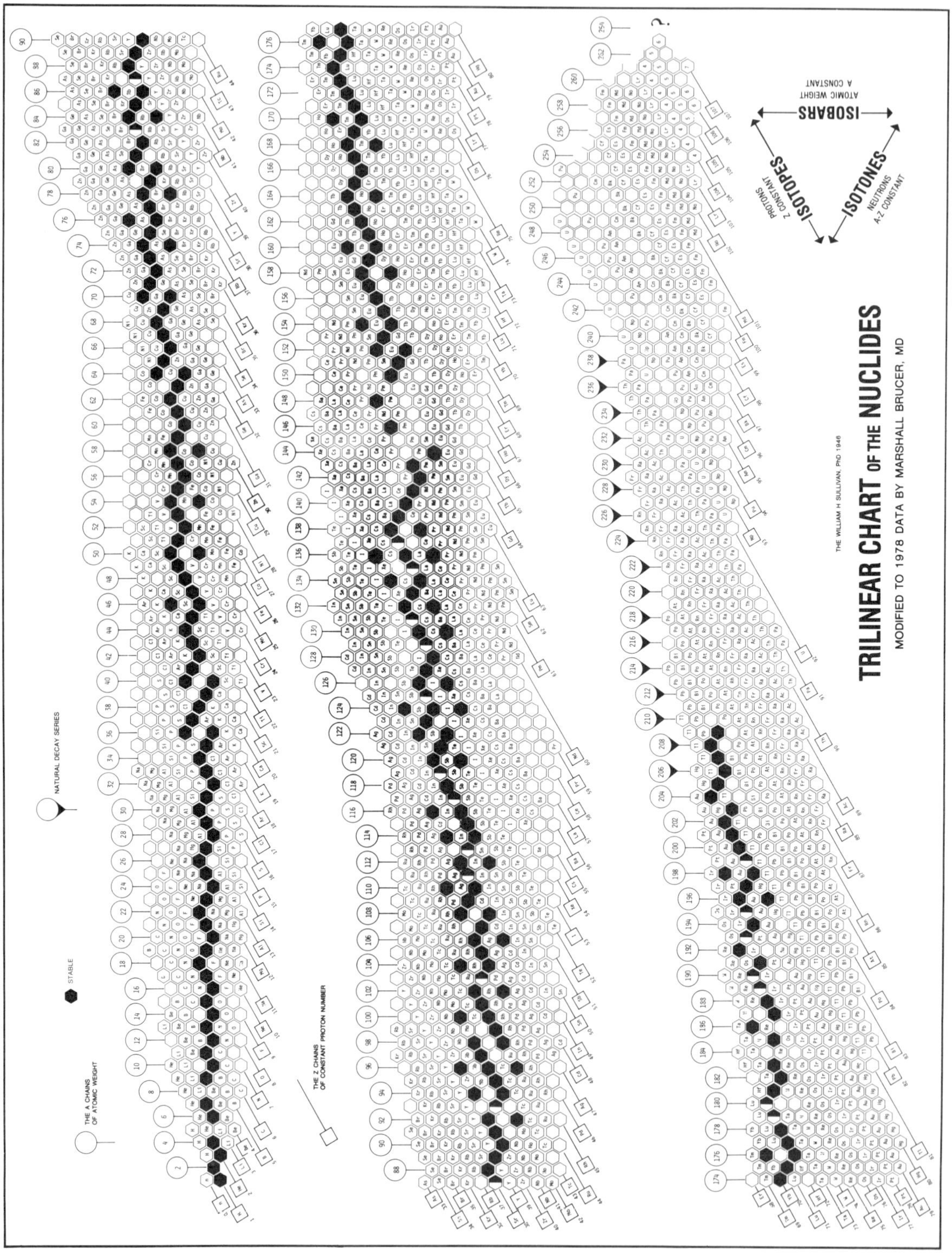
TRILINEAR CHART OF THE NUCLIDES
MODIFIED TO 1978 DATA BY MARSHALL BRUCER, MD
THE WILLIAM H SULLIVAN, PhD 1946
ISOBARS
ATOMIC WEIGHT
A CONSTANT
ISOTOPES
PROTONS
Z CONSTANT
ISOTONES
NEUTRONS
A-Z CONSTANT
NATURAL DECAY SERIES
STABLE
THE A CHAINS
OF ATOMIC WEIGHT
THE Z CHAINS
OF CONSTANT PROTON NUMBER

HOW MANY ELEMENTS (NUCLIDES) ARE THERE?

(It depends upon your birthday, and how you define "element, species, nuclide.")

Year	HOW MANY NUCLIDES	Year	EVENTS THAT CHANGED THINGS

1660-Boyle defines a chemical element.
1789-Lavoisier lists **33** elements.
1803-Dalton weighs a few elements.
1814-Wallaston, table of "Equivalent Weights."
1815-Prout says hydrogen is "protyle."
1860-Avogadro's 1811 Molecule/Atom accepted.
1863-Newland's "octaves" in **62** elements.
1864-Crookes says Equivalents are Atomic Wts.
1869-Mendeleev, Periodic Table of **67** elements.
1876-Crookes' meta-elements are first isotopes.
1894-Ramsay adds noble gases, **74** elements.
1896-Becquerel discovers U is radioactive.
1897-Thomson announces the electron.
1898-Curies discover Po, Ra.
1899-Rutherford finds 3 (4?) "active deposits."
1902-Rutherford announces "transmutation."
1905-Hahn says RaTh & Th are identical.
1911-Rutherford announces "nuclear atom."
1912-Fajans discovers the "isotopes."
1913-Moseley proves only **92** numbers to U.
1917-Stewart says "isobars" have constant A.
1918-Rutherford makes artificial transmutation.
1919-Aston devises the mass spectrometer.
1920-Rutherford proposes the "neutron."
1921-Hahn discovers an "isomer."
1930-Lawrence invents a 4-inch cyclotron.
1932-Chadwick discovers the neutron.
1933-Handbook lists **212** stable, **38** °isotopes.
1934-Joliot-Curies discover and make 3 artificial °isotopes.
1935-Guggenheimer names constant A-Z, Isotones.
1936-Grosse lists **404** isotopes.
1939-Meitner discovers fission.
1940-McMillan makes first transuranic element.
1942-Fermi U "pile" (U Chicago) goes critical.
1944-Evans lists **176** stable, **375** °isotopes (551 total).
1945-Marinsky completes Periodic Table with promethium, #61.
1946-Sullivan's first Trilinear Chart lists **935** "species."
1947-Kohman proposes new name, "nuclide."
1961-Sullivan's revised Trilinear Chart lists **1349** "nuclides."
1966-Nuclear Data Group begins "Data sheets."
1968-Brucer revises Trilinear Chart to show **1447** nuclides.
1976-Seaborg redefines "element"; $T_{1/2}$ criterion
1979-New Brucer Trilinear Chart has **2452** nuclides.
1980-IUPAC names all elements over #103 by number only.
1984-German & USSR groups claim elements #108 and #109.
1987-USSR group claims evidence for element #110.

* * * * *

1989-Depending upon your definitions and with limitations on "Decay Time,"
THERE ARE . . . at least **109** chemical elements
. . . or about **2500** nuclides
. . . of which **2200** are radioactive
. . . and **300** are stable or very long-lived.

[See Vig1914 .Mos; Vig1934 .JC]

NUCLEAR ACCIDENTS AND NEWSMEDIA EXAGGERATED INCIDENTS
(Radiation accidents involving either >1Gy or much newsmedia publicity.)

Date	Place/°Source	Accident/Bioeffect	Dead/Injured	Reference
1916 – 1925	Orange County, NJ Radium dial painters	Swallow Ra paint >1 Gy = aplastic anemia	Thousands expos 0.6% bone ca	JAMA, 1929
— — 1944	Hanford, WA Chem explosion, U dust	Inhale 50 mg U dust No effect 38 yrs later	3 exposed Follow up	HP, 1986
Aug 21, 1945	Los Alamos, MED* Critical assembly	Chain react & flash Acute Rad Syndrome	1 dead 310 Rad 1 expos 8 Rad	AnIM, 1952; Ha, 1956; Hu, 1980
Jul 16, 1945	Trinity site, MED* Atom Bomb mfg	First Atom Bomb test exp Fallout on 60 cows	0 dead Beta burns	AEC, 1964
— — 1945	Hanford, WA Pu production	Release 340 kCi °I into atmosphere, std practice	Trivial expos	AP, 1986
May 21, 1946	Los Alamos, MED* Critical assembly	Chain react & flash Acute Rad Syndrome	1 dead 1 k Rad 7 exp 7-166 Rad	AnIM, 1952; Hu, 1980
May 14, 1948	Eniwetok, USAEC Nuclear Test Program	Sloppy °sample handling Beta burns to hand	1 expos 3 trivial	Ha, 1956
Sep 7, 1948	Los Alamos Nat Lab °nuclide laboratory	Unpacking °active nuc Beta burn to ankle	1 expos	Ha, 1956
— — 1949	Hanford, WA Pu production	Release >5 kCi I-131 in atmosphere, std practice	Trivial expos	AP, 1986
Jun 2, 1952	Arg Nat Lab, Chicago Experimental reactor	Workers enter Hot Room Lo-dose, no Acu Rad Syn	4 expos 12-189 Rad	ANL-4971; OA, 1968
Jul 9, 1952	Los Alamos Nat Lab °nuclide laboratory	Handling with torn glove. Pu beta burn to hand.	1 exposed	AJR, 1958
Dec 12, 1952	Chalk River, Canada Exper Power Reactor	Control rods removed Partial meltdown	None No bioeffect	AP, 1952
— — 1953	USSR	? ? ?	2 dead	BJR, 1983
Mar 1, 1954	Bikini Atoll Marshallese USAEC Hydrogen Bomb	Fallout from H Bomb up to 175 Rad no bath US Navy expos with bath	0 dead 239 expos 28 few Rad	
Mar 1, 1954	Japanese fishermen USAEC Hydrogen Bomb	Fallout from H Bomb Exposure + no bath	0 (1 related) 23 ex 80-320 Rad	Hu, 1980
??? — 1957	Moscow, lab device (JAMA 179:241, 1962)	Gamma-neutron exposure 670 & 320 r, AcutRadSyn	0 dead 2 expos	JAMA, 1962
Jun 14, 1957	Rocky Flats, CO AEC Pu processing	Explosion in dry box Pu imbedded in finger	2 expos 1 amputation	AJR, 1958
Oct 4, 1957	Oak Ridge Nat Lab U processing	Worker enters hot area 1 min exp, no bioeffect	1 exposed 63 rad	OA, 1968
Oct 7, 1957	Windscale #1 England Pu production reactor [Renamed "Sellafield"]	Fire in reactor 20 kCi °I released	None see 1982 rep.	Hu, 1980
— — 1957	Kyshtym, Urals, USSR Plutonium prod ????	Explosion ??????? Area evacuated ??	USSR Secret	HP, 1985
May 23, 1958	Chalk River, Canada Exper Power Reactor	Overheated fuel rod Damage to reactor	0 exposed	Nuc, 1958
Jun 16, 1958	Oak Ridge Nat Lab U-235 Processing	Critical excursion sub-lethal Ac Rad Syn	0 dead 6 68-365 Rad	JAMA, 1962, 1964; WHO, 1960; Hu, 1980

Date	Place/°Source	Accident/Bioeffect	Dead/Injured	Reference
Oct 15, 1958	Vinca, Yugoslavia Exper Reactor	Criticality excursion mix n/gamma, Ac Rad Synd	6 exposed 207-436 Rad	WHO, 1960; JAMA, 1962; BJR, 1983
Dec 30, 1958	Los Alamos Nat Lab Fissionable processing	Critical excursion 49 Gy, death in 34h	1 dead 2 expos	APa, 1967; WHO, 1960; OA, 1968
Apr 3, 1959	Moscow ? (Meditis Radiol 5:34, Oct 1960)	Worker drank 4mCi Cs-137 ??? bio effect	1 exposed	US Joint Pub Res Serv, #5761
Mar 29, 1960	Madison, WI, U of Wisc °nuclide laboratory	$12\frac{1}{2}$ min exp Co-60 source 300r Whol Bdy, 3kr abdom	1 exposed AcRadSynd	JLCM, 1962
Nov 8, 1960	Sandia Base, NM USAF testing lab	Electron beam exposure Est 760 rad to face	1 to surgery	Ha, 1961
Nov 8, 1960	Lockport NY Klystron Tube	Unshielded Klystron tube Inhomogen part bod X-ray	9 exposed to 1500 Rad	WHO, 1960; BJR, 1983
Jan 3, 1961	Idaho Falls, ID Exp military reactor	Removing control rod Hi-pres steam explosion	3 dead from blast	AP, 1961; Nuc, 1961
Mar 21, 1962	Mexico City Co-60 radiograph source	Child finds °source Family exp, Ac Rad Synd	4 dead 1 exposed	IRT, 1963; AP, 1962
Apr 7, 1962	Hanford Nat Lab Pu processing	Critical excursion <1 Gy, no Acute Rad Syn	22 exposed to few Rad	OA, 1968
Jul 24, 1962	Puerto Rico Nuc Center Swim pool reactor	Gamma gun accidently ON Mild Ac Rad Sy.	1 1Gy expos 6 Trivial	JAMA, 1965
Jan 11, 1963	Peop Repub China 10 Ci Co-60 source	Family expos to source Acute Rad Syndrome	2 dead 4-8 k Rad 4 2-800 Rad	Hu, 1980
Feb 18, 1964	Rockford, IL Industrial X-Ray	Worker ankle, 29 k rad, hand, 42 k rad; no rad synd	1 exposed Amputation	Hu, 1980
Aug 24, 1964	United Nuc Corp, RI Uranium recovery plant	Critical excursion >10Gy gamma + neutrons	1 dead 5 minor exp	APa, 1967
Sep 24, 1964 — — 1964	Redondo Beach Ochsner Clinic LA	? ?	1 expos 2 expos	OA, 1968
Dec 30, 1965	Mol, Belgium Experimental reactor	Critical excursion Acute Rad Synd	1 dead est, 600 Rad	Hu, 1980
May 28, 1966	Antigua, W Indies	?	0	OA, 1968
Jun —, 1966	Stanford CA Linear accelerator	Film badge shows 150 rad No evidence of rad expos	1 ???	OA, 1968
Oct 5, 1966	Enrico Fermi, Detroit Nuclear power reactor	Loss of coolant Partial meltdown	0 dead 0 injured	AP, 1966
Oct 4, 1967	Pittsburgh, PA VanDeGraaff accelerator	c20min expose to beam Acute Rad Synd	3 expos c3-600 Rad	AP, 1967
1943 – 1967	USAEC publishes list all forms of rad	Exposures >15 r <100 r show no bio effects	25 examples	OA, 1968
May 3, 1968	La Plata, Argentine	?	1	OA, 1968
Aug 1, 1968	Madras, India	?	1	OA, 1968
Aug 28, 1968	Madison Wisc, U of W	°AuCol dose error	1	OA, 1968
Oct 17, 1969	Saint-Laurent, France Nucclear power reactor	Fuel Loading Error Partial meltdown	0 dead 0 injured	AP, 1969
Jan —, 1971	New Haven, Yale U	?	2	AP, 1971
Feb 4, 1971	Oak Ridge, U of Tenn 7.7 kCi Co-60 rad source	40 sec expos to source Acute Rad Syndrome	1 expos 260 R	Hu, 1980
Sep 17, 1971	Chiba-shi, Japan 5.26 Ci Ir-192 rad sor	Finds lost source 5 expos over 5 days	6 expos c10-124 Rad	Hu, 1980

Date	Place/°Source	Accident/Bioeffect	Dead/Injured	Reference
Nov 19, 1971	Monticello, Minn Nuclear power reactor	°Waste disposal (trivial) 50 kgal in Missis River	0 dead 0 injured	AP, 1971
Apr 18, 1972	Texas father gets 5 Ci ? Cs-137 sources	Attempts sterilize son Local rad necrosis	1 expos >k Rad local	Hu, 1980
Dec 21, 1972	Poughkeepsie NY	?	1	AP, 1972
Dec 17, 1973	Prague hospital, CSSR 110 tBq Co-60 source	Pick up dropped source Amputate hand, eye cat	2 expos 159 rad	HP, 1986
Feb 4, 1974	NY Health & Safety Lab	?	1	AP, 1974
Jun 13, 1974	Parsippany, NJ 120 kCi Co-60 rad source	10 sec expos to source Acute Rad Syndrome	1 expos c410 Rad	Hu, 1980
Mar 21, 1974	Peoria, IL	?	?	AP, 1974
May —, 1974	Savannah River, DOE Pu & H-3 production	479 kCi H-3 released Maintenance problem	Trivial Exposure	Hu, 1980
Sep 27, 1974	Amarillo, TX	?	1	AP, 1974
Jan —, 1975	Brescia, Italy ?	? Hi-dose to brain Acute Rad Syndrome	1 dead 12 Gy	Hu, 1980
Mar 22, 1975	Browns Ferry, Alabama Nuclear power reactor	Maint man starts fire in control cables	None Trivial	AP, 1975
Apr 16, 1975	Louisville, KY	?	?	AP, 1975
May 13, 1975	Northern Italy Co-60 cereal irrad	Minutes expos to source Acute Rad Syndrome	1 dead 1-2.5 k Rad	Hu, 1980
Dec —, 1975	Savannah River, DOE Pu & H-3 production	182 kCi H-3 released Maintenance problem	Trivial Exposure	Hu, 1980
Aug 30, 1976	Hanford, WA, DOE Am ion exc col explos	3.3 mCi face, 0.4 lungs 200 rad to lung by 1979	1 blast injury	Hu, 1980
Aug 30, 1976	Hanford, WA, DOE Am recovery	Ion-exch col explodes 300 μCi chron Am contam	1 expos c860 Rad	AJR, 1958; Hu, 1980
Sep 23, 1977	Rockaway, NJ 500 kCi Co-60 rad source	c10 sec expos to source Mild Acute Rad Syndrome	1 expos c200 Rad	Hu, 1980
Dec 16, 1977	Hanford, WA	?	4	Hu, 1980
— — 1977	Berkeley, CA	?	1	Hu, 1980
May 1978	W. Monroe, LA 100 Ci °Ir radiog source	Sloppy handling Finger & hand burns	1 expos Hi-D local	Hu, 1980
May 1978	Algeria Lost 25 Ci Ir-192 source	Child found source Family expos c35 days	4 hosp est c1 + k Rad	Hu, 1980
Jan 4, 1979	Winston Salem, NC X-ray diffraction unit	Puts fingers in beam Local X-ray burns	1 expos >500 Rad	Hu, 1980
Mar 28, 1979	Three Mile Island, PA Nuclear power reactor	Valve stuck, part melt 17 Ci °I release (trivial)	None but mass hysteria	Hu, 1980 [See Vig1979 .TMI]
May —, 1979	Ship on Gulf Coast, LA kiloCi °Ir radiog source	Wave ups pipe weld photo Local burns & mild ARS	3 expos 8-100 Rad	Hu, 1980
May 1, 1979	Am Atomics Corp, Tucson Tritium lumines signs	Minor spills of H-3 Az AEC charges error	Trivial but Corp. dead	AP, 1979
May 22, 1979	CA Div Occ Safe Adm 28 Ci °Ir radiog source	Sloppy handling of rad Mild ARS + local burns	11 expos 1-100 Rad	Hu, 1980
	Hundreds of such accidents might be unreported.			
Aug 7, 1979	Erwin, TN, US Army U processing plant	Release of enriched U Trivial overexposures	0 dead 0 injured	AP, 1979
Aug 29, 1979	Baton Rouge, LA	?	1	AP, 1979
Feb 11, 1981	TVA TN, Sequoyah I Nuclear power reactor	°Coolant water leak 8 workers, trivial expos	0 dead 0 injured	AP, 1981
Mar —, 1981	Savannah River, DOE Pu & H-3 production	33 kCi H-3 released Minor maintenance prob	Trivial exposure	AP, 1981

Date	Place/°Source	Accident/Bioeffect	Dead/Injured	Reference
Mar 8, 1981	Tsuruga, Japan Nuclear waste storage	Leak in °water tank Workers try to mop up	a few are overexposed	SN, 1981
Jan 25, 1982	Rochester, NY, Ginna Nuclear power plant	°Steam tube rupture Trivial release to air	0 dead 0 injured	AP, 1982
Feb 8, 1983	Gulf Webster Plant, TX Am-241 oil well probe	Worker cuts source in 1/2 No med care for six wks	9 exposed dose ????	AJR, 1985; AP, 1983
Jul 19, 1983	Savannah River, DOE Pu & H-3 production	56 kCi H-3 released Minor maintenance prob	Trivial exposure	AP, 1983
Jan 18, 1984	Juarez, Mexico 400 Ci Co-60 scrapped	°Co melted into 4 k tons Shipped °steel worldwide	>6 get LD_{50} >200 lo-dose	Sc, 1984
Early, 1984	Hebron, OH 1.4 Ci Cs-137 °graphy	Drill thru °graphy sorce Injested °Cs followed	3 expos est 0.05 Rad	Rad, 1985
Mar 23, 1984	Savannah River, DOE Pu & H-3 production	7.5 kCi H-3 released Est 0.2 mrad/y maximum	Trivial exposure	AP, 1984
Apr 19, 1984	TVA TN, Sequoyah I Nuclear power reactor	Superheated °water Minor maintenance prob	0 dead 0 injured	AP, 1984
Jul —, 1984	Morocco °Ir radiography source	Source found by child (?) Family & neighbors irrad	6 (?) dead 20 (?) expos	Sc, 1984
Jun 9, 1985	Oak Harbor, Ohio Nuclear power reactor	Loss of cooling water Caught in time, no effect	0 dead 0 injured	AP, 1985
Jan 4, 1986	Kerr-McGee, Gore, OK Uranium processing	Chemical explosion Minor release of °act	1 caustic chem death	AP, 1986
Apr 26, 1986	Chernobyl, Ukraine Graphite power reactor 100,000 evacuated;	Graphite fire Massive FisProd release Greenpeace "scientists" predict 10,000 ca in 20y. (AP, 86)	31 dead + ? 80 + crit exp	HPN, Feb, 1987 [See Vig1986 .Che]
1988	Review estimate ~15 pBq	Cs-137 0-neg cancers		Sc Dec 1988
Feb 1987	US Trans U Registry Chemistry lab exposure	Inhale Am-241, Pu-239 1945–57 expos, no effect	Autopsies in 1986.	HP, 1987
Sep 13, 1987	Goiânia, Brazil 1.4 kCi Cs-137 TeleRx source	Cs source sold as junk, sawed open, played with, rubbed on body, broken up, eaten	4 dead ?? 244 expos 54 to Hosp	Sc 11/20/87

References for the Nuclear Accidents appendix:
(See also, Key to the Reference Code)

AEC, date — Atomic Energy Commission, news release and reports.
AJR, year — Am J Radiology.
ANL — Argonne National Lab, report or news release.
AP, year — Many items are from AP (or other) press releases day after event.
APa, year — Am J Pathology.
BJR, year — British J Radiology.
Ha, 1956 — D. Hayes; Summary of Accidents . . . TID5360, '56; Supp 1, 2, 3: '57 '59 '61.
HP, year — Health Physics journal.
HPN, year — Health Physics Newsletter.
Hu, 1980 — F. Hubner, S.A. Fry; Med Basis for Rad Accid Prep . . . Elsevier, NY, 1980.
JAMA, year — Journal of the AmericanMedical Association.
JAMA, 1982 — P.R. Larsen, et al; Thyroid Hypofunction After . . . JAMA 247:1571, 1982.
JAMA, 1986 — H. Geiger; Accident at Chernobyl & Medical . . . JAMA 256:609, 1986.
— L. Anspaugh; Global Impact of Chernobyl . . . Science 242:1513, Dec 1988.
JLCM, year — J Lab and Clinical Medicine
OA, 1968 — Operational Accidents & Rad Expos within AEC, 1946–1967; AEC 1968.
Rad, year — Radiology.
Sc — Science.
SN — Science News.
USJPRS — US Joint Pub Research Service, Russian translations, date.
WHO, 1960 — World Health Org, Dx & Rx of Acute Rad Injury. Columbia U, NY, 1961.

* MED = Manhattan Engineering District.

CHRONOLOGY OF SI RADIATION UNITS

1781- Articles of Confederation (Continental Congress) Art 9, ¶ 4: "... establish standards of weights and measures throughout the United States."

1789- Constitution of the United States Sec 8, Art 1: "... Congress shall have the power ... to fix Standards of Weights and Measures."

1795- French Academy of Sciences defines the "metre."

1866- Thirty-ninth Congress authorizes the metric system in the USA.

1875 BIPM-Treaty of the Metric Convention (17 nations) creates Bureau International des Poids et Mesures.

1889 CGPM-First Conférence Générale des Poids et Mesures defines metre and kilogram Pt-Ir prototypes, second as fraction of mean solar day, centigrade temperature scale.

1903- Third CGPM corrects kg to "mass," not "weight"; adopts liter.

1903 NBS-National Bureau of Standards established in USA.

1908 IEC-International Electricity Congress adopts ampere and ohm.

1910- Brussels Radiology Congress adopts gram radium as standard curie.

1925 ICRU-First International Congress of Radiology (**ICR**) appoints Internatl Commission on Radiological Units and Measurements, defines the roentgen (r).

1927- Seventh CGPM redefines the meter; considers electric standards; defines newton, joule, coulomb, watt, etc.

1928- Second ICR adopts roentgen, appoints Internatational Committee on Radiological Protection (**ICRP**).

1933- Eighth CGPM considers photometry standards.

1934- Third ICRU sets a "permissible" exposure level (0.2 r/day).

1946 CIPM-Committee Internatl des Poids et Mesures adopts photometric standards and MKS unit system.

1948- Ninth CGPM tells CIPM to study system of units; adopts symbols N, J, cd, triple point of water for 0°C.

1950- ICRP wants Health Physicists only, no physicians, on ICRP, splits off ICRU.

1953- ICRU adopts 100 ergs/gram as rad unit of dose.

1954- Tenth CGPM adopts 6 base units and many coherent derived units for new system; defines temperature scale around 0° celsius.

1956- ICRP uses rem unit without standard, not accepted by ICRU until 1962.

1960- Eleventh CGPM adopts **SI** (Systéme International), pica to tera prefixes, 2 geometry supplemental units; redefines meter as a wavelength, second as fraction of tropical year, hertz as s^{-1}; questions cc vs ml.

1964- Twelfth CGPM adopts atto & femto prefixes, defines curie & hertz, abrogates the liter.

1967- Thirteenth CGPM redefines second as Cs-134 decay; adopts kelvin as -273.16°C; redefines candella, adds many derived units.

1969- CIPM accepts rad, curie, roentgen as temporary Gy, Bq, C/kg.

1971- Fourteenth CGPM adopts mole as seventh basic unit, adds exa & peta prefixes, accepts "special name" derived units pascal (N/m^2), siemans (1/ohm); proposes **TIA** (International Atomic Time) scale.

1975- Fifteenth CGPM adopts becquerel (Bq), s^{-1} (for curie), gray (Gy) as J/kg for rad; accepts °C as temperature scale.*

1977- ICRU, goaded by ICRP fanatics, accepts sievert (Sv) unit of dose, J/kg times 2 fudge factors calibrated by the Tooth Fairy. [See Vig1976 .Rem]

1985- ICRP dabbles in dose limits in background range; adjusts Q factor to match mathematical manipulations.

*Here "°" means "degree," not "radioactive."

* * *

References

LeMaraic AL, Ciaramella JP; Metric Encyclopedia. Abbey Books, Sommers, NY, 1975

NBS Special Publication 330; International System of Units (SI). US Dept of Commerce, NBS, Aug 1977

ICRU Report 33; Radiation Quantities and Units. 15 Apr 1980. ICRU, 7910 Woodmont, Washington, DC 20014

CONVERSION OF UNITS OF RADIOACTIVITY

curies to becquerels
(1 Ci = 3.7×10^{10} Bq)
(1 curie = 37 gigabecquerels)

1	attocurie	=	37.0	nBq
10	attocuries	=	370.0	nBq
100	attocuries	=	3.7	μBq
1	femtocurie	=	37.0	μBq
10	femtocuries	=	370.0	μBq
100	femtocuries	=	3.7	mBq
1	picocurie	=	37.0	mBq
10	picocuries	=	370.0	mBq
100	picocuries	=	3.7	Bq
1	nanocurie	=	37.0	Bq
10	nanocuries	=	370.0	Bq
100	nanocuries	=	3.7	kBq
1	microcurie	=	37.0	kBq
10	microcuries	=	370.0	kBq
100	microcuries	=	3.7	MBq
1	millicurie	=	37.0	MBq
10	millicuries	=	370.0	MBq
100	millicuries	=	3.7	GBq
1	**curie**	**=**	**37.0**	**GBq**
10	curies	=	370.0	GBq
100	curies	=	3.7	TBq
1	kilocurie	=	37.0	TBq
10	kilocuries	=	370.0	TBq
100	kilocuries	=	3.7	PBq
1	megacurie	=	37.0	PBq
10	megacuries	=	370.0	PBq
100	megacuries	=	3.7	EBq
1	gigacurie	=	37.0	EBq
10	gigacuries	=	370.0	EBq

becquerels to curies
(1 Bq = 27.027×10^{-12} Ci)
(1 becquerel = 27 picocuries)

10	nanobecquerels	=	0.3	aCi
100	nanobecquerels	=	2.7	aCi
1	microbecquerel	=	27.0	aCi
10	microbecquerels	=	270.3	aCi
100	microbecquerels	=	2.7	fCi
1	millibecquerel	=	27.0	fCi
10	millibecquerels	=	270.3	fCi
100	millibecquerels	=	2.7	pCi
1	**becquerel**	**=**	**27.0**	**pCi**
10	becquerels	=	270.3	pCi
100	becquerels	=	2.7	nCi
1	kilobecquerel	=	27.0	nCi
10	kilobecquerels	=	270.3	nCi
100	kilobecquerels	=	2.7	μCi
1	megabecquerel	=	27.0	μCi
10	megabecquerels	=	270.3	μCi
100	megabecquerels	=	2.7	mCi
1	gigabecquerel	=	27.0	mCi
10	gigabecquerels	=	270.3	mCi
100	gigabecquerels	=	2.7	Ci
1	terabecquerel	=	27.0	Ci
10	terabecquerels	=	270.3	Ci
100	terabecquerels	=	2.7	kCi
1	petabecquerel	=	27.0	kCi
10	petabecquerels	=	270.3	kCi
100	petabecquerels	=	2.7	MCi
1	exabecquerel	=	27.0	MCi
10	exabecquerels	=	270.3	MCi
100	exabecquerels	=	2.7	GCi

GLOSSARY of SYMBOLS, ABBREVIATIONS, & JARGON

See also the Key to the Reference Code.
Standard chemical element symbols are used.
°Drug acronyms are listed under °I & °Tc in the Index of Subjects.
Many shortened words were necessitated by space limitation in the original manuscript.

Nuc Med = Nuclear Medicine
°X = "radioactive" X
a < b = a is "less than" b
a > b = a is "greater than" b
[1999] = Refer to year enclosed in [ ]
# = number of

m milli = 10^{-3}
μ micro = 10^{-6}
n nano = 10^{-9}
p pico = 10^{-12}
f femto = 10^{-15}
a atto = 10^{-18}

k kilo = 10^{3}
M mega = 10^{6}
G giga = 10^{9}
T tera = 10^{12}
P peta = 10^{15}
E exa = 10^{18}

A = atomic weight, protons + neutrons
ABC = American Broadcasting Co
ABCC = Atom Bomb Casualty Commission
abd = abdomen, abdominal
absorp = absorption
AEC = Atomic Energy Commission
AERE = Atomic Energy Research Establishment
AfP = Atoms-for-Peace
ALARA = As Low As Reasonably Achievable
Am = American
amput = amputation
amt = amount
anat = anatomy
angios = angiograms
ANL = Argonne National Laboratory
Ap = anterior projection (scan)
ARS = Acute Radiation Syndrome
art = artery, arterial, article
arth = arthritis
artif = artificial
asst = assistant
atmos = atmosphere
At Wt = atomic weight
°AuCol = radioactive gold colloid
Aus = Austria
Austr = Australia
A/V = arterio/venous
ave = average

B^+ B^- = beta particles, positron & negatron
BEI = butanol extractable iodine
Belg = Belgian, Belgium
bio = biology, -ological, -gist
BIPM = Bureau Int Poids et Mesures
Bk = book
bkgd = background level of °activity
bld = blood
BM = bone marrow
b-marrow = bone marrow
BMR = basal metabolic rate
BNL = Brookhaven National Laboratory
BP = blood pressure
Bq = Becquerel unit of activity
bronc = bronchial, bronchus
bronco = bronchograms
BRS = British Roentgen Society
brst = breast
burd = burden (as in bdy burd)

ca = cancer, carcinoma
Ca = calcium
calc = calculation
Can = Canada, Canadian
capil = capillary
card = cardiac
CAT = computerized axial tomography
cath = catheter
CBF = cerebral blood flow
CEA = carcino embryonic antigen
cent = central
cer = cerebral
cereb = cerebral
CGLeuk = chronic granulocytic leukemia
CGPM = Conférence Générale des Poids et Mesures
chem = chemistry, chemical, chemist
chemoRx = chemotherapy
child = childhood, children
chm = chairman
Ci or c = curie unit (c before 1954)
circ = circulation
clear = clearance
clin = clinical
CLLeuk = chronic lymphocytic leukemia
CMLeuk = chronic myelogenous leukemia
CNM = A Chronology of Nuclear Medicine
coll = collimator(s)
collats = collateral blood vessels
Com = committee
Comm = commission
comp = competitive (binding)
conc = concentration
conf = conference
cong = congestive, congress
COPD = chron obstruct pulmonary disease
coron = coronary
cret = cretinism
CSF = cerebrospinal fluid
CRT = cathode ray tube
CT = computerized tomography
Cutie Pie = ion chamber survey meter
CVA = cardiovascular accident

d = day (as in 5d = 5 days)
DAR = differential absorption ratio
DDx = differential diagnosis
defic = deficiency, -ent
Den = Denmark, Danish

dens = density
dept = department
deriv = derivative
descrip = description
desic = desiccate, -ed, -tion
Df = definition
D°If = fluorescent brain scan agent
diff = difference, -t
dis = disease
DISIDA = IDA-class biliary scan agent
dist = distribute, ed, tion
Div = Division
div-con = diverging/converging
doc = documented, documents
DOE = Department of Energy
DP = diphosphate-class scan agent
DTPA = diethyl triaminepentaacetic
DVT = deep venous thrombosis
Dx = diagnosis, diagnostic

E = energy
ECAT = emission comp axial tomography
ECG = electrocardiogram, -graphy
EDTA = edetic acid metal complexer
EEG = electroencephalogram
EF = ejection fraction
effus = effusion
elec = electric, electricity
em = electromagnetic
emf = electromotive force
Eng = England, English
ENIAC = first digital computer
EPA = Enviromental Pollution Agency
equip = equipment
er = equivalent roentgen
esp = especially
est = estimate, -s, -tion
eu = energy unit
exp = exposure
expr = experiment
ext = external (to body)
extr = extract

FDA = Food and Drug Administration
fib = fibrinogen
filt = filtration
Fr = France, French
FRC = Federal Radiation Council
fulm = fulminating
func = function

Ger = Germany, German
GFR = glomerular filtration rate
GI = gastrointestinal
glob = globulin
GM = Geiger-Mueller tube
G-pig = guinea pig
grad = graduate
Grt Brit = Great Britain (see UK)
Gy = gray unit = 100 Rad

h = hour (as in 5h = 5 hours)
HAM = human albumin microspheres
Hb = hemoglobin
HEW = Health Education & Welfare
hepat = hepatic
HGH = human growth hormone
HHS = Health & Human Services
hi- = high (as in hi-dose)
HIDA = IDA-class biliary scan agent
HIDPM = brain scan agent
Hipp = Hippuran, -ate
hist = history
HP = health physics
HSA = human serum albumin
ht = heart
Ht = hematocrit
Hrt = heart
hum = human
Hun = Hungary, -ian
HVL = half value layer
hyper(s) = hyperthyroid, pts or disease
hypo(s) = hypothyroid, pts or disease

IAEA = Internat Atomic Energy Agency
IC = intracarotid injection
ICap = intracapillary infusion
ICC = Interstate Commerce Commission
ICR = Internat College of Radiology
ICRP = Internat Comm Rad Protection
ICRU = Internat Comm Radiation Units
IDA = iminodiacetic acid (bile agent)
IgG = immunoglobulin G (or other symb)
°IHSA = °iodine human serum albumin
°IMAA = °iodine macroaggregated albumin
inj = inject, -d, -ion
int = internal
Int = international
intracav = intracavitary
instr = instrument
insuf = insufficiency
ioniz = ionizing, ionization
IP = intraperitoneal injection
Ir = Irish
IR = infrared
irrad = irradiate, -ed, -ion
It = Italian
IT = intrathecal injection
IUPAC = Inter Union of Pure & Applied Chem
IV = intravenous injection

J or Jr = Journal

keV = kilo electron volts
KI = potassium iodide
kid = kidney
kVp = kilovolt potential
Ky = Kentucky

L nodes = lymph nodes
LAO = left ant oblique projection
LATS = long acting thyroid stimulator
LD_{50} = lethal dose to 50% of population
LET = linear energy transfer
leuk(s) = leucocyte(s), leukemia
Lin = linear
lo- = low (as in lo-dose)
LV = left ventricle of heart

m = minute (as in 5m = 5 minutes)
m = meter (in proper context)

μ = greek lower case mu for micro
MAA = macroaggregated albumin
μAA = microaggregated albumin
mag = magnet, magnetic
malig = malignant
Man Dist = Manhattan Engineering District
max = maximum, maximal
mCi = millicurie (also mc pre 1954)
MDP = diphos-class bone scan agent
med = medical, medicine
MED = Manhattan Engineering District
metab = metabolism
mets = metastases
MeV = mega (million) electron volts
MGH = Mass General Hospital
MIBG = pheochromocytoma scan agent
microsp = microspheres
min = minimal, minimum
MIRD = Med Internal Rad Dose Com
MIT = Mass Institute of Tech
mo = month (not used in Nuc Med)
molec = molecular, molecule
MPC = maximum permissible concentration
MPD = maximum permissible dose
MRC = Med Research Council (Eng)
MRI = magnetic resonance imaging
musc dys = muscular dystrophy
MW_e = megawatts electric
myocard = myocardial (-ium)
myx = myxedema

n = neutron or nano (10^{-9})
nAA = neutron activation analysis
NAS = National Acad of Science
NBS = National Bureau of Standards
NCAB = National Cancer Advis Board
NCC = Nuc Consult Corp (to Mallinckrodt)
NCI = National Cancer Institute
NCRP = National Comm Rad Protection
necro = necrosis
neg = negative as in scan neg
NIH = National Institutes of Health
NMR = nuclear magnetic resonance
nod = nodule, nodular
norm = normal
NRC = National Research Council or
= Nuclear Regulatory Commission
°nuc(s) = nuclide, radionuclides, nuclear

op = operation (surgical)
OR = Oak Ridge
ORINS = Oak Ridge Inst Nuc Studies (ORAU)
ORNL = Oak Ridge National Laboratory
osteo = osteogenic

p = proton
part = particle
path = pathology, -ological
PBI = protein bound iodine
PE = pulmonary embolus, -ism
perf = perfusion
PET = positron emission tomography
photo = photography, -graph
Phys = physics, physical
Physiol = physiology, physiological
pic(s) = picture (s)
PIC = plasma iron clearance
PIPIDA = IDA-class biliary agent
PIT = plasma iron turnover
pl = pool
Pols = politics, -ians
pop = population
Pp = posterior projection (scan)
ppt = precipitate
press = pressure
prob = probable, probability
prost = prostate, -ic gland
protect = protection
pt(s) = patient (s)
PTT = pulmonary transit time
pub (s) = publish, publications
pulm = pulmonary
PV(PVA) = polycythemia vera (acuta)
PYP = polyphosphate bone scan agent

Q = quality factor (RBE)

r or R = roentgen unit (rules change)
rad = radiation
Rad = radiation absorbed dose unit
radiol = radiology, radiologist
RAO = right ant oblique (scan)
°RB = radioactive Rose Bengal
RBC = red blood cells
RBE = relative biological effect
RCG = radiocardiogram, -graph
RCIC = red cell iron clearance
RCIT = red cell iron turnover
RDA = recommended daily allowance
reg(s) = regulation(s)
rejuv = rejuvenate, -tion
Rem = radiation equivalent mouse (man)
Rep = roentgen equivalent physical
RERF = Rad Effects Res Foundation
RERF (J) = Rad Effects Res Foundation (Japan)
res = research
RES = reticulo endothelial system
rhm = roentgens/hour at a meter
RIA = radioimmunoassay
ROC = receiver operat characteristic
RoI = region-of-interest
Roy Soc = Royal Society
RSNA = Rad Soc of North America
Rx = therapy, treatment

s (sec) = second (as in 5s = 5 seconds)
sarc = sarcoma
scan + = scan positive
scint = scintillation
Scot = Scottish, Scotland
sens = sensitive
SI = Systéme International
sig = significant
SNM = Society of Nuclear Medicine
Socs = Societies
sol = solitary
SOL = space occupying lesion
soln = solution
Sp Act = specific activity
SPECT = Single Photon Emission Computerized Tomography
spont = spontaneous
SQ = subcutaneous injection

std(s) = standard (s)
subarach = subarachnoid
subdur = subdural
subQ(SQ) = subcutaneous injection
surg = surgery, surgeon
Sv = Sievert unit
Swe = Sweden, Swedish
Swis = Switzerland, Swiss
syst = systolic or system

$T_{1/2}$ = °half-life or °half-time
$T_{B1/2}$ = biological half-time
T1,2,3 = mono, di, triiodothyronines
TBC = tuberculosis
temp = temperature
testos = testosterone
°TcHSA = °Tc human serum albumin
°TcIDA = °Tc biliary agent
°TcSC = °Tc sulfur colloid
°TcPP = °Tc polyphosphate
°TcRBC = °Tc red blood cells
tech = technician, technic
thyr = thyroid
TIA = transient ischemic attack
TMI = Three Mile Island
tng = training
tox = toxicity, toxic
trans-U = elements over U, #92

μ = Greek lower case mu for micro
U = University
U Chi = University of Chicago
μCi = microcurie (also μc pre-1954)
UCLA = Univ Cal at Los Angeles
UCSF = Univ Cal at San Fransico
UK = United Kingdom
UN = United Nations
US = United States of America
USC = Univ of Southern Calif
USSR = Union of Social Soviet Republics
UV = ultra violet light

vasc = vascular
VB_{12} = vitamin B_{12}
ven = venous
vent = ventricle
vis = visible, visual
Vit A = vitamin A
vol = volume
V/P(VP) = ventilation-perfusion lung scan
vs = versus

W = energy to produce ion pair
WBC = white blood cells
WBody = whole body
WHO = World Health Organization
WL = working level (HP calculation)
WW I = World War One
WW II = World War Two

X-ray = electromagnetic rad (photons)
X-Ray = picture taken with X-rays
xtal = crystal

y = year (as in 5y = 5 years)

Z = atom ordinal number (protons)

KEY TO THE REFERENCE CODE

Official journal abbreviations are too long. I use a code of few letters. Exact references are in yearly indices of the journals listed. To save space I name only the first author, and journal names are abbreviated here for brevity. Books and biographies are by or of the named author. The Dictionary of Scientific Biography, autobiographies, some news articles are accepted as prime sources. My Vignettes in Nuclear Medicine are referred to for stories that require many references.

MED refers to declassified Manhattan Engineering District documents. AEC refers to Atomic Energy Commission reports found in depository libraries. Semiannual Reports of AEC's Isotopes Division were USGPO publications.

AAF	Arch Arb z Fortschr (Ger)
ABB	Arch Biochem & Biophys
ABCC	Atom Bomb Casualty Comm
AC	Anal Chem
ACB	Acta Cardiol (Brux)
ACG	Ann Chir Gyn Fenniae
ACR	Am Coll Radiology
ACS	Am Cancer Soc Report
ACSd	Acta Chir Scand
AD	Arch Dermatology
AdP	Ann d'Physik (Ger)
ADS	Arch Derm et Syph (Fr)
AE	Acta Endocrinologica
AEA	UK Atom Energy Auth
AEC	Atom Energy Comm reports
AEM	Arch d'Elect Med (Fr)
AEPP	Arch Exp Path & Pharm
AERE	Atom Ener Res Estab (UK)
Aero	Aerospace Medicine
AeS	Arch of Skiagraphy (Lon)
AfE	Arch f Electrotech (Ger)
AFMJ	Armed Forces Med J
AfP	First Peace Use of AE Proc
AfP2	Second Atoms for Peace conf
AG	Arch Gynecology (Ger)
AH	Arch Hematol (Basel)
AHJ	Am Heart J
AIC	Arch Ital Chir (It)
AIP	Arch Ital Physiol
AJB	Am J Botany
AJC	Am J Cancer
AJCN	Am J Clin Nutrition
AJCP	Am J Clin Path
AJCr	Am J Cardiology
AJD	Am J Digestive Dis
AJDC	Am J Dis Children
AJE	Am J Epidemiology
AJEB	Austr J Exp Biol Med
AJM	Am J Medicine
AJMS	Am J Med Science
AJO	Am J Ophthalmology
AJOG	Am J Obst & Gyn
AJP	Am J Public Health
AJPa	Am J Pathology
AJPh	Am J Physiology
AJPr	Am J Pharmacology
AJPy	Am J Physics
AJR	Am J Roentgenology
AJS	Am J Science
AJSM	Am J Sports Med
AJSr	Am J Surgery
AJTM	Am J Tropical Med
AK	Arch Kinderheilk (Ger)
AKC	Arch Klin Chir (Ger)
AM	American Magazine
AmJR	Am J Radiology
AmM	American Medicine
AMP	Advances in Med Physics
AMS	Acta Med Scand
AN	Arch Neurology
AnN	Ann Neurology
ANG	Abb Nature Ges (Halle)
AnIM	Ann Internal Med
ANM	Advances in Nuc Med
ANP	Arch Neurol & Psychiat
AnP	Ann Physik (Ger)
AnR	Anatomical Record
ANS	Acta Neurol Scand
AnS	Ann Surgery
ANZJ	Austr & N Zea J Surg
ANZM	Austr & N Zea J Med
AO	Arch Ophthalmology
AORL	Ann Otol Rhin & Laryn
AOS	Acta Orthoped Scand
APS	Acta Physiol Scand
AP	Associated (or United) Press
APa	Arch of Pathology
APC	Ann Phys Chem (Ger)
APe	Arch of Pediatrics
APg	Ann Physik (Gilbert)
APL	Ann Physik (Leipzig)
ApR	Applied Radiology
AQR	Am Quarterly Roentgen
AR	Acta Radiologica
A&R	Arthritis & Rheum
ARD	Am Rev Respiratory Dis
ARE	Arch Radiol & Electrther
ArF	Arkiv Fysik (Swed)
ArIM	Arch Internal Med
ARR	Adv in Radiso Res (Hevesy)
ArRR	Arch Roentgen Ray
ARS	Acta Rheum Scand
AS	Arch of Surgery
ASAT	Am Surg Assoc Trans
ASM	Abstracts Soviet Med
ASS	Am Standards Assoc Reports
AtE	Access to Energy
ATS	Ann Thoracic Surgery
AuR	Australian Radiology
AXJ	American X ray J
B	Brain
BACS	Bull Am Chem Soc
BAEC	Bull Ass Fr l'Etude Ca
BAM	Bull Acad de Med (Fr)
BANM	Bull Acad Nat Med (Fr)
BAP	Beibl Ann Physik (Ger)
BAPS	Bull Am Physical Society
BAR	Bull Acad Roy (Belg)
BAW	Berlin Akad Wsnschf (Ger)
BB	Berlin Berichte (Ger)
BDB	Berichte Deutsch Botany
BDCG	Ber Deutsch Chem Ges
BHJ	Brit Heart J
BHJD	Bull Hosp Joint Dis
BHM	Bull Hist of Med
BICR	Bull Inst Chem Res
Bio	Biography of person named
BJ	Biochem J
BJC	Brit J Cancer
BJEM	Brit J Exp Med
BJEP	Brit J Exp Path
BJHH	Bull Johns Hopkins Hosp
BJIM	Brit J Indust Med
BJN	Brit J Nursing
BJR	Brit J Radiology
BJS	Brit J Surgery
BJU	Brit J Urology
Bk	Book by person named
BKC	Beit Klin Chirg (Ger)
BKW	Berlin Klin Wchnschr
Bl	Blood
BMB	Brit Medical Bull
BMJ	Brit Medical J
BMSJ	Boston Med Surg J
BNYA	Bull NY Acad Med
BSA	Bull Swed Acad Med
BSIM	Bull Soc Imp Nat Moscow
BSMH	Bull Soc Med Hosp (Paris)
C	Chest
ca	Cancer
CaR	Cancer Research
Card	Cardiologia (Basel)
CB	Chemische Berichte
CC	Clinical Chemistry
CDD	Clas Descrip Dis (Major)
CDDR	Clas Descrip Dx Rad (Brewer)
CdR	Cardiac Research
CE	Clin Endocrinology (Eng)
CEA	Comm l'En Atom (French AEC)
CFM	Ninth Con Franc Med d'Paris
Ch	Chest
Chi	Chirurgia (Ger)
CI	Clinical Investigation
Cir	Circulation
CirR	Circulation Research
CJR	Canada J Research
CJS	Canada J Surgery
ClR	Clinical Radiol (Eng)
CM	California Medicine

CMAJ	Canada Med Assoc J
CMJ	China Med J
CN	Chem News (London)
CNM	Clinical Nuc Medicine
CNT	Canada Nuc Technology
COE	Clin Obst & Gyn (Eng)
CPT	Clin Pharm & Therapy
CR	Cardiovasc Radiology
CRB	Compt Rend Soc Biol (Fr)
CRP	Clinical Research Proc
CRS	Compt Rend Acad Sc (Fr)
CS	Clinical Science
CT	Current Therapy
CvR	Cardiovasc Research
CZ	Chemiker Zig (Karlsruhe)
DAKM	Deutsch Akad Klin Med
DC	Dental Cosmos
DCS	Dynamic Clin Studies (AEC)
DD	Digestive Disease
DGIM	Deutsch Ges f Inn Med
DGP	Deutsch Ges Physic
Dis	Dissertat of person named
DLP	Deutsch Landwerk Presse
DMG	Dros Melan Genetics
DMW	Deutsch Med Wchnschr
DoE	Discovery of Elements (Weeks)
DPL	Development of Period Law (Venabel)
DSB	Dict of Scientific Biography
DSM	Dover Sourcebk Math (Smith)
DVS	Danske Vid Sels Bio Med
E	Endocrinology
EB	Encycl Britannica (close date)
Ec	Ecology
EE	Electrical Engineer
EIF	Euratom Information Service
EJC	European J Cancer
EJNM	Europ J Nuc Med
Elm	Electromedica (Ger)
EM	English Mechanic
EMJ	English Mining J
ENM	European J Nuc Med
ER	Electric Review
Eve	Eve's Rutherford Biography
EW	Electrical World
Ex	Experientia
5CN	Fifth Congresso Nuclearc (It)
FGR	Fortschr Geb Roentgstr (Ger)
FM	Fortschr Med (Ger)
FP	Federation Proc
FR	Federal Register
FS	Fertility & Sterility
FV	Fire in Valley (Freiberg)
G	Gastroenterology
GMM	German Medical Monthly
GMP	Glasser's Medical Physics
GSA	Glasstone's Sourcebk of AE
GSR	Glasser's Science of Radiol
Gut	Gut
GW	Ges Wurzburg (Ger)
Gyn	Gynaecologia
Haf	Harefuah (Israel)
HCP	Handbk of Chem Phys (date)
HGS	Handbk der Gesam Strahl (Ger)
HIR	Hormesis w Ioniz Rad (Luckey)
His	Histochemie (Ger)
HL	Harvey Lectures
HNM	Heritage of Nuc Med (SNM)
HP	Health Physics
HPN	Health Physics Newsletter
HRC	Historic Research (T. Chalmers)
Ht	Heart
IAEA	Int Atomic Energy Agency
IC	International Clinics
ICRE	Int Cong Rad et Elec (Fr)
ICS	Int Clinical Surgery
IEE	Inst Elec Eng Trans NS
IJAR	Int J App Radiol & Isotopes
IJG	Ital J Gastroenterology
IJO	Int J Radiation Oncology
IJRB	Int J Radiation Biol
IMJ	Illinois Med J
Inj	Injury
INM	Int J Nuc Med & Biol
IRET	Inst Radio Eng Trans
IRT	Isotopes & Radiation Technol
IU	Investig Urology
IUCC	INT Union Contra Ca Acta
JA	J Anatomy (Eng)
JAAS	J Am Acoustics Society
JACS	J Am Chem Society
JAMA	J Am Medical Assoc
JAP	J Applied Physics
JA&P	J Anatomy & Physics (Eng)
JAPh	J Applied Physiology
JaR	Jahrbh Radioaktivitat (Ger)
JAT	J Advanced Therapeutics
JB	J Bacteriology
JBC	J Biol Chem
JBJS	J Bone & Joint Surgery
JCA	J Comput Assisted Tomogr
JCAE	Joint Comm Atom En (hearing)
JCAR	J Canada Assoc Radiol
JCC	J Cell Comp Physiology
JCE	J Chem Education
JCEM	J Clin Endo & Metab
JCEn	J Clin Endocrinology
JChS	J Chemical Soc
JCI	J Clin Invest
JCP	J Chem Phys
JCPa	J Clin Pathology
JCR	J Cancer Res (Eng)
JCS	J Cardiovasc Surg (It)
JdP	J d'Physics (Fr)
JDR	J Dental Research
JE	J Endocrinology
JEB	J Exper Biology
JEM	J Exper Medicine
JEZ	J Exper Zoology
JFI	J Franklin Inst
JFR	J Faculty of Radiol
JGP	J General Physiology
JH	J of Hygiene
JHHB	Johns Hopkins Hosp Bull
JHJ	Japanese Heart J
JI	J Immunology
JID	J Infectious Dis
JIHT	J Indust Hyg & Tox
JIU	J Investig Urology
JJC	J Chem Soc Japan
JJN	Japan J Nuc Med
JLCM	J Lab & Clin Med
JMAG	J Med Assoc Georgia
JMC	J Med Canada
JMR	J Mag Resonance Med
JMRe	J Med Research
JMS	J Michigan Med Soc
JNB	J Nuc Biol & Med (It)
JNCI	J Nat Cancer Inst
JNM	J Nuc Med
JNMD	J Nerv & Mental Disease
JNN	J Neurol Neurosurg Psyc
JNs	J Neurosurgery
JOGB	J Obst & Gyn Brit Emp
JOM	J Oklahoma Med Assoc
JOS	J Oral Surgery
JP	J Pediatrics
JPB	J Path & Bacteriology
JPCC	J Phys Colloid Chem
JPET	J Pharm & Exp Therapy
JPh	J J Physiology (Eng)
JPS	J Polymer Science
JPSr	J Pediat Surgery
JR	J of Radiology
JRC	J Russian Chem Soc (Rus)
JRE	J Radiol et d'Electr (Fr)
JRS	J Roentgen Society (Eng)
JSH	J Mt Sinai Hosp (NYC)
JSO	J Surgical Oncology
JT	J Trauma
JTAS	J Tenn Acad Science
JU	J Urology
JUN	J Urology Nephrol (Fr)
KDB	Kgl Danske V Biol Med
KDS	Kgl Danske V Selsk
KI	Kidney Int
KM	Klin Med Moskova (USSR)
KP	Kinderarztl Praxis (Ger)
KW	Klin Wochschr (Ger)
La	Lancet
LI	Laboratory Investigation
LPC	Lehrbh d Phys Chem (Ger)
LPM	La Presse Med (Fr)
LPP	Lehrbh Prakt Physik (Ger)
LRB	Letters Rutherford-Boltwood
Ly	Laryngoscope
M	Metabolism
MAE	Moscow Atom Energy
MCJ	Mitt Med Chirg (Jena)
MCNA	Med Clinics of North Am
MCP	Mayo Clinic Proc
MED	Manhat Eng Dist (1942-47)
Med	Medicine

MJA	Med J Australia
MK	Münch Klin (Ger)
MKl	Med Klinic (Ger)
MM	Minerva Medica (It)
MMR	Methods in Med Research
MMW	Münch Med Wchnschr (Ger)
MN	Minerva Nucleare (It)
MnM	Minnesota Med
MO	Minerva Oncologica (It)
MoM	Modern Med
MP	Medical Physics
MR	Med Record
MRC	Med Research Council (Eng)
MRM	Med Radiol (Moscow)
MRNY	Med Research of New York
MS	Military Surgeon
MW	Med Welt (Ger)
N	Neurology
Na	Nature (London)
NAS	Nat Acad Sci - Nat Res Council
NBS	Nat Bur Of Stand Reports
NCM	N Carolina Med J
NEJM	New Eng J Med
NIM	Nuc Instruments & Methods
NIR	Nat Inst Rad Sci (Jap in Eng)
NM	Northwest Medicine
NMG	Nuklear Med (Germany)
NMJ	Nebraska Med J
NMS	Nuk Med Stuttgart (Ger)
NNE	Nat Nuc Energy Ser (McGraw-Hill)
Np	Nephron
NPL	National Phys Lab (Eng NBS)
Nr	Neuroradiology
NRCC	Nat Research Coun Canada
NS	New Scientist
Ns	Neurosurgery
NT	Nutrition Today
NTIS	Nat Tech Info Service
Nuc	Nucleonics
NUT	Natur und Technik (Ger)
NYAS	New York Acad Sci
NYMJ	New York Med J
NYMR	New York Med Record
Nw	Naturwissenschaften
O	Orthopedics
OG	Obstetrics & Gyn
ONR	Off Naval Res Review
ORNL	Oak Ridge Nat Lab News
P	Pediatrics
PAP	Pfluger's Arch Physiol
PAPS	Proc Am Philos Soc
PASA	Proc Acad Sc Amsterdam
PCD	Prog Cardiovasc Dis
PCPS	Proc Cambridge Phil Soc
PEM	Prob Endokrin Moscow
PgM	Postgraduate Med
PHBG	Public Health Bull (GA)
PHR	Public Health Reports
PhR	Physiology Review
PHSB	Public Health Serv Bull
PICC	Proc Int Cancer Conf
PIEE	Proc Inst Elec Engineers
PIM	Proc Inst Med Chicago
PJR	Proc Japan Radioiso Assn
PL	Personal Letter (Brucer)
PLC	Proc Laurentian Conf
PM	Philosophical Mag (London)
PMB	Phys Med & Biol
PMJ	Pennsylvania Med J
PMW	Prag Med Wochnsch (Ger)
PNAS	Proc Nat Acad Sci
PoR	Photogr Rundschau (Ger)
PR	Physical Review
PrM	Presse Med (Fr)
PRS	Plastic & Reconst Surg
PRSL	Proc Roy Soc (London)
PRSM	Proc Roy Soc Med
PS	Picker Scintillator
PSEB	Proc Soc Exp Biol Med
PSR	Proc VII Symp Neurorad
PT	Physics Today
PTRS	Phil Tran Roy Soc (London)
PZ	Physik Zeitschr
QJM	Quart J Medicine
QJP	Quart J Exp Physiol
QJPh	Quart J Physiology
QRB	Quart Rev Biol
RA	Roux' Archives
RAC	Rev Argentina Cirur (Sp)
Rad	Radiology
RadB	Radiologica (Berlin)
RAE	Rev Argen Endo Metab (Sp)
RAP	Rep f Anat Physiol (Ger)
R&R	Radiophys & RadioRx
RB	Roentgen Blätter (Ger)
RBo	Radiation Botany
RERF	Rad Eff Res Found (Jap)
RFC	Rev Franc Clin Biol (Fr)
RH	Rev Hematology
Ri	Radioisotopes (Jap)
RIM	Radioisotopes in Med
RITP	Rev Int d'Ther Phys (Fr)
RM	Revista Med (Sp)
RMP	Rev Modern Physics
RMT	Radiol Med Torino (It)
RP	Radiologia Practica (Sp)
RPh	Radioact Pharmaceu (AEC)
RR	Radiation Research
RS	Rev Science (Paris)
RSI	Rev Scientific Instr
S	Surgery
Sa	Sang (Fr)
SA	Scientific American
SAb	Stat Abstract of USA
SAP	Scand Arch Physiology
Sc	Science
Sem	Seminars in Nuc Med
SF	Surgical Forum
SGO	Surg Gyn & Obstet
SGR	Schwarz Geb Roentgen (Ger)
SHP	Sem Hop Paris
SIP	Smithsonian Inst Pub
SJCL	Scand J Clin Lab Invest
SJG	Scand J Gastroenterol
SJR	Scand J Resp Dis
SJU	Scand J Urol & Neph
SM	Sem Med (Buenos Aires)
SMJ	Southern Med J
SMW	Schwz Med Wchnschr (Ger)
SN	Science News
SNM	Soc Nuc Med Newsletter
SR	Skeletal Radiology
SRC	Second Radioisotope Conf
St	Stroke
Str	Strahlentherapie (Ger)
T	Transfusion
TAA	Trans Am Gen Uri Soc
TAAP	Trans Assn Am Phys
TAGA	Trans Am Goiter Assn
TAM	Trans Am Ob & Gyn Soc
TANA	Trans Am Neurol Assn
TARR	Trans Am Roent Ray Soc
TAUA	Trans Am Urology Assn
TC	Trilinear Chart of Nuc
TEL	The Engineer (London)
Tex	Texas Medicine
Tho	Thorax
TI	Table of Isotop (Lederer)
TNL	T Norsk Laegeforen (Nor)
TNW	The New World (Penn St P Pr)
TRBM	Texas Reports Biol Med
TRDS	Trans Roy Dublin Soc
TRSC	Trans Roy Soc Canada
TSMJ	Texas State Med J
TUM	Thyr Uptake Measurement
U	Urology
VDPG	Verh Deutsch Phys Ges (Ger)
VDRG	Verh Deutsch Roent Ges (Ger)
VN	Voposy Nierokh (USSR)
VPG	Verh Phys Ges
V##	Vignettes in Nuc Med
WAP	Wied Ann Physik (Ger)
WJM	Western J Medicine
WJS	Western J Surgery
WKW	Wiener Klin Wchnschr
WMJ	Wisconsin Med J
WMP	Wiener Presse (Ger)
WoA	World of Atom, Boorse
WZN	Wiss Ztschr Natur (Ger)
YB	Yearbook of Nuc Med
YJBM	Yale J Biol & Med
Z	all German
ZAC	Ztschr Anorg Chem
ZE	Ztschr Electrochem
ZfC	Zentralblt f Chir
ZfP	Ztschr f Physik
ZGL	Ztschr Gynak (Leipzig)
ZGNP	Ztschr f Neur u Psych
ZIM	Ztschr Inner Med
ZKM	Ztschr f Klin Med
ZN	Ztschr Naturforsch
ZPC	Ztschr f Phys Chem
ZPh	Zentbl f Physiol
ZPT	Ztschr Exp Path Therap

INDEX OF NAMES

[For articles with multiple authors, only the first author is listed in this document.]

* * * * *

INDEX OF SUBJECTS

[Nuclear Science terminology changed after 1940. *Isotope Medicine* became Nuclear Medicine; *radioisotopes* became *radionuclides*. The millicurie unit was an *mc*, then *mC*, then *mCi*; a mandatory change to *MBq* began in 1985. In this Index, terms and symbols used by the authors, at the time quoted, are maintained throughout the text.]

The Index of Subjects was originally arranged by years. Changing this data to page numbers introduced occasional small numerical inaccuracy: Ed.

* * * * *